AF738633

Textbooks in Contemporary Dentistry

This textbook series presents the most recent advances in all fields of dentistry, with the aim of bridging the gap between basic science and clinical practice. It will equip readers with an excellent knowledge of how to provide optimal care reflecting current understanding and utilizing the latest materials and techniques. Each volume is written by internationally respected experts in the field who ensure that information is conveyed in a concise, consistent, and readily intelligible manner with the aid of a wealth of informative illustrations. *Textbooks in Contemporary Dentistry* will be especially valuable for advanced students, practitioners in the early stages of their career, and university instructors.

Saman Warnakulasuriya • Kannan Ranganathan
*Editors*

# Oral Submucous Fibrosis

A Guide to Diagnosis and Management

*Editors*
Saman Warnakulasuriya
Faculty of Dentistry
Oral and Craniofacial Sciences
King's College London
London, UK

Kannan Ranganathan
Oral and Maxillofacial Pathology
Ragas Dental College and Hospital
The TN Dr MGR Medical University
Chennai, Tamil Nadu, India

ISSN 2524-4612 ISSN 2524-4620 (electronic)
Textbooks in Contemporary Dentistry
ISBN 978-3-031-12854-7 ISBN 978-3-031-12855-4 (eBook)
https://doi.org/10.1007/978-3-031-12855-4

© The Editor(s) (if applicable) and The Author(s), under exclusive license to Springer Nature Switzerland AG 2023
This work is subject to copyright. All rights are solely and exclusively licensed by the Publisher, whether the whole or part of the material is concerned, specifically the rights of translation, reprinting, reuse of illustrations, recitation, broadcasting, reproduction on microfilms or in any other physical way, and transmission or information storage and retrieval, electronic adaptation, computer software, or by similar or dissimilar methodology now known or hereafter developed.
The use of general descriptive names, registered names, trademarks, service marks, etc. in this publication does not imply, even in the absence of a specific statement, that such names are exempt from the relevant protective laws and regulations and therefore free for general use.
The publisher, the authors, and the editors are safe to assume that the advice and information in this book are believed to be true and accurate at the date of publication. Neither the publisher nor the authors or the editors give a warranty, expressed or implied, with respect to the material contained herein or for any errors or omissions that may have been made. The publisher remains neutral with regard to jurisdictional claims in published maps and institutional affiliations.

This Springer imprint is published by the registered company Springer Nature Switzerland AG
The registered company address is: Gewerbestrasse 11, 6330 Cham, Switzerland

"We dedicate this book to our families, teachers, and colleagues without whose support neither of us would be where we are"

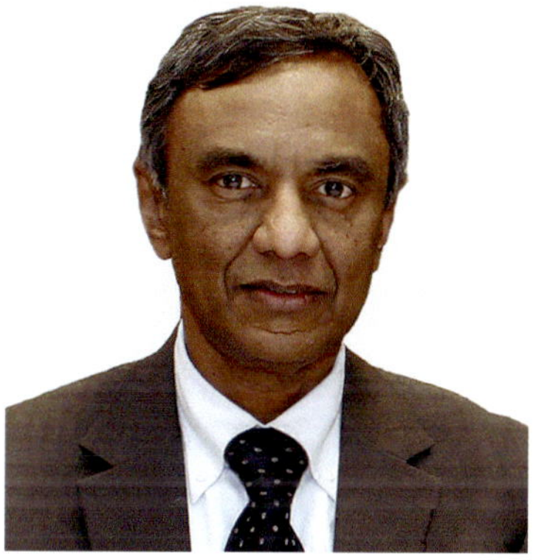

Prof. Saman Warnakulasuriya

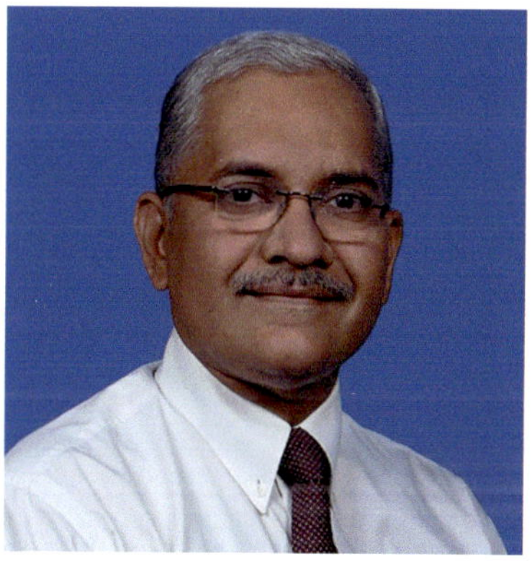

Prof. Kannan Ranganathan

# Foreword

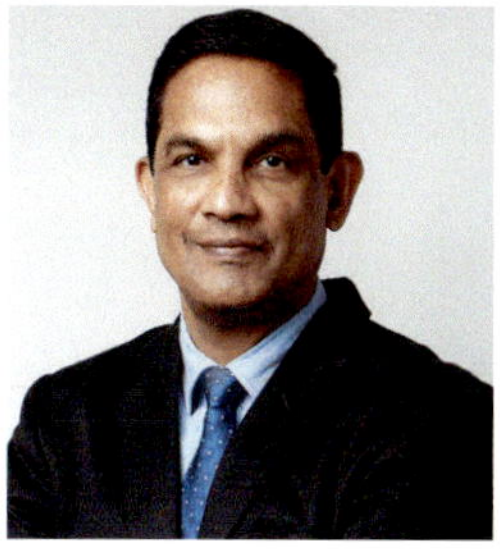

I am privileged and honored to write the foreword for the book titled "Oral Submucous Fibrosis: Guide to Diagnosis and Management." This comprehensive text covers all aspects of this deadly disease mostly prevalent in South and Southeast Asia. The text describes the disease in detail, from its historical aspects to its etiology, pathogenesis, clinical presentation, classification systems, diagnostic methods, histopathological aspects, mechanisms of malignant transformation, and treatment. It also includes sections on areca nut cessation and various other interventions. It has been a long-felt need to compile all the different aspects of this common health problem in South and Southeast Asia under a single title. This affords a unique opportunity for undergraduates, postgraduates, researchers, and other relevant health professionals to read about every aspect of the disease in one place. The chapters describe a complex subject matter in a simple form accessible to any kind of audience.

The textbook is edited by two eminent globally recognized academics in the field of oral cancer and oral potentially malignant disorders (OPMDs). Professor Saman Warnakulasuriya from King's College, London, is a world-renowned professor who has spent many decades of his academic career conducting extensive research on oral cancer and OPMD. His in-depth knowledge on the subject of oral submucous fibrosis is unparalleled, and this would have certainly helped in bringing this book to the highest standards. Professor K. Ranganathan from Ragas Dental College, Chennai, India, is a well-respected oral pathologist who has contributed immensely to the subject both nationally and internationally. In addition, his vast clinico-pathological knowledge on submucous fibrosis would have contributed immensely to editing this book. They have brought together a well-experienced group of academics, clinicians, and researchers to share their enormous experience in compiling this historic text on oral submucous fibrosis.

While congratulating the editors and contributors for this timely contribution to medical literature, I highly recommend this book for anyone who wants to gain in-depth knowledge on oral submucous fibrosis.

**Prof. W. M. Tilakaratne**
Department of Oral Pathology, Faculty of Dentistry
University of Malaya
Kuala Lumpur, Malaysia

Department of Oral Pathology, Faculty of Dentistry
University of Peradeniya
Peradeniya, Sri Lanka

# Preface

Oral submucous fibrosis was first described in early 1950s, and since its discovery, much has been written about this disease. Some early theories about its causation are now outdated, and there is sufficient evidence that areca nut consumption is the major cause of this disease. Because of the important recent developments on many aspects of oral submucous fibrosis (OSF), it is our goal to provide an accurate up-to-date textbook that has a comprehensive coverage on this disease and to reflect on the latest advances that are important to the clinicians for the diagnosis and management of OSF and to the pathologists who contribute to the diagnostic services. The precancerous nature of this disease has been known for several decades, and based on the WHO nomenclature developed in 2005, OSF was established as an oral potentially malignant disorder (OPMD). In fact, epidemiological surveys indicate that oral submucous fibrosis is the most prevalent OPMD in South Asia and the western Pacific region, and hence we recognize its importance as a clinical entity.

This comprehensive textbook consisting of 22 chapters is written by invited experts in the field. The contributors are well-known teachers in dental schools, mostly from South Asia, and this book has drawn them together in a unique collaboration to provide an all-encompassing review of the current state of knowledge on this disease.

For didactic purposes, the chapters in the textbook are organized into six parts. The first set of chapters (▶ Chaps. 1–7) focus on the historical and clinical aspects of the disease. The second and third sets of chapters (▶ Chaps. 8–12) explore the etiology and etiopathogenesis. The fourth set of chapters (▶ Chaps. 13–15) describe the investigative techniques, and the fifth set of chapters (▶ Chaps. 16–18) examine the current concepts on the management of OSF. The final set (▶ Chaps. 19–21) deals with the management of addiction to areca nut to facilitate interventions on the cause of this disease. In the final chapter, we also provide a comprehensive bibliography for additional reading and in the appendix some historical aspects of authors who made contributions to our current understanding of this disease.

The book is primarily intended for undergraduate and graduate students in dentistry and could act as a handy reference book to primary care physicians in Southeast Asia, who regularly see areca nut chewers in their clinical practice. We hope that the readers will appreciate the multidisciplinary prospective of the textbook, extending the book's usefulness to a wider audience of caregivers.

We thank Alison Wolf for commissioning this textbook and Sivachandran Ravanan for the assistance received, who acted as the Project Coordinator for Springer Nature. Editorial assistance given to us by Kavitha Loganathan during numerous occasions throughout this book project is greatly appreciated.

**Saman Warnakulasuriya**
London, UK

**Kannan Ranganathan**
Chennai, Tamil Nadu, India

June 2022

# Contents

## IV Investigative Techniques for Oral Submucous Fibrosis



## V Management of Oral Submucous Fibrosis



## VI Areca Nut Addiction and Treatment

# Contributors

**Anura Ariyawardana** College of Medicine and Dentistry, James Cook University, Cairns, Australia

School of Medicine and Dentistry, Griffith University, Gold Coast, Australia

Metro South Oral Health, Logan Road Woolloongabba, Queensland, Australia

**Radhika Manoj Bavle** Department of Oral and Maxillofacial Pathology, Krishnadevaraya College of Dental Sciences and Hospital, Bangalore, India

**Rajiv S. Desai** Department of Oral Pathology and Microbiology, Nair Hospital Dental College, Mumbai, Maharashtra, India

**Upul Dissanayake** Department of Oral Pathology, Faculty of Dental Sciences, University of Peradeniya, Peradeniya, Sri Lanka

**Sosmitha Girisa** Cancer Biology Laboratory and DBT-AIST International Center for Translational and Environmental Research (DAICENTER), Department of Biosciences and Bioengineering, Indian Institute of Technology (IIT) Guwahati, Guwahati, Assam, India

**Madhura Murittige Gopalakrishna** Department of Oral Pathology and Microbiology, D A Pandu Memorial R V Dental College, Bengaluru, Karnataka, India

**A. Hapangama** Department of Psychiatry, University of Kelaniya, Kelaniya, Sri Lanka

**Vinay K. Hazarey** Department of Oral Pathology, Datta Meghe Institute of Medical Sciences, Wardha, Maharashtra, India

**Thaddeus A. Herzog** Population Sciences Program, University of Hawaii Cancer Center, Honolulu, HI, USA

**Majdy Idrees** UWA Dental School, The University of Western Australia, Perth, WA, Australia

**Ruwan Jayasinghe** Department of Oral Medicine and Periodontology, Faculty of Dental Sciences, University of Peradeniya, Peradeniya, Sri Lanka

Centre for Research in Oral Cancer, Faculty of Dental Sciences, University of Peradeniya, Peradeniya, Sri Lanka

**Primali Jayasooriya** Department of Oral Pathology, Faculty of Dental Sciences, University of Peradeniya, Peradeniya, Sri Lanka

**Newell W. Johnson** Menzies Health Institute Queensland, Griffith University, Gold Coast, Australia

**Kavitha Loganathan** Department of Oral and Maxillofacial Pathology, Ragas Dental College and Hospital, The Tamil Nadu Dr. MGR Medical University, Chennai, Tamil Nadu, India

**Alexander Ross Kerr** Department of Oral and Maxillofacial Pathology, Radiology and Medicine, New York University College of Dentistry, New York, NY, USA

**Paturu Kondaiah** Department of Molecular Reproduction, Development and Gentics, Indian Institute of Science, Bengaluru, Karnataka, India

**Omar Kujan** Oral Pathology Dental School, The University of Western Australia, Perth, WA, Australia

**Aviral Kumar** Cancer Biology Laboratory and DBT-AIST International Center for Translational and Environmental Research (DAICENTER), Department of Biosciences and Bioengineering, Indian Institute of Technology (IIT) Guwahati, Guwahati, Assam, India

**Ajaikumar B. Kunnumakkara** Cancer Biology Laboratory and DBT-AIST International Center for Translational and Environmental Research (DAICENTER), Department of Biosciences and Bioengineering, Indian Institute of Technology (IIT) Guwahati, Guwahati, Assam, India

**Moni Abraham Kuriakose** Department of Head and Neck, Plastic and Reconstructive Surgery, Roswell Park Cancer Institute, Buffalo, NY, USA

Karkinos Healthcare, Kochi, Kerala, India

**K. A. L. A. Kuruppuarachchi** Department of Psychiatry, University of Kelaniya, Kelaniya, Sri Lanka

**Chandramani B. More** Department of Oral Medicine and Radiology, K.M. Shah Dental College and Hospital, Sumandeep Vidyapeeth, Vadodara, Gujarat, India

**Toru Nagao** Department of Maxillofacial Surgery, School of Dentistry, Aichi Gakuin University, Nagoya, Aichi, Japan

**Neal A. Palafox** Department of Family Medicine and Community Health, University of Hawaii, Honolulu, HI, USA

**Deepa Jatti Patil** Department of Oral Medicine and Radiology, K.M. Shah Dental College and Hospital, Sumandeep Vidyapeeth, Vadodara, Gujarat, India

**Vijay Pillai** Head and Neck Surgery, Narayana Healthcity, Bengaluru, Karnataka, India

**Pallavi Priyadarshini** Head and Neck Surgery, Narayana Healthcity, Bengaluru, Karnataka, India

**A. Ramanathan** Department of Oral & Maxillofacial Clinical Sciences, Faculty of Dentistry, University of Malaya, Kuala Lumpur, Malaysia

**Kannan Ranganathan** Department of Oral and Maxillofacial Pathology, Ragas Dental College and Hospital, The Tamil Nadu Dr. MGR Medical University, Chennai, Tamil Nadu, India

**Roopa S. Rao** Department of Oral Pathology and Microbiology Faculty of Dental Sciences M S Ramaiah University of Applied Sciences, Bengaluru, Karnataka, India

**Jay Gopal Ray** Department of Oral Pathology, Dr. R Ahmed Dental College and Hospital, Kolkata, West Bengal, India

**P. Sharada** AECS Maaruti College of Dental Sciences and Research Center, Bangalore, India

**Sumali Sumithrarachchi** Centre for Research in Oral Cancer, Faculty of Dental Sciences, University of Peradeniya, Peradeniya, Sri Lanka

**Saman Warnakulasuriya** King's College London, and the WHO Collaborating Centre for Oral Cancer, London, UK

**Yi-Hsin Connie Yang** National Institute of Cancer Research, National Health Research Institutes, Tainan, Taiwan

**R. B. Zain** Faculty of Dentistry, MAHSA University, Kuala Lumpur, Selangor, Malaysia

Oral Cancer Research & Coordinating Centre, Faculty of Dentistry, University of Malaya, Kuala Lumpur, Malaysia

# Abbreviations

| | |
|---|---|
| 2G | 2-Guanine |
| AA | Adenine adenine |
| AG | Adenine guanine |
| ALK5 | Activin-like kinase 5 |
| AN | Areca nut |
| bFGF | Basic fibroblast growth factor |
| BMP | Bone morphogenetic protein |
| BMP1 | Bone morphogenetic protein 1 |
| BQ | Betel quid |
| C/T | Cytosine/thymine |
| CC | Cytosine cytosine |
| COL1A1 | Collagen 1A1 |
| COL1A2 | Collagen 1A2 |
| COLase | Collagenase-1 |
| CREB3L1 | cAMP response element-binding protein 3-like 1 |
| CST3 | Gene for Cystatin |
| CTG | Connective tissue graft |
| CTGF | Connective tissue growth factor |
| CTLA-4 | Cytotoxic T-lymphocyte-associated antigen 4 |
| CYP-3A | Cytochrome P450 |
| DNA-PK | DNA-dependent protein kinase |
| ECM | Extracellular matrix |
| EGFR | Epidermal growth factor receptor |
| ERK | Extracellular signal-regulated kinase |
| FGF | Fibroblast growth factor |
| GG | Guanine guanine |
| GPx | Glutathione peroxidase |
| GSTs | Glutathione S-transferases |
| HBOT | Hyperbaric oxygen therapy |
| HIF-1α | Hypoxia-inducible factor-1α |
| HIF | Hypoxia-inducible factor |
| HLA | Human leukocyte antigen |
| HNSCC | Head and neck squamous cell carcinoma |
| HPV | Human papillomavirus |
| IFN | Interferon |
| IGF | Insulin-like growth factor |
| IL | Interleukin |
| JAK | Janus kinase |
| LIMK1 | LIM domain kinase 1 |
| LOH | Loss of heterozygosity |
| LOX | Lysyl oxidase |
| LOXL3 | Lysyl oxidase-like 3 |
| MAPK | Mitogen-activated protein kinase |
| MEK | Mitogen-activated protein kinase |
| MHC | Major histocompatibility complex |
| MICA | Major histocompatibility complex class I chain-related gene A |
| MMPs | Matrix metalloproteinases |
| NFK | Nuclear factor kappa |
| NQO1 | NAD(P)H:quinone oxidoreductase 1 |
| OPMDs | Oral potential malignant disorders |
| OSCC | Oral squamous cell carcinoma |
| OSF | Oral submucous fibrosis |
| PAI-1 | Plasminogen activator inhibitor-1 |
| PCR | Polymerase chain reaction |
| PDGF | Platelet-derived growth factor |
| PIK3 | Phosphoinositide 3-kinase inhibitor |
| PLOD2 | Procollagen-lysine, 2-oxoglutarate 5-dioxygenase 2 |
| RFLP | Restriction fragment length polymorphism |
| ROS | Reactive oxygen species |
| SAS | Spindle assembly abnormal protein homolog |
| SMAD | Small worm type, mothers against decapentaplegic |
| SNPs | Single nucleotide polymorphisms |
| SOD | Superoxide dismutase |
| Src | Proto-oncogene c-Src |
| SSCP | Single-strand conformation polymorphism |
| TGF | Transforming growth factor |
| TGF-β | Transforming growth factor-β |

| | |
|---|---|
| TGF-$\alpha$ | Transforming growth factor-$\alpha$ |
| TIMPs | Tissue inhibitors of matrix metalloproteinases |
| TNF | Tumor necrosis factor |
| tPA | Tissue plasminogen activator |
| TT | Thymine thymine |
| uPA | Urokinase plasminogen activator |
| VEGF | Vascular endothelial growth factor |
| XRCC | X-ray cross-complementing |
| αSMA | Alpha smooth muscle actin |

# Introduction to Oral Submucous Fibrosis

Contents

# Oral Submucous Fibrosis: A Historical Perspective

*Vinay K. Hazarey and Newell W. Johnson*

## Contents



© The Author(s), under exclusive license to Springer Nature Switzerland AG 2023
S. Warnakulasuriya, K. Ranganathan (eds.), *Oral Submucous Fibrosis*, Textbooks in Contemporary Dentistry,
https://doi.org/10.1007/978-3-031-12855-4_1

## 1.1 Introduction

Oral cancer has been a significant health issue in the Indian subcontinent and contiguous geographical areas for centuries—possibly for millennia. There are important references to this malady in ancient scripts. In the last century, numerous researchers and clinical groups have undertaken research on oral cancer using contemporary concepts of scientific method and have also studied what were described in the past as oral "precancers": for these, we now use the term oral potentially malignant disorders (OPMDs). Amongst the latter, what is now labeled oral leukoplakia, with its variable definitions, has received most attention. What we now call oral submucous fibrosis (OSF) was, until around the middle of the last century, an entirely enigmatic malady and received little attention. It was not until the Indian otolaryngologists Joshi and De Sa from King Edward VII Memorial (KEM) Hospital, Bombay (Mumbai, India), and the dentist Lal from Central India documented their clinical observations in the 1950s that real progress began to be made. The Basic Dental Research Unit of the Tata Institute for Fundamental Research (TIFR) in Mumbai, India conducted groundbreaking studies on OPMDs and oral cancer throughout the 1960s and 1970s. These brought OSF to the forefront as a critical OPMD in the Indian subcontinent. Thus, there began an understanding of a relationship—potentially causal—with traditional "betel quid" chewing habits, and we now know that it is predominantly the areca nut component in the betel quid which is responsible for the fibrosis. The early twentieth century contains interesting literature by Bentall (1908) and Orr (1933) describing oral cancer in "betel" chewers. Some of these cases had oral symptoms suggestive of OSF [1, 2] (▶ Box 1.1).

**Box 1.1: Learning Objectives**

1. To identify the historical documentation of OSF in South Asia.
2. To appreciate that associations made of OSF with chewing betel quid in the early literature.
3. To correlate the early understanding and descriptions of OSF from the Vedic and Modern era.

## 1.2 A Sweep Across Time

The Indian diaspora has distinguished itself throughout the world. East Africa was one of the earliest countries where Indians migrated. Wherever Indians went, they carried ethnic, cultural, and dietary habits from home: local populations adopted the habits. As a result, the twentieth- and twenty-first-century literature shows reports of OSF studies from, for example, Taiwan, South Africa, Sri Lanka, Nepal, Guam and China.

Areca nut consumption has been an integral part of the sociocultural and religious milieu of India and surrounding countries for millennia. Twentieth-century observations generated interest as to whether betel quid, areca nut in particular, caused the tissue changes seen in OSF—or at least similar signs and symptoms suggestive of the presence of this disease in ancient times. We felt that scrutiny of ancient Indian medical texts and related literature could reveal interesting historical facts and contribute to understanding of pathogenesis. Convincing contemporary evidence has implicated the development of OSF to regular chewing of areca nut, although cases are reported in children after quite short periods of use, as short as several months. The practice of chewing betel quid or *paan* is ancient. Areca nut and betel leaves are often used in Hindu religious and social functions, as in the other major Eastern religions, Islam and Buddhism. The first[1] mention of betel quid dates back to 504 BCE (BC), recorded in a Ceylon historical chronicle of events named "*Mahavamsa*," written in Pali [3]. Mentions of areca nut (*Pugi Phalam*) and betel leaf (*Tambul*) consumption can also be found in the *Sushruta*[1]: *Samhita*[2] of ~600 BCE [4]. The *Chikitsa*[3] *Sthana*[4] of the *Samhita* highlights the benefits and contraindications of *Pugi Phalam* and *Tambul* consumption in various conditions. *Shlokas* 21–24 indicate that the chewing of *Tambul*, in combination with many other ingredients, including areca nut, was wholesome and beneficial for the oral cavity, throat, and face. However, consumption of these mixtures in individuals with "intrinsic hemorrhage, wasting due to chest wound, thirst, fainting, roughness, debility, and mouth dryness" was not advocated. Thus, according to the *Sushruta Samhita*, although betel leaf and areca nut are considered sacred or beneficial, their use by individuals with dry mouth (as observed in OSF) is contraindicated [4].

The *Sushruta Samhita* encompasses all aspects of human disease prevalent in ancient India. The treatise made significant contributions to the principles and techniques of ancient Indian surgery, which are applicable even in the modern era [5]. The Royal Australasian College of Surgeons (RACS) at its headquarters in Melbourne, Australia, has stationed a statue of *Sushruta* as a mark of recognition and respect for his contributions (◘ Fig. 1.1).

1 *Sushruta* was an Indian physician and surgeon who, it is thought, lived around 800–900 years BCE (approx. 2800 years ago). He is revered as the father of Indian (Ayurvedic) medicine. His writings, in Sanskrit, are famous.

2 *Samhita* is a collection of prose, poems, or liturgies compiled under strict rules of style.

3 *Chikitsa* is a method of caring or treating a malady, including cognitive and spiritual approaches.

4 *Sthana* literally means a holy place; here to refer to significant parts of a treatise.

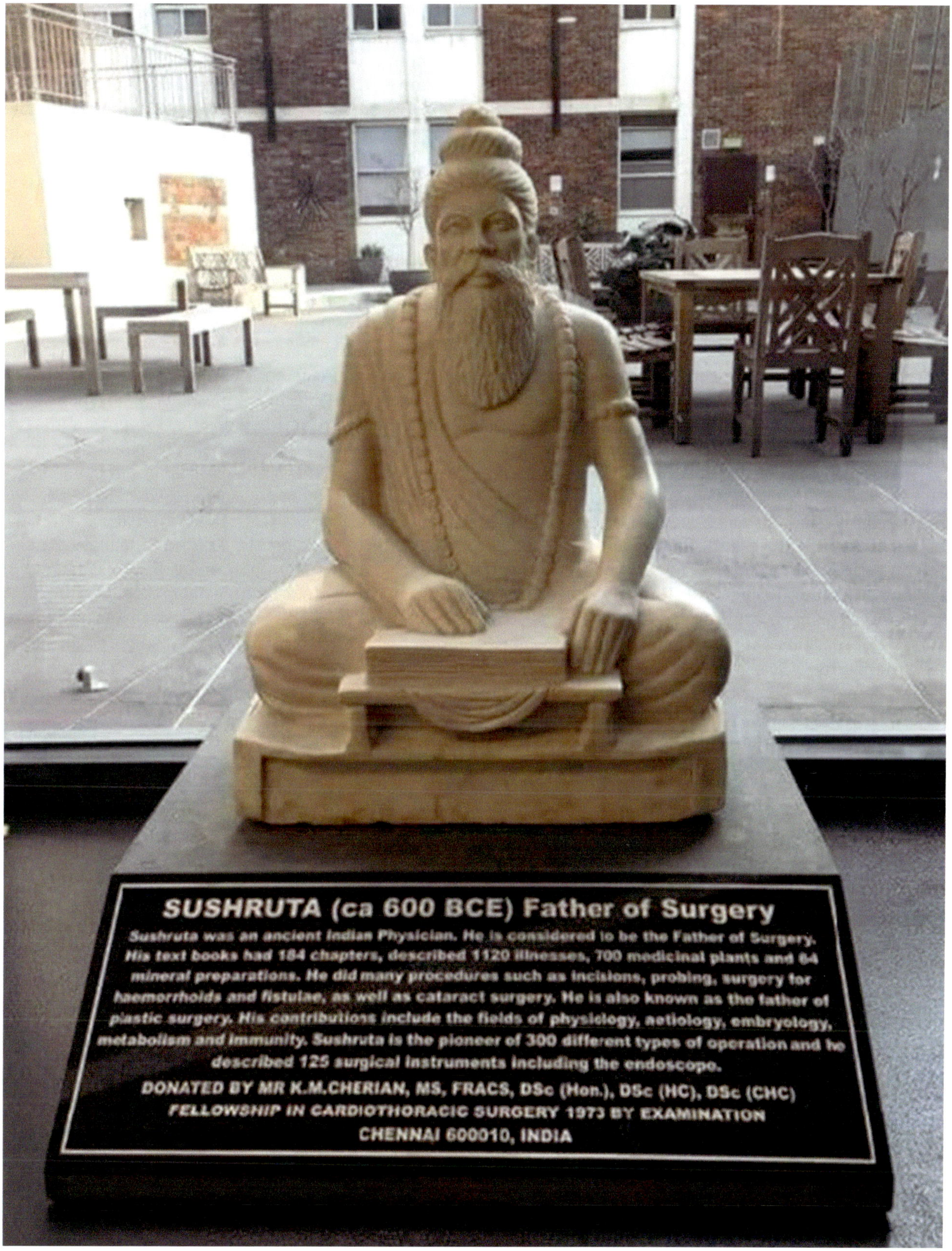


**Fig. 1.1** Statue of *Sushrut*a at the Royal Australasian College of Surgeons (RACS) in Melbourne, Australia

Many twentieth-century researchers, including Mukherjee and Biswas (1972), appear to have compared OSF to a condition known as "*Vidari*" in the Vedic literature [6]. According to them, the features of *Vidari*, as mentioned in the *Sushruta Samhita*, were progressive narrowing of the mouth, depigmentation of the oral mucosa, and pain while taking food, which precisely fit the symptomatology of OSF as we understand it today [6].

We conducted a thorough literature search on "*Vidari*" and scrutinized six *Sushruta Samhitas* published or edited by the eminent Indian Ayurvedic specialists Sharma, Patil, and Rajeshwari, amongst others [7–13]. This search yielded the Sanskrit *shloka* "***Sadahtodam swayathum sarktamantrgale putivishirnsmasaml Pitten Vidhyadwaden Vidarim parsve visheshat sat u yen shete***" (*Shloka* 63). The English translation describes "*a disease in which copper-colored swelling occurs in the throat, featured by pricking and burning sensation, and the flesh of the throat becomes necrosed and falls off and emits a fetid smell.*" The disease was regarded as of *Pittaja* origin and was found to attack the side of the throat on which the patient is lying [9]. The *Samhita* also describes this malady as an incurable disease and recommends that the treatment of *Vidari* should be approached without giving any assurance of cure [10]. Recently edited books on *Sushruta Samhita* confirm the same [7, 13]. Several versions of *Sushruta Samhita* describe *Vidari* as gangrenous stomatitis or "cancrum oris" [12], although today we would recognize cancrum oris (Noma) as an entity distinct from OSF [14]. According to Vidwansa, *Vidari* is synonymous for carcinoma of tonsil and tonsillar fossa [11]. *Vidari* is also translated as *Pitika* (eruptions) by Vagbhata [15].

Thus, according to *Sushruta Samhita*, *Vidari* is a throat disease where copper-colored vesicles are the primary manifestations. The description of *Vidari* mirrored that of gangrenous stomatitis, peritonsillar abscess (quinsy), and carcinoma of the tonsil or tonsillar fossa. Thus, our current understanding of the clinical presentations of OSF is not in agreement with the traditional description of *Vidari*. In our opinion, "*Vidari*" should not be used synonymously for OSF and should be considered a misnomer.

## 1.3 Other Relevant Ayurvedic Literature

According to Ayurveda, diseases of the human body are grouped based on three *Doshas* or principles, namely *Vata* (movement), *Pitta* (transformation), and *Kapha* (lubrication and stability). Vagbhata (in the first century CE (AD)) mentioned a condition with features similar to those of OSF known as "*vataja sarvasara*" [15]. The shlokas mentioned in his compilation are:

*Karonti vadanasyaantvranan sarvasaro nilah/Saccharinorunan rukshnoshto tamro chaltwachow* (*Shloka 66*)

*Jivha shitasaha gurvi sphutita kantakachita/Vivrunoti cha krichchhen mukham pako mukhasya sah* (*Shloka 67*)

*Sloka* 67 translates in English as "*Anila* (*Vata*)" aggravates and moving in all directions produces ulcers inside the mouth, which are mild red in color and dry (non-exudative); the lips are copper colored and unsteady; the tongue is intolerant to cold and is heavy, cracked, and covered with thorns; and the patient opens his mouth with difficulty ("*Vivrinoti cha Krichchhen Mukham*" translated as "mouth opening with difficulty"). This disease is *Mukhapaka of vata* origin [15].

Vidwansa described three pathological conditions that presented with clinical features similar to OSF, namely *Vataja Sarvasara*—herpetic gingivostomatitis/orolabial herpes; *Pittaja Sarvasara* with *Raktaja Sarvasara*—aphthous ulcer/recurrent ulcerative stomatitis; and *Kaphaja Sarvasara*—mild stomatitis [11].

Present-day Ayurveda deals with the management of conditions with clinical features and pathogenesis similar to OSF based on the individual's *prakriti* and associated *Dosha* [16, 17]. Patel et al. compared the clinical features of OSF with *Dosha*-based *mukharogas* and proposed that OSF can be considered a *Vata Pitta Pradhana Sarvasara Mukhroga* [16]. Recently, Patel and Patel, through their work on the Ayurvedic management of OSF, emphasized that one cannot directly equate OSF with any *Mukhrogas* in Ayurvedic classics; instead, it should be considered as *Anukta Vyadhi* or an unexplained disease, which may be managed by methodologies given by *Acharya Charaka*. Studying the above Ayurvedic literature, some Sanskrit terms when translated into English suggest similarities to the clinical symptoms of OSF. These include *Krichchhen Vivrinoti Mukham* (difficulty in opening mouth), *Mukhadaha—Usha* (burning sensation in mouth), *Tishna Asaha* (intolerance to spicy food), *Mukhsosha* (dryness of mouth), *Arasagyata, Alparasagyata, Virasagyata* (defective gustatory sensation), *Mukhantrargata Vrana* (ulceration of oral mucosa), and *Vranavastu, Durudha Vrana* (scar-fibrosis) [16, 17]. Thus, it seems probable that OSF existed in the *Sushruta* or Vedic era (~800–900 BCE) (▶ Box 1.2).

**Box 1.2: Appellations Used for Oral Submucous Fibrosis**

**Vedic Era:**

*Vidari*—Sushruta Samhita (800 BCE) [*Cited by Mukherjee& Biswas (1972)*]

*Vataja Sarvasara*—Waghbatta (first century CE (AD))

**Modern Era:**

Atrophica Idiopathica (Trophica) mucosae oris—Schwartz J (1952)

Submucous Fibrosis of Palate and Pillars—Joshi S (1953)

Diffuse Oral Submucous Fibrosis—Lal D (1953)

Idiopathic Scleroderma of the Mouth—Su I (1954)

Oral Submucous Fibrosis—Pindborg J. (1965)

## 1.4 Studies on OSF During the Past Century

OSF is common in India and elsewhere in South and SE Asia including Sri Lanka, Micronesia, Indonesia, and the Philippines [18–23] (▶ Box 1.3, ◘ Maps 1.1 and 1.2, ◘ Table 1.1). Enclaves are found outside these areas: in Africa, cases are being reported from Zanzibar, Tanzania, Madagascar, Kenya, and South Africa, and in the United Kingdom amongst the ethnic Indian diaspora. Because of modern travel, the use of areca nut and cases of OSF are now found in many continents. Six hundred million users are reported throughout the globe [23], ranking areca nut to fourth place amongst addictive substances after tobacco, alcohol, and caffeine [24, 25].

**Box 1.3: Bibliographic Data on Oral Submucous Fibrosis**

Keyword search on "oral submucous fibrosis" undertaken in the following databases on 8th November 2021:

- Web of Science: 1279 results
- Scopus: 1809 results
- Pubmed: 1638 results

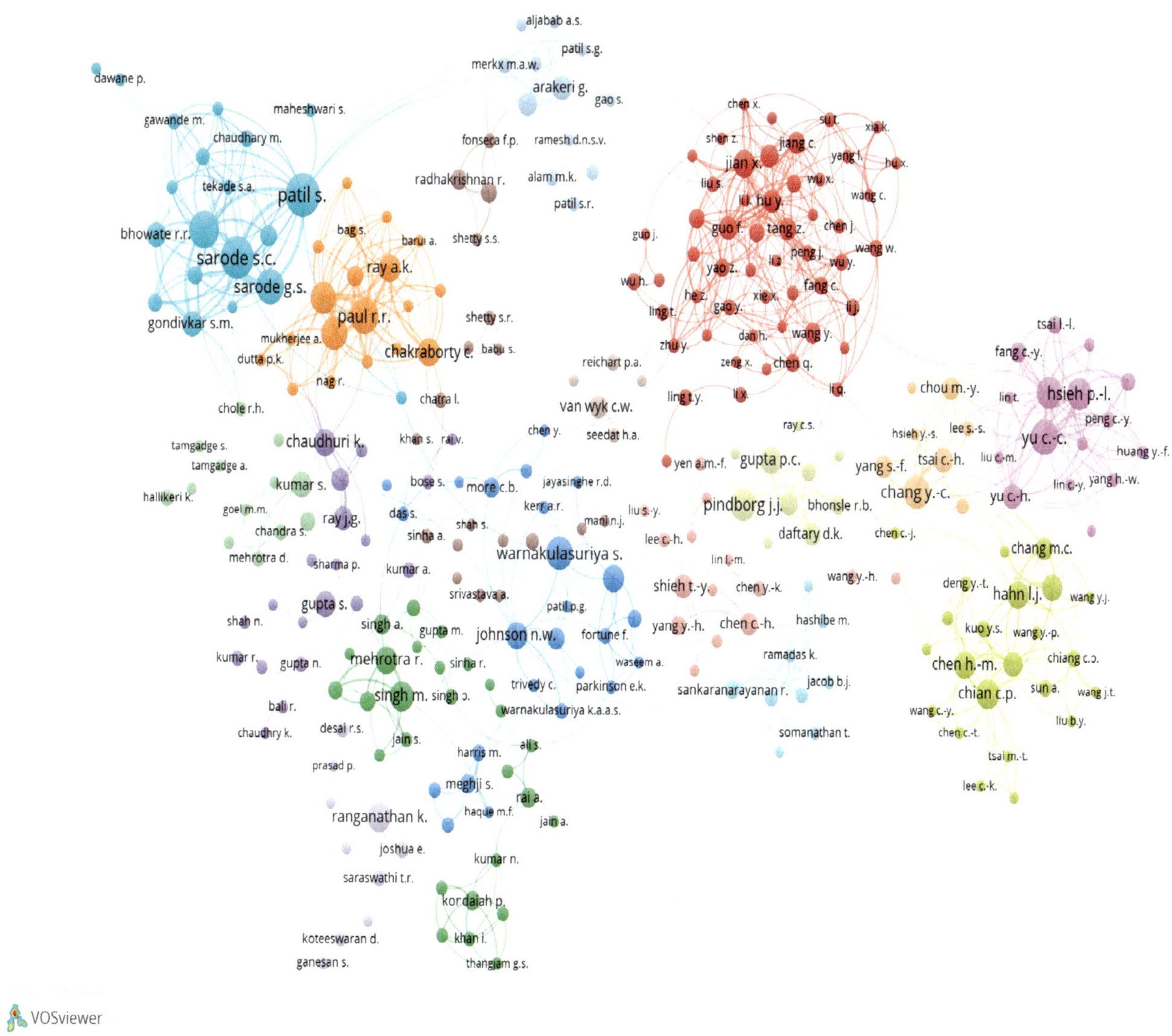


◘ **Map 1.1** Co-authorship data map on oral sub mucous fibrosis. Four or more articles per author = 359 authors. 304 authors were connected

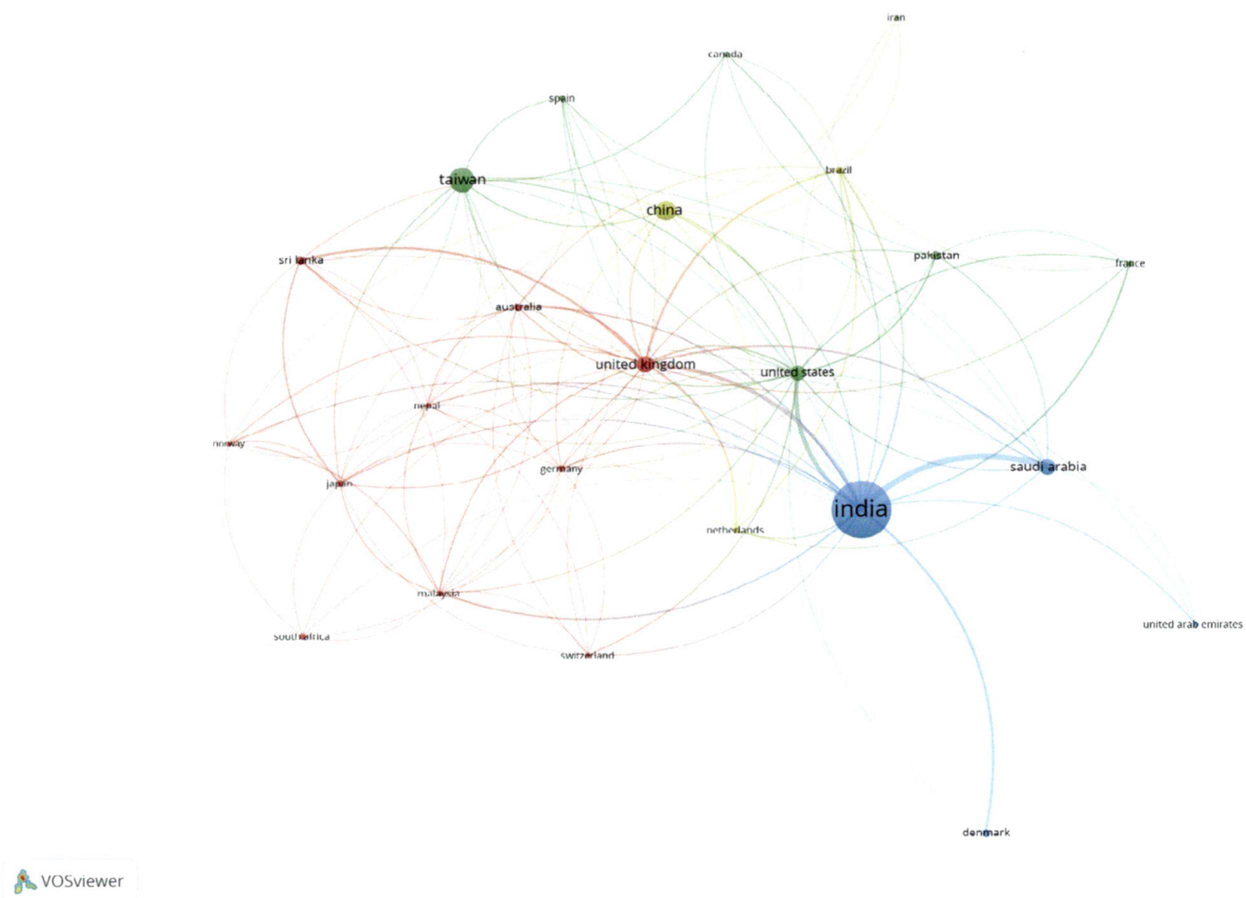


**Map 1.2** Co-authorship map on oral submucous fibrosis-based geographic location—5 or more articles per country = 25 countries; 24 are connected

### 1.4.1 Studies from South and SE Asia

#### 1.4.1.1 India

OSF is an OPMD with an important historical background in India. As summarized above, the earliest studies on OSF have their roots in Bombay in the late 1940s and 1950s. The disease was studied by Joshi and De Sa from around 1949 at the ENT Department of KEM Hospital, Mumbai. However, almost all subsequent literature attributes the first published reference to "idiopathica atrophica (trophica) mucosae oris" by Schwartz, in five Indian Gujarati females from Kenya, with the habit of chewing supari (areca nut). This was referenced as a "demonstration" at the 11th International Dental Congress (of the Federation Dentaire Internationale (FDI)), London, July 1952 [26]. This reference has been quoted scores of times in subsequent literature, but it is clearly quoted secondarily—without sight of the original. We cannot locate original copy in spite of searches through libraries of many institutions throughout the world and online. Quoting material without sight of the original is bad practice.

Thus, the first detailed description of this disease in the modern era should be attributed to Joshi in April 1953, who studied 41 cases from Mumbai and called the condition "submucous fibrosis of palate and pillars" [27]. Lal, an Indian dental graduate with licentiate qualifications from the United Kingdom, working at the Govt. Medical College, Gwalior (Central India), reported in May 1953 the clinicopathological findings of 20 cases. All his cases had supari (areca nut) chewing habits. He classified his cases into clinically early, advanced, and extreme. He describes, in histological sections, diffuse subepithelial fibrosis of the oral mucous membrane, with complete replacement of normal lamina propria by dense acellular nonelastic fibers, together with focal collections of lymphocytes and plasma cells. He termed the disease "diffuse oral submucous fibrosis." He suggested physicochemical irritation or an allergen in supari (areca nut) as causation and discussed the condi-

**Table 1.1** Co-authorship data on oral submucous fibrosis-based geographic location

Create Map ×

**Verify selected countries**

| Selected | Country | Documents | Citations | Total link strength |
|---|---|---|---|---|
| ✓ | india | 1140 | 15407 | 241 |
| ✓ | taiwan | 210 | 6222 | 27 |
| ✓ | china | 141 | 1481 | 33 |
| ✓ | united kingdom | 97 | 5275 | 118 |
| ✓ | saudi arabia | 86 | 530 | 104 |
| ✓ | united states | 82 | 2259 | 95 |
| ✓ | sri lanka | 32 | 1307 | 32 |
| ✓ | pakistan | 31 | 724 | 15 |
| ✓ | australia | 25 | 1618 | 32 |
| ✓ | denmark | 23 | 1830 | 16 |
| ✓ | germany | 19 | 854 | 19 |
| ✓ | south africa | 19 | 595 | 6 |
| ✓ | japan | 18 | 1019 | 29 |
| ✓ | brazil | 17 | 233 | 37 |
| ✓ | malaysia | 16 | 639 | 32 |
| ✓ | france | 14 | 711 | 18 |
| ✓ | netherlands | 13 | 1552 | 31 |
| ✓ | canada | 9 | 215 | 8 |
| ✓ | nepal | 9 | 288 | 19 |
| ✓ | spain | 9 | 194 | 9 |

< Back | Next > | Finish | Cancel

tion as a mucous membrane counterpart of scleroderma [28]. There is, however, no subsequent evidence of which we are aware that OSF occurs as part of a wider fibrotic disease. Nevertheless, despite Lal's probably erroneous linkage to wider scleroderma, his original descriptions and attributes fit closely to our present understanding of the disorder.

Otolaryngologists in India studied the condition comprehensively [27, 28]. Rao and Raju (1954) reported five cases, which had slowly progressive incompetence to mouth opening associated with an inability to eat food and which were treated using oral cortisone tablets [29]. They described pallor of the oral mucosa and palpable, thick vertical fibrous bands on both cheeks.

At KEM Hospital, Bombay, a detailed study of almost 100 cases was undertaken. De Sa presented the investigations, treatment, and outcomes of 64 cases in his 1957 publication [30]. The group there performed extensive research exploring etio-pathological aspects and relationships with other diseases and attempted to provide relief to patients using then current concepts of treatment. They grouped cases with predominantly palatal, faucial, and/or buccal involvement. They described histopathological detail and sought to correlate this with treatment outcomes. They concluded that "submucous fibrosis of the palate and cheek" is a new connective tissue disorder with biological similarity to the other collagen diseases but localized to the oral cavity. These were noteworthy contributions for the time. George shared, in 1958, another report on treatment with cortisone injections [31].

Paymaster (1956) was the first to raise submucous fibrosis as a "precancerous lesion." Neoplasms of the oral cavity and pharynx accounted for 45 percent of all malignancies seen in Indian patients at the Tata Memorial Hospital, Mumbai, at that time—the 1950s [32]. Paymaster described mucosal melanin pigmentation and localized submucosal fibrosis. He described clinical variations, treatment approaches, and 5-year follow-up results of his cases. One-third of his 650 patients with "precancers" developed slow-growing carcinomas in affected areas: another remarkable observation for the time [32].

Many early studies from India were conducted under the guidance of the late, great Professor Jens Pindborg from Copenhagen, working with several government dental colleges in North, Central, and South India. Amongst these was the research conducted at a dental college in Trivandrum, in which 40 out of 100 cases of oral cancer had clinical signs of OSF [33].

Pindborg and Chawla examined 10,000 patients at the Dental Department of King George's Medical College in Lucknow, during 1964/1965 [34, 35]. All diagnoses were made on clinical grounds. Fifty-one patients (1.48%) had OSF: 25 cases of OSF were found in a cohort of patients seeking treatment in the clinics of dental colleges in Lucknow [35]. A detailed demographic analysis of these OSF patients contributed significantly to our understanding of initial and presenting symptoms of OSF. In 7 cases, concomitant leukoplakia was observed in patients with a history of tobacco abuse: this was the first report of such an association [35].

In parallel, the TIFR, Mumbai, established itself as the central hub for designing and executing epidemiological and translational studies on oral cancer and "precancer." Studies by Joshi, Lal, Sirsat, and Pindborg between 1952 and 1964 led to the monumental epidemiological surveys of the Basic Dental Research Unit of TIFR, which began in 1966 and lasted almost 30 years. Professor Fali Mehta was the principal investigator with Pindborg and Dr. James Hamner III from the University of Tennessee, USA, was the National Institute of Health (NIH) project officer—the studies were largely funded by the US NIH. Dinesh Daftary (oral pathologist), Prakash Gupta (statistician), Mira Aghi (behavioral scientist), and Ramesh Bhonsle, Paluri Ram Murti, Pessi Sinor, Peshotan Jalnawalla, and Late Rohinton Irani (dentists) formed the core team camping at rural areas in five districts of different states and conducting oral examinations of close to two hundred thousand people and coordinating with headquarters at TIFR (▶ Box 1.4).

**Box 1.4: Contributions from Tata Institute of Fundamental Research (TIFR), Mumbai**

**Duration: 1966–1995**

1. **Pindborg et al.—1968**

   Epidemiological survey

   Population studied: 50,915 individuals

   Inference: Evidence in support of OSF as a "Precancerous Condition"
2. **Gupta et al.—1980**

   Observational study with 10 years follow-up

   Inference: Association between tobacco and betel quid habits and incidence of oral mucosal lesions.
3. **Murti et al.—1985**

   Observational study with 17 years follow-up of 66 individuals with OSF

   Malignant transformation rate studied over 10, 15 and 17 years (7.6%)
4. **Bhonsle et al.—1987**

   A cohort of 64 and 24 OSF in a survey of 27,000 villagers in Ernakulum and at Pune.

   Regional variations and associations of areca nut habit with OSF in Ernakulum and Pune
5. **Murti et al.—1995**

   Review: The role of areca nut in the etiology of oral submucous fibrosis.

A substantial literature was generated by the team, covering prevalence, incidence, and natural history of a range of OPMD, including OSF and outlining the development of malignancy, over more than a decade of intensive study.

The Pindborg and Mehta 1968 paper presented epidemiological surveys amongst Indian villagers. Amongst 50,915 persons studied, OSF was more prevalent in South than in North India, the prevalence ranging from 0% to 0.4%. Clinical data were analyzed from 63 cases of OSF. Atrophy of tongue papillae was a prominent feature with a prevalence of 60%. Heavy and frequent consumption of chilies was often associated with the disorder, but chilies are an almost universal component of South Asian food, and it is no longer thought that they play a significant role in the pathogenesis of OSF. These findings did, however, support OSF as a "precancerous" condition [36].

Simultaneously, many institutions in India and some overseas instituted research on OSF. Those from India included the Government Dental College and Hospital, Mumbai, and Nair Hospital Dental College, Mumbai. Both these institutes started postgraduate courses in oral pathology (then known as Dental Pathology and Bacteriology) in 1962–1964. Mani was amongst the first to complete a Master's dissertation at the University of Bombay. In 1964–1966, under the supervision of Singh, he evaluated 38 cases of OSF and published four papers in Indian and international journals. Clinical and cytological aspects were published in 1968 and 1976 [37, 38]. Subsequently, Mani and Singh reported on the epithelial features of OSF and observed hyperkeratosis, atrophy, increased mitoses, and glycogen in various grades of OSF. They hypothesized that parakeratosis, increased mitosis, and atrophic epithelium could indicate "premalignant change" and supported the "precancerous" nature of OSF [39]. In 1977, Mani further compared the connective tissue changes of OSF with those of collagen diseases like scleroderma. They found inflammation and progressive collagen deposition in the lamina propria with increasing clinical severity of the condition [40]. These studies highlighted the need to explore whether the epithelial-connective tissue changes occur concomitantly or as independent responses to common irritants or other, still unknown, factors implicated in the pathogenesis of OSF.

Akbar, a postgraduate student of Dholakia (who was the first recognized postgraduate guide for "dental research" in India), completed his dissertation, which focused on the clinical and histopathological features of OSF in partial fulfillment of his Master's degree from the University of Bombay, 1964–1966. Amongst the 30 patients studied, he reported one elderly female with OSF and concurrent scleroderma of the skin. The case showed extensive involvement of the skin of legs, hands, chest, and face; the jaw deviated to the left on opening. Subepithelial hyalinization was noted in 50% of his oral biopsies [41, 42].

Renowned Indian cancer researcher and microbiologist, Sirsat, was the first to employ electron microscopy to study OSF. She completed her doctoral thesis entitled "Biological studies with the electron microscope with special reference to submucous fibrosis of the palate" in 1958 from the University of Bombay [43]. Sirsat, in another collaboration with Pindborg and Padma Bhushan awardee Khanolkar V, studied cases of OSF and established a model in Wistar rats—the first ever animal experiment on then condition (▶ Box 1.5).

**Box 1.5: First Animal Model for OSF—Sirsat and Khanolkar (1960, 1962)**

Study Animal: Wistar Rats

Features evaluated: Histological and Electron Microscopic changes in collagen fibers of rat oral mucosa after treatment with Capsiacin and Arecoline.

Sirsat and Khanolkar (1960) described histological and electron microscopic features and studied the effect of trypsin, collagenases, hyaluronidase, and elastase on the collagen fiber structure in their rat model [44]. They studied the effects of arecoline and capsaicin on rat oral mucosa and noted "elastic degeneration of collagen." They hypothesized that persistent mild injury over a prolonged period led to fibrosis of the lamina propria [45–47].

Pindborg and Sirsat (1966) reviewed the etiological factors, clinicopathological features, and potential treatment approaches [48]. They defined: "Oral submucous fibrosis is an insidious, chronic disease affecting any part of the oral cavity and sometimes the pharynx. It is occasionally preceded by a juxta-epithelial inflammatory reaction followed by a fibroelastic change of lamina propria with epithelial atrophy leading to stiffness of oral mucosa and trismus and inability to eat." They also described mast cell counts and vascular changes in both early and advanced stages of OSF (1967) [49, 50]. They opined that reduced vascularity was responsible for epithelial atrophy [50]. They graded disease into very early, early, moderately advanced, and advanced stages based on the histological features of edema, physical state of collagen, fibroblastic response, vascularity, and number and type of inflammatory cells present [51].

The TIFR team contributed to the understanding of prevalence and incidence and of the timing and proportion of cases, which developed oral cancer, and of the risk factors involved. In 1985, a population-based house-to-house survey examined two lakh (2,00,000) Indian villagers. This project delivered over 100 reports and expanded the knowledge of tobacco and areca nut consumption practices prevalent in India, as well as the pathogenesis of a range of OPMD and the risks of subsequent malignancy.

Murti et al. (1985) followed up 66 cases of OSF for 17 years and found that oral cancer developed in 0.4% of cases at the end of 10 years, in 4.5% at the end of 15 years, and in 7.6% at the end of 17 years [52]. Gupta et al. (1980) reported a 10-year follow-up study, wherein they quantified OSF, oral cancer, and other "precancerous lesions" in Ernakulam, Bhavnagar, and Srikakulam. They associated social habits with the prevalence and incidence of oral lesions: OSF did not occur amongst those who did not practice chewing habits, nor in smoking-only subjects [53].

The etiological role of chewing areca nut by itself was shown in a study of regional variations of this condition in Ernakulam and Pune districts of India by Bhonsle et al. (1987) [54]. This study showed that part of the oral cavity most involved depends on the consumption pattern, i.e., where the quid is customarily held and whether or not the areca nut juice or quid is swallowed.

Hypotheses regarding the role of copper and the cuproprotein, lysyl oxidase (LO), in the pathogenesis of OSF were generated by collaborative work between researchers at King's College London; the Government Dental College, Nagpur; and the Department of Dental Sciences at the Royal College of Surgeons of England. Trivedy et al. (1997) proposed that copper in areca nut upregulates LO leading to cross-linking of collagen and subsequent fibrosis [55]. They proposed that oxidative deamination of lysine residues of collagen and elastin fibers rendered them resistant to physiological degradation. Further, considering the carcinogenic potential of OSF, Trivedy et al. (1998) studied the immunoexpression and mutations of the p53 gene in OSF, oral squamous cell carcinoma (OSCC) arising in OSF, and OSCC not associated with OSF. In a large sample of OSF tissues collected from Karachi, Pakistan, they proposed that the high copper content of areca nut bound to p53 and inhibited its tumor suppressive properties [56]. They demonstrated that fibroblasts in OSF showed intense immunoexpression of LO in the early stages of disease and in the stroma surrounding invading epithelial islands in carcinomas arising in OSF [57].

#### 1.4.1.2 Sri Lanka

In early 1980s, Warnakulasuriya et al. conducted a large-scale oral cancer and precancer screening program in Central Sri Lanka. Close to 30,000 adults aged over 20 years were screened by house-to-house visit by primary healthcare workers. 4.2% of the subjects screened positive, and amongst them 15 were reported with a OSF diagnosis [58].

#### 1.4.1.3 Taiwan

Su (1954) described reduced mouth opening in three Chinese men from Taiwan aged 30–40 years who were "betel nut" chewers. The author showed pale atrophic oral mucosa and limited tongue movement. Microscopic examination of their oral mucosa revealed fibrous "degeneration" of subepithelial layers. Su suggested the term "stromal scleroderma" as the author found the condition similar to systemic scleroderma and reported it with the title "idiopathic scleroderma of the mouth" [59].

Thirty-five cases of OSF were studied by Shiau and Kwan from 1971 to 1976 in Taiwan. All patients had a history of one or more habits of heavy liquor consumption, smoking, and/or "betel nut" chewing with a strong correlation between habitual areca nut consumption and occurrence of OSF [60].

In subsequent decades, Taiwanese scientists have made a significant contribution to the field.

#### 1.4.1.4 China

Apart from Taiwan, areca (betel) nut chewing was traditionally practiced in Hainan Island of the People's Republic of China. In 1983, Pindborg surveyed 100 villagers with "betel nut" chewing habits and habit/s of smoking cigarettes and water pipes. He reported three women areca nut chewers with clinical and histologic changes of OSF [61].

Areca nut chewing was also common in southeast provinces of China. In Xiangtan, a big city of Hunan province, this habit can be traced back to the beginning of the Qing dynasty. In Yuhu, one of the five urban districts of Xiangtan city, 57 units independent of each other were randomly selected for an epidemiological survey wherein 11,046 individuals were examined. OSF was found in 335 individuals (3.03%), all of whom were areca nut chewers. OSF prevalence correlated to habit duration [62].

#### 1.4.1.5 Burma

The leaf of the Piper betel vine is called "*Kun-yet*" in Burmese. A quid containing betel nut/areca nut and other ingredients is called "*Kun-ya*" or simply "*Kun.*" *Kun* finds frequent mention in Burmese literature emphasizing its religious and cultural importance with the tradition dating back at least several hundred years. A marble inscription from 1248 AD refers to betel nut, revealing connections to royal regalia. A host's social status or official rank was ascertained based on the areca nut type and quality he or she provided to his or her guests. A comprehensive survey of 11 villages on the island of Bilugyun, Chuang-zone township, Mon State of southeastern Burma, was carried out for finding the prevalence of "oral precancerous lesions" and chewing and smoking in which 6000 villagers above 15 years were examined. This study, published in 1982, reported for the first time on five patients with OSF from Burma [63].

#### 1.4.1.6 Nepal

Nepal, sharing many cultural and dietary habits with the rest of South Asia, has documented cases of OSF from as early as 1954. Lalchand reported 15 cases during a 25-day stay in Nepal in 1954 [29].

#### 1.4.1.7 Malaysia

An early contribution to OSF came from Malaysia by Krishnappa in 1967 [64]. Subsequently, Ramanathan (1981) observed iron-deficiency anemia in 10 out of 13 OSF cases in Malaysia and hypothesized the disease to be a form of sideropenic dysphagia [65]. All OSF patients were of Indian ethnicity maintaining Indian dietary habits.

#### 1.4.1.8 Papua New Guinea

Consumption of "betel nut" with betel "mustard" and lime is prevalent in Papua New Guinea, but early literature only shows associations with oral cancer [20]. The first documented case of OSF by Barnes and Duke

(1975) was in a Chinese woman residing in Papua New Guinea who had no history of betel consumption [19]. Areca nut is known as *buii* in PNG. Its use is ubiquitous. There are high rates of oral squamous cell carcinomas [66], but no reports of OSF have been found after extensive searches. We have this enigma under investigation.

#### 1.4.1.9 South Africa

Consumption of areca nut was introduced into South Africa by Indian immigrants in 1860 [67]. In what is now the Republic of South Africa, there were soon about one million South Africans of Indian descent concentrated mainly in Durban and environs. First amongst South African studies are those by Shear and Lemmer in 1967 [68], who found a prevalence of use of 0.5% amongst 1000 subjects of Indian ethnicity.

Seedat worked extensively on the epidemiological aspects of OSF in Durban, Natal, and submitted this work for his Ph.D. at Stellenbosch University in 1985 [69].

In 1988, Seedat and Van Wyk conducted an epidemiologic survey of 2058 Indian subjects settled in South Africa and found 71 cases of OSF—a remarkably high prevalence of 3.45% [70]. They revealed the strong association with "betel nut" chewing. Women chewers predominated with a ratio of 13:1. The habit was common in the elderly, with 30.6% of women over 65 years being users. 38% of chewers exhibited features of imminent or overt OSF, with female predominance of 70:1. The majority (12.9%) of affected persons were in the 45-54-year age group; 46% demonstrated fibrous bands in the mouth. The investigators concluded that at that time 5% of the entire Indian population in South Africa could be chewers, of which 2.3% may develop OSF [70].

Seedat and van Wyk (1988) found typical clinical and histopathological features of OSF in six non-betel nut-chewing subjects raising the possibility of genetic predisposition and of other etiological agents in Indian cultural practices [71]. They reported 14 cases of ex-"betel nut" chewers with characteristic clinical and histological features of OSF, which persisted even 13 years after stopping the habit [72].

Van Wyk (1997) reviewed OSF amongst South Africans of Indian origin and found that the betel quid use was more common amongst women. 60% of chewers preferred a betel quid with other "classical" ingredients, while others consumed only nut. Most chewers preferred the baked (black) nut variety, and few added tobacco to their chew. This pattern was reflected in the distribution of OSF. Their OSF subjects were younger with shorter chewing histories compared to chewers without OSF [73].

## 1.5 Summary of Recent History

In the later decades of the previous century, there have been numerous reviews on OSF describing epidemiology and pathogenesis [74, 75]. Pindborg et al. [36] assembled the early information on OSF

**Table 1.2** Distribution of OSF by geographic location, sex, and age in early investigations (1952–1964) [34]

| Investigator | Year | Country | Cases | Percentage women | The age range in years |
|---|---|---|---|---|---|
| Schwartz | 1952 | East Africa (Indians) | 5 | 100 | – |
| Lal | 1953 | India (Madhya Pradesh) | 20 | – | – |
| Joshi | 1953 | India (Bombay) | 41 | 54 | 10–60 |
| Su | 1954 | Taiwan | 3 | 0 | 30–40 |
| Rao and Raju (Lalchand in discussion to Rao and Raju) | 1954 | India<br>Nepal | 7<br>15 | 86<br>– | 18–40<br>– |
| De Sa | 1957 | India | 64 | 53 | 10–55 |
| Sharan | 1959 | India | 21 | Males predominated | 12–62 |
| Rao | 1962 | India (Hyderabad) | 46 | 63 | 12-64 |
| | 1962 | India (Bombay) | 85 | 53 | 10–58 |
| Pindborg | 1964 | India (Lucknow) | 25 | 60 | Female: 22–65<br>Average: 33.7 years<br>Male: 40–70<br>Average: 53.6 years |

1

(Table 1.2) according to geographic location, gender, and age.

In 1978, a working group of the WHO defined OSF as a "probable precancerous" condition, along with leukoplakia [76]. In 2005, the WHO Collaborating Center for Oral Cancer and Precancer at King's College London recommended the term "oral potentially malignant disorders," which included OSF [77]. This list, and definitions of OPMDs, has recently been updated [78].

**Summary**

Evolution of OSF from Vedic to early modern-day literature.

Correlation of dosha/prakruti-based diseases in Ayurveda with OSF.

Early research from South Asian countries and their contributions pertaining to etiology, clinical, histological as well as electron microscopic features of OSF.

Contemporaries—Joshi, De Sa and Lal described OSF in 1952–53 under different terms, to the evolution of existing knowledge of what is now known as OSF.

**Acknowledgements** We thank the following for their enthusiastic support in literature searching, especially in accessing ancient publications:

Dr. Supriya Kheur, Professor and Head, Department of Oral Pathology and Microbiology, Dr. D.Y. Patil Dental College and Hospital, Dr. D.Y. Patil Vidyapeeth, Pune, India.

Dr. Karishma M Desai, Assistant Professor, Department of Oral Pathology and Microbiology, Dr. D.Y. Patil Dental College and Hospital, Dr. D.Y. Patil Vidyapeeth, Pune, India.

Dr. Pankaj M Shirsat, Associate Professor, Department of Oral Pathology and Microbiology, Nair Dental Hospital and Dental College, Mumbai, India.

Dr Pankaj Chande, Former Vice Chancellor, Kavikulaguru Kalidas Sanskrit University Ramtek, Nagpur. India.

Dr Kiran Tawalare, Assistant Professor Shri Ayurved College, Nagpur, India.

Miss. Maria Connor, Information Services at Griffith University, Australia.

Dr. Vinay Hazarey was a research dentist at the Basic Dental Unit of TIFR 1978–1980. He wishes to acknowledge his long-term associations with Dr. Dinesh Daftary, Dr. PC Gupta, Dr. RB Bhonsle, and Dr. PR Murti formerly of TIFR.

## References

1. Bentall WC. Cancers in travancore. South India. Br Med J. 1908;2:1428–31.
2. Orr IM. Oral cancers in betel nut chewers. Lancet. 1933;222(5741):570–80.
3. IARC Monographs on the Evaluation of Carcinogenic Risks to Humans. Betel-quid and Areca-nut Chewing and Some Areca-nut-derived Nitrosamines (Vol. 85) Lyon, 2004. pp. 33
4. Sharma PV. Sushruta-Samhita with English translation of text and Dalhana's commentary along with critical notes. Haridas Ayurveda Series 9. Vol II (Nidana, Sarira and Cikitsasthana), Chapter XXIV, Varanasi: Chowkhambha Visvabharati 2000; p. 493.
5. Singh V. Sushruta: the father of surgery. Natl J Maxillofac Surg. 2017;8(1):1–3. https://doi.org/10.4103/njms.NJMS_33_17.
6. Mukherjee AL, Biswas SK. Oral submucous fibrosis—a search for aetiology. Ind J Otol. 1972;24:11–5. https://doi.org/10.1007/BF02991934.
7. Sharma PV. Susruta-Samhita with English translation of text and Dalhana's commentary along with critical notes. Haridas Ayurveda Series 9. Vol II (Nidana, Sarira and Cikitsasthana), Varanasi: Chowkhambha Visvabharati 2000; p 113–114.
8. Patil VC, Rajeshwari NM. Sushruta Samhita of Maharsi Sushruta with English translation of Text and Dalhana's commentary with critical notes, vol. II. New Delhi: Chaukambha Publications; 2018. p. 110.
9. Bhishagratna Kaviraj Kunjalal. An English translation of the Sushruta Samhita with a full and comprehensive introduction, additional texts, different readings, notes, comparative views, index, glossary and plates (Volume II—Nidana-sthana, Sarira-sthana, Chikitsita-sthana and Kalapa-sthana) Chapter XVI Mukha-Roga, Bhattacharyya, Bharat Mihir Press, Calcutta. 1911; p. 111.
10. Bhishagratna Kaviraj Kunjlal. An English translation of the Sushruta Samhita with a full and comprehensive introduction, additional texts, different readings, notes, comparative views, index, glossary and plates (Volume II—Nidana-sthana, Sarira-sthana, Chikitsita-sthana and Kalapa-sthana) Chapter XXII Chikitsa Sthana. Bhattacharyya, Bharat Mihir Press, Calcutta. 1911; p. 462-474.
11. Vidwansa NJ. Text book of Shalakya Tantra (Ayurvedic E.N.T and Oro-Dental Diseases) (Shiro-Karna-Nasa-Mukh & Dant Rog Vigyan) Vol. II, 1st ed. Chaukhamba Surbharti Publications Varanasi; 2016, p. 241.
12. Shastri Kaviraja Ambikadutta. Sushruta Samhita (The Kashi Sanskrit Series 156) Chaukhambha Sanskrit Sansthan Varanasi. vol 1, Chapter 16, 2010, p.361.
13. P. Himasagara Chandra Murthy. Susruta Samhita of Maharishi Susruta (Translation of Text and Nibandha Sangraha Commentary Of Sri Dalhana), (Banaras Ayurvedic Series 77) Vol II Nidanasthana – Chikitsasthana. Chowkhamba Sanskrit Series Office Varanasi. Chapter 16, 1st ed., 2021, p. 146–147.
14. Ashok N, Tarakji B, Darwish S, Rodrigues JC, Altamimi MA. A review on Noma: a recent update. Glob J Health Sci. 2015;8(4):53–9. https://doi.org/10.5539/gjhs.v8n4p53.
15. Srikantha Murti K R, Astanga Samagra of Wagbhatta (Text English translation, notes etc.) (Jaikrishandas Ayurveda Series 79) Vol III Uttarsthana, Chaukhamba Orientia Varanasi India Reprint edition 2016 Chapter 25, p. 222.
16. Patel PJ, Waghela DB, Maniyar H. Study on Ayurvedic management of Sarvasara Mukharoga Wsr Oral Submucous Fibrosis (OSMF). Int Ayurvedic Med J. 2017;5(6):1825–37.
17. Patel KR. A pilot study on Ayurvedic management of oral submucous fibrosis. Ayu. 2015;36:34–40.
18. Amarasinghe HK, Usgodaarachchi US, Johnson NW, Lalloo R, Warnakulasuriya S. Betel-quid chewing with or without tobacco is a major risk factor for oral potentially malignant disorders in Sri Lanka: a case-control study. Oral Oncol. 2010;46(4):297–301. https://doi.org/10.1016/j.oraloncology.2010.01.017.
19. Barnes P, Duke P. Submucous fibrosis. P N G Med J. 1975;18(1):66–70.
20. Paissat DK. Oral submucous fibrosis. Int J Oral Surg. 1981;10(5):307–12.

21. Oakley E, Demaine L, Warnakulasuriya S. Areca (betel) nut chewing habit among high-school children in the Commonwealth of the Northern Mariana Islands (Micronesia). Bull World Health Organ. 2005;83(9):656–60. Epub 2005 Sep 30. PMID: 16211156; PMCID: PMC2626335
22. Kerr AR, Warnakulasuriya S, Mighell AJ, Dietrich T, Nasser M, Rimal J, et al. A systematic review of medical interventions for oral sub mucous fibrosis and future research opportunities. Oral Dis. 2011;17:42–57.
23. Trivedy CR. The legislative issues related to the sale and consumption of areca (betel) nut products in the UK: Current status and objectives for the future. J Indian Med Assoc. 2001;1:10–6.
24. Marshall M. An overview of drugs in oceania. In: Lindstrom L, editor. Drugs in Western Pacific societies: relations of substance (ASAO Monograph No. 11). Boston, MA: University Press of America; 1987. p. 1–49.
25. Sullivan RJ, Hagen EH. Psychotropic substance-seeking: evolutionary pathology or adaptation? Addiction. 2002;97:389–400.
26. Schwartz J. Atrophica Idiopathica (Tropica) mucosae oris. Demonstrated at the Eleventh International Dental Congress London, 1952. [Cited multiple times since then, including by Rajendran R. Oral submucous fibrosis: etiology, pathogenesis, and future research. Bull World Health Organ. 1994; 72(6): 985-96].
27. Joshi SG. Submucous fibrosis of the palate and pillars. Ind J Otolaryngol. 1953;4:1–4. [Cited by Pindborg JJ, Chawla TN, Srivastava AN, Gupta D, Mehrotra ML. Clinical Aspects Of Oral Submucous Fibrosis. Acta Odontologica Scandinavica, 1964; 22, 679–691]
28. Lal D. Diffuse oral submucous fibrosis. J All India Dent Assoc. 1953;26:1–3.
29. Rao VR, Raju PR. A preliminary report of treatment of oral submucous fibrosis of oral cavity with cortisone. Ind J Otolaryngol. 1954;2:81–3.
30. De Sa JV. Submucous fibrosis of the palate and cheek. Ann Otol Rhinol Laryngol. 1957;66:1143–59.
31. George AT. Oral submucous fibrosis of palate and buccal mucosa. J Indian Med Assoc. 1958;30912:489–90.
32. Paymaster JC. Cancer of the buccal mucosa; a clinical study of 650 cases in Indian patients. Cancer. 1956;9:431–5.
33. Pindborg JJ, Zachariah J. Frequency of oral submucous fibrosis among 100 South Indians with oral cancer. Bull WHO. 1965;32:750–3.
34. Pindborg JJ, Chawla TN, Srivastava AN, Gupta D, Mehrotra ML. Clinical aspects of oral submucous fibrosis. Acta Odontol Scand. 1964;22:679–91.
35. Pindborg JJ, Chawla TN, Misra RK, Nagpaul RK, Gupta VK. Frequency of oral carcinoma, leukoplakia, leukokeratosis, leukoedema, submucous fibrosis, and lichen planus in 10,000 Indians in Lucknow, Uttar Pradesh, India; Preliminary report. J Dent Res. 1965;44:61.
36. Pindborg JJ, Mehta FS, Gupta PC, Daftary DK. Prevalence of oral submucous fibrosis among 50,915 Indian villagers. Brit J Cancer. 1968;22(4):646–54.
37. Mani NJ, Singh B. Studies on oral submucous fibrosis 1. Clinical aspects. J Indian Acad Dent. 1968;9:27–36.
38. Mani NJ, Singh B. Studies on oral submucous fibrosis--exfoliative cytology. J Indian Dent Assoc. 1976;48(2):87–91.
39. Mani NJ, Singh B. Studies on oral submucous fibrosis. III. Epithelial changes. Oral Surg Oral Med Oral Pathol. 1976;41(2):203–14.
40. Mani NJ. Studies on oral submucous fibrosis. IV. Connective tissue changes. J Oral Med. 1977;32(3):70–4.
41. Akbar M. Oral submucous fibrosis. MDS dissertation. University of Bombay; 1966.
42. Akbar M. Oral submucous fibrosis—a clinical study. JIDA. 1978;48(9):365–73.
43. Sirsat SM. Biological studies with the electron microscopic study of sub mucous fibrosis of palate. PhD thesis. University of Bombay; 1958.
44. Sirsat SM, Khanolkar VR. Histological, electron-microscope and enzyme studies of submucous fibrosis of the palate. J Pathol Bacteriol. 1960;79:53–8. https://doi.org/10.1002/path.1700790107.
45. Sirsat SM, Khanolkar VR. Submucous fibrosis of the palate. Induction by local painting of capsaicin in Wistar rats treated with desoxycorticosterone acetate—an optical and electron microscopic study. Arch Pathol. 1960;70:180–7.
46. Sirsat SM, Khanolkar VR. The effect of arecoline on the palatal and buccal mucosa of the Wistar rat. An optical and electron microscope study. Indian J Med Sci. 1962;16:198–202.
47. Sirsat SM, Khanolkar VR. Submucous fibrosis of the palate and pillars of the fauces. Indian J Med Sci. 1962;16:189–97.
48. Pindborg JJ, Sirsat SM. Oral submucous fibrosis. Oral Surg Oral Med Oral Pathol. 1966;22(6):764–79. https://doi.org/10.1016/0030-4220(66)90367-7.
49. Sirsat SM, Pindborg JJ. Mast cell response in early and advanced oral submucous fibrosis. Acta Pathol Microbiol Scand. 1967;70(2):174–8. https://doi.org/10.1111/j.1699-0463.1967.tb01279.x.
50. Sirsat SM, Pindborg JJ. The vascular response in early and advanced oral submucous fibrosis. Acta Pathol Microbiol Scand. 1967;70(2):179–84. https://doi.org/10.1111/j.1699-0463.1967.tb01280.x.
51. Sirsat SM, Pindborg JJ. Subepithelial changes in oral submucous fibrosis. Acta Pathol Microbiol Scand. 1967;70(2):161–73. https://doi.org/10.1111/j.1699-0463.1967.tb01278.x.
52. Murti PR, Bhonsle RB, Pindborg JJ, Daftary DK, Gupta PC, Mehta FS. Malignant transformation rate in oral submucous fibrosis over a 17-year period. Commun Dent Oral Epidemiol. 1985;13(6):340–1.
53. Gupta PC, Mehta FS, Daftary DK, Pindborg JJ, Bhonsle RB, Jalnawalla PN, et al. Incidence rates of oral cancer and natural history of oral precancerous lesions in a 10-year follow-up study of Indian villagers. Commun Dent Oral Epidemiol. 1980;8(6):283–333.
54. Bhonsle RB, Murti PR, Daftary DK, Gupta PC, Mehta FS, Sinor PN, et al. Regional variations in oral submucous fibrosis in India. Commun Dent Oral Epidemiol. 1987;15(4):225–9.
55. Trivedy C, Baldwin D, Warnakulasuriya S, Johnson N, Peters T. Copper content in Areca catechu (betel nut) products and oral submucous fibrosis. Lancet. 1997;349(9063):1447.
56. Trivedy C, Warnakulasuriya KA, Tavassoli M, Steingrimsdottir H, Penhallow J, Maher R, Johnson NW. p53 aberrations in oral submucous fibrosis and oral squamous cell carcinoma detected by immunocytochemistry and PCR-SSCP. J Oral Pathol Med. 1998;27(2):72–7.
57. Trivedy C, Warnakulasuriya KA, Hazarey VK, Tavassoli M, Sommer P, Johnson NW. The upregulation of lysyl oxidase in oral submucous fibrosis and squamous cell carcinoma. J Oral Pathol Med. 1999;28(6):246–51.
58. Warnakulasuriya KA, Ekanayake AN, Sivayoham S, Stjernswärd J, Pindborg JJ, Sobin LH, Perera KS. Utilization of primary health care workers for early detection of oral cancer and precancer cases in Sri Lanka. Bull World Health Organ. 1984;62(2):243–50.

59. Su IP. Idiopathic scleroderma of the mouth; report of three cases. AMA Arch Otolaryngol. 1954;59(3):330–2. https://doi.org/10.1001/archotol.1954.00710050342011.
60. Shiau YY, Kwan HW. Submucous fibrosis in Taiwan. Oral Surg Oral Med Oral Pathol. 1979;47:453–7.
61. Pindborg JJ. Oral submucous fibrosis on Hainan Island. Comm Dent Oral Epidemiol. 1984;12:195–6.
62. Tang JG, Jian XF, Gao ML, Ling TY, Zhang KH. Epidemiological survey of oral submucous fibrosis in Xiangtan City, Hunan Province, China. Commun Dent Oral Epidemiol. 1997;25(2):177–80.
63. Lay KM, Sein K, Myint A, Ko SK, Pindborg JJ. Epidemiologic study of 600 villagers of oral precancerous lesions in Bilugyun: preliminary report. Commun Dent Oral Epidemiol. 1982;10(3):152–5.
64. Krishnappa A. Oral submucous fibrosis. Dent J Malaysia Singapore. 1967;7(2):32–9.
65. Ramanathan K. Oral submucous fibrosis—an alternative hypothesis as to its causes. Med J Malaysia 1981;36(4), 243–245.
66. Kelwaip RA, Fose S, Siddiqui MS, Molumi CP, Apaio LM, Conway DI, Johnson NW, Thomas SJ, Lambert DW, Hunter KD. Oral cancer in Papua New Guinea: looking back and looking forward. Oral Surg Oral Med Oral Pathol Oral Radiol. 2020 Sep;130(3):292–7.
67. Choonoo AG. Indentured Indian immigration into Natal 1860–1911 with particular reference to its role in the development of the Natal Sugar Industry, MA Thesis, Durban, University of Natal, 1967; p. 27
68. Shear M, Lemmer J, Dockrat I. Oral submucous fibrosis in South African Indians: an epidemiological study. South Afr J Med Sci. 1967;32(1):41–6.
69. Seedat, H.A. Oral submucous fibrosis in Durban, Natal: A study of its epidemiology, aetiology and morphological features (Ph.D. Thesis), Stellenbosch, University of Stellenbosch, South Africa. 1985.
70. Seedat HA, van Wyk CW. Betel-nut chewing and submucous fibrosis in Durban. South Afr Med J. 1988;74(11):568–71.
71. Seedat HA, van Wyk CW. Submucous fibrosis in non-betel nut chewing subjects. J Biol Buccale. 1988;16(1):3–6.
72. Seedat HA, van Wyk CW. Submucous fibrosis (SF) in ex-betel nut chewers: a report of 14 cases. J Oral Pathol. 1988;17(5):226–9. https://doi.org/10.1111/j.1600-0714.1988.tb01529.x.
73. VanWyk CW. Oral submucous fibrosis. The South African experience. Indian J Dent Res. 1997;8(2):39–45.
74. Prabhu SR, Wilson DF, Daftary DK, Johnson NW, editors. Oral diseases in the tropics. Oxford University Press; 1993. Chapter 36. p. 417–21.
75. Murti PR, Bhonsle RB, Gupta PC, Daftary DK, Pindborg JJ, Mehta FS. Etiology of oral submucous fibrosis with special reference to the role of areca nut chewing. J Oral Pathol Med. 1995;24:145–52.
76. Kramer IR, Lucas RB, Pindborg JJ, Sobin LH, World Health Organization Collaborating Center for Oral Precancerous Lesions. Definitions of leukoplakia and related lesions: an aid to studies on oral precancer. Oral Surg. 1978;46:518–39.
77. Warnakulasuriya S, Johnson NW, van der Waal I. Nomenclature and classification of potentially malignant disorders of the oral mucosa. J Oral Pathol Med. 2007;36(10):575–80.
78. Warnakulasuriya S, Kujan O, Aguirre-Urizar JM, Bagan JV, Gonzalez-Moles MA, Kerr AR, et al. Oral potentially malignant disorders: a consensus report from an international seminar on nomenclature and classification, convened by the WHO Collaborating Centre for Oral Cancer. Oral Dis. 2021;27(8):1862–80. https://doi.org/10.1111/odi.13704.

# Epidemiology of Oral Submucous Fibrosis: Prevalence and Trends

*Chandramani B. More and Deepa Jatti Patil*

## Contents



© The Author(s), under exclusive license to Springer Nature Switzerland AG 2023
S. Warnakulasuriya, K. Ranganathan (eds.), *Oral Submucous Fibrosis*, Textbooks in Contemporary Dentistry,
https://doi.org/10.1007/978-3-031-12855-4_2

2

## 2.1 Introduction

Oral submucous fibrosis (OSF) belongs to the group of oral potentially malignant disorders (OPMDs) and is characterized by fibrosis of the oral mucosa extending to the submucosa [1]. OSF is a complex, crippling, debilitating, irreversible, persistent progressive, scarring, potentially malignant condition and is a collagen metabolic disorder [2]. Chewing of areca nut-related products is the single most important risk factor for the development of OSF [3]. Despite several advances in diagnostics and therapeutics, OSF is associated with a significant risk of malignant transformation (7–13%), necessitating the development of preventive measures for controlling the condition in the future.

Epidemiological studies provide information on the distribution of diseases, the factors that contribute to their onset and progression, and the strategies used to control them. Analyzing and examining such distributions aid in the compilation of descriptive data that provides an understanding of the scope of the problem as well as understanding the high-risk and low-risk populations. It also aids in comparing the burden of disease and assess resource allocation for researchers, prevention, treatment, and support services. Cross-sectional and observational studies are the epidemiological studies that help in assessing the prevalence of the disease [4].

**Definition**

Prevalence is the proportion of a population who have a specific characteristic in a given time period.

Prevalence studies are used to provide information regarding disease burden to researchers and policymakers, assisting in the identification of healthcare needs, guidelines for prevention, and development of policy [5]. As a result of the rising usage of commercially prepared areca nut preparations, the prevalence of OSF is on the rise in the Indian subcontinent and in Southeast Asia [6].This chapter outlines the findings of the research studies undertaken across the world to determine the prevalence of OSF and to better understand the demographics, risk factors, and sociocultural factors that influence OSF development. In published studies, prevalence of OSF may vary depending on the definition used, the lifestyle of the population studied, and the criteria used to detect OSF.

**Learning Goals**

- To understand the significance of epidemiological studies
- To know the prevalence of OSF globally
- Risk factors associated with the development of OSF
- To explore the demographic and sociocultural behavior influencing the development of the condition

## 2.2 Epidemiology of OSF

OSF has intrigued researchers since many decades, and several epidemiological studies have been undertaken to determine disease prevalence in several countries worldwide [7].

According to estimates by Cox and Walker, the number of people affected by this condition was 2.5 million in 1996 [8]. The World Health Organization (WHO) reported more than six million OSF patients worldwide in 2002 [9]. OSF is now universally acknowledged as an Indian disease that can be seen throughout the Indian subcontinent and Southeast Asia as well as among the diaspora from these countries [7]. ◘ Figure 2.1 depicts the countries with reported observational data and the estimated prevalence of OSF in each country.

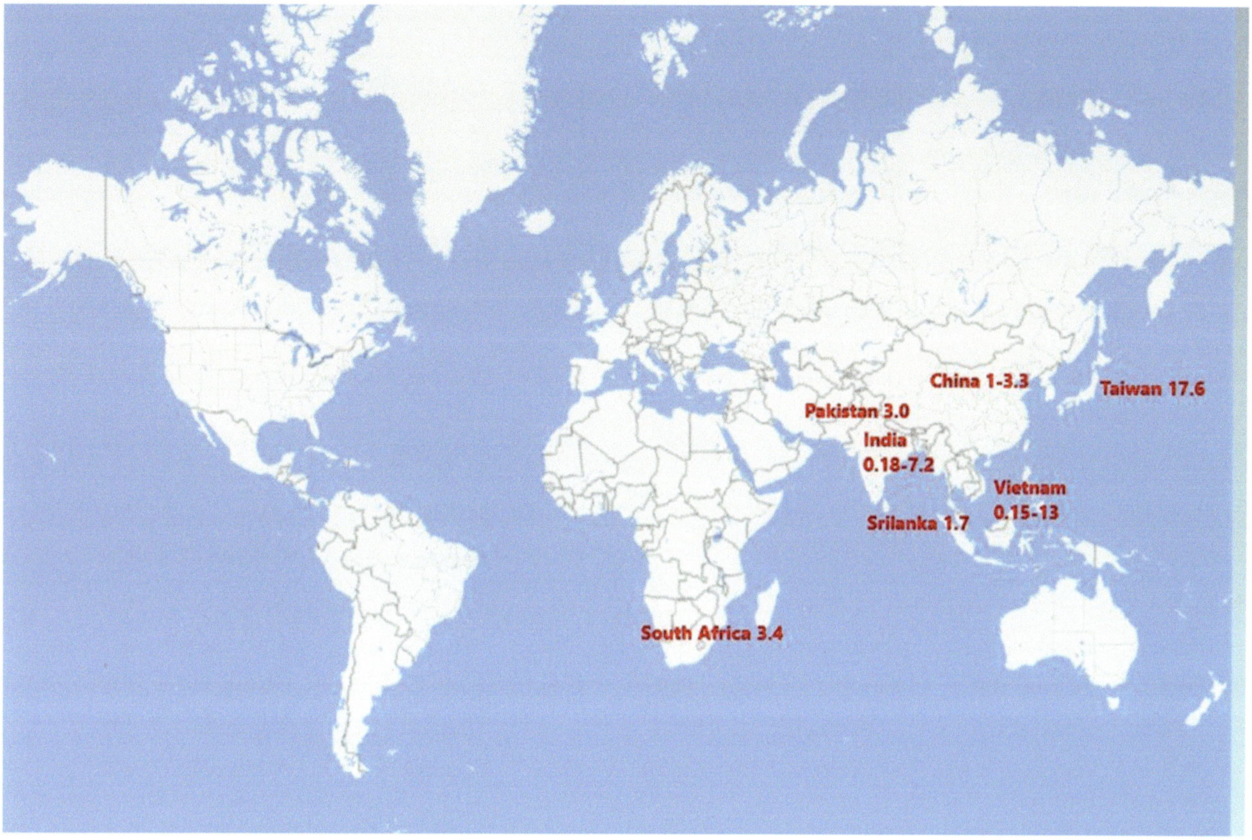
China 1-3.3
Taiwan 17.6
Pakistan 3.0
India
0.18-7.2
Vietnam
0.15-13
Srilanka 1.7
South Africa 3.4

■ **Fig. 2.1** Map depicting the prevalence of OSF among various countries

## 2.3 Prevalence Data from the Indian Subcontinent

Chiu et al. estimated that the population living with OSF in the Indian continent was around 5 million persons (0.5% of the population) [10]. In India, the prevalence of OSF is estimated to be between 0.2% and 2.3% in males and 1.2–4.6% in females, with the disease affecting a wide age range of 11–60 years [7]. ■ Table 2.1 lists published data of OSF prevalence, which range from 0.1% to 7.2%. A marked variation in the prevalence data reported from India is noted (■ Fig. 2.2) depending on the geographic area, sample size, and sampling methods.

The earliest prevalence studies on OSF were performed by Jens Pindborg, a Danish oral pathologist, working with several Indian collaborators [11–21].

**Table 2.1** Indian prevalence studies of OSF

| Year | Authors | Study type | Sample size | Country | City/district | State/ Province | Prevalence (%) |
|---|---|---|---|---|---|---|---|
| 1965 | Pindborg et al. [11] | Observational | 10,000 | India | Mumbai | Maharashtra | 0.50 |
| 1965 | Pindborg et al. [12] | Cross sectional | 10,000 | India | Lucknow | Uttar Pradesh | 4.1 |
| 1966 | Pindborg et al. [13, 14] | Observational | 10,000 | India | Bengaluru | Karnataka | 0.18 |
| 1966 | Zachariah et al. [20] | Observational | 5000 | India | Thiruvananthapuram | Kerala | 1.22 |
| 1968 | Pindborg et al. [21] | Observational | 50,915 | India | Srikakulam | Andhra Pradesh | 0.04 |
| | | | | | Darbhanga | Bihar | 0.07 |
| | | | | | Bhavnagar | Gujarat | 0.16 |
| | | | | | Ernakulum | Kerala | 0.36 |
| 1970 | Wahi et al. [22] | Observational | | India | Mainpuri | Uttar Pradesh | 0.59 |
| 1972 | Mehta et al. [17] | Survey | 101,761 | India | Pune | Maharashtra | 0.03 |
| 2012–13 | Patil et al. [23] | Cross sectional | 2400 | India | Dharwad | Karnataka | 7.08 |
| 2000–2004 | Hazarey et al. [24] | Cross sectional | 2,66,418 | India | Nagpur | Maharashtra | 6.42 |
| 2008 | Mathew et al. [25] | Observational | 1190 | India | Manipal | Karnataka | 2.01 |
| 2012 | Sharma et al. [ 27] | Cross sectional survey | 6800 | India | Jaipur | Rajasthan | 3.39 |
| 2012 | Agarwal et al. [28] | Observational | 750 | India | Dehradun | Uttarakhand | 5.4 |
| 2013 | Bhatnagar et al. [29] | Survey | 8866 | India | Modinagar | Uttar Pradesh | 1.97 |
| 2005–2007 | Burungale et al. [30] | Cross sectional | 800 | India | Jaitala, Nagpur | Maharashtra | 2.62 |
| 2014 | Nigam et al. [31] | Observational | 1000 | India | Moradabad | Uttar Pradesh | 6.3 |
| 2016 | Singh et al. [32] | Cross sectional survey | 132 | India | Nagpur | Maharashtra | 2.9 |
| 2018 | Tyagi et al. [33] | Cross sectional | 1167 | India | Nashik | Maharashtra | 3.51 |
| 2019 | More et al. [34] | Cross sectional | 13,874 | India | Vadodara | Gujarat | 7.21 |
| 2002–2004 | Ahmad et al. [35] | Cross sectional | 3000 | India | Patna | Bihar | 1.16 |
| 2015–17 | Pandaet al [36] | Cross sectional | 36,000 | India | Sambalpur | Odisha | 1.26 |
| 2016–18 | Srivastav et al. [37] | Cross sectional-survey | 31,570 | India | Kanpur | Uttar Pradesh | 2.72 |

Pindborg et al. [11, 12] and Zachariah et al. [20] studied 35,000 urban Indians presenting in admission clinics at dental institutes in Lucknow, Mumbai, Bengaluru, and Trivandrum and found prevalence estimates of 0.5%, 0.5%, 0.2%, and 1.2% respectively. Pindborg later fully characterized many aspects of this condition throughout his diverse and extended journeys as a WHO consultant to the south and far east of the globe in his quest for tropical oral diseases. Pindborg and the team led by Fali S. Mehta at the Tata Institute of Fundamental Research (TIFR) in Mumbai conducted a comprehensive investigation on the natural history of

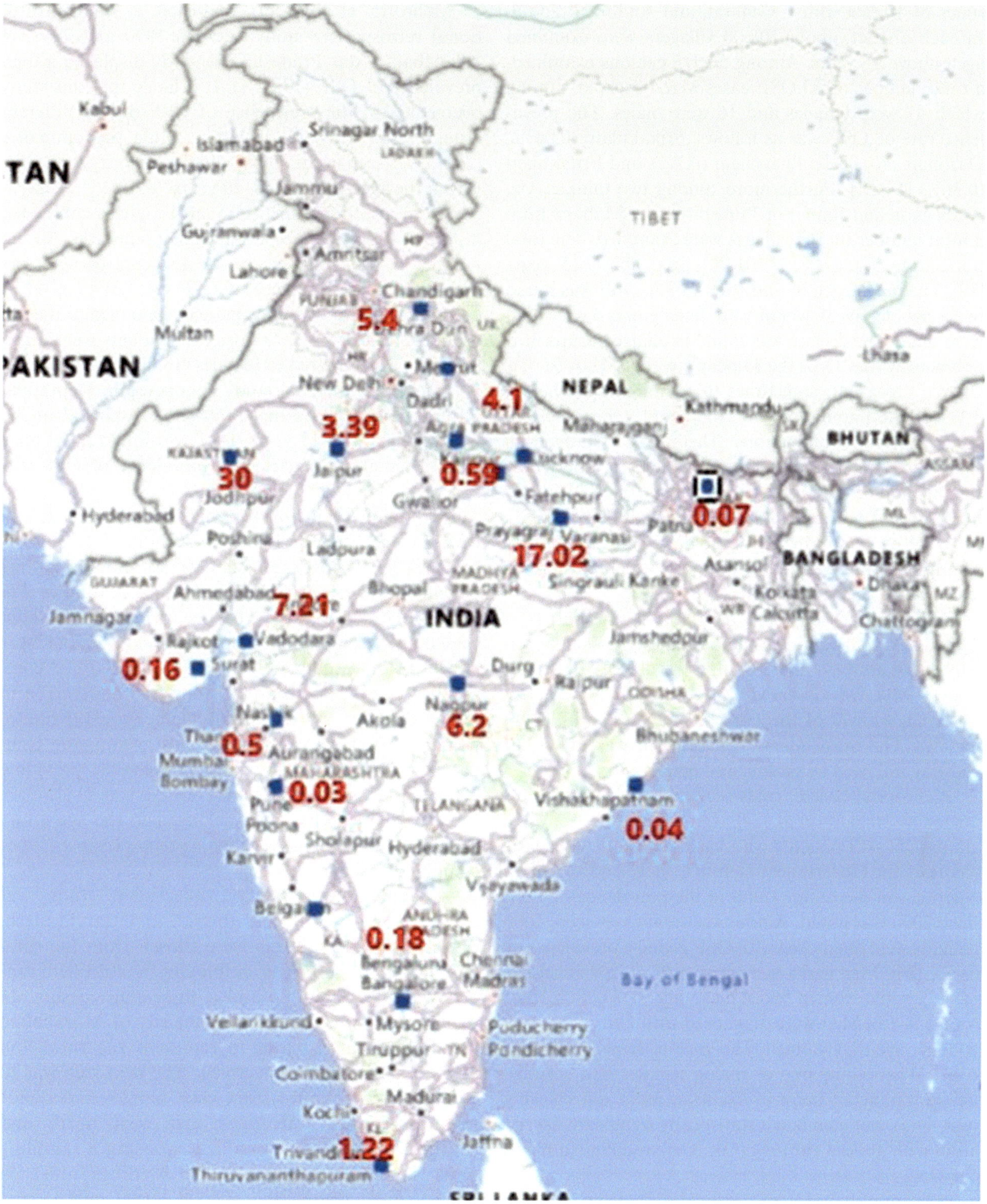

Fig. 2.2 Map depicting the prevalence of OSF from various surveys among Indian populations

oral precancer among five rural Indian populations (see ► Chap. 1 in this book) that resulted in a spectacular study that included the examination of nearly 200,000 Indian villagers [11–21].

The TIFR team conducted epidemiological surveys among villagers in India and compared the findings among urban and rural Indians. House-to-house surveys were conducted in four districts of Indian states of Kerala, Bihar, Gujarat, and Andhra Pradesh. In each district, about 10,000 villagers were examined aged above 15 years. Among 50,915 persons examined, a total number of 63 OSF cases were observed, among which 47 were females and 16 were males. The prevalence rate of OSF was as follows: Srikakulam (0.04%), Darbhanga (0.07%), Bhavnagar (0.2%), and Ernakulam (0.36%) [14–21]. Furthermore, among two talukas, viz. Ambegaon and Junnar of Pune district in Maharashtra, a total number of 169 villages were examined. The total population studied was 101,761 aged above 15 years [17]. The prevalence of OSF was 0.03%. OSF was found in 33 people, 29 of whom were female and 4 of whom were male. The disease was found in all age groups. It is noteworthy that 17 of the 33 people with OSF, or 51.5%, chewed areca nut, sometimes in combination, whereas 2.1% of the population, or 2165 people, chewed areca nut, including combinations. There was a statistically significant association that chewing areca nut may be a significant factor in the development of OSF. The buccal mucosa was reported as the most affected site with OSF.

Wahi et al. conducted an epidemiological study in Mainpuri, Uttar Pradesh, and reported that OSF prevalence was 0.59% [22].

A hospital-based, cross-sectional study was conducted in Dharwad, Karnataka, among 2400 participants aged above 15 years. A high prevalence of OSF, 85 cases (7.8%), was observed [23]. A male preponderance was seen, with 77 of the cases being males and 8 being females. The most common habit seen was areca nut chewing followed by gutkha and betel quid.

A hospital-based, cross-sectional study was conducted by Hazarey et al. [24], over a duration of 5 years among 266,418 patients who visited outpatient departments of the Government Dental College and Hospital, Nagpur. An increasing trend in the prevalence of OSF since 2000 was noted. Among the total cases seen, 1000 patients were diagnosed with OSF giving a prevalence of 6.42% [24]. Men had a mean age of 27.60 ± 9.58 (range 12–75), while women had a mean age of 34.78 ± 12.21 (range 9–75). Men were diagnosed with OSF at a much younger age than women. The male-to-female ratio was 4.9:1. When compared to males, females had a statistically significant habit of exclusive areca nut chewing (OR 44.5), but men had a statistically significant association with gutkha chewing (OR 3.69) and kharra/mawa chewing.

A hospital-based cross-sectional study was conducted in Manipal for a duration of 3 months from March 2005 to June 2005. A total number of 1190 patients reporting for dental treatment were examined. The prevalence of OSF was 2.1% (23 males and 1 female) [25].

Mehrotra et al. [26] conducted a single-institutional retrospective study between 1990 and 2007, in Allahabad, Uttar Pradesh. The study displayed a high prevalence of OSF (17.02%). It is likely that this study overestimated the prevalence of OSF due to different criteria used for case detection. Male predominance (2.4:1) was seen in the study, and the majority with OSF was in the age group of 20–29 years.

A cross-sectional institutional study was conducted in Jaipur, Rajasthan, for a duration of 6 months. A total number of 6800 subjects above 18 years of age were examined. The prevalence of OSF was 231 (3.39%). A considerable proportion of patients belonged to the age group of 15–24 years. Majority of patients were males (81.38%) as compared to females (18.62%) [27].

In a cross-sectional study conducted in Dehradun, Uttarakhand, 750 participants were examined ranging in age from 13 to 19 years. OSF was found in 29 male and 12 female teenagers. The prevalence of OSF was 5.4% [28].

According to an institutional study conducted in Modinagar, Uttar Pradesh (North India), a total number of 8866 were examined over six months among patients aged between 15 and 75 years. A total of 177 cases (1.97%) with OSF were recorded, 146 of whom were males (1.66%) and 31 were females (0.01%). [29]

Between December 2005 and June 2007, a community-based cross-sectional study was undertaken in Jaitala, Nagpur. Out of a total number of 3195 households in Jaitala, a random systematic sampling technique was used to survey 199 households, providing 800 individuals. The prevalence of OSF was 21 (1.62%). Most of the positive cases belonged to the age group of 20–39 years. There was a male preponderance [19] as compared to females [30].

A community-based cross-sectional study was conducted in Moradabad district in Uttar Pradesh. A total of 1000 subjects were chosen from the rural and urban populations employing a stratified random sample technique and a three-stage design. In the first step, four villages and the city of Moradabad were chosen at random to represent the rural and urban populations, respectively. The next step was to choose three colonies from each hamlet and divide Moradabad into four zones: east, west, north, and south. The third stage entailed choosing a sampling unit, which was a colony of 40–50 dwellings from each village/zone. Among the 1000 habitual gutkha and areca nut chewers (678 males and 322 females), the prevalence of OSF was found to be 6.3% with a male-to-female ratio of 7:1. According to the demographics, out of 63 OSF patients, 42 (66.7%) were gutkha chewers, 14 (22.2%) were pan chewers, and 7 (11.1%) were areca nut-only chewers [31].

Singh et al. [32] conducted a cross-sectional study among various schools in the rural areas of Nagpur, Maharashtra. A total of 2132 school-going children between the age group of 8 and 17 years were studied. 62 children showed clinical symptoms of OSF; the prevalence of OSF was calculated to be 2.9%. These 62 children were identified among 156 children (7.3%) who reported chewing areca nut in the form of sweet supari, gutkha, and kharra.

A cross-sectional study was conducted among the patients reporting to an ENT outpatient department in Nasik, Maharashtra, over 8 months from November 2016 to June 2017. OSF was identified in 41 individuals (3.51%), with 21 (51.2%) chewing gutkha, 12 (29.3%) chewing areca nut plus tobacco, and 8 (19.5%) chewing areca nut only [33].

A prospective hospital-based study was conducted by More et al. [34], among 13,874 individuals in Vadodara, Gujarat state. All patients aged over 17 years who presented to the department in 2017 and 2018 were included in the study. The estimated prevalence of OSF was 7.21%. The average age of habit initiation was 28.2 ± 11.7 years. Gutkha followed by mawa chewing were found to be the common behaviours adopted at all initiation ages.

A prospective institution-based study was conducted in Patna, Bihar. A stratified random selection strategy was used to select 3000 people between the ages of 16 and 60 years from both the rural and urban populations. OSF was observed in 243 patients with a prevalence of 1.6%. The frequency of OSF was found to be 2.6% among males and 1.2% among females. A large proportion of young patients were seen, who were between the ages of 20 and 30 [35].

A cross-sectional study was conducted in an outpatient department of a dental hospital in Burla, Sambalpur, Odisha, among 36,000 patients over a period of 3 years (January 2015 to December 2017). Out of the 36,000 people who were screened, 457 were found to have OSF. The prevalence of OSF was 1.26%. Among the study subjects, 453 were males and 4 were females. Out of the 457 cases, 305 had gutkha chewing habit, 57 had betel and areca nut chewing habit, and 95 had gutkha chewing along with smoking habits [36].

An institutional study was conducted in Kanpur, Uttar Pradesh, for a duration of two years from January 2016 to December 2018. A total number of 31,570 patients were examined. 860 patients were diagnosed with OSF with a prevalence of 2.7%. When classified by age group, 30- to 40-year-old patients had a higher prevalence of OSF than the older age groups [37].

All these data corroborate the evidence of high prevalence of OSF in the Indian subcontinent.

## 2.4 Prevalence Data from Other Countries in the South Asian Region

**Burma**: The Union of the Socialist Republic of Burma is India's next-door neighbor, with common oral habits such as smoking and chewing with a similar incidence of oral cancer. To examine the prevalence of OPMDs, a preliminary house-to-house survey was conducted by a local team directed by Jens Pindborg in the island of Bilugyun, Burma. Among the 45 villages, 10 villages were randomly selected for the study. 600 villagers were examined and 5 were detected with OSF; 4 were females and 1 was a male. The prevalence of OSF was 0.1%. Areca nut chewing was the most common habit associated with OSF [38].

**Sri Lanka**: The Ministry of Health in 2009 reported from a national database a prevalence of 4% for OSF. In 2010, a cross-sectional community door-door survey was conducted in the Sabaragamuwa Province by Amarasinghe et al., among urban, rural, and estate-employed people. 1029 individuals were surveyed with questionnaires and clinical examinations. The prevalence of OSF was 1.7%. The estate sector had a higher prevalence of areca nut and betel quid use compared to other sectors [39].

**Pakistan:** A multicentric cross-sectional study conducted in Karachi over a period of 8 years examined 765 cases of OSF. There was a slight male predominance (51.8%) compared to females (48.2%). Consumption of areca nut and its derivatives showed a statistically significant association with the severity of OSF. The mean age was 29.2 years [40].

In a tertiary care hospital in Karachi, Pakistan, a study was conducted for a duration of 1 year. The prevalence of OSF was 3%. Areca nut was the most common habit (79.5%), followed by pan (22%) and gutkha chewing (17%) [41].

**Vietnam:** Cuc et al. [42] conducted a study of 152 betel quid chewers and 137 non-chewers. The prevalence of OSF was 13%. In another study by Khanh [43], in a sample of 9000 individuals from southern provinces of Vietnam (4534 women and 4466 men) with an age range between 50 and 75 years, the prevalence of oral mucosal lesions was 19.8%. In this study, OSF was seen in 0.15% of the patients. Nguyen [44] conducted a survey at Ba Diem Commune from May 2005 to February 2006 on 150 betel quid chewers and 200 non-chewers. Among chewers, OSF was seen in 14.6% of the patients.

2

**China:** The growth of the betel quid (BQ) processing sector in Hunan has boosted the use of this substance, which could have serious health implications. However, there is a scarcity of recent data on the prevalence of betel quid chewing and its impact on OSF. An epidemiological survey was conducted by Tang et al. [45] in Yuhu District, Xiangtan city of Hunan province. 57 independent units were surveyed, and the study population was selected randomly and included participants from shops, schools, and factory workers. A total number of 11,046 individuals were examined. OSF was found in 335 individuals (252 males and 83 females). The prevalence was 3%. All 335 OSF patients were areca nut chewers.

A population-based survey was conducted by Zhang et al. [46] to investigate the prevalence of betel quid chewing and OSF in Hunan. A total of 2356 people took part in the survey, with a response rate of 78.5%. OSF was found to be present in 1.0% of the population. In comparison to the non-OSF respondents (1.7–23.2%), a considerably higher proportion of OSF patients were current chewers. In Hunan, betel quid chewing is a significant risk factor for OSF. The high frequency of betel quid chewing in the younger cohort (15–49 years old) is a serious warning sign for the future.

**Taiwan:** A large-scale nationwide retrospective study in Taiwan showed an increase in OSF prevalence from 8.3 per 10,000 people in 1996 to 16.2 per 10000 people in 2013 (p 0.0001). From 1996 to 2013, the average age of OSF patients increased. Men had a significantly higher OSF prevalence than women ($p < 0.001$). People who lived in rural regions had a higher risk of OSF than those who lived in cities [relative risk (RR) 1.10; 95% CI 1.07–1.13]. When compared to the lower income group, the higher income group had a lower risk of OSF (RR, 0.76; 95% CI, 0.73–0.80) [47, 48].

## 2.5 International Prevalence Studies

Oral submucous fibrosis has become a public health hazard in many parts of the world, including the United Kingdom and South Africa, due to the migration of endemic betel quid chewers [7].

### 2.5.1 Western Countries

Due to the increasing immigration of Indians in the last four to five decades, OSF cases have been reported in the United Kingdom, Canada, Germany, and France. Many cases of OSF have been documented in Bangladeshi [49] and Pakistani origin patients in the United Kingdom and the United States. A single case of OSF was reported in a Greek female [50].

According to a 2007 Census Bureau, South Asians comprised of 0.9% of US population. Thereafter, there has been an increasing trend of migration of Southeast Asians to North America. Studies indicated that South Asian immigrants of lower socioeconomic status or those with minimal English proficiency inclined to consume betel nut at higher rates than those of other immigrants [51, 52].

### 2.5.2 South Africa

Shear et al. (1967) observed a frequency of OSF of 0.5% among 1000 Indians in South Africa [53].

The prevalence of betel nut chewing and the resulting OSF was found to be relatively high in a stratified random sample of South African Indians living in Durban. The prevalence of OSF was 3.4%. In a 13:1 ratio, female chewers predominated. The practice became more common as women became older, with 30.6% of women over 65 years old doing so; 38% of chewers showed symptoms of early and established OSF; women outnumbered men by 70:1, and most patients were between the ages of 45 and 54 [54, 55].

## 2.6 Gender

OSF has a male-to-female ratio that varies by region, and in early studies, females often outnumbered males according to various studies. A male-to-female ratio of 1:13 was found in an earlier study from Durban, South Africa undertaken in 1980s, indicating a clear female predominance [54]. In this region, there was a female predominance in areca nut chewing.

A male-to-female ratio of 1:2.3 was found in studies in Pakistan [40, 41]. A case-control study of 185 people in Chennai, India, found a male-to-female ratio of 9.9:1 [56]. The male-to-female ratio was 2.7:1 in Patna, Bihar (India) [36].

A cross-sectional multicenter study was conducted in Karachi, Pakistan, to monitor the progression of OSF to malignancy over a duration of 8 years. The study showed a female predominance and higher rate of malignant transformation in females [57].

In a retrospective study conducted in Taiwan, the prevalence of OSF was substantially higher in men than in women (p 0.001) [48]. Recent studies indicate a higher prevalence in men compared with women.

## 2.7 Age

Patients with OSF vary by age, and it is noted to be common among teenagers and adolescents in India but the presenting age ranges from 11 to 60 years old. It occurs at any age but is most commonly seen in young adults between 25 and 35 years (2nd–4th decade). Onset of this disease is insidious and may take many years to manifest clinically [24–37].

### 2.7.1 Prevalence of OSF Among Children and Adolescents

A trend of increasing prevalence of OSF is seen occurring in young children and adolescents. Ali et al. [58] reported a 7.4% prevalence of OSF among school-aged males in their study. Cai et al. [59] found 2.37% prevalence in the age category of 10–19 years in a clinicopathological investigation of 647 cases of OSF among the Chinese population.

Oral submucous fibrosis was discovered in 8.8% of teenagers with an average age of 16.3 years (±1.5 years) in research conducted in Saipan [60].

The first case of OSF in a very young child was reported by Hayes [61] in a 4-year-old girl. Although no sex predilection has been demonstrated in children, a small number of studies have found that boys chew areca nuts more than girls.

Areca nut use by children as young as ten years old has been observed in British investigations. Betel nut products were popular among South Asian teens in East London because they provided a link to their cultural history as well as a convenient means to get tobacco-containing items. The most common reasons cited for starting a habit at a young age are peer pressure, attractive packaging, and lucrative advertisement of areca nut-related products, to avoid study pressure, influence by actors, to improve social interaction, and to distract themselves from domestic violence by parents. The case studies emphasize the dangers that children confront when they use these products that are plainly marketed to them [62].

More et al. [63] described a case series of 36 children and adolescents with areca nut chewing habits and OSF symptoms who were treated at a tertiary care facility in Vadodara, Gujarat, India. There were 75% ($n$ = 27) males and 25% ($n$ = 9) females among the 36 children diagnosed with OSF, with the majority falling between the age group of 12 and 14. Eighty-one percent ($n$ = 29) were diagnosed with stage I, while the rest were diagnosed with stage II disease. Majority of the patients initiated their habit at a young age of 4–5 years old followed by 10–11 years old and reported chewing/consumption of flavored areca nut ($n$ = 18, 50%), followed by pan masala ($n$ = 5, 14%), mawa ($n$ = 4, 11%), betel quid with areca nut excluding tobacco ($n$ = 4, 11%), baked areca nut products ($n$ = 3, 8%), and gutkha ($n$ = 3, 8%).

Shah et al. [49] reported a case of 11-year-old Bangladeshi female from the United Kingdom diagnosed with OSF. The parents regularly consumed areca nut and tobacco-related products and were ignorant about their ill-effects. They consumed these substances as natural products to aid in digestion. Kariya et al. [64] reported a case of OSF in a 5-year-old male who was habituated to chewing areca nut since the age of 2 years and chewed two to three packets per day.

## 2.8 Trends in Etiology

Chewing areca nut, genetic predisposition, and immunologic processes have all been postulated as potential triggers for the condition [65, 66].

Areca nut chewing and commercial formulations (gutkha, mawa, pan masala, flavored supari, etc.) are a common and widespread practice in Asian countries, regardless of age or gender [67, 68]. OSF has become more common in recent years, possibly due to an increase in the popularity of commercial areca nut preparations and their increased use [69, 70, 71]. Several case studies of Asian immigrants to the United Kingdom [52], the United States [53], and Africa [54] have been published. Among recent literature from European and Western countries, isolated cases of OSF in non-Asians have also been recorded [49].

## 2.9 Discussion

Various studies conducted globally and within the Indian subcontinent show that the prevalence of OSF varies by region, which can be linked to a variety of sociocultural characteristics, environmental risk factors, data collection methods, and clinical criteria used for case detection. Even within each region, OSF prevalence appears to vary by age and gender.

The published literature has found a link between OSF and use of areca nut or betel quid. According to the current WHO estimates, while tobacco usage is decreasing in industrialized countries, tobacco consumption (particularly smokeless tobacco use) is increasing in developing countries. Areca nut is often mixed in packaged smokeless tobacco products [72].

There have been numerous publications on the various characteristics of OSF since it was originally described in the modern literature in 1952 by Schwartz, who discovered OSF in five Indian women in Kenya [73]. Since then, OSF has been a topic of research among various epidemiologists and clinicians.

According to the prevalence studies outlined here, OSF has a specific geographic distribution and predominantly affects people of South Asia and Southeast Asia—India, Bangladesh, Sri Lanka, Pakistan, Taiwan, and southern parts of China. According to previous reports globally, about 2.5 million people suffer from OSF, but Indian studies in 2002 have reported that over 5 million people are affected in India alone (0.5% of the Indian population). As a result of the traditional usage of betel quid native to these locations, OSF occurs in the Indian subcontinent, among other Asian citizens and Pacific Islanders and among Indian and Pakistani immigrants to Western countries [7, 8, 10].

Tables 2.1 and 2.2 list the prevalence of OSF globally and in the Indian subcontinent. The epidemiological studies conducted in the late nineteenth century by Fali S. Mehta [17], Jens Pindborg [11–15, 21], and Zachariah et al. [20] showed a high prevalence of OSF in various districts of Maharashtra, Gujarat, Karnataka, Kerala, and Uttar Pradesh. The highest prevalence was observed in Lucknow (4.1%) [12] followed by Thiruvananthapuram in Kerala (1.22%) [21]. Most of the studies were conducted among rural population and involved house-to-house surveys among the villagers. A high prevalence of OSF was observed, and areca nut chewing was the significant factor in the development of OSF. In recent years, the trend of OSF with respect to prevalence has emerged, and widespread occurrence of OSF was seen spanning all cities of India as depicted in Table 2.1 and Fig. 2.1. The prevalence rates have increased in various cities of Uttar Pradesh, Bihar, Rajasthan, Gujarat, Karnataka, Maharashtra, Tamil Nadu, and Kerala ranging from 2% to 7.2% according to various studies [22–37]. This has been attributed to the commercialization of areca nut and tobacco products in the recent years. The increasing use of these products globally substantiates the increasing prevalence of OSF among the South Asian countries and among the migrants from these countries to Europe and America.

The prevalence of OSF in the early studies was higher in the middle-aged groups. The recent trends show an increased prevalence among the youth including adolescents. Interestingly, the rural and urban divide in India has also decreased. Both these factors are due to widespread commercialization of smokeless tobacco mixed with areca nut products and uptake in consumption among the youth.

There was a female predominance in the surveys conducted in the late nineteenth century as females during those decades had a habit of consuming areca nut. Studies conducted in Kerala [21], Burma [38], and Durban [54] showed a female predominance. Male pre-

**Table 2.2** Global prevalence studies of OSF

| Year | Authors | Study type | Sample size | Country | City/district | Prevalence (%) |
|---|---|---|---|---|---|---|
| 1982 | Lay et al. [38] | Cross sectional | 6000 | Myanmar | Bilugyun, Mon | 0.1 |
| 1988 | Seedat et al. [53] | Cross sectional | 2400 | South Africa | Durban, KwaZulu-Natal | 3.4 |
| 1996 | Yang et. al. [47] | Population based survey | 312 | Taiwan | Mutan, Ping-tong | 17.6 |
| 1997 | Tang et al. [45] | Population based survey | 11046 | China | Xiangtan City Hunan, | 3.3 |
| 2012 | Zhang et al. [46] | Cross sectional | 2356 | China | Hunan | 1.0 |
| 2004–2012 | Mohiuddin et al. [56] | Cross-sectional, multi-centre study | 1774 | Pakistan | Karachi | 3.0 |
| 2005 | Nguyen et al. [44] | Survey among Betel quid chewers | 150 | Vietnam | Ba Diem Commune | 14.0 |
| 2006 | Amarsinghe et al. [39] | Cross sectional community survey | 1029 | Srilanka | Sabaragamuwa province | 1.7 |
| 2006 | Cuc et al. [42] | Survey among Betel quid chewers | 152 | Vietnam | | 13.0 |
| 2006 | Khanh et al. [43] | Cross sectional survey | 9000 | Vietnam | Southern Province | 0.15 |
| 2018 | Tariq et al. [41] | Cross sectional study | 4405 | Pakistan | Karachi | 3.6 |
| 2018 | Yang et al. [48] | Cross sectional | 23,373,51 | Taiwan | Taiwan | 16.2 |

dominance was seen in more recent studies and particularly in Taiwan [47, 48].

Two studies conducted in India, one in Allahabad [26] in Uttar Pradesh and a second in Jodhpur [74], Rajasthan, reported a high prevalence of OSF (17% and 30%, respectively). It is likely that these two studies used clinical criteria very different to the rest of the studies or had poor calibration among the investigators. These factors need careful control in planning prevalence studies on OSF in the future.

Most of the data from the prevalence studies conducted from the late 1990s till date is from hospital-based cross-sectional studies, and only a few are from community-based surveys. The data from the Northeastern Indian states is particularly scarce. Future studies should focus on multicentric large-scale community-based surveys, especially in areas with high consumption of betel quid and areca nut-related products.

## 2.10 Conclusion

Existing data reveal an increasing trend of OSF in both urban and rural populations, subjects with low education proficiency and socioeconomic status. Measures should be taken to curb the sale of areca nut containing products and increase the awareness among the population regarding their ill-effects especially among teenagers and adolescents to reduce the prevalence of OSF in the future.

**Summary**

- OSF is prevalent in the Indian subcontinent, its neighboring countries in the region, and among the Pacific Islanders.
- Despite the high prevalence of OSF seen among rural communities and among population with low literacy rate, the rural-urban gap is narrowing.
- Adolescents are at a high risk of developing the condition due to commercialization of areca nut mixed with smokeless tobacco products.

## References

1. Warnakulasuriya S, Johnson N, van der Waal I. Nomenclature and classification of potentially malignant disorders of the oral mucosa. J Oral Pathol Med. 2007;36(10):575–80.
2. Rajalalitha P, Vali S. Molecular pathogenesis of oral submucous fibrosis—a collagen metabolic disorder. J Oral Pathol Med. 2005;34:321–8.
3. IARC Working Group on the Evaluation of Carcinogenic Risks to Humans. Personal habits and indoor combustions. volume 100 E. A review of human carcinogens. IARC Monogr Eval Carcinog Risks Hum. 2012;100:1–538.
4. Anon. Epidemiology is a science of high importance. Nat Commun. 2018;9:1703.
5. Harder T. Some notes on critical appraisal of prevalence studies: Comment on: "The development of a critical appraisal tool for use in systematic reviews addressing questions of prevalence". Int J Health Policy Manag. 2014;3:289–90.
6. Gupta PC, Sinor PN, Bhonsle RB, Pawar VS, Mehta HC. Oral submucous fibrosis in India: a new epidemic? Natl Med J India. 1998;11:113–6.
7. Rao NR, Villa A, More CB, Jayasinghe RD, Kerr AR, Johnson NW. Oral submucous fibrosis: a contemporary narrative review with a proposed inter-professional approach for an early diagnosis and clinical management. J Otolaryngol Head Neck Surg. 2020;49(1):3.
8. Cox SC, Walker DM. Oral submucous fibrosis. A review. Aust Dent J. 1996;41(5):294–9.
9. IARC Working Group on the Evaluation of Carcinogenic Risks to Humans. Betel-quid and areca-nut chewing and some areca-nut derived nitrosamines. IARC Monogr Eval Carcinog Risks Hum. 2004;85:1–334.
10. Chiu CJ, Lee WC, Chiang CP, Hahn LJ, Kuo YS, Chen CJ. A scoring system for the early detection of oral submucous fibrosis based on a self-administered questionnaire. J Public Health Dent. 2002;62:28–31.
11. Pindborg JJ, Chawla TN, Srivastava AN, Gupta D, Mehrotra ML. Clinical aspects of oral submucous fibrosis. Acta Odontol Scand. 1964;22:679–91.
12. Pindborg JJ, Sirsat SM. Oral submucous fibrosis. Oral Surg Oral Med Ora Pathol. 1966;22:764–79.
13. Pindborg JJ, Mehta FS, Daftary DK. Occurrence of epithelial atypia in 51 Indian villagers with oral submucous fibrosis. Br J Cancer. 1970;24:253–7.
14. Pindborg JJ. Is submucous fibrosis a pre-cancerous condition in the oral cavity? Int Dent J. 1972;22:474–80.
15. Pindborg JJ, Bhonsle RB, Murti PR, Gupta PC, Daftary DK, Mehta FS. Incidence and early forms of oral submucous fibrosis. Oral Surg Oral Med Oral Pathol. 1980;50:40–4.
16. Bhonsle RB, Murti PR, Daftary DK, et al. Regional variations in oral submucous fibrosis in India. Commun Dent Oral Epidemiol. 1987;15:225–9.
17. Mehta FS, Gupta PC, Daftary DK, Pindborg JJ, Choksi SK. An epidemiologic study of oral cancer and precancerous conditions among 101,761 villagers in Maharashtra. India Int J Cancer. 1972;10(1):134–41.
18. Murti PR, Gupta PC, Bhonsle RB, Daftary DK, Mehta FS, Pindborg JJ. Effect on the incidence of oral submucous fibrosis of intervention in the areca nut chewing habit. J Oral Pathol Med. 1990;19:99–100.
19. Gupta S, Jawanda MK. Oral submucous fibrosis: An overview of a challenging entity. Indian J Dermatol Venereol Leprol. 2021;23:768–77.
20. Zachariah J, Mathew B, Varma NAR, Iqbal AM, Pindborg JJ. Frequency of oral mucosal lesions among 5000 individuals in Trivandrum, South India. J All India Dent Assoc. 1966;38:290–6.
21. Pindborg JJ, Mehta FS, Gupta PC, Daftary DK. Prevalence of oral submucous fibrosis among 50,915 Indian villagers. Br J Cancer. 1968;22(4):646–54.
22. Wahi PN, Mittal VP, Lahiri B, Luthera UK, Seth RK, Arma GD. Epidemiological study of precancerous lesions of the oral cavity: a preliminary report. Ind J Med Res. 1970;50:1361–91.
23. Patil PB, Bathi R, Chaudhari S. Prevalence of oral mucosal lesions in dental patients with tobacco smoking, chewing, and mixed habits: a cross sectional. J Fam Commun Med. 2013;20(2):130–5.

24. Hazarey VK, Erlewad DM, Mundhe KA, Ughade SN. Oral submucous fibrois: study of 1000 cases from central India. J Oral Pathol Med. 2007;36:12–7.
25. Mathew AL, Pai KM, Sholapurkar AA, Vengal M. The prevalence of oral mucosal lesions in patients visiting a dental school in southern India. Indian J Dent Res. 2008;19(2):99–103.
26. Mehrotra R, Pandya S, Chaudhary AK, Kumar M, Singh M. Prevalence of oral pre-malignant and malignant lesions at a tertiary level hospital in Allahabad, India. Asian Pac J Cancer Prev 2008;9(2):263–265.
27. Sharma R, Raj SS, Miahra G, Reddy YG, Shenava S, Narang P. Prevalence of oral submucous fibrosis in patients visiting dental college in rural area of Jaipur, Rajasthan. J Indian Acad Oral Med Radiol. 2012;24(1):1–4.
28. Agarwal A, Chandel S, Singh N, Singhal A. Use of tobacco and oral sub mucous fibrosis in teenagers. J Dent Sci Res. 3(3):1–4.
29. Bhatnagar P, Rai S, Bhatnagar G, Kaur M, Goel S, Prabhat M. Prevalence study of oral mucosal lesions, mucosal variants, and treatment required for patients reporting to a dental school in North India: in accordance with WHO guidelines. J Fam Community Med. 2013;20(1):41–8.
30. Burungale SU, Durge PM, Burungale DS, Zambare MB. Epidemiological study of premalignant and malignant lesions of the Oral cavity. J Acad Ind Res. 2014;2(9):519–23.
31. Nigam NK, Aravinda K, Dhillon M, Gupta S, Reddy S, Srinivas RM. Prevalence of oral submucous fibrosis among habitual gutkha and areca nut chewers in Moradabad district. J Oral Biol Craniofac Res. 2014;4(1):8–13.
32. Singh P, Mittal R, Chandak S, Bhondey A, Rathi A, Chandwani M. Prevalence of oral submucous fibrosis in children of rural area of Nagpur, Maharashtra, India. Int J Prev Clin Dent Res. 2016;3(4):243–5.
33. Tyagi VN, More MD. Prevalence of Oral submucous fibrosis at OPD of ENT department of SMBT Institute of Medical Sciences, Nasik. J Appl Med Sci. 2018;6(1F):395–8.
34. More C, Rao NR, More S, Johnson NW. Reasons for initiation of areca nut and related products in patients with oral submucous fibrosis within an endemic area in Gujarat, India. Subst Use Misuse. 2020;55(9):1413–21.
35. Ahmad MS, Ali SA, Ali AS, Chaubey KK. Epidemiological and etiological study of oral submucous fibrosis among gutkha chewers of Patna, Bihar, India. J Indian Soc Pedod Prev Dent. 2006;24(2):84–9.
36. Panda S, Panda BK, Pattnaik B, Naik C, Dany SS, Avijeeta A. Prevalence of oral submucous fibrosis in a tertiary care hospital of Odisha: a cross-sectional study. J Evid Based Med Health. 2020;49:2903–6.
37. Srivastava R, Jyoti B, Pradhan D, Siddiqui Z. Prevalence of oral submucous fibrosis in patients visiting dental OPD of a dental college in Kanpur: a demographic study. J Family Med Primary Care. 2019;8(8):2612.
38. Lay KM, Sein K, Myint A, Ko SK, Pindborg JJ. Epidemiologic study of 600 villagers of oral precancerous lesions in Bilugyun: preliminary report. Commun Dent Oral Epidemiol. 1982; 10(3):152–5.
39. Amarasinghe AAHK, Usgodaarachchi US, Johnson NW, Warnakulasuriya S. High prevalence of lifestyle factors attributable for oral cancer, and of oral potentially malignant disorders in Rural Sri Lanka. Asian Pac J Cancer Prev. 2018;19(9):2485–92.
40. Hosein M, Mohiuddin S, Fatima N. Association between grading of oral submucous fibrosis with frequency and consumption of areca nut and its derivatives in a wide age group: a multi-centric cross-sectional study from Karachi. Pakistan J Cancer Prev. 2015;20(3):216–22.
41. Tariq H, Ahmed S, Naz M, Naureen A. Frequency of oral sub mucous fibrosis and its correlation with the level of education in patients coming to a tertiary care hospital of Karachi from January 2018 to December 2018. Asian Pac J Cancer Care. 2020;5(3):157–60.
42. Cuc TTK, Nguyen BN, Nguyen TH. Oral mucosa and oral health status of betel chewers in Ba De Hoc Mon- Ho Chi Minh City (in Vietnamese). University of Medicine and Pharmacy; 2008. p. 91–7.
43. Khanh ND. Oral Cancer and Precancer Survey in Southern Provinces of Vietnam (1998). Cited by Huy`nh Anh Lan, 2006. In: Proceedings, oral cancer in the Asia Pacific—a regional update and networking. Kuala Lumpur: Faculty of Dentistry, University of Malaya, 2006. pp. 17–19.
44. Nguyên TBN (2006). Oral mucosa, denture and paradentitis of betel chewers in BàĐiêm Commune, Hóc Môn District, HôChí Minh City (in Vietnamese). Thesis, Faculty of Odontology, University of Medicine and Pharmacy, HôChí Minh City, 2006, pp. 15–7.
45. Tang JG, Jian XF, Gao ML, Ling TY, Zhang KH. Epidemiological survey of oral submucous fibrosis in Xiangtan City, Hunan Province, China. Commun Dent Oral Epidemiol. 1997;25(2):177–80.
46. Zhang SS, Li W-H, Gao Y-J, et al. Betel-quid and oral submucous fibrosis: a cross-sectional study in Hunan province, China. J Oral Pathol Med. 2012;41:748–54.
47. Yang PY, Chen YT, Wang YH, Su NY, Yu HC, Chang YC. Malignant transformation of oral submucous fibrosis in Taiwan: a nationwide population-based retrospective cohort study. J Oral Pathol Med. 2017;46(10):1040–5.
48. Yang S-F, Wang Y-H, Su N-Y, et al. Changes in prevalence of pre- cancerous oral submucous fibrosis from 1996 to 2013 in Taiwan: a nationwide population-based retrospective study. J Formos Med Assoc. 2018;117(2):147–52.
49. Shah B, Lewis MA, Bedi R. Oral submucous fibrosis in a 11-yearold Bangladeshi girl living in the United Kingdom. Br Dent J. 2001;191(3):130–2.
50. Laskaris G, Bovopoulou O, Nicolis G. Oral submucous fibrosis in a Greek female. Br J Oral Surg. 1981;19(3):197–201.
51. Aziz SR. Coming to America: betel nut and oral submucous fibrosis. J Am Dent Assoc. 2010;141(4):423–8.
52. McGurk M, Craig GT. Oral submucous fibrosis: two cases of malignant transformation in Asian immigrants to the United Kingdom. Br J Oral Maxillofac Surg. 1984;22(1):56–64.
53. Shear M, Lemmer J, Dockrat IS. Oral submucous fibrosis in South African Indians. An epidemiological study. S Afr J Med Sci. 1967;32:41–6.
54. Seedat HA, van Wyk CW. Betel-nut chewing and submucous fibrosis in Durban. S Afr Med J. 1988;74(11):568–71.
55. VanWyk CW. Oral submucous fibrosis. The South African experience. Indian J Dent Res. 1997;8(2):39–45.
56. Ranganathan K, Devi MU, Joshua E, Kirankumar K, Saraswathi TR. Oral submucous fibrosis: a case-control study in Chennai, South India. J Oral Pathol Med. 2004;33(5): 274–7.
57. Mohiuddin S, Fatima N, Hosein S, Hosein M. High risk of malignant transformation of oral submucous fibrosis in Pakistani females: a potential national disaster. J Pak Med Assoc. 2016;66(11):1362–6.
58. Ali SM, Qureshi R, Jamal S. Prevalence of oral submucous fibrosis and use of tobacco and related products amongst school going males. Pak Oral Dent J. 2013;31:384–7.

59. Cai X, Yao Z, Liu G, Cui L, Li H, Huang J. Oral submucous fibrosis: a clinicopathological study of 674 cases in China. J Oral Pathol Med. 2019;48:321–5.
60. Oakley E, Demaine L, Warnakulasuriya S. Areca (betel) nut chewing habit among high-school children in the Commonwealth of the Northern Mariana Islands (Micronesia). Bull World Health Organ. 2005;83(9):656–60.
61. Hayes PA. Oral submucous fibrosis in a 4-year-old girl. Oral Surg Oral Med Oral Pathol. 1985;59(5):475–8.
62. South Asian Public Health Association. The health of South Asians in the United States: a brown paper. Berkeley, CA: South Asian Public Health Association; 2002.
63. More CB, Rao NR, Hegde R, Brahmbhatt RM, Shrestha A, Kumar G. Oral submucous fibrosis in children and adolescents: analysis of 36 cases. J Indian Soc Pedod Prev Dent. 2020;38(2):190–9.
64. Kariya P, Khobragade V, Sura S, Singh S. No age predilection for a disease like OSF. A case report of 5-year-old child. J Oral BiolCraniofac Res. 2020;10(2):153–7.
65. Peng Q, Li H, Chen J, Wang Y, Tang Z. Oral submucous fibrosis in Asian countries. J Oral Pathol Med. 2020;49(4):294–304.
66. Tilakaratne WM, Ekanayaka RP, Warnakulasuriya S. Oral submucous fibrosis: a historical perspective and a review on etiology and pathogenesis. Oral Surg Oral Med Oral Pathol Oral Radiol. 2016;122(2):178–91.
67. Gupta PC. Areca nut use in India. Ind J Med Sci. 2007;61:317–9.
68. Gupta PC, Warnakulasuriya S. Global epidemiology of areca nut usage. Addict Biol. 2002;7:77–83.
69. More CB, Rao NR. Proposed clinical definition for oral submucous fibrosis. J Oral Biol Craniofac Res. 2019;9(4):311–4.
70. Babu S, Bhat RV, Kumar PU. A comparative clinicopathological study of oral submucous fibrosis in habitual chewers of pan masala and betel quid. Clin Toxicol. 1996;34:317–22.
71. Maher R, Lee AJ, Warnakulasuriya KA, Lewis JA, Johnson NW. Role of areca nut in the causation of oral submucous fibrosis: a case-control study in Pakistan. J Oral Pathol Med. 1994;23(2):65–9.
72. World Health Organization. (2021) WHO report on the global tobacco epidemic 2021: addressing new and emerging products. Geneva, Switzerland.
73. Schwartz J. AtrophiaIdiopathica Mucosae Oris. London: Demonstrated at the 11th Int Dent Congress; 1952. London.
74. Patil S, Doni B, Maheshwari S. Prevalence and distribution of oral mucosal lesions in a geriatric Indian population. Can Geriatr J. 2015;18(1):11–4.

# Clinical Features: Oral Submucous Fibrosis

*Saman Warnakulasuriya*

## Contents



© The Author(s), under exclusive license to Springer Nature Switzerland AG 2023
S. Warnakulasuriya, K. Ranganathan (eds.), *Oral Submucous Fibrosis*, Textbooks in Contemporary Dentistry,
https://doi.org/10.1007/978-3-031-12855-4_3

3

## 3.1 Introduction

Oral submucous fibrosis (OSF) develops insidiously, and as the early signs and symptoms are rather non-specific, the clinical presentation can be easily overlooked. As the diseases progresses, OSF may present with a wide range of signs and symptoms affecting several subsites of the oral cavity, the pharynx and the upper part of oesophagus. The sites mostly affected are the lips, buccal mucosa, tongue, and palate. Fibrosis of oral tissues leading to limitation of mouth opening remains the hallmark of this disease. This chapter presents a comprehensive description of clinical manifestations to enable a health professional to make a clinical diagnosis during an initial consultation.

**Learning Goals**

The primary goal of this chapter is to educate dentists and physicians in the detection of the early stages of oral submucous fibrosis by learning the signs and symptoms of the disease.

The chapter also lists the essential clinical criteria for patient selection when planning field surveys on oral submucous fibrosis.

## 3.2 Brief Review of the Literature

This disorder was first reported by Schwartz in 1952 [1], in five Indian women living in Kenya but as stated in Chap. 1 this description is no longer accessible in the published literature. Subsequently, the clinical features of OSF were reported, by three Indian clinicians, Joshi [2], Lal [3] and Desa [4], and three cases of OSF were described by Su from Taiwan [5]. A comprehensive clinical and pathological description of OSF was first published by Pindborg during his travels to India [6–9]. The establishment of a large-scale epidemiological investigation by Fali Mehta's group based at the Basic Dental Research Unit of the Tata Institute of Fundamental Research that investigated and reported on 50,915 villagers from five different regions in India [10, 11] contributed largely to enhance the knowledge of the international research community on this disorder. Around the same period, a further impetus to the study of OSF came from investigations on Indian residents in South Africa in Durban by Shear's group [12, 13] and by van Wyk's group [14, 15].

Staging of OSF based on clinical signs and symptoms, and taking into account degrees of mouth opening, functional aspects and presence or absence of a malignancy, has been presented by various authors [16–21], and some modifications to the Kerr classification were done by More [22, 23], and the latest by Arakeri et al. [24]. See details of OSF staging in this volume, ▶ Chap. 6.

Clinical aspects of OSF have been a subject discussed at several international conferences. In 1992, the first Asia-Pacific Workshop on Oral Mucosal Disorders was held in Nagoya, Japan [25]. In 1997, two expert symposia on OSF were held, one in London [26] and the other in Kuala Lumpur [27]. Criteria for diagnosis of OSF were published following the Kuala Lumpur Symposium [27, 28]. The Fifth World Workshop on Oral Medicine included OSF as a topic to develop a systematic review on the disease [21] and the WHO Collaborating Centre's Working Group on Oral Potentially Malignant Disorders recently enumerated the criteria for diagnosis of OSF [29].

**Definition**

A definition of clinical features should include the presence of fibrous bands in lips, buccal mucosa, soft palate and fauces as the hallmark of the disease that leads to marked limitation of mouth opening.

## 3.3 General Aspects: Age and Sex

OSF is a disease found in population groups from South and Southeast Asia and South Pacific islands or among the migrants from these countries to East and South Africa, Europe and North America. The initial literature referred to a female preponderance, but later studies reported that males are more affected by the disease see ▶ Chap. 2. The proportion of males affected in China and in Taiwan appears to be significantly higher than that in India [30, 31]. The common age range at presentation is between 20 and 40 years. Oral submucous fibrosis in a 4-year-old girl whose parents had moved from India to Canada was reported by Hayes [32]. The disease has been described in all ages ranging from 4 to 89 years.

## 3.4 Signs and Symptoms

The signs and symptoms of OSF could be broadly divided to early, intermediate and advanced stages of the disease and are listed in ◘ Table 3.1. The anatomical sites affected by OSF are listed in ◘ Table 3.2.

The most common early symptom is a burning sensation of the mouth, often noted at mealtimes while consuming spicy food. Appearance of transient vesicles, diffuse blanching of the mucosa and loss of tongue papillae have been found in population surveys as early forms of submucous fibrosis [33].

**Table 3.1** Clinical presentation of oral submucous fibrosis by stages of development

| Early stage | Intermediate stage (additional features) | Advanced stage (additional features) |
|---|---|---|
| Burning sensation | Sore mouth<br>Sensitivity to hot and cold foods | Stomatitis |
| Blanching of oral mucosa | Depigmentation | Marble-like appearance of oral mucosa |
| Leathery mucosa | Palpable fibrous bands in lips, buccal mucosa, retromolar trigone and soft palate | Thick and broad fibrous bands of buccal mucosa |
| No limitation in mouth opening | Limited mouth opening (20–40 mm) | Limited mouth opening (<20 mm) |
| Depapillation of tongue | Limited movement of tongue | Fixed tongue |
| | | Sunken cheeks |
| | | Dysphagia, rhinolalia, loss of hearing |
| | | Weight loss |

**Table 3.2** Morphological features noted in different anatomical sites

| Sites | Presenting Features |
|---|---|
| Lips | Thinning and distortion of lips<br>Depigmentation |
| Cheeks | Sunken appearance, Vertical skin folds |
| Buccal mucosa | Vesicles, blanching, marble-like appearance, fibrous bands, patchy hyperpigmentation |
| Tongue | Depapillation of dorsum, later fixation |
| Soft palate | Petechia, fibrous banding, distorted uvula |
| Fauces | Fibrous banding |

As the disease progresses, the oral mucosa becomes more blanched, and whitish areas appear in discrete locations giving the appearance of depigmentation of the mucosa. The mucosa develops a leathery feeling, and fibrous bands first appear around the faucial pillars.

The pathognomonic features of OSF are the presence of palpable fibrous bands, tongue becoming progressively immobile and fibrous bands in the buccal mucosa and retromolar regions leading to limited mouth opening.

As the disease extends inwards from the oral cavity to the pharynx and the upper third of the oesophagus, additional symptoms may be noted during advanced stages. These include dysphagia, deafness, rhinolalia and loss of weight. Characteristic facial features include sunken cheeks and presence of multiple vertical perioral skin folds.

OSF could coexist with several associated oral mucosal lesions [34]. These presentations are discussed further in ► Chap. 4 (see ► Sect. 4.3).

> **Important**
>
> Key features of the disease include
>
> 1. Palpable fibrous bands in the buccal mucosa and retromolar regions.
> 2. Tongue becoming progressively immobile.
> 3. Limited mouth opening.

## 3.5 Burning Sensation

Burning sensation is a universal feature of OSF and can be present spontaneously but is more commonly reported during consumption of spicy foods. This important early symptom is often disguised as a feature of anaemia, and the disease is overlooked by general practitioners during routine consultations. Many patients with OSF tend to reduce the consumption of chillies and spicy food over the evolution of the disease. An OSF patient could suffer from burning sensation for the rest of the life, and this does affect the quality of life. The cause is not well understood but is attributed to the atrophy and flattening of rete ridges of the oral epithelium that could be present from the very early stages of the disease.

## 3.6 Blanching of the Mucosa

Blanching of the oral mucosa was first described as an early feature of OSF by Pindborg et al. [11] based on a field study undertaken in Ernakulam district in India in their baseline survey of 10,169 subjects in 1967. Blanching is characterised by loss of the pink colour and mucosa appearing whitish in discrete areas of the oral mucosa. This feature appears even before the onset of fibrosis and is often under-recognised. Figure 3.1 illustrates a blanched mucosa in a 30-year-old man—an areca nut chewer—who later developed fibrous bands on follow-up. This could often be mistaken for pallor often observed in deficiency states such as anaemias.

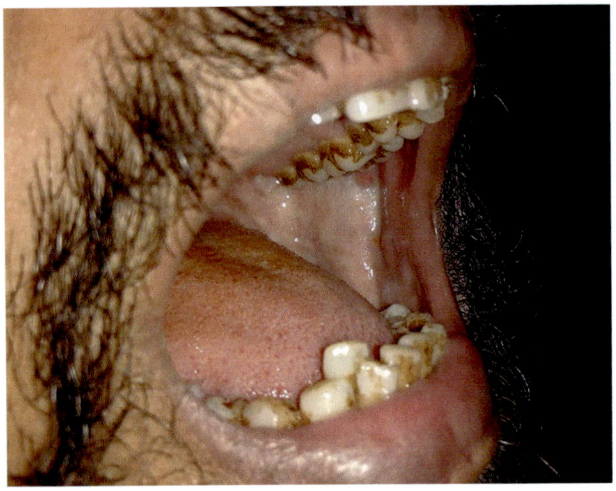

Fig. 3.1 Blanching of buccal mucosa in an areca nut chewer—an early feature of OSF

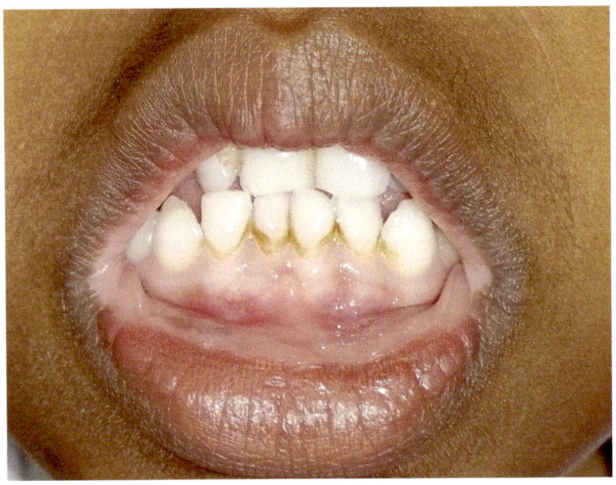

Fig. 3.2 Depigmentation of labial mucosa and the commissure in a child

## 3.7 Depigmentation

Loss of pigmentation of the oral mucosa (Fig. 3.2) has been reported in several studies. Depigmentation near the vermilion border of the lip in five young children aged 2–3 years as the sole clinical feature and as the earliest sign of OSF was reported by Sitheeque et al. [35].

The authors claim that depigmentation is different from blanching referred to above. Depigmented sites retain a glossy appearance, while blanched mucosa exhibits a matt appearance. In cases with loss of pigmentation, several conditions should be considered in the differential diagnosis before confirming OSF: These include focal type of vitiligo, localised scleroderma and lichen sclerosus particularly when affecting the lip.

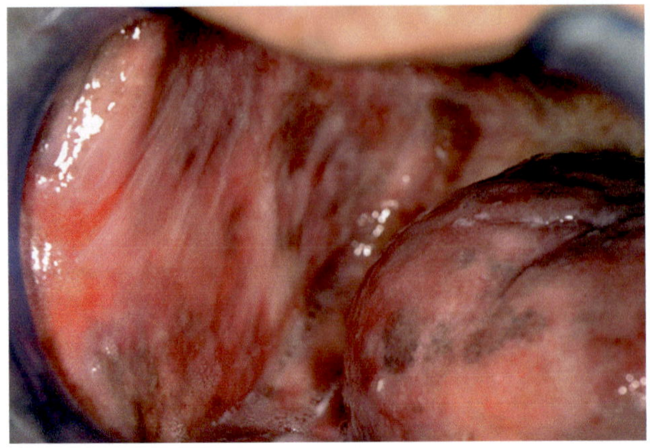

Fig. 3.3 Patchy hyperpigmentation of buccal mucosa and dorsal tongue in an adult patient

In advanced cases along with loss of pigmentation, there may be patchy hyperpigmented areas (Fig. 3.3) of the oral mucosa [33].

## 3.8 Leathery Mucosa

Another early feature of the disease is a leathery consistency that is observed during palpation of lips and buccal mucosa. This feature often precedes the development of fibrous bands and is an indication of the early loss of fibroelasticity of the mucosa. The leathery feeling is fairly well generalised over the lining surfaces of the mucosa. The process is somewhat similar to a tanned skin changing to leather and gives a tough feel to the oral mucosa.

## 3.9 Marble-Like Appearance

Due to increased blanching, pallor and loss of pigmentation, the oral mucosa takes up a characteristic generalised marble-like appearance (Fig. 3.4), particularly affecting the buccal mucosa bilaterally.

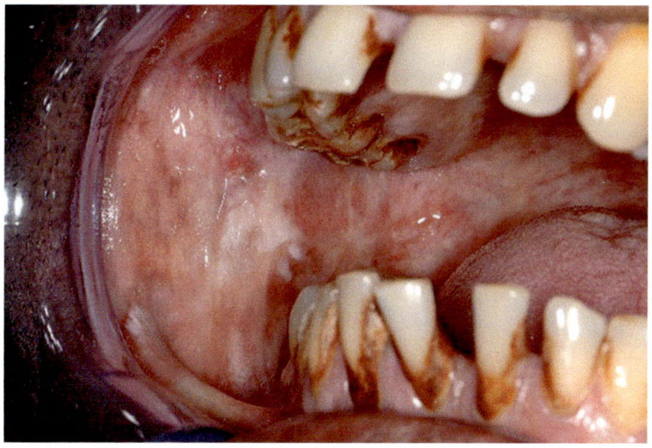

Fig. 3.4 Marble-like appearance of buccal mucosa in moderately advanced OSF

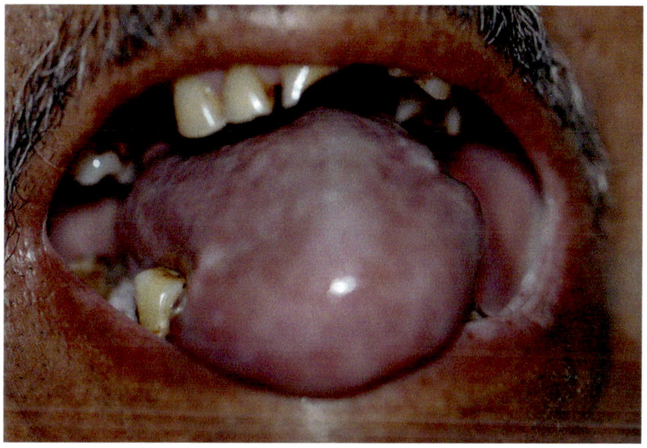

Fig. 3.5 Totally depapillated tongue giving a glossy appearance

## 3.10 Depapillation of Tongue

Loss of filiform papillae from the dorsum of tongue (Fig. 3.5) is another common feature found in OSF patients. Initially, the feature is noted as a partial loss, and as the disease evolves, there is almost complete loss of tongue papillae. This results in a glazed tongue with or without any erythema. Figure 3.5 illustrates the feature of a glazed tongue in OSF due to loss of papillae. This appearance could masquerade glossitis. The differential diagnosis should include erythema migrans and glossitis found in iron-deficiency anaemia and Plummer-Vinson syndrome.

## 3.11 Vesicles

Vesicles that may last up to few days may appear during any stage of OSF but are more common in the early stages of the disease. In OSF, vesicles are usually located on the soft palate and the anterior pillars of fauces but may also be found on other areas of lining mucosa. Vesicles are subepithelial and retain the normal surface colour of the oral mucosa. They usually rupture within 24 to 72 hours discharging an aseptic fluid [36] leaving small ulcers.

## 3.12 Petechia

Tiny, circular red or blue spots on the oral mucosa, caused by minor vascular dilatations or a minor bleed from broken capillary blood vessels, were reported by Bhonsle et al. [37]. The authors found blue spots in 22% of 40 patients with OSF in India.

## 3.13 Ulceration and Stomatitis

Mouths of OSF patients may demonstrate superficial ulceration especially in the area of retromolar trigone. A sore mouth and stomatitis are common findings.

## 3.14 Fibrous Bands

The most outstanding feature and the important reliable sign of OSF is the presence of palpable bands in the oral mucosa. The soft palate and fauces are first affected by fibrosis (Fig. 3.6), and as the disease advances, fibrosis gradually involves the retromolar region, buccal mucosa (Fig. 3.7) and lips. Haider et al. [19] based their clinical staging on the location of fibrous bands in the mouth and grouped clinical stages by (1) faucial bands only, (2) faucial and buccal bands and (3) faucial, buccal and labial bands. They concluded that bands are common at the back of the mouth in mild cases of OSF and, as the disease increases in severity, are more likely

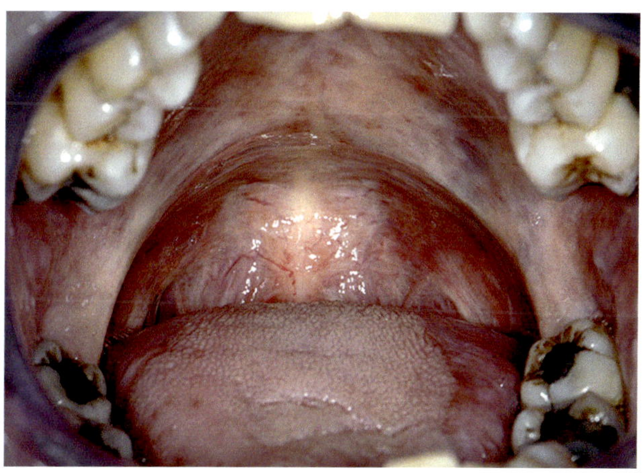

Fig. 3.6 Horizontal fibrous band across the soft palate

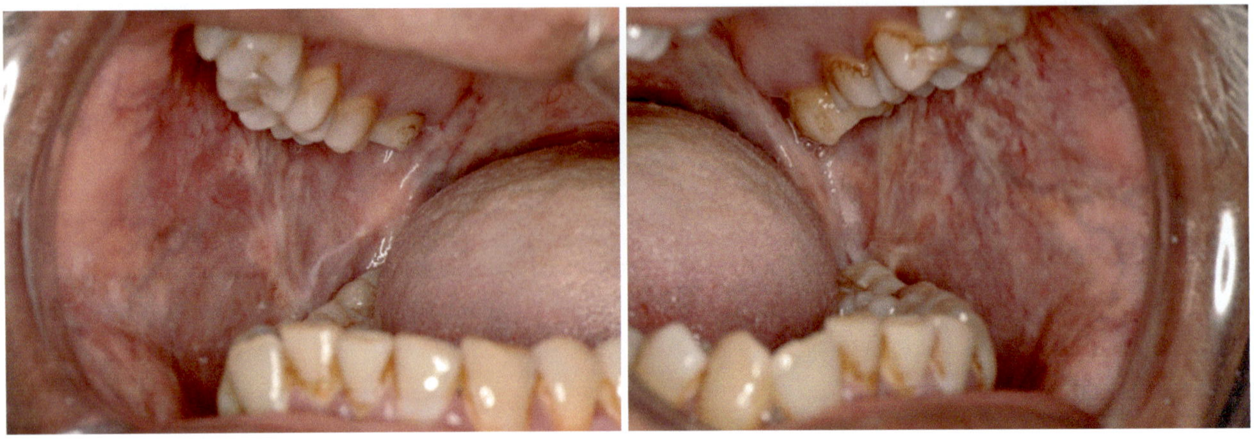

Fig. 3.7 Vertical fibrous bands bilaterally on the buccal mucosa

to be found anteriorly. However, a study from Taiwan reported that only a quarter of their OSF patients presented with fibrosis of palate [38]. More frequent affliction of posterior parts of the mouth has been attributed to the habit of pure areca nut consumption (without betel quid) as noted in Maharashtra state in India [39]. The degree of fibrosis can be semi-quantitatively assessed in the buccal mucosa by the presence of a single band, multiple bands or a broad band when it extends over two cm in width [16]. The extent and severity of fibrous banding found in the retromolar region (around the pterygomandibular raphe) or the buccal mucosa have a significant correlation with the function of mouth opening. Though fibrous bands may be visible on opening the mouth during a systematic oral examination, it is important to palpate both sides of the buccal mucosa to find any palpable fibrous bands. In the field surveys conducted by Fali Mehta's group, the demonstration of fibrous bands was mandatory for the diagnosis of OSF [33, 40, 41]. The expert group that met in Kuala Lumpur also included this as an essential inclusion criterion for diagnosis of OSF [28].

## 3.15 Distorted Uvula

As a component of fibrosis of the palatal arch, the shape and size of the uvula could be affected and could appear shrunken or bud-like. The uvula may also show deviations [42]. The uvula may point anteriorly instead of downward pointing and present as inverted or in the shape of a hockey stick (Fig. 3.8).

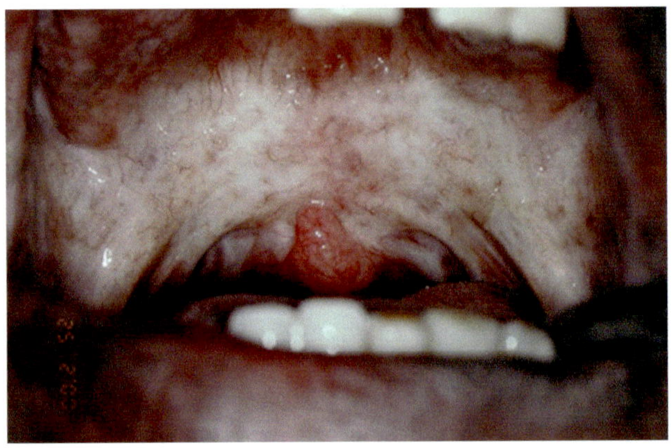

Fig. 3.8 Anteriorly pointing uvula due to palatal fibrosis

> **Tip**
>
> Observing a deformed uvula should raise the suspicion of patient presenting with OSF.

## 3.16 Limited Mobility of Tongue

Fibrosis generally affects the tongue during intermediate and advanced stages (Table 3.1). This leads to limited mobility of the tongue. On protrusion, a normal tongue could reach beyond the mucocutaneous junction of the lower lip. However, when affected by fibrosis, mobility may be restricted and the tongue cannot be protruded beyond the incisal edges (Fig. 3.9). Lateral movement will also be restricted. In advanced cases, the tongue remains in a fixed position and limits the rolling movement. Once the fibrosis involves the striated muscle, the tongue structure will demonstrate hardness on squeezing the tongue during palpation.

## 3.17 Limited Mouth Opening

As fibrosis advances, one of the main consequences of OSF relates to the restriction of mouth opening (◘ Fig. 3.10). In an Indian survey, 90.8% of the survey subjects reported inability to open the mouth wide as their chief complaint [39]. Degree of mouth opening measured as interincisal distance has been used as an objective criterion to stage the disease [16] and in many subsequent systems (e.g. [23, 29, 43]). As a reference guide, the average size of the mouth opening of South Indian males was reported as 47.5 mm, and 44.6 mm in females [44]. The majority of OSF patients present with a mouth opening <40 mm and > 20 mm [45]. An opening of less than 20 mm is considered as a presentation of advanced disease. A device useful to measure the interincisal distance is illustrated in ◘ Fig. 3.11.

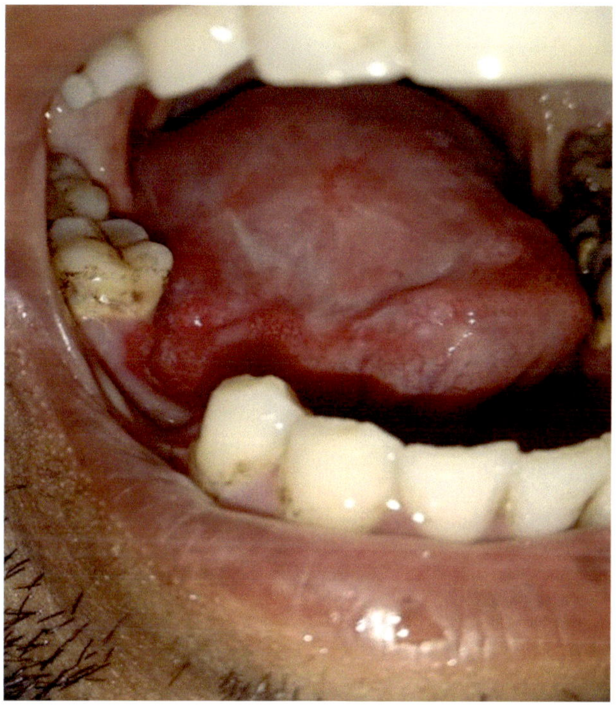

◘ **Fig. 3.9** Limited mobility of tongue. On attempting to protrude, the tongue does not reach lower incisors

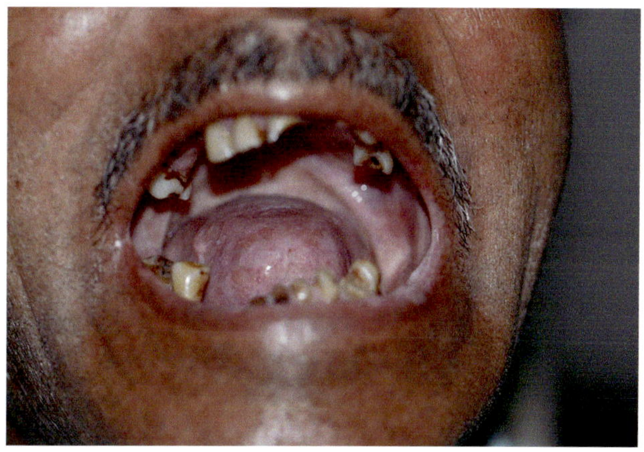

◘ **Fig. 3.10** Limited mouth opening in a moderately advanced OSF patient. Vertical skin fold on cheeks is also seen

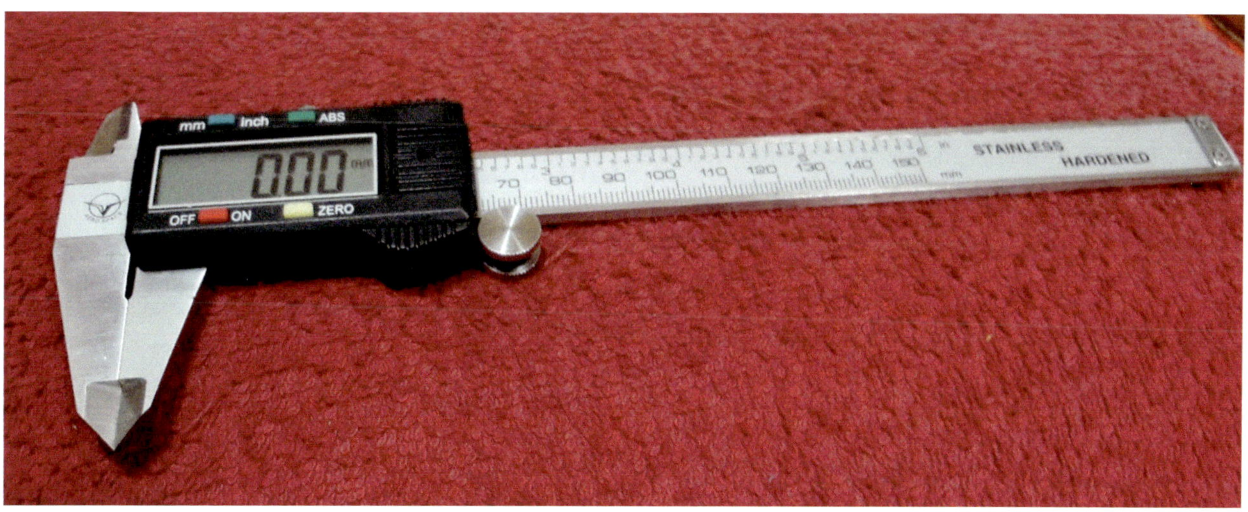


◘ **Fig. 3.11** Callipers to measure mouth opening (Courtesy Prof. Vinay Hazarey)

3

## 3.18 Other Associated Clinical Conditions

OSF could coexist with several associated oral mucosal lesions, some that are also potentially malignant [29, 46], e.g. oral leukoplakia, erythroplakia, erythroleukoplakia, exophytic verrucous hyperplasia [47] betel quid-associated oral lichenoid lesions [48, 49], Oral squamous cell carcinoma arising from OSF may be found in patients with poor access to care [50]. These presentations are discussed further in ▶ Chap. 4.

Oesophageal subepithelial fibrosis as an extension of OSF leading to thickening and narrowing of the oesophagus was first reported by Maher et al. [51] and by taking endoscopic biopsies by Misra et al. [52].

## 3.19 Mastication and Deglutition

The ability to masticate food is affected due to reduced oral opening and generalised stomatitis. Moreover, the mucosa becomes extremely sensitive to hot, cold and spicy food that makes it difficult to tolerate any form of food in the mouth. In advanced stages, the patient may have to be tube fed. Loss of suppleness of tongue severely affects the formation of a bolus of food, and due to fibrosis and narrowing of the upper digestive tract, deglutition may be affected (Maher et al. [51]). Dysphagia could be a presenting symptom particularly among rural populations who have not had access to early diagnosis. Defective gustatory sensation was reported by Seedat and van Wyk [15].

## 3.20 Extraoral

Thinning or distortion of lips is visible extraorally. Chaturvedi referred to sunken cheeks in people affected by OSF as a part of what he coined as Gutka syndrome [53]. Ranganathan et al. [44] referred to reduced cheek flexibility. Other aspects include the presence of multiple peri-oral skin folds instead of a single deep naso-labial fold. Due to stiffening of cheeks, inability to whistle or to blow out a candle is reported [6]. Referred pain in the ears and deafness due to occlusion of Eustachian tubes were reported in Indian studies. Speech may be affected due to difficulty in the pronunciation of words as a result of fixation of the tongue muscles.

**Summary**

Oral submucous fibrosis is a generalised condition that presents with a plethora of signs and symptoms involving the whole oral cavity and the upper digestive track. An understanding of the initial signs and symptoms could help a healthcare provider to make an early diagnosis and to institute interventions, primarily advice on the cessation of areca nut that could halt the progression of the disease. Presence of fibrous bands in lips, buccal mucosa, soft palate and fauces is the hallmark of the disease that leads to marked limitation of mouth opening. In advanced stages, the oral health and quality of life are severely compromised leading to loss of weight and a cachexic state.

**Acknowledgement** I thank Prof. Ruwan Jayasinghe for providing ◘ Figs. 3.1 and 3.2 for this chapter and Prof. Vinay Hazarey for supplying ◘ Fig. 3.11.

## References

1. Schwartz J. Atrophia idiopathica (tropical) mucosae oris. In: Proceedings of the 11th International Dental Congress, London. 1952.
2. Joshi SG. Fibrosis of the palate and pillars. Ind J Otolaryngol. 1953;4:1.
3. Lal D. Diffuse oral submucous fibrosis. J All India Dent Assoc. 1953;26:1–3.
4. Desa JV. Submucous fibrosis of the palate and cheek. Ann Otol Rhinol Laryngol. 1957;66(4):1143–59.
5. Su P-I. Idiopathic scleroderma of the mouth. Arch Otolaryngol. 1954;59:330–2.
6. Pindborg JJ, Chawla TN, Srivastava AN, Gupta D, Mehrotra ML. Clinical aspects of oral submucous fibrosis. Acta Odontol Scand. 1964;22:679–91.
7. Pindborg JJ, Sirsat SM. Oral submucous fibrosis. Oral Surg Oral Med Oral Pathol. 1966;22:764–79.
8. Zachariah J, Mathew B, Varma NA, Iqbal AM, Pindborg JJ. Frequency of oral mucosal lesions among 5000 individuals in Trivandrum, South India. Preliminary Rep J Indian Dent Assoc. 1966;38(11):290–4.
9. Mehta FS, Gupta PC, Daftary DK, Pindborg JJ, Choksi SK. An epidemiologic study of oral cancer and precancerous conditions among 101,761 villagers in Maharashtra. India Int J Cancer. 1972;10(1):134–41.
10. Pindborg JJ, Mehta FS, Gupta PC, Daftary DK. Prevalence of oral submucous fibrosis among 50,915 Indian villagers. Brit J Cancer. 1968;22:646–54.
11. Gupta PC, Mehta FS, Daftary DK, et al. Incidence rates of oral cancer and natural history of oral precancerous lesions in a 10-year follow-up study of Indian villagers. Commun Dent Oral Epidemiol. 1980;8(6):283–333.

12. Dockart I, Shear M. Oral submucous fibrosis in Natal. In: Cahn L, editor. Fourth Proceedings of the International Academy of Oral Pathology. Gordon & Breach Scientific Publishing: New York; 1969. p. 57–63.
13. Shear M, Lemmer J, Dockhart I. Oral submucous fibrosis in South African Indians. S Afr J Med Sci. 1967;32:41–6.
14. van Wyk CW, Staz J, Farman AG. The prevalence of oral mucosal lesions among a random sample of Asian residents in Cape Town. J Dent Assoc S Afr. 1977;32:589–92.
15. Seedat HA, Van Wyk CW. Betelnut chewing and sub mucous fibrosis in Durban. South Africa Med J. 1988;74(3):568–71.
16. Warnakulasuriya S. Semi-quantitative clinical description of oral submucous fibrosis. Ann Dent. 1987;46:18–21.
17. Khanna JN, Andrade NN. Oral submucous fibrosis: a new concept in surgical management. Report of 100 cases. Int J Oral Maxillofac Surg. 1995;24(6):433–9.
18. Maher R, Sankaranarayanan R, Johnson NW, et al. Evaluation of inter-incisal distance as an objective criterion of the severity of oral submucous fibrosis. Eur J Cancer B Oral Oncol. 1996;32B:362–4.
19. Haider SM, Merchant AT, Fikree FF, Rahbar MH. Clinical and functional staging of oral submucous fibrosis. Br J Oral Maxillofac Sur. 2000;38(1):12–5.
20. Ranganathan K, Mishra G. An overview of classification schemes for oral submucous fibrosis. J Oral MaxFac Pathol. 2006;10:55–8.
21. Kerr AR, Warnakulasuriya S, Mighell AJ, Dietrich T, Nasser M, Rimal J, et al. A systematic review of medical interventions for oral submucous fibrosis and future research opportunities. Oral Dis. 2011;17(Suppl. 1):42–57.
22. More C, Gupta S, Joshi J, Varma S. Classification system for oral submucous fibrosis. J Ind Acad Oral Med Radiol. 2012;24(1):24–9.
23. More CB, Das S, Patel H, Adalja C, Kamatchi V, Venkatesh R. Proposed clinical classification for oral submucous fibrosis. Oral Oncol. 2012;48(3):200–2.
24. Arakeri G, Brennan PA. TFM classification and staging of oral submucous fibrosis: a new proposal. J Oral Pathol Med. 2018;47(5):539.
25. Warnakulasuriya S. Clinical and pathological criteria for diagnosis of oral submucous fibrosis. In: Proceedings of the First Asia-Pacific Workshop for Oral Mucosal Lesions. 1992; Nagoya: Japan.
26. Meghji S, Warnakulasuriya S. Oral submucous fibrosis: an expert symposium. Oral Dis. 1997;3:276–91.
27. Zain RB, Gupta PC, Warnakulasuriya S, et al. Oral lesions associated with betel quid and tobacco chewing habits. Oral Dis. 1997;3:204–5.
28. Zain RB, Ikeda N, Gupta PC, Warnakulasuriya S, van Wyk CW, Shrestha P, Axell T. Oral mucosal lesions associated with betel quid, areca nut and tobacco chewing habits: consensus from a workshop held in Kuala Lumpur, Malaysia, November 25-27, 1996. J Oral Pathol Med. 1999 Jan;28(1):1–4.
29. Warnakulasuriya S, Kujan O, Aguirre-Urizar JM, Bagan JV, González-Moles MÁ, Kerr AR, Lodi G, Mello FW, Monteiro L, Ogden GR, Sloan P, Johnson NW. Oral potentially malignant disorders: a consensus report from an international seminar on nomenclature and classification, convened by the WHO Collaborating Centre for Oral Cancer. Oral Dis. 2021;27(8):1862–80.
30. Cai X, Yao Z, Liu G, Cui L, Li H, Huang J. Oral submucous fibrosis: a clinicopathological study of 674 cases in China. J Oral Pathol Med. 2019;48(4):321–5.
31. Shih YH, Wang TH, Shieh TM, Tseng YH. Oral submucous fibrosis: a review on etiopathogenesis, diagnosis, and therapy. Int J Mol Sci. 2019;20(12):2940.
32. Hayes PA. Oral submucous fibrosis in a 4-year-old girl. Oral Surg Oral Med Oral Pathol. 1985;59:475.
33. Pindborg JJ, Bhonsle RB, Murti PR, Gupta PC, Daftary DK, Mehta FS. Incidence and early forms of oral submucous fibrosis. Oral Surg. 1980;50:40–4.
34. Warnakulasuriya S. Clinical features and presentation of oral potentially malignant disorders. Oral Surg Oral Med Oral Pathol Oral Radiol. 2018;125(6):582–90.
35. Sitheeque M, Ariyawardana A, Jayasinghe R, Tilakaratne W. Depigmentation of oral mucosa as the earliest possible manifestation of oral submucous fibrosis in Sri Lankan preschool children. J Investig Clin Dent. 2010;1(2):156–9.
36. Hamner JE 3rd, Looney PD, Chused TM. Submucous fibrosis. Oral Surg Oral Med Oral Pathol. 1974;37(3):412–21.
37. Bhonsle RB, Murti PR, Pindborg JJ, Daftary DK, Mehta FS. Focal vascular dilatations and petechiae in oral submucous fibrosis. Scand J Dent Res. 1981;89(3):270–4.
38. Shiau YY, Kwan HW. Submucous Fibrosis Taiwan Oral Surg. 1979;47:453–7.
39. Hazarey VK, Erlewad DM, Mundhe KA, Ughade SN. Oral submucous fibrosis: Study of 1000 cases from central India. J Oral Pathol Med. 2007;36:12–7.
40. Gupta PC, Sinor PN, Bhonsle RB, Pawar VS, Mehta FH. Oral submucous fibrosis in India: a new epidemic. Nat Med J India. 1998;11:113–6.
41. Pindborg JJ. Oral submucous fibrosis: a review. Ann Acad Med. 1989;18:603–7.
42. Rao NR, Villa A, More CB, Jayasinghe RD, Kerr AR, Johnson NW. Oral submucous fibrosis: a contemporary narrative review with a proposed inter-professional approach for an early diagnosis and clinical management. J Otolaryngol Head Neck Surg. 2020;49(1):3.
43. Warnakulasuriya S, Kerr AR. Oral submucous fibrosis: a review of the current management and possible directions for novel therapies. Oral Surg Oral Med Oral Pathol Oral Radiol. 2016;122(2):232–41.
44. Ranganathan K, Davi U, Joshua E, Bhardwaj A, Rooban T, Viswanathan R. Mouth opening, cheek flexibility and tongue protrusion. Parameters of 800 normal patients in Chennai. South India J Indian Dent Assoc. 2001;72:78–80.
45. Kiran Kumar K, Saraswathi TR, Ranganathan K, Uma Devi M, Elizabeth J. Oral submucous fibrosis: a clinico-histopathological study in Chennai. Indian J Dent Res. 2007;18:106–11.
46. Warnakulasuriya S, Tilakaratne WM, Kerr A. Oral submucous fibrosis. In: Kuriakose MA, editor. Chapter 8 Contemporary oral oncology. Switzerland: Springer; 2017. p. 329–53.
47. Zain RB, Kallarakkal TG, Ramanathan A, et al. A consensus report from the first Asian regional meeting on the terminology and criteria for verruco-papillary lesions of the oral cavity held

in Kuala Lumpur, Malaysia, December 15–18, 2013. Annal Dent Univ Malaya. 2013;20(2):1–3.
48. Yanduri S, Kumar VB, Suma S, Madhura MG. Lichenoid features and fibrosis: coexistence in quid-induced oral lesions. J Contemp Dent Pract. 2015;16:389–93.
49. Reichart PA, Warnakulasuriya S. Oral lichenoid contact lesions induced by areca nut and betel quid chewing: a mini review. J Investig Clin Dent. 2012;3(3):163–6.
50. Chaturvedi P, Vaishampayan SS, Nair S, Nair D, Agarwal JP, Kane SV, et al. Oral squamous cell carcinoma arising in background of oral submucous fibrosis: a clinicopathologically distinct disease. Head Neck. 2013;35:1404–9.
51. Maher R, Ahmed W, Qureshi H, Zuberi SJ, Syed S. Oesophageal changes in oral submucous fibrosis using fibreoptic endoscopy—a pilot study. J Pak Med Assoc. 1991;41:312–3.
52. Misra SP, Misra V, Dwivedi M, Gupta SC. Oesophageal subepithelial fibrosis; an extension of oral submucous fibrosis. Postgrad Med J. 1998;74:733–6.
53. Chaturvedi P. Gutka or areca nut Chewer's syndrome. Indian J Cancer. 2009;46:170–2.

3

# Associated Conditions of Oral Submucous Fibrosis

*A. Ramanathan and R. B. Zain*

## Contents



© The Author(s), under exclusive license to Springer Nature Switzerland AG 2023
S. Warnakulasuriya, K. Ranganathan (eds.), *Oral Submucous Fibrosis*, Textbooks in Contemporary Dentistry,
https://doi.org/10.1007/978-3-031-12855-4_4

## 4.1 Introduction

OSF is one of the oral potentially malignant disorders (OPMDs) that occur due to areca nut chewing. Many changes to the teeth and oral mucosa occur in OSF due to the effects of areca nut and betel quid chewing with or without tobacco. These effects from areca nut chewing, which could be both physical and chemically induced, can be divided into three types: (i) effects on the dental hard tissues and periodontium, (ii) effects on the soft tissue lining the oral cavity and (iii) effects on extraoral structures such as temporomandibular joint [1].



**Learning Objectives**

To recognise the clinical features and histopathological features of various associated conditions of oral submucous fibrosis with emphasis on verrucopapillary lesions.

## 4.2 Conditions Affecting the Dental Hard Tissues and Periodontium

Habitual chewing of areca nut may result in extrinsic staining of the dental hard tissues, i.e. the teeth (Fig. 4.1). The mechanical abrasiveness of chewing areca nut can affect the teeth and result in dental attrition (Fig. 4.2). Chronic habitual chewing of areca nut causes increased masticatory load on the teeth and results in root fractures. Some studies have indicated an inverse relationship between the caries experience and the intensity of areca nut chewing [2]. However, others have reported no difference in the caries prevalence between areca nut chewers and non-chewers [3, 4]. It has been reported that quid chewers with areca nut have increased injury to the periodontal tissues leading to bleeding gums, increased incidence of gingival recession and periodontal damage when compared to subjects without quid-chewing habits. As there is sparse literature on the conditions affecting the dental hard tissues and periodontium in OSF, this chapter primarily focuses on oral mucosal or soft-tissue lesions.

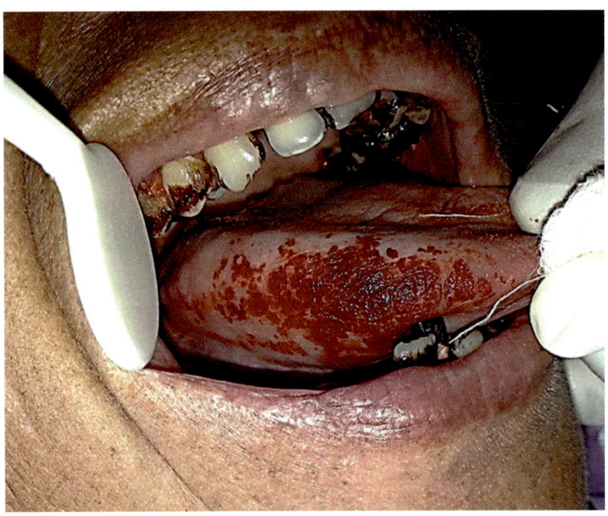

**Fig. 4.1** Intraoral photograph showing areca nut quid staining on the teeth and tongue

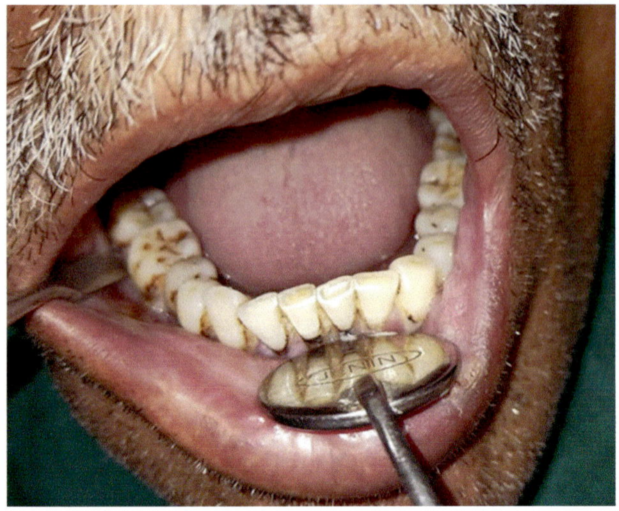

**Fig. 4.2** Intraoral photograph showing dental attrition in an areca nut chewer (Courtesy: Dr Bhavikumar Dholia)

## 4.3 Conditions Affecting the Soft-Tissue Lining of the Oral Cavity

### 4.3.1 Quid Stain on Oral Mucosa

Habitual areca nut quid chewing results in extrinsic staining of the oral mucosa (Fig. 4.1) similar to that occurring on dental hard tissues. This is due to the deposition of the quid contents on the oral mucosa especially in places where the quid is placed. The staining may be enhanced by lack of good oral hygiene prophylaxis and minimal oral healthcare. Quid chewing can also impart generalised extrinsic staining of the oral mucosa especially on the dorsal surface of the tongue. Prevalence of quid staining has not been extensively studied.

### 4.3.2 Chewer's Mucosa

The definition of the chewer's mucosa was first given by Mehta et al. (1971) [5] and reported later by others including Reichart et al. (1996) [6].

**Definition-Chewer's mucosa**

A condition of the oral mucosa where, either because of direct action of the quid or due to traumatic effect of chewing, or both, there is a tendency to desquamation or peeling off of the oral epithelium. Loose and detached tags of the tissue can also be seen and felt. The underlying area assumes a pseudomembranous or wrinkled appearance. The area may also show evidence of incorporation of the quid in the form of yellowish encrustations and can be scraped off.

However, Zain et al. (1999) have suggested to expand the above definition by adding additional criteria [7]:

**Definition**

Yellowish or reddish-brown wrinkled encrustations on the oral mucosa that can be scraped off, leaving behind non-elevated mucosal alterations such as a whitish area.

The authors recommend the above definition to differentiate chewer's mucosa from other similar lesions which are discussed below:

There are no studies in the literature on the prevalence of chewer's mucosa in OSF patients. Thus, the discussion below is again based on the understanding that chewer's mucosa may be seen in OSF as both conditions share the same aetiological agent, i.e. areca nut chewing.

Clinically, chewer's mucosa presents as a brownish-red discolouration of the oral mucosa. The quid ingredients get attached to the mucosa giving it the brownish-red colour (◘ Fig. 4.3). These quid ingredients contain calcium hydroxide and polyphenols. The number and composition of the quid influence the discolouration of the oral mucosa. Buccal mucosa seems to be the most common site to be affected; however, the appearance of chewer's mucosa depends on the place where the quid is placed during chewing. It is usually unilateral but sometimes can be bilateral. Apart from the brownish-red discolouration seen in the chewer's mucosa, the affected oral mucosa is irregular and shows a rough, macerated surface, with epithelial tags. Due to partial or total loss of epithelium, and underling hyperaemia, the desquamated areas appear red. The mucosa is diffusely affected and may show a dried-out appearance. The continued presence of the discolouration of the oral mucosa following cessation of the chewing habit is presently unknown.

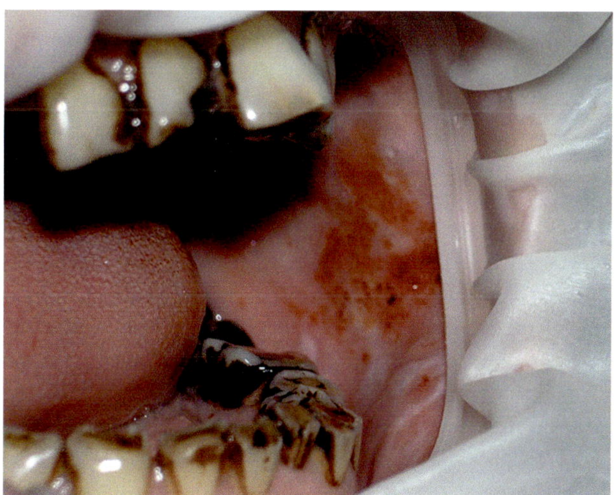

◘ **Fig. 4.3** Intraoral photograph shows chewer's mucosa of the left buccal mucosa (Courtesy: Dr. Fairuz Abdul Rahman)

Aetiology of chewer's mucosa is due to constant chewing of the areca nut quid. The suppleness of the mucosa and the presence of teeth with attrition and sharp edges can result in the traumatisation of the mucosa. Thus, the development of chewer's mucosa may be due to the traumatic, mechanical and/or chemical injuries that the mucosa is subjected to in an areca nut quid chewer. Substance such as lime present in the betel quid may also be involved in the causation of chewer's mucosa. The presence or absence of tobacco in the quid does not influence the causation of chewer's mucosa.

Prevalence of chewer's mucosa is 0.2% in the Cambodian general population [8], 1.6% in Malaysian population [9], 56.1% in the Sri Lankan tea estate workers [10] and as high as 60.8% in Cambodian elderly women [6]. The variation in prevalence may be due to various factors such as the sampling methods (highly selected versus unselected populations), age profile of the population studied, different interpretation of the definition of the chewer's mucosa and insufficient calibration of examiners. Chewer's mucosa more commonly affects women than men and occurs commonly in the elderly above 60 years of age. The most common site affected by chewer's mucosa is the buccal mucosa since the most common place where the areca nut quid is placed is in the lower buccal sulcus. Buccal mucosa and lower buccal sulcus are followed by lateral borders of the tongue, hard palate and upper lip. The edentulous alveolar ridges are also commonly affected.

The clinical appearances of cheek biting (i.e. morsicatio buccarum) and/or lip biting (i.e. morsicatio labiorum) are similar to chewer's mucosa except that they are without the quid stain [11]. Moreover, these lesions are also histologically similar, thus leading to difficulty in differentiation between these lesions [12]. However, chewer's mucosa occurs from an intentional habit in older adults above 50 years of age, whereas cheek biting in an unintentional habit usually occurs in a younger adult (20–35 years) [13].

Chewer's mucosa shows histologically encrusted betel quid ingredients on the surface epithelium (◘ Fig. 4.4). These ingredients are derived from the fragments of betel quid that are adherent to the oral mucosa. These ingredients may be present in small pits or attached to the outermost cell layer of the epithelium. They are seen as brownish amorphous substances that are unstained in haematoxylin

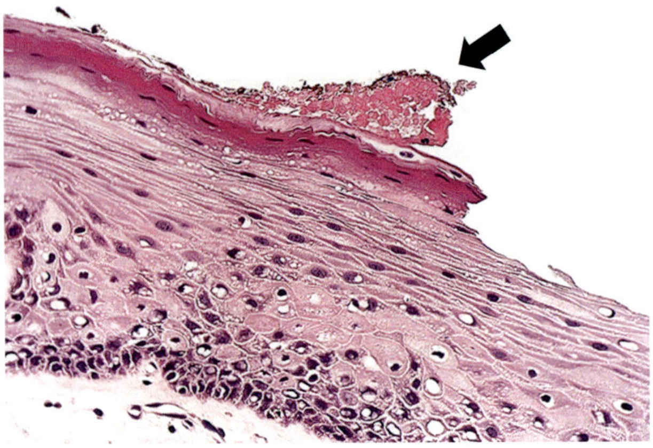

**Fig. 4.4** Photomicrograph showing brownish encrusted betel quid ingredients attached to the keratinised surface epithelium in chewer's mucosa with oral submucous fibrosis (Courtesy: Dr. Fairuz Abdul Rahman)

and eosin (H&E) staining. The encrustation reacts positively to von Kossa stain, which indicates that they contain calcium hydroxide which is derived from the slaked lime. Surface epithelium is hyperplastic with sub-epithelial inflammatory infiltrate. In some areas, the surface epithelium may be hyperkeratotic, and in other places, they may have ballooning epithelial cells. In the zones of ballooning cells, there is presence of small, dust-like von Kossa-positive granules seen both intra- and inter-cellularly [14, 15]. This is also observed in electron microscopy [16].

Chewer's mucosa has not been included as part of an OPMD. It can be present along with other lesions which do not have any potential for malignant transformation such as leukoedema and with OPMD such as oral leukoplakia and oral submucous fibrosis. The prevalence of chewer's mucosa in OSF patients has not been studied but has been generally noted.

**Chewer's Mucosa**

- It is not considered as part of the OPMD.
- It is caused due to either direct action of the quid or traumatic effect of chewing, or both.
- Areca nut chewing alone does not cause chewer's mucosa.
- Presence or absence of tobacco does not influence the causation of chewer's mucosa.
- Clinically, it presents as a brownish-red discolouration of the oral mucosa.
- Brownish-red discolouration is due to quid ingredients that are adherent to the mucosa.
- Histologically encrusted betel quid ingredients are present in small pits or attached to the outermost cell layer of the surface epithelium.
- These quid ingredients are seen as brownish amorphous substances that are left unstained in H&E staining.

### 4.3.3 Oral Candidiasis

Similar to other disorders mentioned in the earlier section, there are no reports on candidiasis and OSF. However, there are a few studies that have reported on oral candidiasis in areca nut chewers. One of the first studies to report the presence of angular cheilitis in 20 betel quid chewers is from Sri Lanka [17], where *Candida albicans* was isolated, from the affected region. There was no difference in the *Candida* species that were isolated from these 20 areca nut (betel quid) chewers with angular cheilitis when compared to other studies that had reported on angular cheilitis in patients without areca nut (betel quid)-chewing habits. There are two studies by Reichart et al. (2002 and 2005) on women betel quid chewers in Cambodia and North Thailand [18, 19]. *Candida albicans* (27.1%) was the most common species isolated in Cambodian women with areca nut-chewing habit, whereas *Candida parapsilosis* (46%) was most commonly isolated in Northern Thailand. *Candida tropicalis* (22.9%) was the second most common to be isolated from areca nut chewers in Cambodian women, whereas in Northern Thailand, it was *Candida albicans* (24%). The other yeasts isolated from areca nut chewers in these two studies were *Candida glabrata, Candida krusei, Candida parapsilosis, Candida utilis, Candida inconspicua, Candida famata, Candida guilliermondii, Candida lusitaniae, Pichia ohmeri, Saccharomyces cerevisiae, Trichosporon asahii and Kloeckera spp.* However, the authors failed to observe any cases of oral candidiasis [18, 19]. This might be due to the antimicrobial activity of the areca nut (betel quid). However, there are no studies that have reported on oral candidiasis in OSF patients.

### 4.3.4 Oral Lichenoid Contact Reactions to Betel Quid

Oral lichenoid contact reactions to betel quid were first reported in a large population-based study in India. It was termed as 'oral lichen planus (OLP) like lesion' as it looked clinically similar to OLP but arose on the oral mucosa that was in contact with the betel quid. These were lesions reported apart from OLP seen in that study [5]. The first detailed descriptions of this lesion were given by Daftary et al. (1980) and Gupta et al. (1980) [20, 21]. OLP should be distinguished from lichenoid contact reactions to betel quid. The main feature to distinguish lichenoid contact reactions to betel quid is that the lesion has a direct topographical relation to the placement of the betel quid/areca nut. The prolonged retention of areca nut/betel quid against the oral mucosa (buccal mucosa or buccal sulcus) causes these lesions.

The prevalence of lichenoid contact reactions to betel quid is 0.7–5.9% [20–22]. One hospital-based study from India reported a high prevalence rate of 9.5% [23] with all lesions occurring in individuals with betel quid-chewing habit or mixed habit having betel quid chewing. Peak incidence was seen in females aged 45–54.

Lichenoid contact reactions to betel quid have been reported in the background of OSF [21, 24]. Arya et al. (2017) also reported that females tend to have a greater number of other lesions (OLP and OSF) associated with lichenoid contact reactions to betel quid compared to males [23]. Individuals using quid containing both areca nut and tobacco were nine times more likely to have lichenoid contact reactions to betel quid and other lesions (OLP and OSF) than individuals chewing quid with tobacco alone, therefore suggesting that tobacco and areca nut act synergistically to affect the oral mucosa.

Clinically, lichenoid contact reactions to betel quid resemble OLP and it is difficult to distinguish between them. Both present as white lesions that cannot be scrapped off, with thin, wavy, linear, parallel, non-elevated striae that may radiate from the central erythematous area. However, in lichenoid contact reactions to betel quid, these white striae do not crisscross or overlap. Moreover, they tend to occur on the oral mucosa that is in contact with the betel quid. Individuals using quid containing both areca nut and tobacco were seven times more likely to have lichenoid contact reactions to betel quid than individuals chewing quid with tobacco alone [23]. Processed areca nut and tobacco products was associated with higher incidence of lichenoid contact reactions to betel quid [23].

Histopathological features of OLP and lichenoid contact reactions to betel quid are similar having signs of vacuolar degeneration of the basal and/or suprabasal cell layers (◘ Fig. 4.5) with keratinocyte apoptosis and presence of a well-defined band-like lymphocytic infiltrate that is confined to the superficial part of the connective tissue except that there will be presence of plasma cells in lichenoid contact reactions to betel quid (◘ Fig. 4.5).

**Oral Lichenoid Contact Reactions to Betel Quid**

- Oral lichenoid contact reactions to betel quid were first described in betel quid chewers as OLP-like lesions.
- Now they are considered as oral lichenoid reactions or lesions.
- Clinically, it is difficult to distinguish between OLP and oral lichenoid contact reactions to betel quid.
- Both cannot be scrapped off and present with thin, wavy, linear, parallel, non-elevated strikes that may radiate from the central erythematous area.
- In oral lichenoid reactions to betel quid, the white striae do not crisscross or overlap.
- Oral lichenoid reactions to betel quid occur on the oral mucosa that is in contact with the betel quid.
- Both oral lichenoid reactions and OLP can occur in betel quid chewers and in the background of OSF.

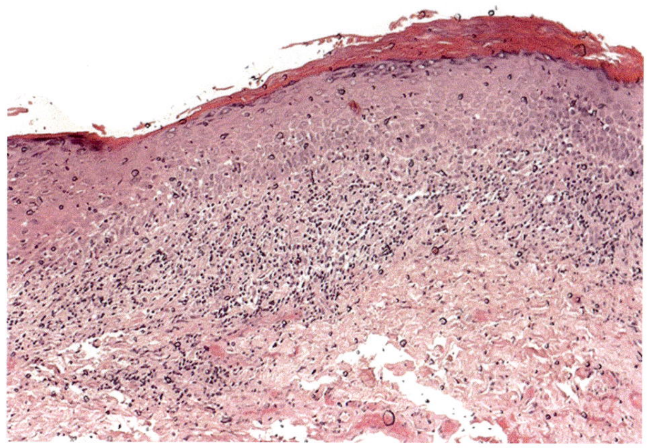

◘ **Fig. 4.5** Photomicrograph of lichenoid mucositis consistent with clinical diagnosis of oral lichenoid contact reactions to betel quid in oral submucous fibrosis showing vacuolar degeneration of the basal cell layer and a well-defined, sub-epithelial band-like predominantly lymphocytic infiltrate (Courtesy: Dr. Fairuz Abdul Rahman)

### 4.3.5 Oral Lichen Planus (OLP)

OLP is a chronic inflammatory condition of unknown aetiology that is mediated by T-lymphocytes. OLP affects approximately 1–3% of the population. Clinically, it presents as a white lesion that cannot be scrapped off, with thin, wavy, linear, parallel, non-elevated striae that may radiate from the central erythematous area. It is present bilaterally and manifests in as white or red lesions. The white lesions can be further sub-divided into reticular, papular and plaque-like (◘ Fig. 4.6) types, and the red form of lesions can be sub-divided into erosive, atrophic and bullous types. Buccal mucosa, tongue and gingiva are commonly affected locations in the oral cavity [25]. The clinical criteria for the diagnosis of OLP are (i) presence of bilateral, symmetrical white lesions affecting buccal mucosa, and/or tongue, and/or lip and/or gingiva; (ii) presence of white papular lesions and lace-like network of slightly raised white lines (reticular, annular or linear pattern) with or without erosions and ulcerations; and (iii) desquamative gingivitis. The histopathological criteria for its diagnosis include (i) presence of a well-defined band-like lymphocytic infiltrate that is confined to the superficial part of the connective tissue, (ii) signs of vacuolar degeneration of the basal and/or suprabasal cell layers with keratinocyte apoptosis (◘ Fig. 4.7) and (iii) epithelial thinning and sometimes ulceration in the atrophic type caused by failure of epithelial regeneration as a result of basal cell destruction where a mixed inflammatory infiltrate may be found. The diagnosis of OLP is made using both clinical and histopathological criteria [26].

OLP has been reported to occur in the background of OSF with a prevalence of 0.30–5.9% [21, 23, 27–31]. All these reports are from India and China. Clinically, these lesions resemble non-scrapable white or mixed

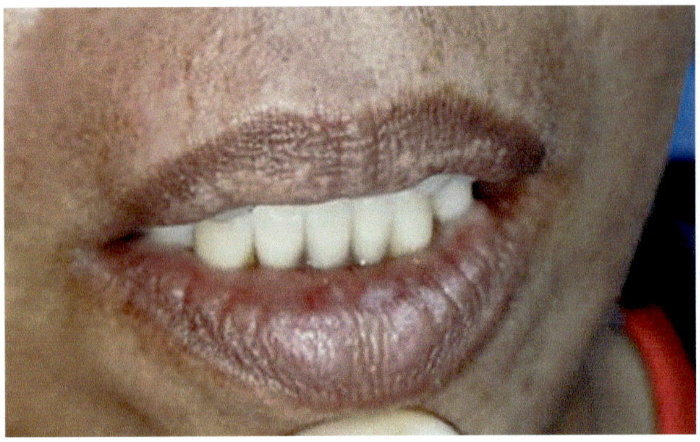

Fig. 4.6 Photograph of oral lichen planus on the lower lip of an areca nut chewer (Courtesy: Dr. April Wong Ling Siew)

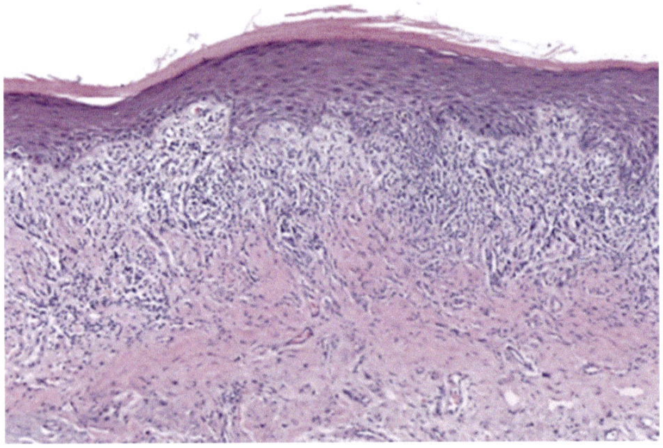

Fig. 4.7 Photomicrograph of oral lichen planus associated with OSF showing features of vacuolar degeneration of the basal cell layer and a well-defined, sub-epithelial band-like predominantly lymphocytic infiltrate (Courtesy: Dr. Sarvambika Kazakydasan)

red and white lesion with striae in the background of blanched mucosa with limited mouth opening and fibrotic bands. They tend to occur bilaterally and need to be distinguished from lichenoid contact reactions to betel quid, which tend to occur in areas of contact with the quid. However, the malignant transformation rate of OLP in the background of OSF has not been reported. Therefore, further research in this area is needed.

### 4.3.6 Oral Leukoplakia

Oral leukoplakia is the most common lesion among the oral OPMDs. It is defined as

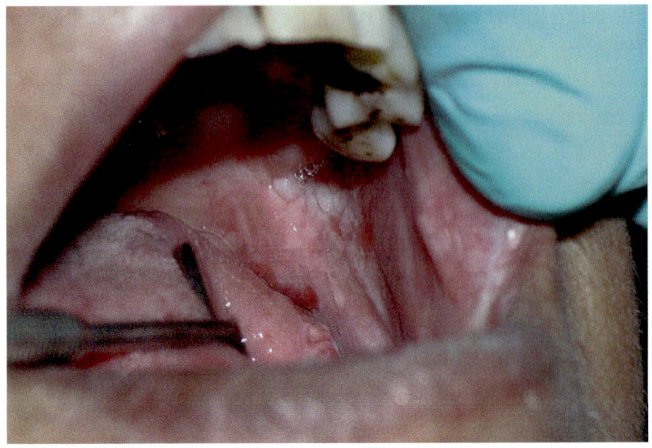

Fig. 4.8 Intraoral photograph of oral leukoplakia on the right buccal mucosa in an OSF patient (Courtesy: Dr. Fairuz Abdul Rahman)

**Definition-oral leukoplakia**

A predominantly white plaque of questionable risk having excluded (other) known diseases or disorders that carry no increased risk for cancer [32].

Oral leukoplakias are classified as homogenous type (Fig. 4.8) and the non-homogenous type, which include nodular, erythro-leukoplakia and verrucous types. Oral leukoplakia has been reported in patients with various risk habits such as smoking tobacco, smokeless tobacco, areca nut chewing, alcohol drinking and various combinations of these habits and also in persons with no habits (idiopathic). Oral leukoplakia seems to occur more in patients with mixed habits than those with only areca nut-chewing habit (Table 4.1). The malignant transformation rate of oral leukoplakia has been reported as 9.8% (95% CI: 7.9–11.7) in a recent meta-analysis [33].

Oral leukoplakia has been reported to occur along with OSF (Table 4.2) by Yang et al. [44]. The incidence of oral leukoplakia with OSF ranges from 4.8% to 24.6%. A recent meta-analysis reported the malignant transformation of OSF as 4.2% (95% CI: 2.7–5.6%) [45]. The malignant transformation rate of OSF alone (4.6–7.2% see table below) seems to be lower when compared to cases having oral leukoplakia in the background of OSF (11.1–18.5%, see Table 4.2). Therefore, patients with both conditions

**Table 4.1** Studies that have reported on the prevalence of oral leukoplakia in areca nut chewers and mixed habits

| Author (year) | Country | Total number of subjects (*n*) | Habit | No. or percentage of leukoplakia *N* (%) |
|---|---|---|---|---|
| Reichart et al. (1987) [13] | North Thailand | 1866 (BQ and non-BQ) | Areca nut | 21 (1.1%) |
| Reichart et al. (2002) [18] | Cambodia | 48 (all BQ) | Areca nut | 4 (8.3%) |
| Chung et al. (2005) [34] | South Taiwan | 1075 (mixed habits) | Areca nut, smoking and alcohol | 17 (1.6%) |
| | | | Areca nut and smoking | 5 (0.5%) |
| | | | Areca nut and alcohol | 2 (0.2%) |
| | | | Areca nut only | 1 (0.1%) |
| Pindborg et al. (1984) [35] | China | – | Areca nut | 2.1% |
| Liu et al. (1988) [36] | China | | ANS | 20.3% |
| Tang et al. (1993) [28] | China | – | Areca nut | 0.5% |
| Jian et al. (1989) [37] | China | – | Areca nut | 0.1% |
| Lin et al. (1988) [38] | China | – | Areca nut | 2.5% |
| Tran et al. (2006) [39] | Vietnam | 152 BQ<br>137 non-BQ | Areca nut | 3.8% |
| Nguyen et al. (2006) [40] | Vietnam | 150 BQ<br>200 non-BQ | Areca nut | 3.8% |
| Ngo et al. (2006) [41] | Vietnam | 9000 (all) | Mixed | 3.8% |
| Lee et al. (2011) [42] | Indonesia (I)<br>Taiwan (T)<br>China (C)<br>Sri Lanka (SL)<br>Nepal (N)<br>Malaysia (M) | | Areca nut or betel quid | Indonesia 6.6% male, 9.1% female<br>Taiwan 6.4% male<br>China 0.6% male<br>Sri Lanka 0.8% male<br>Nepal 1.6% male |
| Sujatha et al. (2012) [43] | India | 1028 (all habits) | Areca nut<br>Smokeless tobacco | 7 (0.7%)<br>38 (3.7%) |

have a higher risk of transformation and need careful follow-up. However, more research in this aspect is required to know about the risk habits and its influence on the occurrence of oral leukoplakia in the background of OSF. The type of oral leukoplakia that occurs more often in the background of OSF and the type that shows more malignant transformation need to be explored. As the duration of chewing areca nut is extended, the risk of OSF with associated lesions increases.

### Oral Leukoplakia in the Background of OSF

- Oral leukoplakia has been reported to coexist along with OSF.
- Malignant transformation rate of OSF alone (4.6–7.2%) seems to be lower when compared to cases having oral leukoplakia in the background of OSF (11.1–18.5%).
- Therefore, patients with both conditions need to be followed up closely.

4

**Table 4.2** Prevalence of oral leukoplakia in the background of OSF and their malignant transformation rate

| Author (year) | Country | No. of OSF | MTR of OSF alone | No. of OL in OSF | MTR of OL in OSF |
|---|---|---|---|---|---|
| Hazarey et al. (2007) [46] | India | 1000 | – | 48 (4.8%) | – |
| Angadi et al. (2011) [47] | India | 205 | – | 13 (6.3%) | – |
| Lian et al. (2013) [48] | Taiwan | 829 | 5.0% | 104 (12.6%) | 15.0% |
| Yang et al. (2017) [49] | Taiwan | 778 | 7.2% | 191 (24.6%) | 15.2% |
| Wang et al. (2018) [50] | Taiwan | | 4.7% | 180 | 11.1% |
| Cai et al. (2019) [31] | China | 647 | – | 101 (14.5%) | – |
| Chiang et al. (2020) [51] | Taiwan | 145 | 4.6% | 27 (18.6%) | 18.5% |
| Xiao et al. (2020) [52] | China | 30 | - | 3 (10%) | - |

*OSF* Oral submucous fibrosis, *MTR* malignant transformation rate, *OL* oral leukoplakia

### 4.3.7 Proliferative Verrucous Leukoplakia (PVL)

**Definition PVL**

A distinct form of multifocal oral leukoplakia characterised by having a progressive clinical course, changing clinical and histopathological features.

PVL has the highest malignant transformation rate (49.5%; 99% CI 26.7–72.4%) when compared to other OPMDs [53]. Clinically, it presents as multiple or sometimes as an OLL at one or more sites in the oral cavity. Later, it develops to include multiple locations in the oral cavity either by gradual spread of individual focus or by the fusion of adjacent foci [54]. The diagnosis of PVL is made by a combination of clinical and histological features as stated first by Hansen et al. [55]. Cerero-Lapiedra et al. [56], Carrard et al. [57] and Villa et al. [54] have proposed specific clinical criteria for the diagnosis of PVL, which includes the initial presence of oral leukoplakia, (Fig. 4.9) OLLs (non-verrucous) in two different sites of the oral cavity and the existence of a verrucous area (Fig. 4.10). The histopathological features include a spectrum from normal epithelium to hyperkeratosis, to verrucous hyperplasia, to any grades of oral epithelial dysplasia to verrucous carcinoma (VC) or papillary variant of SCC or conventional SCC. PVL in the gingiva seems to show the highest malignant transformation when compared to other sites [58].

Mechery et al. (2015) in their case report describe a case of PVL in the background of OSF on the right buccal mucosa of a 33-year-old male patient having the habit of chewing pan (tobacco, lime and areca nut) for 15 years [59]. The histopathological features described by the authors seemed to be that of verrucous carcinoma. However, the photomicrographic features do not show fibrosis in the underlying connective tissue. Moreover, the presence of

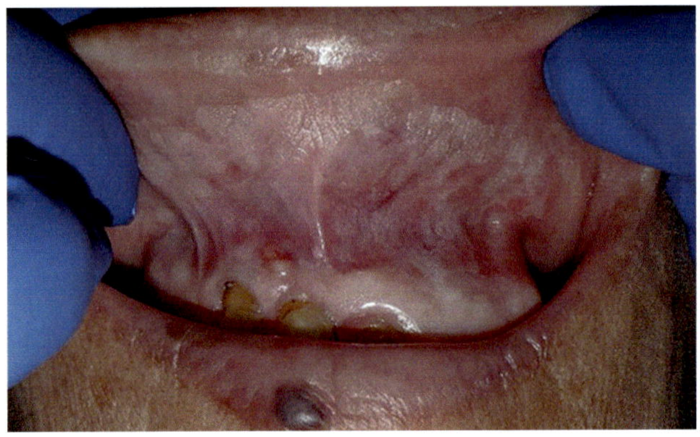

**Fig. 4.9** Intraoral photograph shows a large flat leukoplakic lesion on the upper labial mucosa as one of the multifocal lesions in PVL in an OSF patient (Courtesy: Dr. Fairuz Abdul Rahman)

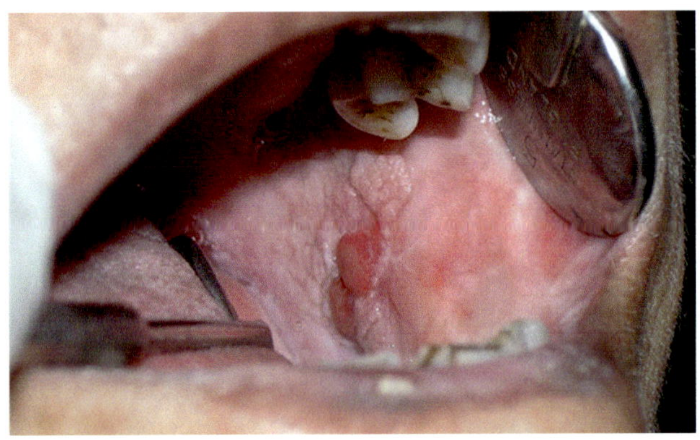

**Fig. 4.10** Intraoral photograph shows an exophytic blunt whitish pink papillary lesion (exophytic verrucous hyperplasia—EVH) on the left buccal mucosa as one of the multifocal lesions in PVL in an OSF patient. In addition, there is also a red erythroplakic lesion adjacent to the EVH. (Courtesy: Dr. Fairuz Abdul Rahman)

oral leukoplakia in multiple sites in the oral cavity over a period of time was not established in this case. Therefore, if we are to discount this case report, then there are no cases of PVL in OSF so far reported in the literature. This raises the question whether PVL can occur with OSF. Thus, more research is required in this area.

### 4.3.8 Erythroplakia

Erythroplakia is a solitary lesion:

> **Definition-erythroplakia**
>
> A predominantly fiery red patch that cannot be characterised clinically or pathologically as any other definable disease.

It is a well-defined lesion which is flat or slightly depressed. It has a matt appearance. Chung et al. (2005) have reported erythroplakia in areca nut chewers and those with mixed habits in Taiwan [34]. Subjects with mixed habits tend to have a higher frequency of erythroplakia ($n = 3$) than those with only areca nut-chewing habit ($n = 1$).

Erythroplakia has been reported in the background of OSF in one study from India, in a cohort of 205 OSF patients [47]. The prevalence of erythroplakia in OSF patients was reported as 3.41% (7 cases). No other studies have reported the incidence or prevalence of erythroplakia in the background of OSF.

Clinically, there might be difficulty in differentiating erythroplakia and atrophic oral mucosa in the background of OSF. Therefore, further research with detailed clinical criteria to differentiate between atrophic oral mucosa and erythroplakia needs to be carried out to obtain the prevalence and incidence of erythroplakia in OSF. The malignant transformation rate of erythroplakia in OSF was not reported by Angadi et al. (2011) [47]. Therefore, further research is required in this area.

### 4.3.9 Verrucopapillary Lesions

Verrucopapillary lesions (VPLs) of the oral cavity can range from benign lesions to carcinomas. The spectrum of VPLs that occur in the oral cavity include oral squamous papilloma, verruca vulgaris, exophytic verrucous hyperplasia (EVH), focal epithelial hyperplasia, condyloma, PVL, verrucouc carcinoma (VC), conventional carcinoma (SCC) with verrucopapillary features and papillary squamous cell carcinoma (papillary SCC). It is possible for various VPLs to occur in the background of OSF. The following section describes these VPLs and their occurrence in the background of OSF.

#### 4.3.9.1 Oral Squamous Papilloma

Oral squamous papillomas are solitary pedunculated verrucopapillary lesions with finger-like projections seen in the oral cavity. They can affect any age group but are more common between 30 and 50 years. Clinically, oral squamous cell papilloma is less than 1 cm in size. The histopathological features that are present in the oral squamous papilloma are the presence of keratinised exophytic verrucopapillary processes, hyperplastic epithelium (basal cell hyperplasia and acanthosis) and prominent fibrovascular core.

Oral squamous papilloma (6.5%) has been reported to occur in areca nut chewers by Chang et al. (2002) in Taiwan among 153 subjects [60]. However, their occurrence in OSF has not been reported, thus requiring further research.

#### 4.3.9.2 Exophytic Verrucous Hyperplasia (EVH) (Oral Verrucous Hyperplasia—OVH)

The term verrucous hyperplasia was first introduced by Ackerman and McGavran [61]. Adkins and Monsour (1976) reviewed cases of verrucous leukoplakia and reported that some of them might be verrucous hyperplasia [62]. Shear and Pindborg (1980) described the clinical and histopathological features of verrucous hyperplasia of oral mucosa [63]. Clinically, there are two types of verrucous hyperplasia: (i) sharp variety: white lesions having heavily keratinised verrucous process that are long and narrow, and (ii) blunt variety: lesions that do not have heavily keratinised verrucous process and are broader and flatter.

Chung et al. (2005) reported in areca nut chewers from Taiwan a new type of verrucous lesion, which was an exophytic with pink mucosa, and foci of granular surface of similar to the blunt variety of verrucous hyperplasia [34]. Wang et al. (2009) described two types of verrucopapillary lesion: (i) plaque-type and (ii) mass-type lesions based on their histopathological features. The mass type are whitish pink verrucous lesions that are single or multiple lesions and were termed as OVH both clinically and histopathologically, whereas the plaque type are whitish verrucous plaques and termed as oral verruciform leukoplakia clinically and as verruciform hyperplasia histopathologically [64].

Due to this various terminology used in the literature, there existed confusion regarding OVH until the 1st Asian regional meeting on the terminology and criteria for verrucopapillary lesions of the oral cavity held in Kuala Lumpur, Malaysia [65]. Clear clinical and histopathological criteria for all verrucopapillary lesions were proposed at this meeting. The term EVH was proposed for the clinical entity of those verrucopapillary lesions whether they are sharp or blunt variety, or plaque type (whitish) (◘ Fig. 4.11) or mass type (whitish pink) (◘ Fig. 4.12).

The clinical criteria for EVH and its various histopathological features are given in ◘ Table 4.3 [65].

The histopathological differential diagnosis that should be considered while considering a diagnosis of OVH is oral VC, papillary squamous cell carcinoma, conventional squamous cell carcinoma and oral squamous cell papilloma. A detailed histopathological difference between these lesions is given in ◘ Table 4.4 [66]. The most important histopathological feature that differentiates between oval verrucous hyperplasia and oral VC is the absence of down growth when compared to the adjacent normal mucosa.

From Sri Lanka, a case series has reported five cases of verrucopapillary lesions (clinically can be re-termed as EVH) in the background of OSF out of which four cases were histologically OVH with no dysplasia (1 case), mild dysplasia (2 cases) and moderate dysplasia (1 case) in the background of OSF. One EVH was early invasive SCC. The malignant transformation rate is 20%. All these five cases were in areca nut chewers [67].

A single-centre study from India reported 13 cases (1.96%) of verrucopapillary lesions (clinically can be termed as EVH) among 662 OSF patients. Of the 13 EVH cases, only 9 were biopsied and 6 (0.9%) were histopathologically diagnosed as EVH without dysplasia [68] (◘ Table 4.5). The malignant transformation rate of EVH was 23.07%.

Of these 18 cases of EVH in OSF from these two studies [67, 68], all cases were in males with an age range from 19 to 75 years and predominantly affecting the buccal mucosa. Two cases were reported on the tongue and one each on the gingiva and labial mucosa. The follow-up period was limited to only few cases in these two studies. One case in [67] showed early invasion in OSF area, and malignant transformation was seen in three cases (two OVC and one OSCC) in the study by Shah et al. [68]. However, more studies are required to find the incidence and prevalence of EVH in OSF and its malignant transformation rate.

In areca nut chewers who are non-OSF patients, Chang et al. (2002) reported 24.6% ($n = 57$) verrucous hyperplasia among 153 areca nut chewers in Taiwan [60]. Based on their case description, it is clear that these Taiwan authors were referring to cases that could be considered EVH clinically and OVH histopathologically. Wang et al. (2009) reported that 91% (60 cases) of OVH, which are clinically described as plaque-type and mass-type OVH (which again can be re-termed as EVH clinically and OVH histopathologically), were associated with areca nut chewers [64] (◘ Table 4.5). Out of these 60 EVH cases, 4 underwent malignant transformation (6.67%).

In conclusion, EVH with or without OSF has the potential for malignant change, and thus exophytic verrucous hyperplasia (EVH) (in our opinion as well as from the expert group discussion at the regional meeting held in KL) can be considered as a potentially malignant disorder. However, in the recent publication from the WHO Collaborating Centre for Oral Cancer, EVH has been considered as a disorder with limited evidence needing more longitudinal studies to ascertain its potentially malignant behaviour [26].

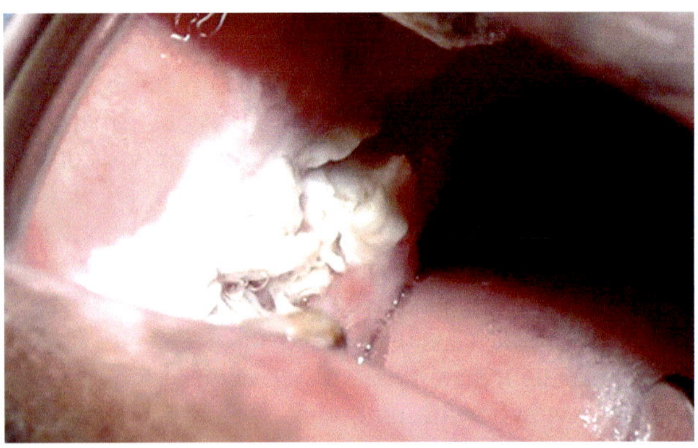

◘ **Fig. 4.11** Photograph of an exophytic verrucous hyperplasia (EVH) , the sharp, plaque type (whitish and has also been termed verrucous leukoplakia in earlier publications) on the right buccal mucosa (Courtesy: Dr. Juliana Khairi)

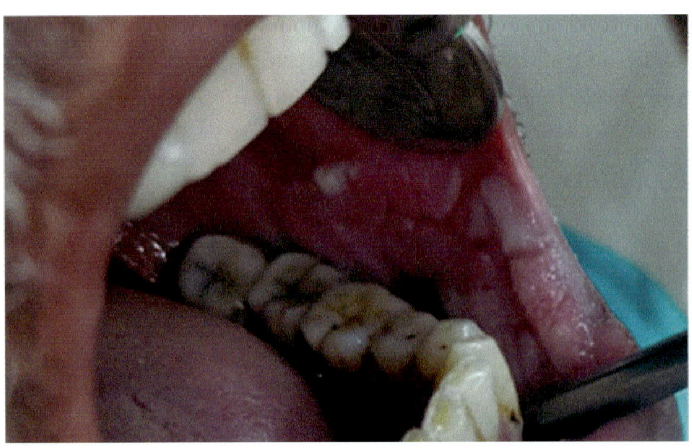

◘ **Fig. 4.12** Photograph of an exophytic verrucous hyperplasia (EVH), the blunt, mass type (whitish pink) on the left commissure and left buccal mucosa (Courtesy: Dr Bhavikkumar Dholia)

### Exophytic Verrucous Hyperplasia (EVH)

1. EVH is a clinical diagnosis.
2. EVH clinically present in two forms: (1) as an exophytic, fleshy verrucopapillary outgrowth with a white and/or pink surface colour and (2) as a white, plaque-like exophytic verrucous lesion. The latter has been previously termed verrucous leukoplakia. In both instances, the clinical term 'EVH' should be used.
3. Malignant transformation rate of EVH in areca nut chewers is 6.67%.
4. Malignant transformation rate of EVH in the background of OSF ranges from 20% to 23.07%.

**Table 4.3** The clinical criteria of EVH and histopathological criteria of OVH [65]

| Terminology | Criteria |
| --- | --- |
| EVH (clinical diagnosis) | These lesions clinically present in two forms: (1) as an exophytic, fleshy verrucopapillary outgrowth with a white and/or pink surface colour and (2) as a white, plaque-like exophytic verrucous lesion. The latter may mimic verrucous leukoplakia. In both instances, the clinical term 'EVH' should be used.<br>EVH may occur in any anatomical site in the oral cavity and in general would be more than 1 cm in size.<br>Unlike PVL, EVH is a discrete and solitary lesion.<br>EVH may coexist in a patient presenting with oral submucous fibrosis.<br>The clinical presentation of EVH could masquerade as a squamous cell carcinoma or VC. Absence of induration is a cardinal feature of EVH. |
| OVH (Histopathological diagnosis) | 1. Keratinised exophytic verrucopapillary processes seen. Keratin plugging may be present.<br>2. Epithelium is hyperplastic with both basal cell hyperplasia and acanthosis.<br>3. Absence of downward growth of the hyperplastic epithelium into the lamina propria when compared with the level of the basement membrane of the adjacent normal epithelium.<br>4. Epithelial dysplasia may or may not be present.<br>5. Sub-epithelial lymphocytic infiltration as a host response may or may not be present.<br>6. Verrucous hyperplasia should be clearly differentiated from VC which exhibits frank downward growth of the epithelial processes below the level of the basement membrane of the adjacent normal epithelium.<br>7. Verrucous hyperplasia should be differentiated from squamous cell papilloma by its size and by the presence of a prominent fibrovascular core in the latter.<br>8. In a small biopsy without adjacent normal mucosal epithelium, particular attention should be paid to exclude other pathologies such as squamous cell papilloma and VC. |

**Table 4.4** Histopathological criteria for the diagnosis of VPLs [66]

| Histological diagnosis | OVC | PSCC | CSCC | OVH | SCP |
| --- | --- | --- | --- | --- | --- |
| Clinical size of lesion | >1 cm | >1 cm | >1 cm | ≥1 cm | <1 cm |
| Histological criteria: | | | | | |
| Keratinized exophytic verruco-papillary processes | Y | Y* | Y | Y | Y |
| Epithelium is hyperplastic (basal cell hyperplasia and acanthosis) | Y | Y | Y | Y | Y |
| Growth of the hyperplastic epithelium into the lamina propria when compared with the level of the basement membrane of the adjacent normal epithelium | Y | Y | Y | N | N |
| Epithelial Dysplasia cellular atypia | N** | Y | Y | Y/N | N |
| Subepithelial lymphocytic infiltration | Y | Y/N | Y/N | Y/N | Y/N |
| Frank downward growth of the epithelial processes below the level of basement membrane of the adjacent normal epithelium showing pushing border effect) | Y | N | N | N | N |
| Prominent fibrovascular core | N | Y | N | N | Y |
| Invasion | N | Y | Y | N | N |
| Keratin plugging | Y | N | Y | Y/N | N |

(ii) A diagnosis of oral verrucous hyperplasia (OVH) should be made only when there is an absence of growth of the hyperplastic epithelium into the lamina propria as compared with the level of the basement membrane of the adjacent normal epithelium, (iii) Oral verrucous hyperplasia (OVH) should he clearly differentiated from oral verrucous carcinoma (OVC) where OVC exhibits frank downward growth of the epithelial processes below the level of the basement membrane of the adjacent normal epithelium. OVC can be differentiated from Papillary squamous cell carcinoma (PSCC)/ Conventional SCC (CSCC) by the presence of invasion and cytologic atypia: (iv) Oral verrucous hyperplasia(OVH) should be differentiated from squamous cell papilloma (SCP) by its size and by the presence of a prominent fibrovascular core in the latter; (v) * Verrucous exophytic processes with minimal or abscence of keratinization; (vi) * *Mild cellular atypia has been reported in cases of OVC

4

**Table 4.5** EVH in OSF and non-OSF patients

| Author (year) | Country | Total number of subjects (n) | Habit | Malignant transformation rate |
|---|---|---|---|---|
| Chang et al. (2002)[a] [60] | Taiwan | 57 EVH/153 of areca nut chewers (non-OSF) | Areca nut chewers | - |
| Wang et al. (2009) [64] | Taiwan | 60 EVH /60 of mixed habit (non-OSF) | Mixed habits | 4/60 (6.67%) |
| Jayasinghe et al. (2016) [67] | Sri Lanka | 5 EVH/5 cases of OSF | Areca nut chewers | 1/5 (20%) |
| Shah et al. (2019) [68] | India | 13 EVH/662 cases of OSF | Areca nut chewers | 3/13 (23.07%) |

[a]Only histopathological diagnosis was given and thus unable to report the malignant transformation rate

**Oral Verrucous Hyperplasia (OVH)**

1. OVH is a histopathological diagnosis which can be present with or without epithelial dysplasia.
2. The most important histopathological feature that differentiates between OVH and oral verrucous carcinoma is the absence of down growth when compared to the adjacent normal mucosa.

### 4.3.9.3 Oral Verruciform Xanthoma (VX)

This is a mucocutaneous verrucopapillary lesion that was first described in the oral cavity by Shafer [69] and later in an extraoral site [70]. The most common intra-oral site of VX is the gingiva followed by tongue, hard palate, buccal mucosa and vestibular mucosa, floor of the mouth and soft palate, whereas the extraoral sites are skin and anogenital mucosa. It occurs most commonly in the middle age with a slight male predilection up to 50 years of age and a female predilection after 50 years of age. Most of the cases have been reported in Caucasians.

The lesions are mostly exophytic white verrucopapillary except a few that have been reported as crateriform or ulcerated. Most of these lesions are yellow in colour true to the meaning of the Greek term "Xanthos". The lesions measure from 0.2 to 2.0 cm. They are usually solitary and may be sessile or pedunculated. The differential diagnosis of VX includes all verrucopapillary lesions such as oral squamous papilloma, verruca vulgaris, condyloma acuminatum, EVH, VC and papillary variant of SCC.

VX has been reported to occur concomitantly with many systemic conditions and oral lesions. It has been reported with OPMDs such as OLP [71–73], chronic graft-versus-host disease with and without leukoplakia and erythroplakia [74–77], discoid lupus erythematosus [78], snuff dipper keratosis [79], carcinoma in situ [80] and SCC [81]. VX has been reported to occur in the background of OSF [81–84]. The age of these patients ranged from 25 to 52 years. The common site for VX to occur in the background of OSF is the buccal mucosa. Most cases have been reported from India. All cases were in male having areca nut or mixed habits. All cases were surgically excised without recurrence (Table 4.6).

Histopathologically, all VX show varying degrees of surface parakeratinisation with uniformly elongated rete processes. There is accumulation of numerous foam cells in the connective tissue papillae between the elongated rete processes. VX can be classified into three types based on the surface epithelium: (i) verrucous type, shows verrucous surface keratinised stratified squamous epithelium with keratin plugs extending from the surface into the crypts formed by epithelial projections, (ii) papillary type, shows papillary projections with keratinised surface epithelium without crypts and keratin plugging and (iii) flat type, has surface-keratinised stratified squamous epithelium [81].

The reason for occurrence of VX in the background of OSF cannot be explained at present and needs further research.

### 4.3.9.4 Oral Verrucous Carcinoma (VC)

Oral VC is a low-grade variant of oral squamous cell carcinoma (OSCC). It was first defined by Ackerman in 1948 as a separate pathological entity. Aetiological factors of VC are smokeless tobacco (such as snuff) and areca nut chewing. It is clinically a verrucopapillary lesion and is considered in the differential diagnosis of verrucous leukoplakia, EVH and OSCC. Histopathological feature of oral VC is the presence of downward growth of the epithelial processes below the level of basement membrane of the adjacent normal epithelium showing pushing border effect but without breach in the basement membrane zone. The surface shows keratinised exophytic verrucopapillary processes with keratin plugging. VC shows minimal/no epithelial dysplasia/cellular atypia.

**Table 4.6** Cases of verruciform xanthoma (VX) reported in the background of OSF

| Author (year) | Age and gender | Habits | Site and clinical features | Diagnosis | Tx | Prognosis |
|---|---|---|---|---|---|---|
| Yu et al (2007) [81] | 28 years Male | Areca nut chewing, smoking and alcohol drinking | Right buccal mucosa - verrucopapillary lesion 2.0 × 1.0 | VX in the background of OSF | Surgical excision | No recurrence |
| Gosh et al (2014) [82] | 25 years Male | Tobacco chewing, six packets per day for the past 6 years | Right buccal mucosa—whitish-yellow papillary lesion | VX in the background OSF | Surgical excision | No recurrence |
| Hegde et al (2015) [83] | 39 years Male | - | Left buccal mucosa | VX in the background of OSF | - | - |
| Gannepalli et al (2019) [84] | 52 years Male | Alcohol three times per week and chewing paan-zarda (betel nut + tobacco + slaked lime) 10 times a week | Attached gingiva—solitary, sessile lesion with a rough surface and yellowish white in colour. Size: 0.8 × 2.0 cm | VX concomitantly with OSF | Surgical excision | No recurrence |

VC has been reported in areca nut chewers. Chang et al. (2002) reported about 2.1% of areca nut chewers to have VC in a study in Taiwan [60]. Yang et al. (2005) reported about 1.4% of VC in areca nut chewers and smokers, whereas a higher percentage (3.6%) of VC was reported in areca nut chewers only [85] (Table 4.7).

There are a few case reports of VC arising in OSF, from India. All these cases are in male, except for one. The age ranges from 24 to 60 years. Majority of the cases occurred on buccal mucosa (6 cases) followed by lower labial mucosa (2 cases) and one case on the buccal gingiva. Only a few report on the treatment received by the patient and their prognosis (Table 4.8). Therefore, further research is required to determine the actual prevalence of oral VC in OSF.

**Oral Verrucous Carcinoma (VC)**

- Oral VC is a low-grade variant of oral squamous cell carcinoma (OSCC).
- Clinically, oral VC is a verrucopapillary lesion with a differential diagnosis of EVH (the white variety has been termed verrucous leukoplakia) and OSCC.
- Histopathologically, there is presence of downward growth of the epithelial processes below the level of basement membrane of the adjacent normal epithelium showing pushing border effect but without the breach in the basement membrane zone.

**Table 4.7** Verrucous carcinoma (VC) reported in areca nut chewers and mixed habits

| Author (year) | Country | Total number of subjects (n) | Habit | No. of VC |
|---|---|---|---|---|
| Chang et al (2002) [60] | Taiwan | 153 | Areca nut | 5 (2.1%) |
| Yang et al (2005) [85] | Taiwan | 102 | Areca nut + smoking<br>Areca nut only | 1.4%<br>3.6% |

### 4.3.9.5 Oral Squamous Cell Carcinoma (OSCC)

OSF is one of the OPMDs which can transform into oral cancer (Fig. 4.13). OSCC arising in OSF can present clinically as a verrucopapillary lesion. Histopathologically, it may be conventional OSCC with verrucopapillary surface feature or the papillary variant of OSCC. The papillary variant of OSCC and the conventional OSCC differ from the VC by the presence of cytological atypia and the frank invasion of the tumour epithelial cells into the underlying connective tissue. The histopathological difference between the papillary variant of the OSCC and the conventional OSCC (Fig. 4.14) is the exophytic

4

**Table 4.8** Verrucous carcinoma (VC) reported in the background of OSF

| Author (year) | Age and gender | Habits | Site | Diagnosis | Tx | Prognosis |
|---|---|---|---|---|---|---|
| Pravadu et al (2011) [86] | 29 years Male | Chewing tobacco for 15 years | Left buccal mucosa | VC in OSF | Surgery + intralesional steroids and hyaluronidase | No recurrence with regular follow-up |
| Komal et al (2015) [87] | 60 years Male | 8–10 packets of gutkha per day for the past 30 years | Right lower labial mucosa | VC in OSF | Cryosurgery | Under follow-up without recurrence |
| Malhotra et al (2016) [88] | 45 years Female | Pan chewing for the past 17 years | Right lower labial mucosa and vestibule | VC in OSF | Not reported | Not reported |
| Ramani et al (2016) [89] | 24 years Male | Chewing mawa for the past 3 years | Left buccal mucosa | VC in OSF with early invasive SCC | Surgery | Not reported |
| Yunus et al (2016) [90] | 26 years Male | Chewing gutkha and tobacco with lime 10-15 times a day and was an occasional alcoholic | Left buccal mucosa | VC in OSF | Not reported | Not reported |
| Popli et al (2018) [91] | 35 years Male | Gutka and khaini chewing for the past 10 and 15 years with a frequency of 4–5 gutka per day and khaini 1–2 times a day | Right buccal mucosa | VC in OSF | Not reported | Not reported |
| Shah et al (2019) [68] | 49 years Male | Areca nut chewer | Right buccal gingiva | VC in OSF | Not reported | Not reported |
| Shah et al (2019) [68] | 35 years Male | Areca nut chewer | Right commissure extending onto right buccal mucosa | VC in OSF | Not reported | Not reported |
| Tyagi et al (2021) [92] | 35 years Male | 5–6 pouches of gutkha for 7–8 years, 5–6 times a day and 2–3 cigarettes/day for 2–3 months | Left buccal mucosa | VC in OSF | Referred to oral surgery | Not reported |

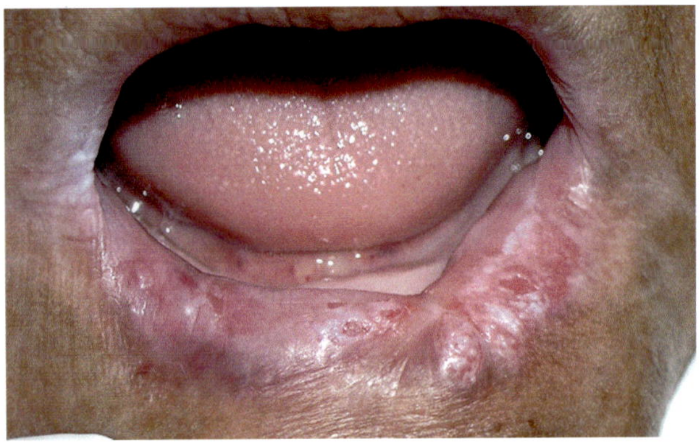

**Fig. 4.13** Photograph shows a mixed white and red lesion on the lower lip with induration, which is indicative of oral cancer in an OSF patient having limited mouth opening (Courtesy: Dr. Fairuz Abdul Rahman)

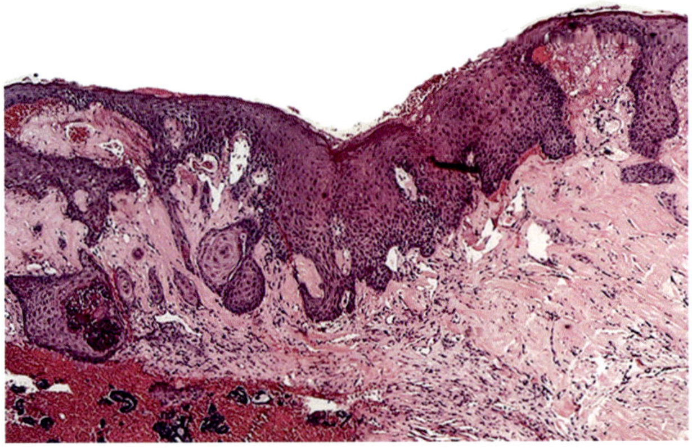

**Fig. 4.14** Photomicrograph showing invasion of the dysplastic epithelial tumour cells into the underlying connective tissue, which has dense collagen fibres indicative of oral submucous fibrosis (Courtesy Dr. Fairuz Abdul Rahman)

growth and presence of prominent fibrovascular core in the former and the lack of fibrovascular core in the latter [66].

A recent systematic review reported the pooled proportion malignant transformation rate of OSF in nine observational studies as 4.2% (95% CI: 2.7–5.6%) with an annual transformation rate of 0.73% [45]. OSF with dysplasia had higher potential for malignant transformation. However, the systematic review concluded that there was a high risk of bias in all the studies included with most of them having incomplete demographic and clinicopathological data. Thus, further research to examine the natural history of OSF with or without interventions is required.

**Summary**

There are numerous associated conditions of oral submucous fibrosis affecting the oral mucosa. They may be benign conditions (quid staining on oral mucosa, chewer's mucosa, oral squamous papilloma and verruciform xanthoma) to OPMDs (oral lichenoid reaction to areca nut (betel quid), oral lichen planus, oral leukoplakia, erythroplakia and proliferative verrucous leukoplakia) to cancer (verrucous carcinoma, conventional oral squamous cell carcinoma and papillary squamous cell carcinoma) and verrucopapillary lesions such as exophytic verrucous hyperplasia, which has yet to be recognised as an OPMD due to limited evidence needing more longitudinal studies to ascertain its potentially malignant behaviour. These associated conditions need to be recognised by the clinicians and histopathologists to find their true prevalence and their clinical behaviour.

## References

1. Trivedy CR, Craig G, Warnakulasuriya S. The oral health consequences of chewing areca nut. Addict Biol. 2002;7(1):115–25. https://doi.org/10.1080/13556210120091482.
2. Schamschula RG, Adkins BL, Barmes DE, Charlton G. Betal chewing and caries experience in New Guinea. Community Dent Oral Epidemiol. 1977;5(6):284–6. https://doi.org/10.1111/j.1600-0528.1977.tb01015.x.
3. Reichart P, Gehring F. Streptococcus mutans and caries prevalence in Lisu and Karen of northern Thailand. J Dent Res. 1984;63(1):56–8. https://doi.org/10.1177/00220345840630011301.
4. Williams SA, Summers RM, Ahmed IA, Prendergast MJ. Caries experience, tooth loss and oral health-related behaviours among Bangladeshi women resident in West Yorkshire, UK. Community Dent Health. 1996;13(3):150–6.
5. Mehta FS, Pindborg JJ, Hamner JE III. Oral cancer and precancerous conditions in India. Copenhagen: Munksgaard; 1971. p. 17.
6. Reichart PA, Schmidtberg W, Scheifele C. Betel chewer's mucosa in elderly Cambodian women. J Oral Pathol Med. 1996;25(7):367–70. https://doi.org/10.1111/j.1600-0714.1996.tb00280.x.
7. Zain RB, Ikeda N, Gupta PC, et al. Oral mucosal lesions associated with betel quid, areca nut and tobacco chewing habits: consensus from a workshop held in Kuala Lumpur, Malaysia, November 25–27, 1996. J Oral Pathol Med. 1999;28(1):1–4. https://doi.org/10.1111/j.1600-0714.1999.tb01985.x.
8. Ikeda N, Handa Y, Khim SP, et al. Prevalence study of oral mucosal lesions in a selected Cambodian population. Community Dent Oral Epidemiol. 1995;23(1):49–54. https://doi.org/10.1111/j.1600-0528.1995.tb00197.x.
9. Zain R, Ikeda N, Yaacob MBH. Oral mucosal lesions survey of adults in Malaysia, vol. 44. Kuala Lumpur: Ministry of Health, Malaysia, University of Malaya, Malaysia and Aichigakuin University, Japan; 1995. p. 25–6.
10. Philipsen HP, Ramanathan J, Mendis BRRN. Betel chewer's mucosa in Sri Lankan tea estate workers. (unpublished).
11. Hjorting-Hansen E, Holst E. Morsicatio mucosae oris and suctio mucosae oris. An analysis of oral mucosal changes due to biting and sucking habits. Scand J Dent Res. 1970;78(6):492–9. https://doi.org/10.1111/j.1600-0722.1970.tb02102.x.
12. Van Wyk CW, Staz J, Farman AG. The chewing lesion of the cheeks and lips: its features and prevalence among a selected group of adolescents. J Dent. 1977;5(3):193–9. https://doi.org/10.1016/0300-5712(77)90003-3.
13. Reichart PA, Mohr U, Srisuwan S, Geerlings H, Theetranont C, Kangwanpong T. Precancerous and other oral mucosal lesions related to chewing, smoking and drinking habits in Thailand. Community Dent Oral Epidemiol. 1987;15(3):152–60. https://doi.org/10.1111/j.1600-0528.1987.tb00505.x.
14. Maeda H, Ikeda N, Zain R, et al. Detection of human papillomaviruses in betel chewer's mucosae and leukoplakias of Cambodian patients. The 2nd Asia Pacific Workshop for Oral Mucosal Lesions, 5–8 November 1995, Chiang Mai, Thailand, Program and Abstracts: P3
15. Reichart PA, Philipsen HP, Mohr U, Geerlings H, Srisuwan S. Miang chewing in northern Thai villagers. Trop Geogr Med. 1988;40(1):39–44.
16. Reichart PA, Lenz H, König H, Becker J, Mohr U. The black layer on the teeth of betel chewers: a light microscopic, microradiographic and electronmicroscopic study. J Oral Pathol. 1985;14(6):466–75. https://doi.org/10.1111/j.1600-0714.1985.tb00518.x.
17. Warnakulasuriya KA, Samaranayake LP, Peiris JS. Angular cheilitis in a group of Sri Lankan adults: a clinical and microbiologic study. J Oral Pathol Med. 1991;20(4):172–5. https://doi.org/10.1111/j.1600-0714.1991.tb00915.x.
18. Reichart PA, Schmidtberg W, Samaranayake LP, Scheifele C. Betel quid-associated oral lesions and oral Candida species in a female Cambodian cohort. J Oral Pathol Med. 2002;31(8):468–72. https://doi.org/10.1034/j.1600--0714.2002.00009.x.
19. Reichart PA, Khongkhunthian P, Samaranayake LP, Yau J, Patanaporn V, Scheifele C. Oral Candida species and betel quid-associated oral lesions in Padaung women of Northern Thailand. Mycoses. 2005;48(2):132–6. https://doi.org/10.1111/j.1439-0507.2004.01071.x.
20. Daftary DK, Bhonsle RB, Murti RB, Pindborg JJ, Mehta FS. An oral lichen planus-like lesion in Indian betel-tobacco chewers. Scand J Dent Res. 1980;88(3):244–9. https://doi.org/10.1111/j.1600-0722.1980.tb01221.x.
21. Gupta PC, Mehta FS, Daftary DK, et al. Incidence rates of oral cancer and natural history of oral precancerous lesions in a 10-year follow-up study of Indian villagers. Community Dent Oral Epidemiol. 1980;8(6):283–333. https://doi.org/10.1111/j.1600-0528.1980.tb01302.x.

4

22. Dang V, Nagpal M. Quid-induced lichenoid reactions: a prevalence study. J Indian Acad Oral Med Radiol. 2011;23:39–41.
23. Arya S, Vengal M, Raju B, et al. Betel quid oral lichenoid lesions: a hospital based cross-sectional study. J Investig Clin Dent 2017;8(1):https://doi.org/10.1111/jicd.12180. doi:10.1111/jicd.1218
24. Reichart PA, Warnakulasuriya S. Oral lichenoid contact lesions induced by areca nut and betel quid chewing: a mini review. J Investig Clin Dent. 2012;3(3):163–6. https://doi.org/10.1111/j.2041-1626.2012.00130.x.
25. Roopashree MR, Gondhalekar RV, Shashikanth MC, George J, Thippeswamy SH, Shukla A. Pathogenesis of oral lichen planus—a review. J Oral Pathol Med. 2010;39(10):729–34. https://doi.org/10.1111/j.1600-0714.2010.00946.x.
26. Warnakulasuriya S, Kujan O, Aguirre-Urizar JM, et al. Oral potentially malignant disorders: A consensus report from an international seminar on nomenclature and classification, convened by the WHO Collaborating Centre for Oral Cancer. Oral Dis. 2021;27(8):1862–80. https://doi.org/10.1111/odi.13704.
27. Gao ML, Tang JQ, Zhu ZT, Jian XF. A pathological study of oral submucous fibrosis. Chin J Stomatol. 1990;25:363–5. [in Chinese] (Cross ref Cai et al 2019)
28. Tang JQ, Zhu ZT, Ling TY, Gao ML, Jian XF. A study of 335 cases of oral submucous fibrosis. West China J Stomatol. 1993;11:130–2. [in Chinese] (Cross Ref Cai et al 2019)
29. Tan H, Xie H. The clinical analysis of oral submucous fibrosis. J Oral Sci Res. 2004;20:529–31. [in Chinese] (Cros ref Cai et al 2019)
30. Gao YJ, Ling TY, Yin XM, Yao ZG, Tang JQ. A retrospective study of malignant transformation of oral submucous fibrosis. J Clin Stomatol. 2005;21:119–20. [in Chinese] (Cross ref Cai et al 2019)
31. Cai X, Yao Z, Liu G, Cui L, Li H, Huang J. Oral submucous fibrosis: A clinicopathological study of 674 cases in China. J Oral Pathol Med. 2019;48(4):321–5. https://doi.org/10.1111/jop.12836.
32. Warnakulasuriya S, Johnson NW, van der Waal I. Nomenclature and classification of potentially malignant disorders of the oral mucosa. J Oral Pathol Med. 2007;36(10):575–80. https://doi.org/10.1111/j.1600-0714.2007.00582.x.
33. Aguirre-Urizar JM, Lafuente-Ibáñez de Mendoza I, Warnakulasuriya S. Malignant transformation of oral leukoplakia: systematic review and meta-analysis of the last 5 years. Oral Dis. 2021;27(8):1881–95. https://doi.org/10.1111/odi.13810.
34. Chung CH, Yang YH, Wang TY, Shieh TY, Warnakulasuriya S. Oral precancerous disorders associated with areca quid chewing, smoking, and alcohol drinking in southern Taiwan. J Oral Pathol Med. 2005;34(8):460–6. https://doi.org/10.1111/j.1600-0714.2005.00332.x.
35. Pindborg JJ, Zheng KH, Kong CR, Lin FX. Pilot survey of oral mucosa in areca (betel) nut chewers on Hainan Island of the People's Republic of China. Community Dent Oral Epidemiol. 1984;12(3):195–6. https://doi.org/10.1111/j.1600-0528.1984.tb01438.x.
36. Liu SF, Jian XC, Shen ZH. A study of oral submucous fibrosis. J Clin Stomatol. 1988;4:81–3. [in Chinese]
37. Jian XC, Liu SF, Shen ZH, Cheng HB. A clinical study of oral submucous fibrosis. Chin J Stomatol. 1989;24:299–302. [in Chinese]
38. Lin FX, Kong QR, Lin TC. An epidemiologic study of oral leukoplakia in Hainan Island. Chin J Stomatol. 1985;20:180–2. [in Chinese]
39. Tran TKC, Nguyen TBN, Nguyen TH, Priebe S. Betel chewing and oral mucosal lesions in Vietnamese population sample. In: Proceedings, Oral Cancer in the Asia Pacific—A Regional Update and Networking. Kuala Lumpur: Faculty of Dentistry, University of Malaya, February 17–19, 2006, P.71.
40. Nguyen TBN. Oral mucosa, denture and paradentitis of betel chewers in Ba Diem Commune, Hoc Mon District, Ho Chı Minh City (in Vietnamese). Thesis, Faculty of Odontology, University of Medicine and Pharmacy, Ho Chı Minh City, 2006: pp. 15–7
41. Ngo DK. Oral Cancer and Precancer Survey in Southern Provinces of Vietnam, 1998. Cited by Huynh Anh Lan, 2006. In: Proceedings, Oral Cancer in the Asia Pacific—A Regional Update and Networking. Kuala Lumpur: Faculty of Dentistry, University of Malaya, 17–19 February 2006.
42. Lee CH, Ko AM, Warnakulasuriya S, Yin BL, Sunarjo ZRB, Ibrahim SO, Liu ZW, Li WH, Zhang SS, Kuntoro UB, Rajapakse PS, Warusavithana SA, Razak IA, Abdullah N, Shrestha P, Kwan AL, Shieh TY, Chen MK, Ko YC. Intercountry prevalences and practices of betel-quid use in south, southeast and eastern Asia regions and associated oral preneoplastic disorders: an international collaborative study by Asian betel-quid consortium of south and east Asia. Int J Cancer. 2011;129(7):1741–51. https://doi.org/10.1002/ijc.25809.
43. Sujatha D, Hebbar PB, Pai A. Prevalence and correlation of oral lesions among tobacco smokers, tobacco chewers, areca nut and alcohol users. Asian Pac J Cancer Prev. 2012;13(4):1633–7. https://doi.org/10.7314/apjcp.2012.13.4.1633.
44. Yang X, Wang Z, Zhou L, Liu W. Focus on higher rate of malignant transformation of oral submucous fibrosis and concomitant leukoplakia [published online ahead of print, 2021 Oct 30]. Oral Dis. 2021; https://doi.org/10.1111/odi.14063.
45. Kujan O, Mello FW, Warnakulasuriya S. Malignant transformation of oral submucous fibrosis: a systematic review and meta-analysis. Oral Dis. 2021;27(8):1936–46. https://doi.org/10.1111/odi.13727.
46. Hazarey VK, Erlewad DM, Mundhe KA, Ughade SN. Oral submucous fibrosis: study of 1000 cases from central India. J Oral Pathol Med. 2007;36(1):12–7. https://doi.org/10.1111/j.1600-0714.2006.00485.x.
47. Angadi PV, Rekha KP. Oral submucous fibrosis: a clinicopathologic review of 205 cases in Indians. Oral Maxillofac Surg. 2011;15(1):15–9. https://doi.org/10.1007/s10006-010-0225-x.
48. Lian IB, Tseng YT, Su CC, Tsai KY. Progression of precancerous lesions to oral cancer: results based on the Taiwan National Health Insurance Database. Oral Oncol. 2013;49(5):427–30. https://doi.org/10.1016/j.oraloncology.2012.12.004.
49. Yang PY, Chen YT, Wang YH, Su NY, Yu HC, Chang YC. Malignant transformation of oral submucous fibrosis in Taiwan: a nationwide population-based retrospective cohort study. J Oral Pathol Med. 2017;46(10):1040–5. https://doi.org/10.1111/jop.12570.
50. Wang TY, Chiu YW, Chen YT, et al. Malignant transformation of Taiwanese patients with oral leukoplakia: a nationwide population-based retrospective cohort study. J Formos Med Assoc. 2018;117(5):374–80. https://doi.org/10.1016/j.jfma.2018.01.017.
51. Chiang WF, Liu SY, Lin JF, et al. Malignant development in patients with oral potentially malignant disorders detected through nationwide screening: outcomes of 5-year follow-up at a single hospital. Head Neck. 2020;42(1):67–76. https://doi.org/10.1002/hed.25973.
52. Xiao X, Hu Y, Li C, Shi L, Liu W. DNA content abnormality in oral submucous fibrosis concomitant leukoplakia: a preliminary evaluation of the diagnostic and clinical implications. Diagn Cytopathol. 2020;48(11):1111–4. https://doi.org/10.1002/dc.24469.

53. Iocca O, Sollecito TP, Alawi F, et al. Potentially malignant disorders of the oral cavity and oral dysplasia: a systematic review and meta-analysis of malignant transformation rate by subtype. Head Neck. 2020;42(3):539–55. https://doi.org/10.1002/hed.26006.
54. Villa A, Menon RS, Kerr AR, et al. Proliferative leukoplakia: proposed new clinical diagnostic criteria. Oral Dis. 2018;24(5):749–60. https://doi.org/10.1111/odi.12830.
55. Hansen LS, Olson JA, Silverman S Jr. Proliferative verrucous leukoplakia. A long-term study of thirty patients. Oral Surg Oral Med Oral Pathol. 1985;60(3):285–98. https://doi.org/10.1016/0030-4220(85)90313-5.
56. Cerero-Lapiedra R, Baladé-Martínez D, Moreno-López LA, Esparza-Gómez G, Bagán JV. Proliferative verrucous leukoplakia: a proposal for diagnostic criteria. Med Oral Patol Oral Cir Bucal. 2010;15(6):e839–45. Published 2010 Nov 1
57. Carrard VC, Brouns ER, van der Waal I. Proliferative verrucous leukoplakia; a critical appraisal of the diagnostic criteria. Med Oral Patol Oral Cir Bucal. 2013;18(3):e411–3. https://doi.org/10.4317/medoral.18912.
58. Bagan J, Murillo-Cortes J, Poveda-Roda R, Leopoldo-Rodado M, Bagan L. Second primary tumors in proliferative verrucous leukoplakia: a series of 33 cases. Clin Oral Investig. 2020;24(6):1963–9. https://doi.org/10.1007/s00784-019-03059-9.
59. Mechery R, Kumar M, Arora P, Rajkamal T, Dinakar N. Oral proliferative verrucous leukoplakia with oral submucous fibrosis treated with CO2 laser. J Dent Lasers. 2015;9:100–3.
60. Chang KC, Su IJ, Tsai ST, Shieh DB, Jin YT. Pathological features of betel quid-related oral epithelial lesions in Taiwan with special emphasis on the tumor progression and human papillomavirus association. Oncology. 2002;63(4):362–9. https://doi.org/10.1159/000066227.
61. Ackerman LV, McGavran MH. Proliferating benign and malignant epithelial lesions of the oral cavity. J Oral Surg (Chic). 1958;16(5):400–13.
62. Adkins KF, Monsour FN. Verrucous leukoplakia. N Z Dent J. 1976;72(327):28–32.
63. Shear M, Pindborg JJ. Verrucous hyperplasia of the oral mucosa. Cancer. 1980;46(8):1855–62. https://doi.org/10.1002/1097-0142(19801015)46:8<1855::aid-cncr2820460825>3.0.co;2-#.
64. Wang YP, Chen HM, Kuo RC, et al. Oral verrucous hyperplasia: histologic classification, prognosis, and clinical implications. J Oral Pathol Med. 2009;38(8):651–6. https://doi.org/10.1111/j.1600-0714.2009.00790.x.
65. Zain RB, Kallarakkal TG, Ramanathan A, Kim J, Tilakaratne WM, Takata T, et al. A consensus report from the first Asian regional meeting on the terminology and criteria for verruco-papillary lesions of the oral cavity held in Kuala Lumpur, Malaysia, December 15–18, 2013. Annal Dent Univ Malaya. 2013;20:1–3.
66. Zain RB, Kallarakkal TG, Ramanathan A, Kim J, Tilakaratne WM, Takata T, Warnakulasuriya S, Hazarey VK, Rich A, Hussaini HM, Jalil A. Exophytic verrucous hyperplasia of the oral cavity—application of standardized criteria for diagnosis from a consensus report. Asian Pac J Cancer Prev. 2016 Jan 9;17(9):4491. https://doi.org/10.7314/APJCP.2016.17.(9).4491.
67. Jayasinghe LA, Peiris PM, Tilakaratne WM, et al. Clinically malignant exophytic lesions in the background of oral submucous fibrosis: report of five cases. Oral Surg Oral Med Oral Pathol Oral Radiol. 2016;122(2):210–5. https://doi.org/10.1016/j.oooo.2016.06.001.
68. Shah AM, Bansal S, Shirsat PM, Prasad P, Desai RS. Exophytic verrucous hyperplasia in oral submucous fibrosis: a single-center study. J Oral Maxillofac Pathol. 2019;23(3):393–9. https://doi.org/10.4103/jomfp.JOMFP_276_19.
69. Shafer WG. Verruciform xanthoma. Oral Surg Oral Med Oral Pathol. 1971;31(6):784–9. https://doi.org/10.1016/0030--4220(71)90134-4.
70. Santa Cruz DJ, Martin SA. Verruciform xanthoma of the vulva. Report of two cases. Am J Clin Pathol. 1979;71(2):224–8. https://doi.org/10.1093/ajcp/71.2.224.
71. Hume WJ, Smith CJ, Franklin CD. Verruciform xanthoma. Br J Oral Surg. 1980;18(2):157–61. https://doi.org/10.1016/0007--117x(80)90034-7.
72. Miyamoto Y, Nagayama M, Hayashi Y. Verruciform xanthoma occurring within oral lichen planus. J Oral Pathol Med. 1996;25(4):188–91. https://doi.org/10.1111/j.1600-0714.1996.tb00218.x.
73. Polonowita AD, Firth NA, Rich AM. Verruciform xanthoma and concomitant lichen planus of the oral mucosa. A report of three cases. Int J Oral Maxillofac Surg. 1999;28(1):62–6.
74. Allen CM, Kapoor N. Verruciform xanthoma in a bone marrow transplant recipient. Oral Surg Oral Med Oral Pathol. 1993;75(5):591–4. https://doi.org/10.1016/0030-4220(93)90231-r.
75. Sibaud V, Marit G, Deminière C, Campana F, Taieb A, Fricain JC. Xanthomes verruciformes multiples buccaux au cours d'une maladie du greffon contre l'hôte [Multiple verruciform xanthomas of the oral mucosa associated with graft versus host disease]. Ann Dermatol Venereol. 2006;133(12):995–9. https://doi.org/10.1016/s0151-9638(06)71086-9.
76. Shahrabi Farahani S, Treister NS, Khan Z, Woo SB. Oral verruciform xanthoma associated with chronic graft-versus-host disease: a report of five cases and a review of the literature. Head Neck Pathol. 2011;5(2):193–8. https://doi.org/10.1007/s12105-011-0246-2.
77. Capocasale G, Panzarella V, Tozzo P, et al. Oral verruciform xanthoma and erythroplakia associated with chronic graft-versus-host disease: a rare case report and review of the literature. BMC Res Notes. 2017;10(1):631. Published 2017 Nov. 28. https://doi.org/10.1186/s13104-017-2952-7.
78. Poulopoulos AK, Epivatianos A, Zaraboukas T, Antoniades D. Verruciform xanthoma coexisting with oral discoid lupus erythematosus. Br J Oral Maxillofac Surg. 2007;45(2):159–60. https://doi.org/10.1016/j.bjoms.2005.06.020.
79. Neville BW, Weathers DR. Verruciform xanthoma. Oral Surg Oral Med Oral Pathol. 1980;49(5):429–34. https://doi.org/10.1016/0030-4220(80)90287-x.
80. Drummond JF, White DK, Damm DD, Cramer JR. Verruciform xanthoma within carcinoma in situ. J Oral MaxillofacSurg.1989;47(4):398–400.https://doi.org/10.1016/0278--2391(89)90343-1.
81. Yu CH, Tsai TC, Wang JT, et al. Oral verruciform xanthoma: a clinicopathologic study of 15 cases. J Formos Med Assoc. 2007;106(2):141–7. https://doi.org/10.1016/S0929--6646(09)60230-8.
82. Ghosh S, Gupta S, Singh K, Urs A. Verruciform xanthoma associated with oral submucous fibrosis—a report of an unusual case with literature review. Int J Contemp Med Res. 2014;1:88–91.
83. Hegde U, Doddawad VG, Sreeshyla HS, Patil R. Verruciform xanthoma: a case report with immunohistochemical findings. Aust Road Res Boad. 2015;8:1–4.
84. Gannepalli A, Appala A, Reddy L, Babu DBG. Insight into verruciform xanthoma with oral submucous fibrosis: case report and review of literature. J Oral Maxillofac Pathol. 2019;23(Suppl 1):43–8. https://doi.org/10.4103/jomfp.JOMFP_210_18.

85. Yang YH, Lien YC, Ho PS, et al. The effects of chewing areca/betel quid with and without cigarette smoking on oral submucous fibrosis and oral mucosal lesions. Oral Dis. 2005;11(2):88–94. https://doi.org/10.1111/j.1601-0825.2004.01061.x.
86. Pravda C, Srinivasan H, Koteeswaran D, Manohar LA. Verrucous carcinoma in association with oral submucous fibrosis. Indian J Dent Res. 2011;22(4):615. https://doi.org/10.4103/0970-9290.90329.
87. Komal K, Deshmukh SB, Deshmukh A. Verrucous carcinoma with oral submucous fibrosis: a rare case with brief review. J Clin Diagn Res. 2015;9(8):ED06–ED8. https://doi.org/10.7860/JCDR/2015/10042.6305.
88. Malhotra S, Raghavan V, Kumar A, Singh AK. Verrucous carcinoma on pre-existing oral submucous fibrosis. J Indian Acad Oral Med Radiol. 2015;27:593–7.
89. Ramani P, Krithika C, Ananthalakshmi R, et al. Verrucoid variant of invasive squamous cell carcinoma in oral submucous fibrosis: a clinicopathological challenge. Cureus. 2016;8(11):e862. https://doi.org/10.7759/cureus.862.
90. Yunus SM, Gadodia P, Wadhwani R, Nayyar AS, Patil N, Kumar V, et al. Verrucous carcinoma in association with OSMF: a rare case report. Austin J Dent. 2016;3(3):1039.
91. Popli H, Kumar S. Verrucous carcinoma with oral sub-mucous fibrosis: an uncommon occurrence. Int J Appl Dent Sci. 2018;4(4):01–4.
92. Tyagi M, Mohan V, Gupta R. Verrucous carcinoma in association with oral submucous fibrosis. Univ J Dent Sci. 2021;7(1):111–3.

# Oral Submucous Fibrosis in Childhood

*Anura Ariyawardana*

## Contents



© The Author(s), under exclusive license to Springer Nature Switzerland AG 2023
S. Warnakulasuriya, K. Ranganathan (eds.), *Oral Submucous Fibrosis*, Textbooks in Contemporary Dentistry,
https://doi.org/10.1007/978-3-031-12855-4_5

5

## 5.1 Introduction

Oral submucous fibrosis (OSF) is generally regarded as a disease of the adults where the peak incidence is reported between 20 and 40 years of age [1, 2]. However, in the recent past, cases were reported occurring among paediatric and adolescent population in different geographic locations [3].

With OSF being a progressive and insidious disease, it is highly likely that the condition may have devastating outcomes when the children grow older with more morbidity and likely malignant transformation. Areca nut chewing is the only well-established etiological factor [4]. Older adults who develop OSF in their mouths are generally known to have been exposed to areca nut for a substantial period of time when they develop the condition. This is not the case in very young children who develop OSF. It is therefore likely that these children do have a genetic susceptibility to develop OSF in addition to exposure to areca nut from a young age. This chapter aims to discuss the epidemiology, aetiology, clinical features among children and potential outcomes and avenues for prevention.

**Learning Goals**

The objective of this chapter is to provide readers an insight into the involvement of children with oral submucous fibrosis. Readers will be able to understand the early initiation of areca nut chewing, which is influenced by the socio-economic and cultural practices. It is important to learn the early signs of OSF among children and help the vulnerable children to be screened to detect OSF at its early stage.

## 5.2 Epidemiology

OSF cases have been reported from South and Southeast Asian countries such as India [5], Sri Lanka [6], China [7], Pakistan [8], Bangladesh [9], Taiwan [10], Thailand [11], Malaysia [12] and Cambodia [13] and among migrants to the Western countries [14–16]. The prevalence of OSF varies across children and adolescents, and no exact data are available.

◘ Table 5.1 gives a summary of the cases reported among children and adolescents since 1985. The age range of the children affected varies from country to country

◘ **Table 5.1** Demographic, symptom and habit information among children diagnosed with OSF

| Author, year | Country | Number of cases | Age (y) | Sex | Presenting complaint | Mouth opening | Biopsy findings | Habits |
|---|---|---|---|---|---|---|---|---|
| Hayes, 1985 [15] | Canada | 1 | 4 | F | Restricted mouth opening | 11 mm | Hyperorthokeratotic and atrophic epithelium, subepithelial hyalinization, patchy lymphocytic infiltrate in the deeper tissues | Pan supari since the age of 2 years |
| Anil and Beena, 1993 [37] | Andaman and Nicobar islands | 1 | 12 | F | Difficulty in opening the mouth, protruding the tongue and tolerating spicy food | 17 mm | Atrophic epithelium with absence of rete ridges, connective tissue showed hyalinization and moderate chronic inflammatory cell infiltration | Pan supari chewing since the age of 7 yrs |
| Mundra et al., 1999 [38] | India | 1 | 8 | F | Difficulty in opening the mouth, fever, chills and rigors | 20 mm | Intact squamous epithelium with focal aggregates of chronic inflammatory cell Infiltration. | Betel nut chewing for 6 months |
| Shah et al., 2001 [16] | UK | 1 | 11 | F | Recurrent oral ulceration, discomfort and a burning sensation for spicy foods | N/A | N/A | Regular Supari use since the age of 10 |
| Yusuf and Yong 2002 [39] | Bangladesh | 1 | 12 | M | Difficulty opening his mouth and occasional difficulty in swallowing | 21 mm | N/A | Paan supari since the age of 8 years |

**Table 5.1** (continued)

| Author, year | Country | Number of cases | Age (y) | Sex | Presenting complaint | Mouth opening | Biopsy findings | Habits |
|---|---|---|---|---|---|---|---|---|
| Hazare et al., 2007 [40] | India | 2 | 9 | F | N/A | N/A | N/A | N/A |
| | | | 12 | M | N/A | N/A | N/A | N/A |
| Sitheeque et al., 2010 [29] | Sri Lanka | 5 | 3 | F | White discolouration of lips | Normal | Mildly-atrophic squamous epithelium, with increased amount of collagen in the upper Corium, Fibrosis extends into muscle in a few foci. No inflammatory infiltrate | Areca nut 2–3 times per day |
| | | | 3 | M | Loss of lip pigmentation | Normal | Mild atrophic changes in surface epithelium, features suggestive of OSF, no significant increase in fibrosis of a lesser degree | Areca nut 2–3 times per day |
| | | | 3 | M | Whitish shade of lip | Normal | N/A | Betel with areca nut 1–2 per day |
| | | | 3 | M | Loss of lip colour | Normal | N/A | Betel with areca nut 2–3 per day |
| | | | 2 | F | Loss of lip pigmentation | Normal | N/A | Areca nut only Frequency N/A |
| Agrawal et al., 2011 [41] | India | 1 | 9 | F | Inability to open the mouth for 4 yrs, burning mouth for spicy food | 16 mm | Thick parakeratinized epithelium dense fibrous tissue stroma and chronic inflammation | Areca nut (Sweet Supari) 3–4 per day |
| Dhariwal et al., 2012 [42] | India | 2 | 10 | M | Difficulty in opening mouth and taking spicy food for 3 months | 15 mm | N/A | Chewing gutkha 2–3 per day for 1 year |
| | | | 12 | F | Burning sensation on having food for the last 3–4 years | 19 mm | N/A | Pan masala daily for 7 years |
| Deshpande et al., 2013 [43] | India | 1 | 14 | F | Difficulty in opening the mouth and burning sensation for spicy food | 30 mm | N/A | Chewing flavoured areca nut and scented tobacco, 2 packets/day since 1 year. |

(continued)

5

**Table 5.1** (continued)

| Author, year | Country | Number of cases | Age (y) | Sex | Presenting complaint | Mouth opening | Biopsy findings | Habits |
|---|---|---|---|---|---|---|---|---|
| Gupta et al., 2013 [31] | India | 2 | 11 | F | Reduced mouth opening, discomfort and a burning sensation particularly when eating spicy foods | 14 mm | N/A | Areca nut chewing since seven year |
| | | | 10 | M | Reduced mouth opening, discomfort and a burning sensation particularly when eating spicy foods | 13 mm | N/A | Areca nut chewing since six year |
| Duggirala et al., 2015 [44] | India | 3 | 9 | F | Burning sensation on taking spicy foods was noticed since 1 year with increase in severity and progressive restriction of the mouth opening since 6 months | 14 mm | N/A | Sweetened form of areca nut continuous |
| | | | 13 | M | Progressive inability to open the mouth since 1 year and severe burning sensation on taking spicy foods since 2 years. | 22 mm | N/A | Pan 2–3 times a day since 4 years |
| | | | 15 | F | Recurrent oral ulcers since 6 months and burning sensation in the mouth particularly when eating hot and spicy foods since 1 year | 28 mm | N/A | Sweet supari for several minutes for 6–7 times in a day since 4 years. |
| Khandelwal et al., 2018 [45] | India | 1 | 14 | M | Difficulty in opening the mouth for 3 years, burning sensation for spicy food for 4 months | 14 mm | N/A | Tobacco and areca nut (Gutkha) 3–4 per day for 6 yrs |
| Talla et al., 2019 [46] | India | 1 | 5 | F | Limited mouth opening for 3 months and burning sensation for spicy food | 15 mm | N/A | Areca nut |
| Kariya et al., 2020 [47] | India | 1 | 5 | M | Restricted mouth opening since 3–4 months, Intolerance to spicy food | 6 mm | N/A | Sweet supari for since the age of 3.5 yrs |

**Table 5.1** (continued)

| Author, year | Country | Number of cases | Age (y) | Sex | Presenting complaint | Mouth opening | Biopsy findings | Habits |
|---|---|---|---|---|---|---|---|---|
| More et al., 2020 [28] | India | 36 | 12 | M | Occasional mild burning sensation on eating spicy food | N/A | N/A | Flavoured areca nut/2–3 large sachets per day |
| | | | 11 | F | Nil | N/A | N/A | Flavoured areca nut/1–2 large sachets per day |
| | | | 11 | M | Occasional mild burning sensation on eating spicy food | N/A | N/A | 1–2 nuts per day |
| | | | 14 | M | Burning sensation on eating spicy food<br>Loss of taste sensation<br>Xerostomia | N/A | N/A | Gutkha 2–3 small sachets per day |
| | | | 14 | M | Nil | N/A | N/A | Flavoured areca nut/4–5 large sachets per day |
| | | | 9 | M | Loss of taste sensation | N/A | N/A | Baked arecanut, 1 big nut per day |
| | | | 14 | M | Nil | N/A | N/A | Betel leaf with areca nut but without tobacco 4–5 times per day |
| | | | 10 | F | Occasional mild burning sensation on eating spicy food | N/A | N/A | Flavoured areca nut/2–3 small sachets per day |
| | | | 13 | M | Occasional mild burning sensation on eating spicy food | N/A | N/A | Flavoured areca nut/4–5 small sachets per day |
| | | | 14 | M | Burning sensation on eating spicy food | N/A | N/A | Flavoured areca nut/7–8 large sachets per day |
| | | | 13 | M | Mild burning sensation on eating spicy food | N/A | N/A | Flavoured areca nut/8–9 large sachets per day |
| | | | 14 | M | Mild burning sensation on eating spicy food<br>Xerostomia | N/A | N/A | Flavoured areca nut/8–9 large sachets per day |

(continued)

**Table 5.1** (continued)

| Author, year | Country | Number of cases | Age (y) | Sex | Presenting complaint | Mouth opening | Biopsy findings | Habits |
|---|---|---|---|---|---|---|---|---|
| | | | 15 | M | Mild burning sensation on eating spicy food | N/A | N/A | Pan Masala, 5–6 small sachets per day |
| | | | 10 | F | Loss of taste, excessive salivation | N/A | N/A | Flavoured areca nut/9–10 small sachets per day |
| | | | 15 | M | Occasional mild burning sensation on eating spicy food | N/A | N/A | Mawa 1–2 balls per day |
| | | | 16 | M | Mild burning sensation on eating spicy food excessive salivation | N/A | N/A | Pan Masala, 7–8 large packets |
| | | | 11 | M | Occasional mild burning sensation on eating spicy food | N/A | N/A | Flavoured areca nut/4–5 large sachets per day |
| | | | 16 | M | Loss of taste, xerostomia | N/A | N/A | Betel leaf with areca nut but without tobacco 4–5 times per day |
| | | | 14 | M | Burning sensation on eating spicy food | N/A | N/A | Flavoured areca nut/5–6 large sachets per day |
| | | | 14 | F | Occasional mild burning sensation on eating spicy food | N/A | N/A | Flavoured areca nut/4–5 small sachets per day |
| | | | 12 | M | Nil | N/A | N/A | Flavoured areca nut/4–5 small sachets per day |
| | | | 14 | M | Loss of taste | N/A | N/A | Betel leaf with areca nut but without tobacco 2–3 times per day |
| | | | 13 | F | Occasional mild burning sensation on eating spicy food | N/A | N/A | Flavoured areca nut/5–6 small sachets per day |
| | | | 15 | M | Burning sensation on eating spicy food | N/A | N/A | Mawa 2–3 balls per day |
| | | | 15 | M | Burning sensation on eating spicy food | N/A | N/A | Pan masala 5–6 small packets per day |

■ **Table 5.1** (continued)

| Author, year | Country | Number of cases | Age (y) | Sex | Presenting complaint | Mouth opening | Biopsy findings | Habits |
|---|---|---|---|---|---|---|---|---|
| | | | 11 | M | Burning sensation on eating spicy food | N/A | N/A | Flavoured areca nut, 5–6 large sachets |
| | | | 12 | M | Loss of taste | N/A | N/A | Backed areca nut, 1–2 whole nuts per day |
| | | | 15 | M | Burning sensation on eating spicy food, Loss of taste, excessive salivation | N/A | N/A | Gutkha, 4–5 large sachets per day |
| | | | 13 | F | Occasional burning sensation on eating spicy food | N/A | N/A | Flavoured areca nut/5–6 small sachets per day |
| | | | 14 | M | Burning sensation on eating spicy food | N/A | N/A | Mawa 4–5 balls per day |
| | | | 10 | F | Loss of taste | N/A | N/A | Flavoured areca nut/4–5 small sachets per day |
| | | | 15 | M | Mild burning sensation on eating spicy food | N/A | N/A | Pan masala, 5–6 small packets |
| | | | 13 | M | Loss of taste | N/A | N/A | Betel leaf with areca nut without tobacco 5–6 times per day |
| | | | 12 | F | Nil | N/A | N/A | Flavoured areca nut/2–3 small sachets per day |
| | | | 15 | M | Occasional burning sensation on eating spicy food, excessive salivation | N/A | N/A | Pan masala 4–5 small packets per day |
| | | | 14 | M | Burning sensation on eating spicy food | N/A | N/A | Mawa 4–5 balls per day |

*N/A* Not available

with a mean age of 8.7 years, with the youngest child being 2 years of age. Childhood OSF is more common among male children with a female-to-male ratio of 1:1.8.

## 5.3 Aetiology

The use of areca nut with or without betel quid or tobacco is the only known risk factor [17]. The relationship of areca nut chewing with OSF and pathogenic mechanisms are described in later chapters in this book. Areca nut chewing habit is commonly seen in South and Southeast Asian countries and among Pacific Islanders, where OSF is highly prevalent.

Addiction to areca nut chewing is a serious health concern among South and Southeast Asian populations where about 600 million people are impacted by this substance disorder [18]. Areca nut is the fourth most abused addictive substance after alcohol, caffeine, and tobacco [19]. Among those populations where areca nut use is prevalent, there is a deep-seated cultural link from ancient past to date [18, 19]. Areca nut use is more commonly seen among the middle age to elderly men and women. However, case reports and some studies confirm that children and young adults are also addicted to areca nut [20–26]. ◘ Table 5.2 provides a summary of the prevalence of the areca nut chewing among school children. Among the children studied, males have the higher prevalence of chewing areca nut than females.

It is generally regarded that OSF develops over a long period of time after the initiation of areca nut chewing. However, the reported cases indicate that the children have developed at least the initial signs of OSF after a short exposure. This raises the question if these affected children are genetically more susceptible for the development of OSF.

## 5.4 Vulnerability Factors for Areca Nut Chewing Habits and Developing OSF

A recent review reported that the mean age of initiation of areca nut chewing habit among children was 7.40 years (2–13 years) with some having consumed with a frequency of 15 times a day. The mean duration of areca nut consumption was reported to be 43 months (6–84 months). The presence of clinical features was dependent on the site they kept the quid in the mouth [3].

Multiple social factors influence the children to embark on areca nut chewing, making them more vulnerable to develop OSF at a very young age (◘ Table 5.3). Most children start chewing areca nut due to the influence from their parents, grandparents, siblings and other relatives and through peer pressure. Areca nut chewing is a strongly deep-seated practice with strong cultural bonds. Having parents, grandparents and siblings in family environment who jointly

◘ **Table 5.2** Prevalence of areca nut-chewing habit among children

| Author, year | Country | Population | Sample size | Habit prevalence (%) | | | % of OSF cases |
|---|---|---|---|---|---|---|---|
| | | | | Overall | Males | Female | |
| Lu et al., 1993 [20] | Taiwan | Junior high school | 2367 | 4.7 | 9.2 | 0.9 | NA |
| Ho et al., 2000 [21] | Taiwan | High school | 2083 | 5.4 | NA | NA | |
| Shah et al., 2002 [22] | Pakistan | Preschool children | 159 | 75.0 | 72.0 | 30.0 | NA |
| Oakley et al., 2005 [23] | N. Mariana Island | High school children | 309 | 63.0 | 73.0 | 54.0 | 8.8 |
| Khandalwal et al., 2012 [24] | India | Middle school children | 3896 | 27.0 | 34.6 | 17.8 | NA |
| Singhvi, 2016 [25] | India | Primary school children | 1174 | 34.5 | 35.2 | 33.8 | 3.4 |
| | | High school children | 1672 | 72.8 | 74.6 | 70.7 | |
| Wazir et al., 2017 [26] | Nepal | High school children | 1359 | 30.4 | 38.0 | 23.2 | NA |

*NA* not available

enjoy the use of areca nut would likely influence the children to use the same. Lack of awareness on the harmful effects of areca nut chewing supports the cultural setting to thrive and pass the areca nut chewing to the next generation.

▫ Table 5.4 summarises the reported reasons for initiation of areca nut chewing. In addition to the family influence and peer pressure, various other reasons were reported as determinants for initiation of areca nut chewing. They include the belief that chewing areca nut increases the appetite, aids digestion, reduces tiredness, increases social interaction and helps to look mature. Further, some chewed areca nut due to the attractiveness of packaging, to distract family violence and to avoid pressure of studies.

## 5.5 Clinical Features

Clinical features of OSF in children are not different from that in adults. The most common presenting complaint of children with OSF was mild burning sensation in parts of the oral mucosa. This was followed by restricted mouth opening. A minority of children had presented with a complaint of loss of taste sensation and depigmentation (▫ Fig. 5.1). ▫ Table 5.5 summarises the reported symptoms and signs based on the case histories reported in the literature.

More et al. suggested a classification system for OSF based on the clinical and functional changes [27]. A recent case series from India reported that of the 36 cases, the majority ($n$ = 29, 81%) were stage I cases in which stomatitis and/or blanching of oral mucosa were the prominent clinical features [28]. However, a narrative review of existing literature between 1952 and 2016 on OSF in 18 children reported that over 50% were at the advanced stages (Stage 3/4) of the condition [3].

Restricted mouth opening could perhaps be the most devastating outcome of OSF among children considering the likely further deterioration. ▫ Table 5.1 summarises the reported interincisal mouth opening in the reported cases. Of the 24 cases included in ▫ Table 5.1, the average mouth opening of 16 patients was 17.2 mm (6–30 mm).

Depigmentation of the oral mucosa is one of the early signs of OSF (▫ Fig. 5.1). Sitheeque and colleagues reported five cases presenting with the initial complaint of depigmentation of the lips [29]. None of these children had restricted mouth opening, and hence depigmentation can be considered as a very early sign of the disease among children. This feature is very important as an initial finding to suspect potential OSF in children, and hence all clinicians who provide dental care for children should take a thorough social history on areca nut use through their parents. This will enable for prevention of the condition progressing further.

**Important**

It is important to carefully examine the oral mucosa of vulnerable children to exclude early features of paediatric OSF such as depigmentation. Careful parental social history of areca nut chewing is helpful to identify such vulnerable kids. This will enable practitioners to prevent young children from being affected with devastating advanced OSF later in life.

▫ **Table 5.3** Social circumstances influencing areca nut chewing among children

| |
|---|
| Child labour: to reduce appetite and tiredness when working as housemaid; chewing with peers while watching cows |
| Parents at work: no one at home to look after while parents at work as labourers |
| Influence from friends who chew areca nut |
| Grandparents regularly offered areca nut |
| Family chews after dinner including children |
| Living with multiple families together who consume areca nut |
| Siblings chew areca nut |

Adapted from More et al., 2020; Chitguppi C, Brar T., 2017

▫ **Table 5.4** Reported reasons for chewing areca nut

| |
|---|
| Peer pressure |
| Family influence |
| To avoid pressure of studies |
| Taste of areca nut |
| Distract from domestic violence |
| Attractiveness of packaging |
| To increase social interaction |
| Considered a digestive agent |
| Belief that chewing reduces appetite |
| Belief that chewing reduces tiredness |
| To look mature |

Adapted from More et al. (2020), Chitguppi and Brar (2017)

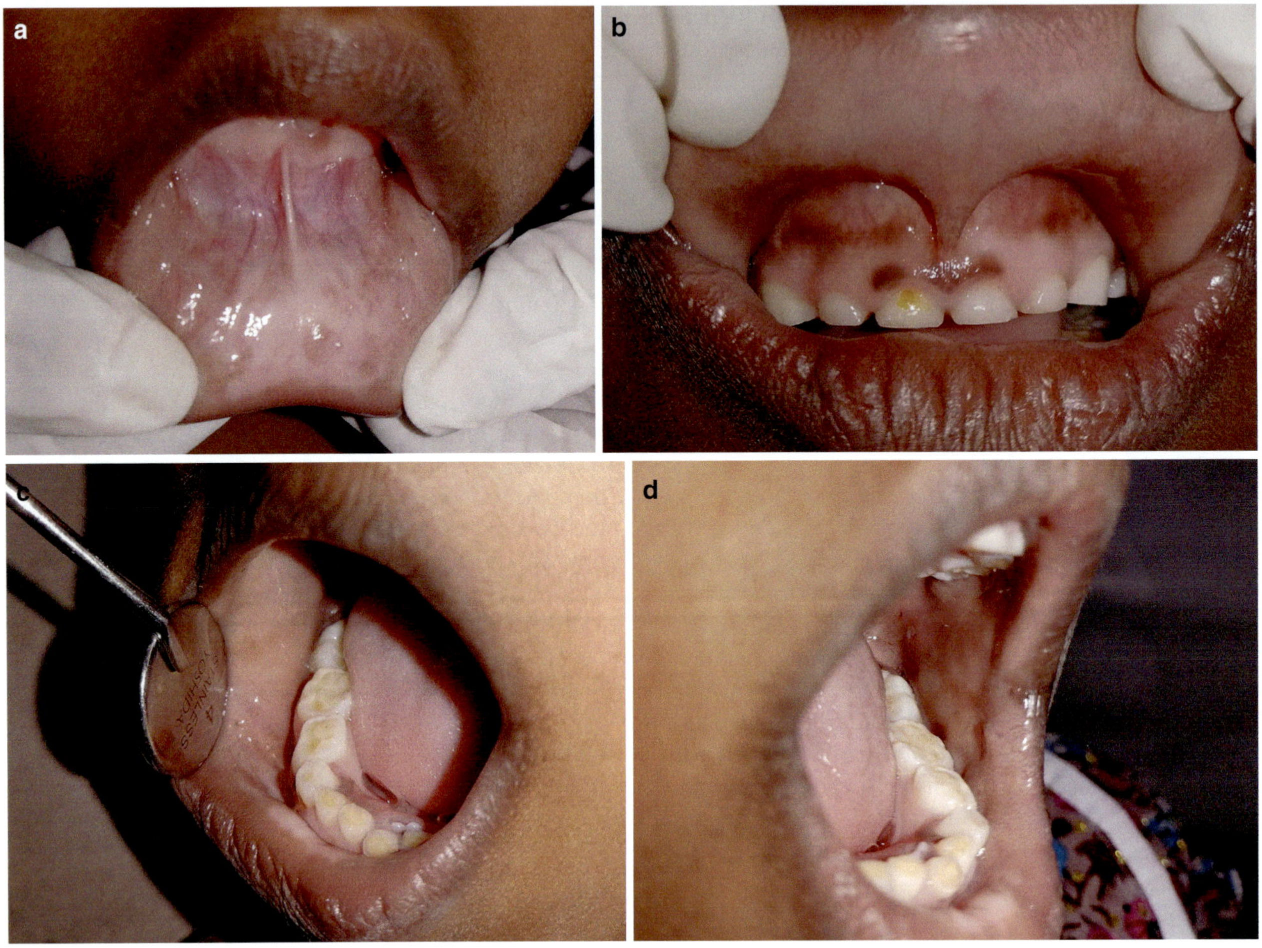

**Fig. 5.1** (**a**) Depigmentation of lower lip, (**b**) Depigmentation of gingiva, (**c**) Depigmentation of the left buccal mucosa and lower lip, (**d**) Depigmentation of right buccal mucosa (Illustrations courtesy of Dr Ruwan Jayasinghe, University of Peradeniya, Sri Lanka)

**Table 5.5** Clinical features of childhood OSF

| |
|---|
| **Symptoms** |
| Burning sensation [16, 28, 31, 42–47] |
| Difficulty in opening the mouth [15, 37–39, 41–47] |
| Oral depigmentation [29] |
| Loss of taste [28] |
| Reduced saliva [28] |
| Excessive salivation [28] |
| **Signs** |
| Restricted mouth opening [15, 37–39, 41–47] |
| Blanching of the oral mucosa [29, 31] |
| Fibrous bands in buccal mucosa [15, 16, 37–42] |
| Leathery mucosa [43] |
| Erosions or ulcerations [16, 44] |
| Altered shape of uvula [3, 38, 42, 44, 45, 47] |
| Depapillation of the tongue [28, 37, 42, 44] |
| Tongue fibrosis [28] |

## 5.6 Diagnosis

Diagnosis of OSF is easy and simple at its advanced stages and can be made based on the clinical presentations alone [28]. In most cases, biopsy might not be necessary and clinical diagnosis is sufficient if no dysplasia is suspected with concomitant potentially malignant lesions such as leukoplakia and erythroplakia. However, diagnosis at early stages may be complex and difficult due to the absence of classic features. In these cases, a thorough history with regard to possible areca nut chewing is needed. Of the cases reported in Table 5.1, only six cases had biopsies performed to confirm the diagnosis, and the rest were diagnosed on the basis of clinical features and history of areca nut chewing habit. The most common histological feature was the atrophic epithelium.

## 5.7 Management

No specific treatment for OSF has been reported to date [30]. Essentially, the management should aim at preventing the disease progression and malignant transformation. The management of children with OSF should be done through a multidisciplinary approach, which includes oral medicine specialists, paediatric dentists, general dentists and dietitians/nutritionists with additional behavioural support if required. All children and their parents should be educated on the strong association between areca nut chewing and development of OSF and potential outcomes. Although no malignant transformation of childhood OSF has been reported, children can be considered a more vulnerable group for malignant transformation due to the fact that they have more years to live. Hence, the affected children need to be followed up carefully for a long period of time while paying attention to the general oral health. Due to the progressive nature of OSF that may lead to restricted mouth opening, their oral health can deteriorate. Hence, regular oral prophylaxis at primary healthcare settings is recommended in view of improving oral health and minimising the morbidity associated with dental diseases.

**Tip**

Depigmentation of oral mucosa or gingiva in young children could be an early sign of OSF that should raise suspicion and needs further investigation.

## 5.8 Prevention

Given that no treatment is currently available for OSF, prevention is the main strategy. It is pivotal to recognise paediatric areca nut chewing and OSF as a public health problem. It is apparent that the children acquire the areca nut chewing habit from sociocultural environment in which they are living. Studies report that the highest risk of children initiating areca nut habit falls between the ages of 5 and 12 years [3, 31]. It is also likely that the children continue areca nut chewing until adulthood and probably the rest of their life thereafter if there is no early intervention. Moreover, daily consumption of areca nut makes the children more vulnerable to develop OSF [32, 33].

As primary prevention, parents should be educated, and grandparents and families consuming areca nut should be encouraged to quit. They should also be encouraged to avoid promoting the use of areca nut among the children. Primary prevention can be done at various levels using primary healthcare workers, schoolteachers, and community and religious leaders to encourage to quit and prevent the areca nut-chewing habit.

Screening at clinical levels, especially paediatric dental clinic and general practitioner level, to identify cases through the history of areca nut use and the presence of early clinical features of OSF should be encouraged. Parents can be educated at this level to improve their awareness on the dangers of areca nut chewing.

Parents and teachers can also play a significant role in the early detection of OSF among vulnerable children. Dentists, oral health therapists and other allied health workers need to be educated regarding paediatric OSF and the early clinical features. Strong links of areca nut chewing with the sociocultural background must be considered in case identification and prevention [30].

**Important**

OSF develops among young children after being exposed to areca nut for a short period. Hence, genetic susceptibility for the development of OSF should be explored in future studies in childhood cases.

## 5.9 Malignant Transformation and Associated Risk Factors of Malignant Transformation

A recent systematic review of adult OSF in 9 longitudinal studies reported that 292 OSF cases developed carcinomas out of 6337 with the pooled proportion of 4.2% (95% CI: 2.7–5.6%) and an annual transformation rate of 0.73% [34]. However, to date, no follow-up studies are available reporting malignant transformation (MT) of childhood OSF [35, 36].

**Summary**

OSF among children is very rare. However, if children are affected with OSF, they are more likely to have advanced disease with significant disability before reaching adulthood. Children can develop OSF at a very early age with a mean age of the disease initiation being 8.7 years. With areca nut being the only known aetiological factor, it is very important to educate the parents to prevent their young children from initiating the chewing of areca nut. The parents and schoolteachers need to be educated on the danger of the habit of areca nut chewing. Vulnerable children should be screened for likely OSF, and prompt action should be taken to prevent further progression of the disease. Dentists and dental specialists need to be aware of early signs and symptoms of childhood OSF and screen the vulnerable children.

## References

1. Punnya V, Angadi PV, Rekha KP. Oral submucous fibrosis: a clinicopathologic review of 205 cases in Indians. Oral Maxillofac Surg. 2011;15:15–9.
2. Desai KM, Kale AD, Punnya VA, Datar UV. Clinicopathological evaluation of oral Submucous fibrosis—a retrospective, single Institute study. Ann Dent Spec. 2021;9(1):27–33.

3. Chitguppi C, Brar T. Paediatric oral submucous fibrosis—the neglected pre-malignancy of childhood. Int J Ped Otorhinolaryngol. 2017;97:55e60.
4. Arakeria G, Brennanb PA. Oral submucous fibrosis: an overview of the aetiology, pathogenesis, classification, and principles of management. Br J Oral Maxillofac Surg. 2013;51:587–93.
5. Mehta FS, Pindborg JJ, Gupta PC, Daftary DK. Epidemiologic and histologic study of oral cancer and leukoplakia among 50,915 villagers in India. Cancer. 1969;24(4):832e849.
6. Ariyawardana A, Sitheeque MAM, Ranasnghe AW, et al. Prevalence of oral cancer and pre-cancer and associated risk factors among tea estate workers in the central Sri Lanka. J Oral Pathol Med. 2007;36:581–7.
7. Tang J-G, Jian X-F, Gao M-L, Ling T-Y, Zhang K-H. An epidemiological survey of oral submucous fibrosis in Xiangtan City, Hunan Province, China. Community Dent Oral Epidemiol. 1997;25:177–80.
8. Jafarey NA, Zaidi SH. Carcinoma of the oral cavity and oropharynx in Karachi (Pakistan). An appraisal. Trop Dr. 1976;6(2):63e67.
9. McCarty KM, Houseman EA, Quamruzzaman Q, et al. The impact of diet and betel nut use on skin lesions associated with drinking-water arsenic in Pabna. Bangladesh Environ Health Perspect. 2006;114(3):334–40.
10. Yang S-F, Wang Y-H, Su N-Y, et al. Changes in prevalence of precancerous oral submucous fibrosis from 1996 to 2013 in Taiwan: a nationwide population-based retrospective study. J Formos Med Assoc. 2018;117(2):147–52. https://doi.org/10.1016/j.jfma.2017.01.012.
11. Reichart PA. Oral cancer and precancer related to betel and Miang chewing in Thailand: a review. J Oral Pathol Med. 1995;24(6):241–3.
12. Zain RB, Fukano H, Razak IA et al. Risk factors for oral leukoplakia: a comparison of two ethnic groups in Malaysia. In: Varma AK, editor. Oral oncology, vol. VI. New Delhi: Macmillan; 1999, pp. 207–10.
13. Reichart PA, Schmidtberg W, Scheifele CH. Betel chewer's mucosa in elderly Cambodian women. J Oral Pathol Med. 1996;25:367e370. https://doi.org/10.1111/j.1600-0714.1996.tb00280.x.
14. Sukumar S, Coleman HG, Cox SC. Areca nut chewing in an expatriate population in Sydney: report of two cases. Aust Dent J. 2012;57:373–8.
15. Hayes PA. Oral submucous fibrosis in a 4-year-old girl. Oral Surg Oral Med Oral Pathol. 1985;59:475–8.
16. Shah B, Lewis MAO, Bedi R. Oral submucous fibrosis in a 11-year-old Bangladeshi girl living in the United Kingdom. Br Dent J. 2001;191:130–2.
17. Tilakaratne WM, Ekanayake RP, Warnakulasuriya S. Oral submucous fibrosis: a historical perspective and a review on etiology and pathogenesis. Oral Surg Oral Med Oral Pathol Oral Radiol. 2016;122:178–91.
18. Papke R L, Brunzell D H, Biasi M. Cholinergic receptors and addiction. In Shoaib M, Wallace TL, editors. Behavioral pharmacology of the cholinergic system. Springer Nature Switzerland. Curr Topics Behav Neurosci 202; 45: 123–152.
19. Gupta PC, Warnakulasuriya S. Global epidemiology of areca nut usage. Addict Biol. 2002;1:77–83.
20. Ho CS, Gee MJ, Tsai CC, Lo CI, Hwang MN. Factors related to betel chewing among junior high school students in Taiwan. Community Dent Oral Epidemiol. 2000;28(2):150–4. https://doi.org/10.1034/j.1600-0528.2000.028002150.x.
21. Lu CT, Lan SJ, Hsieh CC, Yang MJ, Ko YC, Tsai CC, Yen YY. Prevalence and characteristics of areca nut chewers among junior high school students in Changhua county, Taiwan. Community Dent Oral Epidemiol. 1993;21:370–3.
22. Shah S, Merchant AT, Luby SP, Chotani RA. Addicted school children: Prevalence and characteristics of areca nut chewers among primary school children in Karachi. Pakistan J Paediatr Child Health. 2002;28:507–10.
23. Oakley E, Demaine L, Warnakulasuriya S. Areca (betel) nut chewing habit among high schoolchildren in the commonwealth of Northern Mariana Islands (Micronesia). Bull WHO. 2005;83:656–60.
24. Khandelwal A, Khandelwal V, Saha MK, et al. Prevalence of areca nut chewing in the middle school-going children of Indore. India Contemp Clin Dent. 2012;3(2):155–7.
25. Singhvi A, Joshi A, Bagul N, et al. The Insight for Initiation and Maintenance of areca nut chewing habit and its effects on oral health status among School Age Population in Western Rajasthan, India. J Clin Diagn Res. 2016;10(11):ZC15–8.
26. Wazir SS, Arora P, Kapoor S, Jayam R, et al. Prevalence of areca nut chewing habit among high school children of Parsa district of Nepal. J Oral Biol Craniofac Res. 2017;7:161–6.
27. More CB, Das S, Patel H, Adalja C, Kamatchi V, Venkatesh R. Proposed clinical classification for oral submucous fibrosis. Oral Oncol. 2012;48:200–2.
28. More CB, Rao NR, Hegde R, et al. Oral submucous fibrosis in children and adolescents: analysis of 36 cases. J Indian Soc Pedod Prev Dent. 2020;38(2):190–9. https://doi.org/10.4103/JISPPD.JISPPD_173_20.
29. Sitheeque M, Ariyawardana A, Ruwan Jayasinghe R, Tilakaratne W. Depigmentation of oral mucosa as the earliest possible manifestation of oral submucous fibrosis in Sri Lankan preschool children. J Investig Clin Dent. 2010;1(2):156–9. https://doi.org/10.1111/j.2041-1626.2010.00021.x.
30. Rao, et al. Oral submucous fibrosis: a contemporary narrative review with a proposed interprofessional approach for an early diagnosis and clinical management. J Otolaryngol Head Neck Surg. https://doi.org/10.1186/s40463-020-0399-7.
31. Gupta VK, Malhotra S, Patil R, Tripathi A. Oral submucous fibrosis at paediatric age, now time to think: series of two cases. Indian J Med Paediatr Oncol. 2013;34(2):107–10.
32. Maher R, et al. Role of areca nut in the causation of oral K.A. submucous fibrosis: a case-control study in Pakistan. J Oral Pathol Med. 1994;23(2):65–9.
33. Sinor P N, Gupta P C, Murti PR, Bhonsle RB A case-control study of oral submucous fibrosis with special reference to the etiologic role of areca nut. J Oral Pathol Med 1990;19 (2): 94e98.
34. Kujan O, Mello FW, Warnakulasuriya S. Malignant transformation of oral submucous fibrosis: a systematic review and meta-analysis. Oral Dis. 2021; https://doi.org/10.1111/odi.13727.
35. Ariyawardana A. Malignant transformation of potentially malignant disorders. In: Warnakulasuriya S, Greenspan JS, editors. Textbook of oral cancer, textbooks in contemporary dentistry. Springer Nature Switzerland AG; 2020. https://doi.org/10.1007/978-3-030-32316-5_13.
36. Yang PY, Chen YT, Wang YH, Su NY, Yu HC, Chang YC. Malignant transformation of oral submucous fibrosis in Taiwan: a nationwide population-based retrospective cohort study. J Oral Pathol Med. 2017;46(10):1040–5.
37. Anil S, Beena VT. Oral submucous fibrosis in a 12 year old girl: case report. Paed Dent. 1993;16(2):121–3.
38. Mundra RA, Gupta SK, Gupta Y. Oral submucous fibrosis in paediatric age group. Indian J Otolaryngol Head Neck Surg. 1999;51(3):60–2. https://doi.org/10.1007/BF02996533.
39. Yusuf H, Yong SL. Oral submucous fibrosis in a 12-year-old Bangladeshi boy: a case report and review of literature. Int J Paediatr Dent. 2002;12(4):271–6. https://doi.org/10.1046/j.1365-263x.2002.00373.x.

5

40. Hazarey VK, Erlewad DM, Mundhe KA, Ughade SN. Oral submucous fibrosis: study of 1000 cases from central India. J Oral Pathol Med. 2007;36(1):12–7. https://doi.org/10.1111/j.1600-0714.2006.00485.x.
41. Agrawal A, Sarkar PA, Shigli A. Oral submucous fibrosis in a 9-year-old Indian girl. BMJ Case Rep. 2011;2011.:bcr0820114588 https://doi.org/10.1136/bcr.08.2011.4588.
42. Dhariwal R, Ray JG, S, Pattanayak M, Swain N. Oral submucous fibrosis: a report of two pediatric cases and a brief review. J Indian Soc Pedod Prev Dent. 2012;30(1):85–8. https://doi.org/10.4103/0970-4388.95592.
43. Deshpande A, Kiran S, Dhillon S, Mallikarjuna R. Oral submucous fibrosis: a premalignant condition in a 14-year-old Indian girl. BMJ Case Rep. 2013.:bcr2013200786; https://doi.org/10.1136/bcr-2013-200786.
44. Dugirala TL, Marthala M, Gannepalli A, Podduturi SR. Oral submucous fibrosis in children: Report of three cases and review. J Indian Acad Oral Med Radiol. 2015;27:105–11.
45. Khandelwal V, Kambalimath HV, Reddy NB, Khandelwal S, et al. Oral submucous fibrosis in a school-going Indian adolescent boy. Int J Adolesc Med Health. https://doi.org/10.1515/ijamh-2016-0096.
46. Talla H, Reddy PVR, Mudavath M, Bathina T. Oral submucous fibrosis in a 5 year old child. Contemp Clin Dent. 2019;10(4):679–81. https://doi.org/10.4103/ccd.ccd_898_18.
47. Kariya P, Khobragade V, Sura S, Singh S. No age predilection for a disease like OSMF. A case report of 5-year-old child. J Oral Biol Craniofac Res. 2020;10(2):153–7. https://doi.org/10.1016/j.jobcr.2020.03.010.

# Classification Systems for Oral Submucous Fibrosis

*Kannan Ranganathan and Kavitha Loganathan*

## Contents



© The Author(s), under exclusive license to Springer Nature Switzerland AG 2023
S. Warnakulasuriya, K. Ranganathan (eds.), *Oral Submucous Fibrosis*, Textbooks in Contemporary Dentistry,
https://doi.org/10.1007/978-3-031-12855-4_6

## 6.1 Introduction

There are many classification systems, reported for OSF. The classifications are based on clinical signs (mouth opening, tongue protrusion and cheek flexibility), clinical symptoms (vesicle, burning sensation, dry mouth and dysphagia) and histopathological features (epithelial morphology, connective tissue changes, epithelial-connective tissue interface) alone or in combination. The different classification systems used from 1957 to 2018 are presented here.

6

**Properties of a Good Classification**

A good medical classification system should help clinicians stratify the patients to enable appropriate clinical management of the patient and aid in follow-up and prognostication. It should be

- Stable: Based on specific premise or criterion
- Suitable: Relevant to the subject of interest
- Unambiguous: The various groups/classes should be clearly defined
- Complete and mutually exclusive: All terms in each group or class should be distinct without overlap
- Flexible: It should be able to accommodate new entities as our understanding of the subject evolves
- Reproducible and communicable

**Learning Goals**

To familiarise the reader to the published classification systems on OSF to allow the best use of them in future epidemiological surveys and in clinical studies

## 6.2 Oral Submucous Fibrosis (OSF): Classification Systems

All classifications use clinical signs, clinical symptoms and histopathology of OSF either separately or in combination:

- Clinical signs:
  - Restriction in mouth opening (measured in mm/cm/finger width)
  - Limitation of tongue protrusion (measured in mm/cm)
  - Reduced cheek flexibility (measured in mm/cm)
  - Restricted soft palate movement
  - Deformity of uvula
  - Palpable fibrous bands
  - Pallor
  - Xerostomia (measured as salivary flow rate-stimulated/unstimulated saliva)
  - Lingual papillary atrophy
  - Leukoplakia
  - Erythroplakia
- Clinical symptoms:
  - Vesicles
  - Burning sensation
  - Restricted mouth opening
  - Inability to swallow
  - Dry mouth (perception of dryness by the patient)
- Histopathology:
  - Hyperkeratosis
  - Atrophy
  - Dysplasia
- Connective tissue changes:
  - Juxta-epithelial hyalinisation
  - Reduction in vascularity
  - Inflammatory cell infiltrate
  - Fibrosis
  - Muscle degeneration
- Epithelial connective tissue interface:
  - Flattened epithelial-connective tissue interface

The published classification systems are presented below in their chronological order.

### 6.2.1 Desa (1957)

In one of the earliest reports, an otolaryngologist, reported from the King Edward VII Memorial Hospital, Mumbai, India, the clinical presentation, history and the haematological and histological findings in 64 patients with OSF. In their classification system, the patients were divided into three stages, depending on the clinical features as [1]

- Stage I: Stomatitis and vesiculation

  Oral mucosa shows areas of redness on either the entire soft palate, the anterior faucial pillar or the buccal mucous membrane. It is in these areas the vesicles appear first; these vesicles are tender and rupture, leaving small superficial ulcers. Cultures of the vesicular fluid failed to reveal any specific organism.
- Stage 2: Stage of fibrosis

  Characterised by pallor of the mucous membrane together with small "spider-like" areas, due to the fibrosis, at the junction of the faucial pillars with the soft palate.
- Stage 3: Stage of sequelae

  The patients seek relief for the disabling effects produced by the increasing deposition of fibrous tissue in the submucosa. The fibrosis was described as being palatal, faucial or buccal. The mouth opening varied from 0.75 to 4.0 cm, depending on the severity of fibrosis (normal mouth opening was 4.05 cm).

### 6.2.2 Pindborg and Sirsat (1966)

Classified OSF, based on histology, into four stages based on the connective tissue changes, in haematoxylin and eosin-stained sections as follows [2]:

- Very early stage: Fine, fibrillar, dispersed collagen, marked oedema and connective tissue with plump young fibroblasts containing abundant cytoplasm. Blood vessels are normal or dilated and congested. Inflammatory cells seen are mainly polymorphonuclear leukocytes with occasional eosinophils.
- Early stage: There is juxta-epithelial hyalinisation. Collagen is in separate thick bundles. Moderate numbers of plump young fibroblasts are present, the blood vessels are dilated and congested. Inflammatory cells are primarily lymphocytes, eosinophils and occasional plasma cells.
- Moderately advanced stage: Collagen is moderately hyalinised, and this extends from the juxta-epithelial hyalinisation seen in the early stage. Collagen bundles are thick and separated by tissue oedema. Fibroblastic response is less marked, and the cells are predominantly spindle fibrocytes. Blood vessels are either normal or compressed, depending on the tissue fibrosis. Inflammatory exudate consists of lymphocytes and plasma cells.
- Advanced stage: Collagen is completely hyalinised and presents as a smooth sheet with loss of the bundle morphology of collagen. Oedema is absent. The hyalinised areas are devoid of fibroblasts. Blood vessels are completely obliterated or narrowed. Inflammatory cells are lymphocytes and plasma cells.

### 6.2.3 Wahi and Kapur et al. (1966)

Classified OSF based on the clinical features, severity and extent of involvement into three groups as follows [3]:

- Group I: Asymptomatic, focal fibrosis of one or more sites of oral mucosa with pallor or whitish coloration and wrinkling of mucosa with minimal induration.
- Group II: Soreness of mucosa or increased sensitivity to chillies. Oral mucosa is white, and the changes are diffuse and extensive and show induration, involving one or more anatomical sites.
- Group III: Restricted mobility due to trismus, stretching at angles of the mouth, and inability to protrude the tongue. Pronunciation is altered. Firm submucosal bands are palpable. Surface may be fissured or ulcerated.

### 6.2.4 Ahuja and Agarwal (1971)

This classification is discussed by Passi and colleagues in their review of classification systems and is based on the extent and type of clinical fibrosis [4, 5].

- Class I: Localised fibrous bands in the cheek extending from the superior to the inferior fornix on one or both sides. The bands are most commonly found on the lips followed by the premolar region or the second molar region.
- Class II: Generalised diffuse hardening of the subepithelial tissues extending from the cheek and hard palate to the soft palate, uvula and faucial pillars. Occasionally, the hardening might extend to the lining mucosa of the pharynx.
- Class III: Combination of the above two types, where the fibrous bands are associated with a generalised diffuse form of submucous fibrosis.

### 6.2.5 Bhatt and Dholakia (1977)

Clinically grouped OSF patients into three grades based on the subjective assessment of mouth opening and clinical fibrosis as follows [6]:

- Grade I: Mild and early cases with very slight fibrous bands and little difficulty in opening of the mouth.
- Grade II: Moderately pronounced symptoms with fibrous bands extending from the cheek to the palate.
- Grade III: Excessive amount of fibrosis involving the cheek, palate, uvula, tongue and lips with narrow opening of the mouth.

### 6.2.6 Gupta and Golhar (1980)

Classified OSF into four stages based primarily on the severity of trismus as follows [7]:

- Very early stage: No difficulty in mouth opening; the patients have burning sensation in the mouth or ulceration.
- Early stage: Along with burning sensation, the patients complain of slight difficulty in opening the mouth.
- Moderately advanced stage: Trismus is marked to such an extent that the patient cannot open his/her mouth more than two fingers width and has difficulty in mastication.
- Advanced stage: Patient has a marked degree of trismus and is undernourished and anaemic.

### 6.2.7 Warnakulasuriya (1987)

Provided a semi-quantitative grading of the severity of OSF based on mouth opening, fibrous banding and fixation of the tongue. Assessment was based on (a) three groups of mouth opening <20 mm, 20–35 mm and >35 mm; (b) fibrous bands of buccal mucosa grouped as broad single band >2 cm, multiple bands and a single, thin fibrous band; (c) ability to protrude the tongue beyond mucocutaneous (MC) junction: beyond lower incisors but unable to touch MC junction and only up to lower incisors [8].



### 6.2.8 Pindborg (1989)

Divided OSF into three stages based on clinical signs and symptoms. This classification is discussed by Gupta and colleagues in their review of classification systems [9, 10].

- Stage I: Stomatitis - includes erythematous mucosa, vesicles, mucosal ulcers, melanotic mucosal pigmentations and mucosal petechiae.
- Stage II: Fibrosis occurring in the healing vesicles and ulcers is the hallmark of this stage. Early lesions demonstrate blanching of the oral mucosa. Older lesions include vertical and circular palpable fibrous bands in the buccal mucosa and around the mouth opening or lips resulting in mottled marble-like appearance of the mucosa, because of the vertical thick fibrous bands in association with blanched mucosa. Specific findings include reduction of mouth opening, stiff and small tongue, blanched and leathery floor of the mouth, fibrotic and depigmented gingiva, rubbery soft palate with decreased mobility, blanched and atrophic tonsils, shrunken bud-like uvula and sunken cheeks, not commensurate with age or nutritional status.
- Stage III: Sequelae of OSF: Leukoplakia is found in more than 25% of the individuals with OSF. Speech and hearing defects may occur due to involvement of the tongue and Eustachian tubes.

### 6.2.9 Katharia et al. (1992)

In their study on the effects of placenta extract in the management of OSF described a scoring system [11] based on (a) the mouth opening, (b) tongue protrusion measured as the distance between incisal edges of lower anterior teeth and tongue tip protruded to its maximum, (c) colour of oral mucosa, (d) fibrous band and (e) burning sensation.

a. Mouth opening: Measured in mm between upper and lower central incisor edges:
   - Score 0: Mouth opening is greater than 41 mm.
   - Score 1: Mouth opening between 37 and 40 mm.
   - Score 2: Mouth opening between 33 and 36 mm.
   - Score 3: Mouth opening between 29 and 32 mm.
   - Score 4: Mouth opening between 25 and 28 mm.
   - Score 5: Mouth opening between 21 and 24 mm.
   - Score 6: Mouth opening between 17 and 20 mm.
   - Score 7: Mouth opening between 13 and 16 mm.
   - Score 8: Mouth opening between 9 and 12 mm.
   - Score 9: Mouth opening between 5 and 8 mm.
   - Score 10: Mouth opening between 0 and 4 mm.
b. Tongue protrusion: measured in mm as the distance between incisal edges of lower anterior teeth and tip of tongue, protruded to its maximum:
   - Score 0: ≥33 mm
   - Score 1: 30-32 mm
   - Score 2: 27-29 mm
   - Score 3: 24-26 mm
   - Score 4: 21-23 mm
   - Score 5: 18-20 mm
   - Score 6: 15-17 mm
   - Score 7: 12-14 mm
   - Score 8: 9-11 mm
   - Score 9: 5-8 mm
   - Score 10: 0-4 mm
c. Colour of oral mucosa:
   - Score 0: normal pink
   - Score 1: red or deep pink
   - Score 2: pale white
   - Score 3: blanched white
d. Fibrous band:
   - Score 0: no fibrous bands
   - Score 1: one or two solitary fibrous bands
   - Score 2: bands felt nearly in the entire surface
   - Score 3: adherent fibrous band producing binding and rigidity of mucosa
e. Burning sensation:
   - Score 0: no burning sensation
   - Score 1: mild
   - Score 2: moderate
   - Score 3: severe

### 6.2.10 Bailoor (1993)

This classification is discussed by Passi and colleagues in their review of classification systems and is based on a combination of clinical features as follows [5, 12]:

- Stage I: Early OSF:

  Mild blanching. No restriction in mouth opening (normal distance between central incisor tips: males

35–45 mm, females 30–42 mm). No restriction in tongue protrusion (normal mesio-incisal angle of the upper central incisor to the tip of the tongue when maximally extended with the mouth wide open: males 5–6 cm, females 4.5–5.5 cm). Cheek flexibility was measured from a reference point one-third the distance from the angle of the mouth on a line joining the tragus of the ear to the angle of the mouth. The patient is asked to blow his or her cheeks fully, and the distance between the points marked on the cheek indicates cheek flexibility. Mean values for cheek flexibility: males 1.2 cm and females 1.08 cm. Burning sensation on taking spicy or hot foods only.

- Stage II: Moderate OSF

  Moderate-to-severe blanching. Mouth opening reduced by 33%. Cheek flexibility also demonstrably reduced. Burning sensation in the absence of stimuli. Palpable bands felt. Lymphadenopathy either unilateral or bilateral. Demonstrable anaemia on haematological examination.
- Stage III: Severe OSF

  More than 66% reduction in the mouth opening, cheek flexibility and tongue protrusion. Tongue may appear fixed. Severe burning sensation; patient is unable to do day-to-day work. Ulcerative lesions may appear on the cheek. Thick palpable bands. Bilateral lymphadenopathy.

### 6.2.11 Racher (1993)

Classified OSF into three stages based on clinical features. This classification is discussed by Passi and colleagues in their review of classification systems [5].

- Stage I: Stage of stomatitis and vesiculation. Characterised by recurrent stomatitis and vesiculation. Patient complains of burning sensation in the mouth and inability to eat pungent food. The examination reveals vesicles on the palate that may rupture, and superficial ulceration may be seen. Some amount of fibrosis can be seen.
- Stage II: Stage of fibrosis. There is inability to open the mouth completely and stiffness in mastication. As disease advances, there is difficulty in blowing the cheeks and protruding the tongue. On examination, there is increasing fibrosis in the submucosal tissue. Mucosa is blanched and white. Lips and cheeks are stiff. Dorsum of the tongue may show atrophy of papillae. Blanching and stiffness of the mucosa of the floor of the mouth are less marked than those seen in the lips, cheeks and palate. Larynx is free from disease, and respiration is not affected.
- Stage III: Stage of sequelae and complications. Leukoplakia changes in the mucosa. An ulcerating malignant lesion may be seen involving the cheeks, oropharynx or tongue. Patients are predisposed to develop oral cancer under the influence of carcinogens.

### 6.2.12 Khanna and Andrade (1995)

Studied a series of 100 patients prospectively and proposed a group classification system based on both clinical and histopathological features to aid in the surgical management of OSF. OSF was staged into four categories [13]:

- Group I: Very early cases:
  - Clinically: Burning sensation in the mouth, acute ulceration and recurrent stomatitis; not associated with mouth opening limitation.
  - Histology: Fine fibrillar collagen network, oedema, dilated and congested blood vessels, large aggregates of plump young fibroblasts with abundant cytoplasm. Inflammatory cells consist of polymorphonuclear leukocytes with few eosinophils. The epithelium is normal.
- Group II: Early cases
  - Clinically: Limitation of mouth opening; the buccal mucosa is mottled and marble-like; there is palpable fibrosis predominantly involving soft palate and faucial pillars.
  - Histology: Juxta-epithelial hyalinisation; thick bundles of collagen are present that are in separate bundles; dilated and congested blood vessels; and moderate number of young fibroblasts. Inflammatory cells are mainly polymorphonuclear leukocytes with few eosinophils and occasional plasma cell. Epithelial rete pegs are short and flat with varying degrees of keratinisation.
- Group III: Moderately advanced cases
  - Clinically: Trismus with interincisal distance of 15–25 mm. Pale buccal mucosa firmly adherent to underlying tissues with palpable, fibrous bands in the premolar region, the soft palate anterior faucial pillar and the pterygomandibular raphe. The fibrosis has a scar-like appearance. Some cases exhibit atrophy of vermilion border of the lip.
  - Histology: Juxta-epithelial hyalinisation with faintly visible collagen bundles. There is mild oedema, constricted blood vessels and mature fibroblasts with scanty cytoplasm and spindle-shaped nuclei. The inflammatory cells present are lymphocytes and plasma cells. The surface epithelium is markedly atrophic with loss of rete pegs. Muscle fibres exhibit fibrosis and early signs of degeneration such as loss of striae.

- Group IV is subdivided into IVA and IVB.
- Group IVA: Advanced cases:
  - Clinically: Severe trismus with interincisal distance of 2–15 mm; fibrosed faucial pillars compressing the tonsil, shrunken and deformed uvula and restricted tongue movement. There may be diffuse papillary atrophy of the tongue. Fibrosis of the lip occurs leading to constriction of the rima oris and vermilion border atrophy.
- Group IVB: Advanced cases with "premalignant/malignant changes":
  - Clinically: OSF features with potentially malignant lesions such as leukoplakia and/or squamous cell carcinoma.
  - Histology: Hyalinised connective tissue in which the collagen bundles cannot be discerned. Blood vessels are obliterated. Fibroblasts are absent or scanty. The surface epithelium exhibits loss of melanocytes and epithelial rete ridges. Epithelium may show mild-to-moderate atypia or malignant changes in Group IVB. There is extensive degeneration of muscle fibres.



The authors recommend that patients in group I and group II be managed by symptomatic treatment, whereas those in group III and group IV by surgical management.

### 6.2.13 Lai et al. (1995)

Examined a series of 150 patients and divided their cohort of 150 OSF patients into six groups for management: medical (groups A, B, C) and surgical (groups D, E, F). Their classification was based on the interincisal distance as follows [14]:

- Group A: Interincisal distance greater than 35 mm
- Group B: Interincisal distance 30–35 mm
- Group C: Interincisal distance 20–30 mm
- Groups D, E, F: Interincisal distance less than 20 mm

### 6.2.14 Maher et al. (1996)

Their classification of OSF was based on the extent of the clinical disease based on the overall clinical impression. They subdivided intra-oral regions into seven areas: palate, posterior one-third of the buccal mucosa, middle one-third of the buccal mucosa, anterior one-third of the buccal mucosa, upper labial mucosa, tongue and floor of the mouth. These areas were further grouped into three categories [15]:

- Involvement of one-third or less of the oral cavity (three or less of the above zones involved)
- Involvement of one-third to two-thirds of the oral cavity (if four to six intra-oral sites are involved)
- Involvement of more than two-thirds of the oral cavity (if more than six intra-oral sites are involved)

### 6.2.15 Haider et al. (2000)

Their criteria for diagnosis of OSF was the presence of mucosal blanching, mucosal hardness, and palpable intra-oral bands. Following diagnosis, the patients were clinically and functionally staged [16]:

- Clinical staging:
  - Stage 1: Faucial bands only
  - Stage 2: Faucial and buccal bands
  - Stage 3: Faucial, buccal and labial bands
- Functional staging:
  - Stage A: Mouth opening greater than 20 mm
  - Stage B: Mouth opening between 11 and 19 mm
  - Stage C: Mouth opening less than or equal to 10 mm

### 6.2.16 Ranganathan et al. (2001)

Reported normal mouth opening, tongue protrusion and cheek flexibility in 800 patients and proposed the classification for OSF based on mouth opening as follows [17]:

- Group I: Only symptoms with no demonstrable restriction of mouth opening
- Group II: Limited mouth opening 20 mm and above
- Group III: Mouth opening less than 20 mm
- Group IV: OSF advanced with limited mouth opening and precancerous or cancerous changes

### 6.2.17 Rajendran (2003)

Classified OSF based on the clinical features as follows [18].

- Early OSF: Burning sensation in the mouth on consuming spicy food, blisters especially on the palate, ulceration or recurrent generalised inflammation of oral mucosa, petechiae, excessive salivation, defective gustatory sensation, dryness of mouth and pain on palpation of the fibrous bands.
- Advanced OSF: Blanched and slightly opaque mucosa, fibrous bands in the buccal mucosa running in vertical direction. Palate and faucial pillars are the areas first involved with gradual impairment of tongue movement and difficulty in mouth opening due to the fibrosis of the pterygomandibular raphe.

### 6.2.18 Utsonumiya et al. (2005)

Classified OSF based on histological features as follows [19]:

- Early stage: Myxedematous changes in the area corresponding to lamina propria, diffuse lymphocytic infiltration and no fibrosis.
- Intermediate stage: Hyalinisation in sub-epithelial zone, fibrotic changes extending close to the muscles. Blood vessels are compressed by fibrous bundles. Reduced inflammatory cells in sub-epithelial layer are seen.
- Advanced stage: Marked fibrous areas with hyaline changes extending from sub-epithelial to superficial muscle layers are seen. Atrophic, degenerative changes start in muscle fibres. Inflammatory cell infiltrates are hardly seen. Number of blood vessels is dramatically less in the sub-epithelial zone.

### 6.2.19 Bose and Balan (2007)

Classified OSF based on clinical features as follows [20]:

- Group A: Mild cases with occasional symptoms, pallor, vesicles, one or two solitary palpable bands, loss of mucosal elasticity, variable tongue fibrosis with tongue protrusion beyond vermillion border. Mouth opening is greater than 3 cm.
- Group B: Moderate cases with soreness of oral mucosa, increased sensitivity to chillies, diffuse involvement of the mucosa with blanched appearance, buccal mucosa is tough and inelastic with fibrous bands palpable, considerable restriction of mouth opening (1.5–3 cm) and variable tongue movement.
- Group C: Severe cases with symptoms being more severe, broad fibrous bands palpable, blanched opaque mucosa, rigid oral mucosa, severe restriction of mouth opening (less than 1.5 cm), tongue is depapillated with restricted tongue protrusion.

### 6.2.20 Kumar et al. (2007)

Clinical stage of the disease in terms of the ability to open mouth was correlated with histopathological grading. Clinical criteria for the diagnosis of OSF were difficulty in opening the mouth and associated blanched oral mucosa with palpable fibrous bands. The distance between the interincisal edges was measured in mm for assessing the ability to open the mouth [21].

OSF cases were clinically categorised into three clinical stages according to their ability to open mouth as follows:

- Stage I: Mouth opening greater than 45 mm
- Stage II: Mouth opening between 20 and 44 mm
- Stage III: Mouth opening less than 20 mm

The histopathological grading followed in the study is as follows:

- Grade I: Loose connective tissue thick and thin fibres
- Grade II: Loose connective tissue with thick fibres and partial hyalinisation
- Grade III: Complete connective tissue hyalinisation

### 6.2.21 Mehrotra et al. (2009)

The patients were divided into four groups based on their clinical presentations as [22]:

- Grade I: Stomatitis, burning sensation in the buccal mucosa and with no palpable fibrous bands.
- Grade II: Symptoms of grade I, palpable fibrous bands, involvement of soft palate and maximal mouth opening of 26–35 mm.
- Grade III: Symptoms of grade II, blanched oral mucosa, involvement of tongue and maximal mouth opening of 6–25 mm.
- Grade IV: Symptoms of grade III, lip fibrosis and mouth opening of less than or equal to 5 mm. Suggested treatment is abstinence from habit and surgical management.

### 6.2.22 More et al. (2011)

Their classification was based on the common site of occurrence, symptoms, other affected sites and associated lesions as follows [23]:

I. Clinical staging:
   - S1: Stomatitis and/or blanching of oral mucosa
   - S2: Presence of palpable fibrous bands in buccal mucosa and/or oropharynx, with/without stomatitis
   - S3: Presence of palpable fibrous bands in buccal mucosa and/or oropharynx, and in any other parts of oral cavity, with/without stomatitis
   - S4: A: Any one of the above stages along with other potentially malignant disorders, e.g. oral leukoplakia and oral erythroplakia. B: Any one of the above stages along with oral carcinoma

II. Functional staging:
   - M1: Interincisal mouth opening up to or greater than 35 mm
   - M2: Interincisal mouth opening between 25 and 35 mm

- M3: Interincisal mouth opening between 15 and 25 mm
- M4: Interincisal mouth opening less than 15 mm

A combination of the clinical and functional staging was used to stratify patients for management. For example, the final staging may be S1M1, S2M3, S2M4 and so on.

### 6.2.23 Kerr et al. (2011)

Proposed the following grading system for OSF, following the World Workshop on Oral Medicine (WWOM V) as a recommendation for future studies on the various aspects of OSF, based on clinical severity as follows [24]:

- Grade 1: Mild: Any features of the disease triad for OSF (burning, depapillation, blanching or leathery mucosa) may be reported. Interincisal opening greater than 35 mm
- Grade 2: Moderate: Above features of OSF and interincisal limitation of opening between 20 and 35 mm
- Grade 3: Severe: Above features of OSF and interincisal opening less than 20 mm
- Grade 4A: Above features of OSF with other potentially malignant disorders on clinical examination. Grade 4B: Above features of OSF with any grade of oral epithelial dysplasia on biopsy
- Grade 5: Above features of OSF with oral squamous cell carcinoma

### 6.2.24 Patil and Maheshwari (2014)

Diagnosis of OSF was made on clinical symptoms and fibrosis. They proposed that patients with OSF can be further classified based on cheek flexibility, which was measured as "distance in millimetres, from maxillary incisal midline to the cheek retractor during retraction". Their proposed values for normal cheek flexibility were males 35 to 45 mm and females 30 to 40 mm [25]:

- Grade 1 (early): Cheek flexibility of 30 mm and above
- Grade 2 (mild): Cheek flexibility between 20 and 30 mm
- Grade 3 (moderate): Cheek flexibility less than 20 mm
- Grade 4 (severe): Any of the above condition without concurrent presence of potential malignant lesions
- Grade 5 (advanced): Any of the above condition with concurrent presence of oral carcinoma

### 6.2.25 Arakeri et al. (2018)

They proposed a classification based on trismus, fibrosis and presence or absence of malignant changes in the epithelium, which they called TFM classification [26], with recommendations for therapy based on their staging.

| **Parameters of TFM classification** |
|---|
| **Trismus (T)** |
| TX: Trismus cannot be assessed due to the presence of confounding factors such as tooth impingement, temporomandibular join disorders (TMDs) and infection |
| T0: Interincisal distance of more than 36 mm |
| T1: Interincisal distance of 26–35 mm |
| T2: Interincisal distance of 15–25 mm |
| T3: Interincisal distance of less than 15 mm |
| TE: Edentulous (E) state due to either complete or partial loss of anterior teeth |
| TE0: Anterior free space after maximum mouth opening more than 41 mm |
| TE1: Anterior free space after maximum mouth opening of 36–40 mm |
| TE2: Anterior free space after maximum mouth opening of 25–35 mm |
| TE3: Anterior free space after maximum mouth opening of less than 25 mm |
| **Fibrosis (F)** |
| F0: No signs of fibrosis |
| FX: Fibrosis cannot be assessed due to severe trismus |
| F1: Burning sensation in the mouth and/or blanching of oral mucosa and/or acute ulceration and/or recurrent stomatitis |
| F2: Mottled and marble-like oral mucosa, dense, pale, depigmented fibrosed areas alternated with pink normal mucosa, widespread sheets of fibrosis (palpable fibrous bands) involving labial and/or buccal mucosa and/or oropharynx |
| F3: Pale oral mucosa firmly attached to underlying tissues, palpable vertical fibrous bands at the buccal mucosa and in the soft palate-radiating fibrous bands from the pterygomandibular raphe or the anterior faucial pillar in a scar-like appearance, atrophy of the vermilion border, patient unable to blow out cheeks and whistle |
| F4: Thickened faucial pillars, shrunken fibrous bud-like small uvula, narrowed isthmus, restricted tongue movement, diffuse papillary atrophy, palpable circular fibrous band around the entire mouth, obliquity of rima oris, vermilion border atrophy |

| Malignant transformation (M) |
|---|
| M0: No signs of malignant transformation |
| MX: Malignant transformation cannot be assessed due to severe trismus |
| MQ: Lesion in question |
| MP: Associated potentially malignant disorder |
| M1: Histopathological evidence of dysplasia |
| M1a: Low grade |
| M1b: High grade |
| M2: Histopathological evidence of malignant transformation |

| TFM staging of oral submucous fibrosis | |
|---|---|
| **Stages** | **TFM classification** |
| Stage 1 (medical therapy): | $T_{0\text{-}2/\,E0\text{-}E2}$ or $F_{1\text{-}2}$, $M_{0,1a}$ |
| Stage 2 (surgical therapy): | $T_{2\text{-}3/E2\text{-}E3}$ or $F_{3\text{-}4}$, $M_{0,1b}$ |
| Stage 3 (neoplastic disease therapy): | Any T, $F_{1\text{-}4}$, $M_2$ |

## Summary

As discussed, vide supra, each classification is based on a premise which is unique to the aspect being studied in OSF. The features are summarised in ▣ Table 6.1

▣ **Table 6.1** Summary of features used by authors in their classification systems

| Authors | Clinical signs | Clinical symptoms | Histopathological features |
|---|---|---|---|
| 1. Desa (1957) | ✓ | ✓ | ✕ |
| 2. Pindborg and Sirsat (1966) | ✕ | ✕ | ✓ |
| 3. Wahi and Kapur et al. (1966) | ✓ | ✓ | ✕ |
| 4. Ahuja and Agarwal (1971) | ✓ | ✕ | ✕ |
| 5. Bhatt and Dholakia (1977) | ✓ | ✓ | ✕ |
| 6. Gupta and Golhar (1980) | ✓ | ✓ | ✕ |
| 7. Warnakulasuriya (1987) | ✓ | ✓ | ✕ |
| 8. Pindborg (1989) | ✓ | ✓ | ✕ |
| 9. Katharia et al. (1992) | ✓ | ✓ | ✕ |
| 10. Bailoor (1993) | ✓ | ✓ | ✕ |
| 11. Racher (1993) | ✓ | ✓ | ✕ |
| 12. Khanna and Andrade (1995) | ✓ | ✓ | ✓ |
| 13. Lai et al (1995) | ✓ | ✕ | ✕ |
| 14. Maher et al. (1996) | ✓ | ✕ | ✕ |
| 15. Haider (2000) | ✓ | ✕ | ✕ |
| 16. Ranganathan et al. (2001) | ✓ | ✓ | ✕ |
| 17. Rajendran (2003) | ✓ | ✓ | ✕ |
| 18.Utsonumiya et al. (2005) | ✕ | ✕ | ✓ |
| 19. Bose and Balan (2007) | ✓ | ✓ | ✕ |
| 20. Kumar et al. (2007) | ✓ | ✕ | ✓ |
| 21. Mehrotra et al. (2009) | ✓ | ✓ | ✕ |
| 22. More et al. (2011) | ✓ | ✓ | ✕ |
| 23. Kerr et al. (2011) | ✓ | ✓ | ✓ |
| 24. Patil and Maheshwari (2014) | ✓ | ✕ | ✕ |
| 25. Arakeri et al. (2018) | ✓ | ✓ | ✓ |

## 6.3 Conclusion and Recommendations

There are many classification systems that have been suggested [5, 10, 23, 26–29]. Four of the systems recommend using both clinical and histopathological features to classify the disease [13, 21, 24, 26]. The classification by Pindborg and Sirsat [2] is the widely accepted histopathological classification. Khanna and Andrade's [14] classification system includes both clinical and histopathological features and is often used by clinicians. The Fifth World Workshop on Oral Medicine discussed the published studies and emphasised the need for a system that could assess the clinical severity and be used in clinical trials. OSF has a spectrum of features that segue without distinct demarcation as the disease progresses. This makes it difficult to have a classification system that is unambiguous and mutually exclusive. Consequently, the classification system chosen will depend on the variables being studied.



## References


1. Desa JV. Submucous fibrosis of palate and cheek. Otol Rhinol Laryngol. 1957;66:1143–59. https://doi.org/10.1177/000348945706600420.
2. Pindborg JJ, Sirsat SM. Oral submucous fibrosis. Oral Surg Oral Med Oral Pathol. 1966;22:764–79. https://doi.org/10.1016/0030-4220(66)90367-7.
3. Wahi PN, Kapur VL, Luthra UK, Srivastava MC. Submucous fibrosis of the oral cavity. 1. Clinical features, 2. Studies on epidemiology. Bull World Health Organ. 1966;35:789–99.
4. Ahuja SS, Agrawal GD. Submucous fibrosis of the oral mucosa. J Oral Med. 1971;26:35–6.
5. Passi D, Bhanot P, Kacker D, Chahal D, Atri M, Panwar Y. Oral submucous fibrosis: Newer proposed classification with critical updates in pathogenesis and management strategies. Natl J Maxillofac Surg. 2017;8(2):89–94. https://doi.org/10.4103/njms.NJMS_32_17.
6. Bhatt AP, Dholakia HM. Mast cell density in OSMF. J Indian Dent Assoc. 1977;49:187–91.
7. Gupta DS, Gupta MK, Golhar BL. Oral submucous fibrosis: a clinical study and management of physiofibrolysis (MWD). J Indian Dent Assoc. 1980;52:375–8.
8. Warnakulasuriya S. Semi-quantitative clinical description of oral submucous fibrosis. Ann Dent. 1987;46(2):18–21.
9. Pindborg JJ. Oral submucous fibrosis: a review. Ann Acad Med Singapore. 1989;18(5):603–7.
10. Gupta H, Grover N, Tyagi N, Misra A. Classification systems in oral submucous fibrosis patients: a review. TMU J Dent. 2018;5(2):13–9.
11. Katharia SK, Singh SP, Kulshreshtha VP. The effects of placental extract in management of oral sub-mucous fibrosis. Ind J Pharma. 1992;24:181–3.
12. Bailoor DN. Oral submucous fibrosis: the Mangalore study. IAOMR. 1993;4:12–5.
13. Khanna JN, Andrade NN. Oral submucous fibrosis: a new concept in surgical management. Report of 100 cases. Int J Oral Maxillofac Surg. 1995;24:433–9.
14. Lai DR, Chen HR, Huang YL, Tsai CC. Clinical evaluation of different treatment methods for oral submucous fibrosis: a 10-year experience with 150 cases. J Oral Pathol Med. 1995;24:402–6. https://doi.org/10.1111/j.1600-0714.1995.tb01209.x.
15. Maher R, Sankaranarayanan R, Johnson NW, Warnakulasuriya KAAS. Evaluation of inter-incisor distance as an objective criterion of the severity of oral submucous fibrosis in Karachi, Pakistan. Eur J Cancer Part B: Oral Oncol. 1996;32:362–4. https://doi.org/10.1016/0964-1955(96)00009-7.
16. Haider SM, Merchant AT, Fikree FF, Rahbar MH. Clinical and functional staging of oral submucous fibrosis. J Oral Maxillofac Surg. 2000;38:12–5. https://doi.org/10.1054/bjom.1999.0062.
17. Ranganathan K, Uma Devi M, Elizabeth J, Kiran Kumar K, Saraswathi TR. Oral submucous fibrosis: a case control study in Chennai, South India. J Oral Pathol Med. 2004;33:274–7. https://doi.org/10.1111/j.0904-2512.2004.00116.x.
18. Rajendran R. Oral submucous fibrosis. J Oral Maxillofac Pathol. 2003;7:1–4.
19. Utsunomiya H, Tilakaratne WM, Oshiro K, et al. Extracellular matrix remodelling in oral submucous fibrosis: Its stage-specific modes revealed by immunohistochemistry and in situ hybridization. J Oral Pathol Med. 2005;34:498–507. https://doi.org/10.1111/j.1600-0714.2005.00339.x.
20. Bose T, Balan A. OSMF: A changing scenario. JIAOMR. 2007;19:334–40.
21. Kumar K, Saraswathi TR, Ranganathan K, Uma DM, Joshua E. Oral submucous fibrosis: a clinicohistopathological study in Chennai. Ind J Dent Res. 2007;18:106–11. https://doi.org/10.4103/0970-9290.33785.
22. Mehrotra D, Pradhan R, Gupta S. Retrospective comparison of surgical treatment modalities in 100 patients with oral submucous fibrosis. Oral Surg Oral Med Oral Pathol Oral Radiol Endod. 2009;107:e1–10. https://doi.org/10.1016/j.tripleo.2008.12.012.
23. More CB, Das S, Patel H, Adalja C, Kamatchi V, Venkatesh R. Proposed clinical classification for oral submucous fibrosis. Oral Oncol. 2012;48:200–2. https://doi.org/10.1016/j.oraloncology.2011.10.011.
24. Kerr AR, Warnakulasuriya S, Mighell AJ, et al. A systematic review of medical interventions for oral submucous fibrosis and future research opportunities. Oral Dis. 2011;17(Suppl. 1):42–57. https://doi.org/10.1111/j.1601-0825.2011.01791.x.
25. Patil S, Maheshwari S. Proposed new grading of oral submucous fibrosis based on cheek flexibility. J Clin Exp Dent. 2014;6(3):e255–8. Published 2014 Jul 1. https://doi.org/10.4317/jced.51378.
26. Arakeri G, Thomas D, Aljabab AS, Hunasgi S, Rai KK, Hale B, Fonseca FP, Gomez RS, Rahimi S, Merkx MAW, Brennan PA. TFM classification and staging of oral submucous fibrosis: a new proposal. J Oral Pathol Med. 2018;47(4):403–9. https://doi.org/10.1111/jop.12689. Epub 2018 Mar 2
27. Priyadharshni B. Classification system for oral submucous grading: a review. Int J Sci Res. 2014;3(3):740–4.
28. Vikas Berwal V, Khangwal M, Solanki R, Khandeparker R, Savant K, Shetye O. Classification systems for oral submucous fibrosis- from past to present: a review. Int J Dental Health Sci. 2014;1(6):900–13.
29. Shivakumar GC, Sahana S. Clinical staging of oral submucous fibrosis: a review. Int J Oral-Med Sci. 2011;10(3):216–9.

# Malignant Transformation of Oral Submucous Fibrosis

*Omar Kujan and Majdy Idrees*

**Contents**



© The Author(s), under exclusive license to Springer Nature Switzerland AG 2023

S. Warnakulasuriya, K. Ranganathan (eds.), *Oral Submucous Fibrosis*, Textbooks in Contemporary Dentistry,
https://doi.org/10.1007/978-3-031-12855-4_7

## 7.1 Introduction

Oral potentially malignant disorders (OPMDs) include a variety of lesions and conditions with different aetiologies and clinicopathological presentations, but all share an increased risk of malignant transformation [1]. One of the most prevalent OPMDs is oral submucous fibrosis (OSF), which is a relatively widespread disorder in Southeast Asia and in the Pacific [2, 3].

Several chapters in this textbook have addressed significant aspects of this disorder such as epidemiology, aetiology, pathogenesis, clinical and histopathological features, staging, and predictive and prognostic biomarkers. This chapter aims to provide an updated review of the malignant transformation potential of oral submucous fibrosis.

7

Paymaster, in 1956, first described the potential malignant nature of OSF among a cohort of 650 patients [4]. Since then, many reports have been published to describe the malignant transformation rate of OSF, with estimations ranging from 1.2% to 9.1% [3]. However, these reports are associated with a very high level of heterogeneity and a relatively low quality [3, 5], which may indicate that the actual number is underestimated. A recent meta-analysis published in a special issue by the WHO Collaborating Centre for Oral Cancer on OPMDs revealed that the pooled ratio of malignant transformation among patients with OSF is 4.6%, and the annual malignant transformation rate is 0.73% [3].

**Learning Goals**

- Provide a global estimation of the malignant transformation rate of oral submucous fibrosis.
- Discuss the related literature in detail and highlight the major outcomes of each individual study.
- Explain the demographic, pathological, and molecular factors contributing to the malignant transformation of oral submucous fibrosis.

## 7.2 Insight into the Literature

An extensive search of the literature was conducted through various databases (Web of Science, MEDLINE by PubMed, Embase, Scopus) for the period from 1952 to October 2021 using special MeSH terms [3] to find relevant studies that documented the rate and/or risk of malignant transformation of OSF. The search revealed 611 papers, which were screened. Of these, 14 papers underwent further assessment. Of these papers, nine reported the malignant transformation rate of OSF [6–14] (Table 7.1), while the others were either cross-sectional or case-control without further details to assess the malignant transformation rate [15–19] (Table 7.2).

**Table 7.1** General description of relevant studies about the malignant transformation rate and/or risk of OSF

| Authors/year | Country | Design | Total (N) M:F | Mean age (years) | MT (N) | Overall MT ratio | Annual MT rate | Follow-up (years) | General description/main findings |
|---|---|---|---|---|---|---|---|---|---|
| Jian et al. 2021 [14] | China | Prospective | 567 | – | 32 | 5.6% | – | – | An institutional prospective study reported from Hunan province in China. All OSF cases were among areca nut chewers. Patients with verrucopapillary lesions or leukoplakia had higher transformation |
| Chiang et al. 2020 [13] | Taiwan | Prospective | 87 | – | 4 | 4.6% | 0.69% | 6.7 | To assess the MT rate among a group of OPMDs. The independent risk factor for the MT of OPMDs was heavy betel quid chewing. No data were specifically provided for OSF |
| Chuang et al. 2018 [12] | Taiwan | Prospective | 2333 No females | – | 114 | 4.8% | 0.86% | 5.7 | To assess the MT rate among OPMDs and identify risk factors. The estimated annual malignant risk per 1000 was 8.9 for OSF with betel nut chewing. The risk of OSF MT was higher among patients aged more than 50 years |

**Table 7.1** (continued)

| Authors/ year | Country | Design | Total (N) M:F | Mean age (years) | MT (N) | Overall MT ratio | Annual MT rate | Follow-up (years) | General description/main findings |
|---|---|---|---|---|---|---|---|---|---|
| Yang et al. 2017 [11] | Taiwan | Retrospective | 778<br>678:100 | 41.8 ± 11.7 | 71 | 9.1% | 1.4% | 6.5 | To investigate the MT rate of OSF. Patients with OSF are associated with a significantly higher risk of MT than controls. OLK enhances the MT potential when combined with OSF. This risk of MT was higher among the males in comparison to the females |
| Chourasia et al., 2015 [10] | India | Retrospective | 119<br>88:31 | 33.8 | 5 | 4.2% | – | – | The incidence of oral cancer concomitant with OSF was 25.77%. The authors concluded that the malignant potential of OSF is underestimated |
| Wang et al. 2014 [9] | Taiwan | Retrospective | 1180<br>1091:89 | 44.69 ± 12.43 | 46 | 3.9% | – | – | To assess the MT risk among a group of OPMDs. Risk factors were not identified for individual OSF cases. 88.43% and 86.2% of OSF cases were associated with betel quid and smoking, respectively |
| Hazarey et al. 2007 [8] | India | Retrospective | 1000<br>830: 170 | M<br>27.60 ± 9.58<br>F<br>34.78 ± 12.21 | 33 | 3.3% | 0.66% | 5 | OSF MT was significantly associated with increased frequency of betel quid chewing and smoking. The majority of the malignant transformed cases were diagnosed as OSCC, 28 out of 33 cases |
| Hsue et al. 2007 [7] | Taiwan | Prospective | 439 | – | 10 | 2.3% | 0.63% | 3.6 | To assess the rate of OSF MT. The mean time of MT was shorter for cases with epithelial dysplasia; however, it was not significant |
| Murti et al. 1985 [6] | India | Prospective | 66 | – | 5 | 7.6% | 0.76% | 10[a] | To assess the OSF MT rate. All transformed cases were in women who had habits of chewing tobacco and areca nut with betel leaves and lime |
| **Total (studies that assessed the OSF MT rate)** | | | **6569** | – | **320 (4.87%)** | | **0.84%** | **6.25** | |

*M* male, *F* female, *MT* malignant transformation, *OLK* oral leukoplakia, *OLP* oral lichen planus, *OSCC* oral squamous cell carcinoma

[a] Median follow up period

**Table 7.2** Cross-sectional studies with no information on MT

| Authors/year | Country | Design | Total (N) M:F | Mean age (years) | General description/main findings |
|---|---|---|---|---|---|
| Srivastava et al. 2020 [15] | India | Cross-sectional | 2150 1865:285 | Not specified | To assess the prevalence of OPMDs and oral cancers. The major risk factors were tobacco and areca nut, with or without tobacco. The malignant transformation rate of OSF was not assessed |
| Rangaswamy et al. 2019 [16] | India | Prospective case series | 30 23: 7 | 44.5 | To describe the features of oral carcinomas in the background of OSF. No controls. OSF-related carcinomas have distinct clinical presentations The malignant transformation rate of OSF was not assessed |
| Wang et al. 2018 [17] | Taiwan | Retrospective | 181 | Not specified | The aim was to study the MT of OLK alone and OLK with other oral lesions. No data was specified for OSF alone. Patients with both OSF and OLK had 58 more risks for MT. The malignant transformation rate of OSF was not assessed |
| Mohiuddin et al. 2016 [18] | Pakistan | Cross-sectional | 765 OSF 472 OSF-OSCC | Not specified | To assess the risk of MT of OSF. 48.3% of transformed cases were related to betel quid with tobacco. The malignant transformation rate of OSF was not assessed |
| Zhou et al. 2008 [19] | China | Case-control | 40 OSF 42 OSF-OSCC | (OSF-OSCC 45) (OSF 38) | To assess the risk of OSF MT. Odds ratios were older age 12.59, duration of chewing 10.15, smoking 7, OSF with OLK or OLP 8.04. The malignant transformation rate of OSF was not assessed |

*M* male, *F* female, *MT* malignant transformation, *OLK* oral leukoplakia, *OLP* oral lichen planus, *OSCC* oral squamous cell carcinoma

7

The geographic distribution of the reported studies is consistent with the global distribution of OSF, as almost all cases were reported in India and Southeast Asia [20]. Of these studies, six were conducted in India [6, 8, 10, 15, 16, 21] and Taiwan [7, 9, 11–13, 17], followed by two studies in Mainland China [14, 19] and one study in Pakistan [18].

## 7.3 Malignant Transformation Rate among OSF Patients

Iocca et al., in 2019, conducted a systematic review and meta-analysis to assess the malignant transformation rate among a group of OPMDs [5]. They found that out of 3986 OSF patients, 194 patients exhibited malignant transformation (4.8%) [5]. A comparable result was reported in a more recent meta-analysis by Kujan et al. in 2021: out of 6337 OSF patients, 292 patients underwent malignant transformation (4.6%), with an annual malignant transformation rate of 0.73% [3].

In India, the malignant transformation rate of OSF ranges from 3.3% to 7.6% [6, 8, 10], while studies from Mainland China and Taiwan reveal a malignant transformation rate between 2.3% and 9.1% [7, 9, 11–14]. Previous subgroup analysis showed no significant difference in the malignant transformation rate between "Mainland China and Taiwan" and India, at 4.9% and 3.5%, respectively [3]. Likewise, adjusted odds ratios did not report a significant difference between Mainland China and Taiwan [22]. Based on our literature search, we did not find epidemiological information about the malignant transformation rate of OSF in Vietnam, Pakistan, Thailand, Bangladesh, Sri Lanka, or Nepal.

The malignant potential of OSF is higher or comparable to other OPMDs, such as oral leukoplakia and oral lichenoid lesions; hence, OSF is considered a condition with significant morbidity and mortality rates [5, 23]. However, the malignant transformation potential of OSF has gained less attention among researchers because the literature includes only two meta-analyses in this area [3, 5], in comparison to many studies assessing the malignant transformation of other OPMDs. In addition, studies that report malignant transformation of OSF cases are associated with high heterogeneity and low methodological quality [3, 5]. We believe that the reported number of OSF cases in general, and malignant transformation cases in particular, might be much lower than the real situation.

In India, for example, a recent, nationally representative study in 2021 estimated that the number of areca nut users is more than 223 million people, and the majority of them consume areca nut with tobacco [24]. At the same time, the International Agency for Research on Cancer revealed that more than 35% of global oral and lip cancer cases are in India [25]. This is much higher than in China, including Taiwan (7.9%), although the population in both countries is comparable—around 1.4 billion [26]. Nonetheless, the literature includes only three Indian studies that assessed the malignant transformation rate among cohorts of 3500 OSF patients [6, 8, 10].

We found that the global malignant transformation rate of OSF among nine studies including 6569 OSF patients was 4.87% with an annual malignant transformation rate of 0.84%. Of these studies, five studies were retrospective while the other four were prospective as shown in ◘ Table 7.1. The follow-up time ranged from 3 to 10 years with a mean follow-up time of 6.25 years. The age and gender of OSF patients undergoing malignant transformation were only mentioned in one study by Murti et al. [6] The specific descriptions of the included studies with a brief outcome are presented below:

**Murti et al.** [6] followed up 66 Indian patients with OSF for 17 years with a median observation of 10 years. Patients were diagnosed clinically and followed up annually to detect any malignant transformation changes. The authors mentioned that surgical biopsies were performed according to the patient's consent; however, it was not clear how many patients underwent surgical biopsies during the follow-up time. At the end of the observation period, a malignant transformation of OSF lesions was detected among five female patients aged between 48 and 81 years (average age 64.6 years), giving a malignant transformation rate of 7.6%. The time between the initial diagnosis of OSF and the malignant transformation ranged between 3 and 16 years. All patients with malignant transformation had the habit of chewing areca nut with betel leaves and lime and with or without tobacco.

**Hsue et al.** [7] followed up a cohort of 1458 Taiwanese patients with various OPMDs including 439 patients with OSF. The patients were followed up for over 10 years, while the mean follow-up time was 42.6 months (3.5 years). Of the patients with OSF, eight cases progressed to carcinoma (2.3%), and two of them were associated with epithelial dysplasia. The mean duration of malignant transformation of the OSF patients with and without epithelial dysplasia was 40 months (3.3 years) and 52.3 months (4.4 years), respectively. However, this difference was not significant.

**Hazarey et al.** [8] carried out a retrospective hospital-based study among a cohort of 1000 Indian patients with OSF, 830 males, and 170 females. Clinical diagnosis of OSF patients was confirmed by surgical biopsies among a subgroup of cases; however, the number of these cases is unknown. Of the OSF patients, 33 cases (3.3%) transformed to malignancy; most of the malignant cases (28 cases) were diagnosed as OSCCs, while the remaining five cases were diagnosed as verrucous carcinomas. The gender and age of the malignant transformed cases were not mentioned; however, the authors reported significant associations between the malignant transformation of OSF cases and the frequency and duration of smoking and betel quid/tobacco chewing.

**Zhou et al.** [19] conducted a case-control study among a cohort of 82 Chinese patients (40 with OSCC at the background of OSF and 40 with OSF as controls) to assess the risk factors of OSF malignant transformation. The vast majority of the included subjects were males (97.6%). The mean age of patients in the OSF-OSCC group and OSF control group was 45 years and 38 years, respectively. The most common site of carcinoma involvement was the tongue (61.9%), followed by the buccal mucosa (28.6%) and the gingiva (9.5%). The authors reported significant associations between the malignant transformation of OSF and patient age ($p$ = 0.001, OR 12.59), duration of betel quid chewing ($p$ = 0.008, OR 10.15), duration of cigarette smoking ($p$ = 0.025, OR 7), and concomitant presentations with oral leukoplakia or oral lichen planus ($p$ = 0.019, OR 8.04).

**Wang et al.** [9] performed a retrospective study among a cohort of 5071 Taiwanese patients with OPMDs; all cases were associated with histopathological assessments. Of these, 1180 patients were diagnosed with OSF (994 OSF cases without epithelial dysplasia and 186 OSF cases with epithelial dysplasia). The mean age of patients at the time of diagnosis was 44.7 ± 12.4 years for OSF patients without dysplasia and 47.7 ± 11.8 years for OSF patients with epithelial dysplasia. Of all OSF cases, the malignant transformation was reported in 46/1180 cases (3.9%); 40 cases of them were diagnosed as OSCCs, and 6 cases were diagnosed as verrucous carcinomas. The rate of the malignant transformation was higher among OSF patients with epithelial dysplasia than OSF cases without epithelial dysplasia, 4.8% vs. 3.7%. The mean duration of the malignant transformation was higher for OSF patients with epithelial dysplasia (3.6 years) in comparison to those without epithelial dysplasia (3.12 years). Although the authors found that the malignant transformation of OPMDs is statistically significantly associated with patients aged more than 45 years ($p = 0.03$) and male patients ($p = 0.001$), no data were provided specifically for OSF.

**Chourasia et al.** [10], conducted a retrospective study among a cohort of 344 Indian patients (225 patients with OSCC and 119 patients with OSF) to assess the incidence of OSCC arising secondary to OSF as well as the associated risk factors. Of the OSF patients, there were 88 males and 31 females; more than 97% of them had the habit of areca nut/tobacco chewing. Five OSF patients progressed to carcinoma, giving a malignant transformation rate of 4.2%. However, the mean duration taken for malignant transformation was not specified. The incidence of the concomitant presentations of OSCC with OSF was statistically significant ($p < 0.05$), and it was reported in 25.7% of the OSCC cases.

7

**Mohiuddin et al.** [18] carried out a cross-sectional multicentre study among Pakistani patients diagnosed with OSCC and/or OSF between 2004 and 2012 with a major aim to identify the risk factors for the malignant transformation of OSF. The malignant transformation rate of OSF was not assessed in this study. However, a statically significant association between various chewing habits and OSF malignant transformation was reported, $p = 0.001$.

**Yang et al.** [11] performed a retrospective study to assess the malignant transformation rate of OSF among Taiwanese patients. Data were retrieved from Taiwan's National Health Insurance Research Database and included 778 OSF patients in addition to a control group of 43,568 non-OSF individuals. OSF patients were predominantly males (87.1%), while the mean age of patients was 41.8 ± 11.7 years. The hazard ratios (HRs) were calculated to assess the OSF-associated risk of malignancy. The malignant transformation rate among the OSF patients was higher than that of the control group, 9.1% and 0.3%, respectively. The mean duration of the malignant transformation was 2.5 years for the OSF patients and 5.1 years for the controls. The authors concluded that OSF patients were associated with a higher risk of malignancy in comparison to the control group (adjusted HR: 29.3; 95% CI: 20.5–41.7). The risk of malignancy was higher among the male OSF patients in comparison to the female OSF patients (adjusted HR: 14.5; 95% CI: 3.6–58.6). To further stratify the risk of malignancy among OSF patients, the authors reported that the concomitant presence of oral leukoplakia increased the malignant transformation risk by up to 52.5 times in comparison to the non-OSF patients.

**Wang et al.** [17] conducted a retrospective study among a cohort of 11,898 Taiwanese patients with oral leukoplakia. Although this study aimed mainly to assess the malignant transformation risk of oral leukoplakia, the possible synergistic effects between oral leukoplakia and OSF in the malignant transformation were analysed. The authors reported that OSF enhances the malignant transformation of oral leukoplakia and increases the risk of malignancy: adjusted HR 27.1 (95% CI: 18.9–38.6) for oral leukoplakia alone in comparison to controls and adjusted HR 53.4 (95% CI: 34.6–98.5) for oral leukoplakia and OSF in comparison to the controls. However, the mean duration of the malignant transformation was lower for the cases of oral leukoplakia alone than the cases with oral leukoplakia and OSF, 1.8 years and 2.6 years, respectively.

**Chuang et al.** [12] performed a prospective study with an average follow-up time of 5.7 years for a cohort of 8501 Taiwanese patients with OPMDs. Of these, there were 2333 OSF patients and all of them were males. The malignant transformation rate among the OSF patients was 4.9%. The estimated annual malignant transformation risk per 1000 person-years for OSF betel nut chewing was 8.9. This risk was higher for OSF patients with alcohol-drinking habits, 10.0 per 1000. OSF patients aged between 50 and 69 years were associated with a higher annual malignant transformation risk (10.2 per 1000) in comparison to patients in other age groups.

**Rangaswamy et al.** [16] performed a prospective case series to describe 30 cases of OSCC in the background of OSF related to Indian patients. The mean age of patients was 44.5 years. More than four-quarters of the cases were associated with males, and more than 73% of the cases were linked to a previous history of gutkha usage.

**Chiang et al.** [13] retrospectively assessed 555 Taiwanese patients with OPMDs for a mean follow-up period of 6.7 years. Out of the 87 OSF cases in this cohort, four patients developed malignancy (4.6%). The duration of the malignant transformation ranged between 6 and 60 months. Heavy betel quid chewing was reported as a significant independent risk for the malignant transformation of OPMDs; however, no specific data were provided for OSF alone.

**Srivastava et al.** [15] conducted a cross-sectional descriptive study to assess the prevalence of OPMDs among 3735 Indian patients with oral lesions. A group of 9060 healthy subjects without a history of oral lesions were included as a control group. Of the OPMDs group, 2150 patients were diagnosed with OSF. The OSF malignant transformation rate was not assessed in this study;

however, the authors concluded that betel quid chewing, with or without tobacco, is the major risk factor for OPMDs and oral cancers.

**Jian et al.** [14] reported a prospective study conducted in a single institution in Hunan province in China. Among 567 patients enrolled from 1986 to 2017 and diagnosed with OSF, 32 cases transformed into OSCC (32/567, 5.6%). In 1 patient (3%), the malignant transformation was observed 24 years after the initial diagnosis. The presence of oral leukoplakia increased the rate of malignant transformation.

## 7.4 Epithelial Dysplasia and OSF

The presence of epithelial dysplasia increases the malignant transformation risk among OPMDs in general [27] and OSF in particular [3, 28–30]. However, among the studies that assessed the malignant transformation rate of OSF, we found that only two studies included the presence or absence of epithelial dysplasia in their cohorts [7, 9]. None of these studies differentiated between the grades of dysplasia. This may be attributed to the classic presumption that fibrosis in OSF starves the tissue and reduces epithelial thickness as a result of blood vessel construction, which in turn reduces the probability of epithelial dysplasia [29]. However, a more logical presumption hypothesizes that the reduction of blood supply would lead to the accumulation of carcinogens in the epithelium for a longer time, which in turn would increase the genotoxicities of these carcinogens and stimulate epithelial changes and malignant transformation [29].

In 2011, Jayasooriya et al. documented a significant increase in the incidence of epithelial dysplasia as the fibrosis thickness increased ($p = 0.004$), and at the same time found that OSF cases with moderate epithelial dysplasia had a significantly thicker fibrous layer than cases with mild epithelial dysplasia ($p < 0.005$) [28]. On the contrary, another study showed that neither the fibrosis thickness nor the grade of epithelial dysplasia is related to each other [31]. In this respect, it is worth noting that in 2021, Sanjai [32] noted that using the WHO grading system of epithelial dysplasia is not possible with all OSF cases, as some features of atypia are not discernible [33]. Instead, the author recommended using the binary system for grading epithelial dysplasia of Kujan et al. [34], with some modifications relevant to OSF [32].

Epithelial dysplasia has been reported in 2.5–43% of OSF cases in various studies [7, 9, 28, 35]. The meta-analysis by Kujan et al. determined that out of 414 patients with OSF and oral leukoplakia or epithelial dysplasia, 40 patients exhibited malignant transformation (9.7%), in comparison to 78 out of 1963 OSF patients without epithelial dysplasia or oral leukoplakia (4%), $p < 0.005$ [3].

## 7.5 Potential Risk Factors of Malignant Transformation among OSF Patients

### 7.5.1 Areca Nut Usage as a Major Carcinogen

The significance of this disorder is seen from the global epidemiology of areca nut usage, where it is estimated that this substance is regularly consumed by approximately 600 million people worldwide [36]. However, there are challenges in documenting areca nut usage and its role in malignant transformation in OSF because the areca nut is usually wrapped in the leaf of *Piper betle* and masticated in combination with a huge range of additives, including tobacco [37, 38]. These additives vary between countries, communities, and individuals, to a level that may not be easy to qualify.

It is well established that areca nut is the major etiological factor for OSF [39, 40]. In 2004, the International Agency for Research on Cancer Monographs declared areca nut and betel quid as a “group one carcinogen” [40]. This means that there is enough evidence to conclude that it can cause cancer in humans. Areca nut is consumed either alone or as betel quid, where the latter refers to any chewing materials that contain areca nut besides a wide range of additives [38]. One of the significant pathways for carcinogenesis in subjects chewing area nut is oxidative DNA damage [41, 42]. This is supported by statistically significant serum uric acid values in OSF patients compared to controls [43].

While it has been estimated that the risk of malignancy is 35-fold higher among those who smoke and drink alcohol, a report shows that this risk jumps to be 123-fold among those who smoke and drink alcohol besides chewing betel quid [44]. A previous retrospective study revealed that 68% of women with buccal cancer and 84% of women with tongue cancer are non-smokers and only chew betel quid [45]. According to that study, the elimination of chewing habits would substantially reduce this risk of malignancy by up to 91% [45].

In general, areca nut can contribute to malignant transformation through two major pathways: alkaloids and trace elements. Four major alkaloids have been specified in areca nut: arecoline, guvacine, arecaidine, and guvacoline. Of these, arecoline (1,2,4,5-tetrahydro-1-methyl-pyridine carboxylic acid) is the most potent, as it has cytotoxic and genotoxic properties on oral mucosal fibroblasts and keratinocytes. A dose-dependent effect of arecoline in inhibiting gingival fibroblast attachment and migration in vivo was documented [46].

Furthermore, collagen synthesis was significantly inhibited by the action of arecoline [46]. A previous study to identify a possible mechanism of arecoline-induced carcinogenesis found that arecoline downregulated p21 and p27 through the reactive oxygen species/mTOR complex 1 and facilitated G [1]/S transition of the cell cycle, which subsequently led to error-prone DNA replication [47]. Another animal study found that chronic exposure to arecoline downregulates tumour suppressor genes BRCA1 and BRCA2 and increases the risk of cancer formation [48].

On the other hand, a high copper concentration in the areca nut could play a potential role in the malignant transformation of OSF. A previous study reported a higher mean salivary copper level in OSF than oral leukoplakia and oral lichen planus [49]. Another study found a significant increase in serum copper level among patients with OSF and oral cancers in comparison to normal controls [50]. Likewise, it has been reported that the level of serum copper increased gradually from OSF to oral cancer as the duration of areca nut consumption increased [51]. The high copper content of areca nut has been shown to stimulate tumour angiogenesis by activating several angiogenic molecules, such as vascular endothelial growth factor (VEGF), tumour necrosis factor-α (TNF-α), and interleukin-1 (IL-1) [52].



## 7.6 Pathological Mechanisms of the Malignant Transformation of OSF

Although the potential of malignancy of OSF was first described in 1956 [4], the pathological mechanisms implicated have yet to be elucidated. However, the pathogenesis of this disease is believed to be multifactorial, where numerous pathways and molecules are implicated. These pathways are among the hallmarks of cancer, namely hypoxia, angiogenesis, alterations in the cell cycle, and epithelial-mesenchymal transition [52–54].

### 7.6.1 Hypoxia

It is widely accepted that connective tissue fibrosis, as a characteristic pathological feature for OSF, i.e. narrow blood vessels, further results in compromised blood supply and lesional hypoxia. Therefore, several previous reports have highlighted the possible role of hypoxia in the malignant transformation of OSF [55]. Hypoxia-inducible factor 1α (HIF-1α), a known transcription factor induced by hypoxic conditions, is significantly upregulated at both the protein and mRNA levels in OSF cases with epithelial dysplasia [35]. Therefore, HIF-1α was proposed for use as a marker of malignant transformation in OSF cases [35]. Moreover, a previous study by Jayasooriya et al. in 2011 revealed that the severity of epithelial dysplasia grade was significantly associated with the thickness of fibrosis in OSF cases [28]. This finding was attributed to the advancement of fibrosis in OSF, which reduces local vascularity, resulting in hypoxia, and in turn increases the incidence and the grade of epithelial dysplasia [28]. Based on these findings, Ye et al. proposed using hyperbaric oxygen as a supplementary therapy to treat OSF, as it can increase oxygen tension at the cellular level and reduce the expression of HIF-1α at the molecular level [56].

### 7.6.2 Angiogenesis

In environments with reduced oxygen concentrations, HIF-1α activates several hypoxia-related genes and upregulates VEGF, which in turn promotes angiogenesis in an attempt to compensate for the oxygen reduction [57]. However, once the malignant process begins, angiogenesis promotes malignant proliferation by causing normally quiescent vasculature to continue growing to assist growing neoplastic mass [58]. A previous study in 2014 performed computer-aided quantification of immunohistochemical images and proposed using HIF-1α as a strong screening marker of OSF and VEGF for risk stratification [59].

### 7.6.3 Alterations in Cell Cycle

Proliferating cell nuclear antigen (PCNA) acts as a central coordinator of DNA transactions involved in DNA replication, repair, chromatin dynamics, and cell cycle regulation [60]. PCNA is used to assess proliferative activities and is known to be highly expressed in malignancies. However, several previous reports revealed a significantly higher expression of PCNA in OSF cases than in normal tissues, in addition to a significant increase of PCNA expression in dysplastic OSF cases in comparison with non-dysplastic OSF [60].

### 7.6.4 Epithelial-Mesenchymal Transition

Epithelial-mesenchymal transition (EMT) is a complex biological process in which polarized epithelial cells undergo multiple biochemical changes to gain the migratory and invasive properties of mesenchymal stem cells [61]. The most characteristic feature associated with EMT is the loss of E-cadherin expression [61]. E-cadherin is considered an important tumour suppressor gene that is localized on the surfaces of epithelial cells and responsible for adherens junctions [62]. The reduction of E-cadherin expression has been correlated with a poor OSCC prognosis in many previous studies [63]. Transcription factors such as Snail (SNAI1), Slug (SNAI2), and Twist, as known repressors for E-cadherin, are involved in the pathogenesis of areca nut-related OSF. In a recent study (2021), the authors found that the expressions of Snail and Twist were significantly higher in OSF than in normal tissues. This association was concomitant with a significant loss of E-cadherin expressions among OSF with dysplasia [64]. This suggests a possible role for this mechanism in the malignant transformation of OSF [64]. Another study revealed that Twist transcript and protein expression were higher in areca nut-associated OSF than in normal tissues [65]. A previous in vivo experiment reported that treatment of human primary buccal mucosal fibroblasts with arecoline increased the Twist expression transcript and protein levels in a dose-dependent manner, while this phenomenon was reversed by knocking down Twist [65].

## 7.7 Prognosis of OSF Malignant Transformation

OSF is not only a condition with high morbidity and mortality rates; it is believed that OSF-associated malignancy represents a distinctive clinicopathological, morphological, and histological disease [66]. This has been attributed to the distinct biochemical mechanisms of the areca nut [52]. Many studies have shown that OSF-associated malignancy has a younger age of onset than other non-OSF-associated malignancies [16, 66–68]. Moreover, OSF-associated malignancy was associated with more aggressive pathological behaviours, although this association was not significant [67]. The metastasis and recurrence rates of OSF-associated malignancy were 13.5% and 39.1%, respectively, while these rates were lower in non-OSF-associated malignancies, 7.6% and 27.8% [67]. On the contrary, other studies found that regional lymph node metastasis and 3-year disease-free survival were significantly higher in non-OSF-related malignancies compared to OSF-associated malignancies [66, 68]. This was attributed to the potential protective effect of fibrosis in OSF, where collagen with abnormal cross-linking may resist the invasion process. This can also be explained by the ability of fibrosis to reduce and block submucosal lymphatics [66, 68]. Nonetheless, the current evidence is insufficient to support these suppositions.

Regarding the histopathological features, it has been reported that OSF-associated malignancies are significantly associated with a better grade of tumour differentiation, i.e. well-differentiated squamous cell carcinoma. In contrast, non-OSF-related malignancies were significantly associated with moderate- and low-differentiated squamous cell carcinoma [66].

One study found that OSF patients with reduced mouth opening presented with a more advanced tumour stage [16, 69]. Although the evidence is not strong enough to support this association, this can be attributed to the difficulty of earlier diagnosis among patients with limited mouth opening.

## 7.8 Conclusion

OSF is a widespread condition with very limited published data on malignant transformation. While there is reason to suggest that the malignant transformation potential associated with OSF is underestimated, the current malignant transformation rate based on our analyses is around 4.87%. The risk of malignancy is increased substantially by the concomitant presence of oral leukoplakia and epithelial dysplasia with OSF. The risk of malignancy is directly associated with the dose and duration of areca nut chewing. There is an urgent need to conduct well-designed, multicentre longitudinal studies to further investigate the potential malignancy of OSF.

**Summary**

The current evidence indicates that oral submucous fibrosis is associated with a malignant transformation rate of 4.87% while the annual malignant transformation rate is 0.84%. The risk of malignancy is directly linked with the concomitant presentation of oral leukoplakia, as well as the dose and duration of areca nut chewing.

## References

1. Warnakulasuriya S, Kujan O, Aguirre-Urizar JM, et al. Oral potentially malignant disorders: a consensus report from an international seminar on nomenclature and classification, convened by the WHO Collaborating Centre for Oral Cancer. Oral Dis. 2021;27(8):1862–80.
2. Mello FW, Miguel AFP, Dutra KL, et al. Prevalence of oral potentially malignant disorders: a systematic review and meta-analysis. J Oral Pathol Med. 2018;47(7):633–40.
3. Kujan O, Mello FW, Warnakulasuriya S. Malignant transformation of oral submucous fibrosis: a systematic review and meta-analysis. Oral Dis. 2021;27(8):1936–46.
4. Paymaster JC. Cancer of the buccal mucosa; a clinical study of 650 cases in Indian patients. Cancer. 1956;9(3):431–5.
5. Iocca O, Sollecito TP, Alawi F, et al. Potentially malignant disorders of the oral cavity and oral dysplasia: a systematic review

and meta-analysis of malignant transformation rate by subtype. Head Neck. 2019;42(3):539–55.
6. Murti PR, Bhonsle RB, Pindborg JJ, Daftary DK, Gupta PC, Mehta FS. Malignant transformation rate in oral submucous fibrosis over a 17-year period. Community Dent Oral Epidemiol. 1985;13(6):340–1.
7. Hsue SS, Wang WC, Chen CH, Lin CC, Chen YK, Lin LM. Malignant transformation in 1458 patients with potentially malignant oral mucosal disorders: a follow-up study based in a Taiwanese hospital. J Oral Pathol Med. 2007;36(1):25–9.
8. Hazarey VK, Erlewad DM, Mundhe KA, Ughade SN. Oral submucous fibrosis: study of 1000 cases from central India. J Oral Pathol Med. 2007;36(1):12–7.
9. Wang YY, Tail YH, Wang WC, et al. Malignant transformation in 5071 southern Taiwanese patients with potentially malignant oral mucosal disorders. BMC Oral Health. 2014;14:99.
10. Chourasia NR, Borle RM, Vastani A. Concomitant Association of Oral Submucous Fibrosis and Oral Squamous Cell Carcinoma and Incidence of Malignant Transformation of Oral Submucous Fibrosis in a Population of Central India: A Retrospective Study. J Maxillofac Oral Surg. 2015;14(4):902–6.
11. Yang PY, Chen YT, Wang YH, Su NY, Yu HC, Chang YC. Malignant transformation of oral submucous fibrosis in Taiwan: a nationwide population-based retrospective cohort study. J Oral Pathol Med. 2017;46(10):1040–5.
12. Chuang TD, Khorram O. Expression profiling of lncRNAs, miRNAs, and mRNAs and their differential expression in leiomyoma using next-generation RNA sequencing. Reprod Sci. 2018;25(2):246–55.
13. Chiang WF, Liu SY, Lin JF, et al. Malignant development in patients with oral potentially malignant disorders detected through nationwide screening: Outcomes of 5-year follow-up at a single hospital. Head Neck. 2020;42(1):67–76.
14. Jian X, Jian Y, Wu X, et al. Oral submucous fibrosis transforming into squamous cell carcinoma: a prospective study over 31 years in mainland China. Clin Oral Investig. 2021;25(4):2249–56.
15. Srivastava R, Sharma L, Pradhan D, Jyoti B, Singh O. Prevalence of oral premalignant lesions and conditions among the population of Kanpur City, India: a cross-sectional study. J Family Med Prim Care. 2020;9(2):1080–5.
16. Rangaswamy S, Chikkalingaiah RG, Sanjeevarayappa PN, Govindraju P. Carcinoma arising in the background of oral submucous fibrosis. Ann Maxillofac Surg. 2019;9(2):247–52.
17. Wang T, Chiu YW, Chen YT, et al. Malignant transformation of Taiwanese patients with oral leukoplakia: a nationwide population-based retrospective cohort study. J Formos Med Assoc. 2018;117(5):374–80.
18. Mohiuddin S, Fatima N, Hosein S, Fatima N. High risk of malignant transformation of oral submucous fibrosis in Pakistani females: a potential national disaster. J Pak Med Assoc. 2016;66(11):1362–6.
19. Zhou S, Guo F, Li L, et al. Multiple logistic regression analysis of risk factors for carcinogenesis of oral submucous fibrosis in mainland China. Int J Oral Maxillofac Surg. 2008;37(12):1094–8.
20. Tilakaratne WM, Klinikowski MF, Saku T, Peters TJ, Warnakulasuriya S. Oral submucous fibrosis: review on aetiology and pathogenesis. Oral Oncol. 2006;42(6):561–8.
21. Singh AK, Chauhan R, Anand K, Singh M, Das SR, Sinha AK. Prevalence and risk factors for oral potentially malignant disorders in Indian Population. J Pharm Bioallied Sci. 2021;13(Suppl 1):S398–401.
22. Li S, Lee YC, Li Q, et al. Oral lesions, chronic diseases and the risk of head and neck cancer. Oral Oncol. 2015;51(12):1082–7.
23. Shearston K, Fateh B, Tai S, Hove D, Farah CS. Malignant transformation rate of oral leukoplakia in an Australian population. J Oral Pathol Med. 2019;48(7):530–7.
24. Singh PK, Yadav A, Singh L, et al. Areca nut consumption with and without tobacco among the adult population: a nationally representative study from India. BMJ Open. 2021;11(6):e043987.
25. Ferlay J EM, Lam F, Colombet M, Mery L, Piñeros M, Znaor A, Soerjomataram I, Bray F. Global Cancer Observatory: Cancer Today. International Agency for Research on Cancer. https://gco.iarc.fr/today. Published 2020. Accessed September, 2021.
26. The World Bank data. Total Population. https://data.worldbank.org/indicator/SP.POP.TOTL. Accessed 10 September, 2021.
27. Speight PM, Khurram SA, Kujan O. Oral potentially malignant disorders: risk of progression to malignancy. Oral Surg Oral Med Oral Pathol Oral Radiol. 2018;125(6):612–27.
28. Jayasooriya PR, Nadeeka Jayasinghe KA, Mudiyanselage TW. Relationship between thickness of fibrosis and epithelial dysplasia in oral submucous fibrosis. J Investig Clin Dent. 2011;2(3):171–5.
29. Ray JG, Ranganathan K, Chattopadhyay A. Malignant transformation of oral submucous fibrosis: overview of histopathological aspects. Oral Surg Oral Med Oral Pathol Oral Radiol. 2016;122(2):200–9.
30. Ranganathan K, Kavitha L. Oral epithelial dysplasia: classifications and clinical relevance in risk assessment of oral potentially malignant disorders. J Oral Maxillofac Pathol. 2019;23(1):19–27.
31. Illeperuma RP, Ryu MH, Kim KY, Tilakaratne WM, Kim J. Relationship of fibrosis and the expression of TGF-β1, MMP-1, and TIMP-1 with epithelial dysplasia in oral submucous fibrosis. Oral Med Pathol. 2010;15(1):21–8.
32. Sanjai K. Does oral epithelial dysplasia criteria hold true for dysplastic epithelium of oral submucous fibrosis? Oral Surg Oral Med Oral Pathol Oral Radiol. 2021;132(1):e41–2.
33. Barnes L, Eveson J, Reichart P, Sidransky D. Pathology and genetics of head and neck tumours, International Agency for Research on Cancer (IARC), vol. 9. 3rd ed. Lyon: IARC Press; 2005.
34. Kujan O, Oliver RJ, Khattab A, Roberts SA, Thakker N, Sloan P. Evaluation of a new binary system of grading oral epithelial dysplasia for prediction of malignant transformation. Oral Oncol. 2006;42(10):987–93.
35. Tilakaratne WM, Iqbal Z, Teh MT, et al. Upregulation of HIF-1alpha in malignant transformation of oral submucous fibrosis. J Oral Pathol Med. 2008;37(6):372–7.
36. Gupta PC, Warnakulasuriya S. Global epidemiology of areca nut usage. Addict Biol. 2002;7(1):77–83.
37. Warnakulasuriya S, Trivedy C, Peters TJ. Areca nut use: an independent risk factor for oral cancer. BMJ. 2002;324(7341):799–800.
38. Sharan RN, Mehrotra R, Choudhury Y, Asotra K. Association of betel nut with carcinogenesis: revisit with a clinical perspective. PLoS One. 2012;7(8):e42759.
39. Amarasinghe HK, Usgodaarachchi US, Johnson NW, Lalloo R, Warnakulasuriya S. Betel-quid chewing with or without tobacco is a major risk factor for oral potentially malignant disorders in Sri Lanka: a case-control study. Oral Oncol. 2010;46(4):297–301.
40. Humans IWGotEoCRt. Betel-quid and areca-nut chewing and some areca-nut derived nitrosamines. IARC Monogr Eval Carcinog Risks Hum. 2004;85:1–334.

41. Liu TY, Chen CL, Chi CW. Oxidative damage to DNA induced by areca nut extract. Mutat Res. 1996;367(1):25–31.
42. Li YC, Cheng AJ, Lee LY, Huang YC, Chang JT. Multifaceted mechanisms of Areca nuts in oral carcinogenesis: the molecular pathology from precancerous condition to malignant transformation. J Cancer. 2019;10(17):4054–62.
43. Yadav KD, Patil BA, Raheel SA, et al. Serum uric acid levels in patients with oral cancer, leukoplakia and submucous fibrosis: a cross-sectional study. Transl Cancer Res. 2020;9(4):3084–91.
44. Ko YC, Huang YL, Lee CH, Chen MJ, Lin LM, Tsai CC. Betel quid chewing, cigarette smoking and alcohol consumption related to oral cancer in Taiwan. J Oral Pathol Med. 1995;24(10):450–3.
45. van Wyk CW, Stander I, Padayachee A, Grobler-Rabie AF. The areca nut chewing habit and oral squamous cell carcinoma in South African Indians. A retrospective study. S Afr Med J. 1993;83(6):425–9.
46. Jeng JH, Lan WH, Hahn LJ, Hsieh CC, Kuo MY. Inhibition of the migration, attachment, spreading, growth and collagen synthesis of human gingival fibroblasts by arecoline, a major areca alkaloid, in vitro. J Oral Pathol Med. 1996;25(7):371–5.
47. Ji WT, Yang SR, Chen JY, et al. Arecoline downregulates levels of p21 and p27 through the reactive oxygen species/mTOR complex 1 pathway and may contribute to oral squamous cell carcinoma. Cancer Sci. 2012;103(7):1221–9.
48. Choudhury Y, Sharan RN. Altered BRCA1 and BRCA2 responses and mutation of BRCA1 gene in mice exposed chronically and transgenerationally to aqueous extract of betel nut (AEBN). Environ Toxicol Pharmacol. 2011;31(1):57–69.
49. Ayinampudi BK, Narsimhan M. Salivary copper and zinc levels in oral pre-malignant and malignant lesions. J Oral Maxillofac Pathol. 2012;16(2):178–82.
50. Khanna S, Udas AC, Kumar GK, Suvarna S, Karjodkar FR. Trace elements (copper, zinc, selenium and molybdenum) as markers in oral sub mucous fibrosis and oral squamous cell carcinoma. J Trace Elem Med Biol. 2013;27(4):307–11.
51. Hosthor SS, Mahesh P, Priya SA, Sharada P, Jyotsna M, Chitra S. Quantitative analysis of serum levels of trace elements in patients with oral submucous fibrosis and oral squamous cell carcinoma: a randomized cross-sectional study. J Oral Maxillofac Pathol. 2014;18(1):46–51.
52. Ekanayaka RP, Tilakaratne WM. Oral submucous fibrosis: review on mechanisms of malignant transformation. Oral Surg Oral Med Oral Pathol Oral Radiol. 2016;122(2):192–9.
53. Hanahan D, Weinberg RA. Hallmarks of cancer: the next generation. Cell. 2011;144(5):646–74.
54. Kujan O, Huang G, Ravindran A, Vijayan M, Farah CS. The role of cyclin-dependent kinases in oral potentially malignant disorders and oral squamous cell carcinoma. J Oral Pathol Med. 2019;48(7):560–5.
55. Kujan O, Shearston K, Farah CS. The role of hypoxia in oral cancer and potentially malignant disorders: a review. J Oral Pathol Med. 2017;46(4):246–52.
56. Ye X, Zhang J, Lu R, Zhou G. HBO: a possible supplementary therapy for oral potentially malignant disorders. Med Hypotheses. 2014;83(2):131–6.
57. Pouyssegur J, Dayan F, Mazure NM. Hypoxia signalling in cancer and approaches to enforce tumour regression. Nature. 2006;441(7092):437–43.
58. Hanahan D, Folkman J. Patterns and emerging mechanisms of the angiogenic switch during tumorigenesis. Cell. 1996;86(3):353–64.
59. Anura A, Conjeti S, Das RK, et al. Computer-aided molecular pathology interpretation in exploring prospective markers for oral submucous fibrosis progression. Head Neck. 2016;38(5):653–69.
60. Chiang CP, Lang MJ, Liu BY, et al. Expression of proliferating cell nuclear antigen (PCNA) in oral submucous fibrosis, oral epithelial hyperkeratosis and oral epithelial dysplasia in Taiwan. Oral Oncol. 2000;36(4):353–9.
61. Kalluri R, Weinberg RA. The basics of epithelial-mesenchymal transition. J Clin Invest. 2009;119(6):1420–8.
62. Birchmeier W, Behrens J. Cadherin expression in carcinomas: role in the formation of cell junctions and the prevention of invasiveness. Biochim Biophys Acta. 1994;1198(1):11–26.
63. Luo SL, Xie YG, Li Z, Ma JH, Xu X. E-cadherin expression and prognosis of oral cancer: a meta-analysis. Tumour Biol. 2014;35(6):5533–7.
64. Hosur MB, Puranik RS, Vanaki SS, Puranik SR, Sudhakara M, Das S. Evaluation of immunohistochemical expression of epithelial- mesenchymal transition markers E-cadherin, Twist and Snail in oral submucous fibrosis and their possible association with malignant transformation. J Oral Maxillofac Pathol. 2021;25(1):97–104.
65. Lee YH, Yang LC, Hu FW, Peng CY, Yu CH, Yu CC. Elevation of Twist expression by arecoline contributes to the pathogenesis of oral submucous fibrosis. J Formos Med Assoc. 2016;115(5):311–7.
66. Gadbail AR, Chaudhary M, Gawande M, et al. Oral squamous cell carcinoma in the background of oral submucous fibrosis is a distinct clinicopathological entity with better prognosis. J Oral Pathol Med. 2017;46(6):448–53.
67. Guo F, Jian XC, Zhou SH, Li N, Hu YJ, Tang ZG. A retrospective study of oral squamous cell carcinomas originated from oral submucous fibrosis. Zhonghua Kou Qiang Yi Xue Za Zhi. 2011;46(8):494–7.
68. Chaturvedi P, Vaishampayan SS, Nair S, et al. Oral squamous cell carcinoma arising in background of oral submucous fibrosis: a clinicopathologically distinct disease. Head Neck. 2013;35(10):1404–9.
69. Xu H, Lyu FY, Song JY, et al. Research achievements of oral submucous fibrosis: progress and prospect. Biomed Res Int. 2021;2021:6631856.

# Aetiology of Oral Submucous Fibrosis

Contents

# Lifestyle Factors

*Yi-Hsin Connie Yang and Saman Warnakulasuriya*

## Contents



© The Author(s), under exclusive license to Springer Nature Switzerland AG 2023
S. Warnakulasuriya, K. Ranganathan (eds.), *Oral Submucous Fibrosis*, Textbooks in Contemporary Dentistry,
https://doi.org/10.1007/978-3-031-12855-4_8

## 8.1 Introduction

Several factors have been previously considered as contributing to the development of OSF, including chilies, nutritional deficiency, and autoimmune disease [1]. Based on the evidence from several epidemiological studies conducted in India, Murti et al. published a review in 1995 and suggested a possible association between areca nut chewing and OSF [2]. Since then, evidence has been emerging to strengthen this causal relationship [1, 3, 4]. Areca nut is prepared and consumed in many different forms around the world. Many chewers often simultaneously use areca nut with tobacco products and/or alcohol. Therefore, it is important to consider synergistic effects, if any, that may also contribute to the risk of developing OSF.

In this chapter, we review the literature published since the year 1985 that assesses the risk of developing OSF from betel quid and areca nut with or without added tobacco; we also examine any likely synergistic effects with tobacco and/or alcohol and the dose-response effect.



**Learning Goals**

- Identify the methodological issues to assess the risk estimate of betel quid and areca nut chewing for OSF.
- Study the risk of developing OSF from betel quid and areca nut with or without added tobacco.
- Understand the synergistic effects from tobacco and/or alcohol with betel quid as well as the dose-response effect.
- Explore the association between chewing frequency and duration with severity and malignant transformation of OSF.

## 8.2 A Review of Methodological Issues

It is important to understand how epidemiological evidence is collected and analyzed to assess the risk estimate of a substance for a specific disorder. Several study methods could be employed, which include a cross-sectional design, case-control studies, or cohort studies. The principles underlying these different studies are outlined below.

A cross-sectional study is done in a community with a high prevalence of betel quid and areca nut chewing. A community survey is conducted by using a questionnaire to collect lifestyle information and conducting oral mucosal examinations to evaluate disease condition among participants. Odds ratio (OR) and 95% confidence intervals are often presented to show the magnitude of risk. When the OR is computed directly from cross tabulation of OSF status (usually, yes vs. no) and behavior (say, areca nut chewing vs. not chewing), it is considered as an unadjusted (or crude) OR. One may also compute ORs by using multiple (also called multivariable) logistic regression with added covariates to adjust for possible confounding effects from demographic characteristics or other lifestyle habits. This type of OR is referred to as the adjusted OR and is preferrable when tobacco smoking and alcohol drinking habits are also included in the regression analysis.

A case-control study design is used when there is relatively small number of OSF patients in the community and when there are several factors associated with chewing practices. The selection of controls is intended to balance possible demographic and associated confounding factors between cases and controls.

Cohort study is generally a common design in epidemiological studies. In this design, participants are divided into comparison groups based on their exposure status at the beginning of the study. The cohort study design is usually employed in the intervention studies of behavior changes for participants with a risk factor. In these studies, the primary outcome would be changes in chewing behaviors, and the incidence of OSF cases is usually considered as the secondary outcome. Alternatively, one may consider a retrospective cohort study based on the longitudinal data collection from participants. The rate ratios (RR, or relative risk) can be estimated by dividing the rate of new incidences in exposed group compared with the nonexposed group. In addition, when incidence rates are calculated for both exposure groups, the ratio of the two incidence rates is referred to as incidence rate ratio (IRR). In some situations, when time-to-event (disease) data are recorded, the hazard ratios (HR) or hazard rate ratios (HRR) are calculated to present the risk of chewing behavior in developing OSF.

**Definition**

Odds ratio (OR) is a common epidemiological measure for the association between exposure (e.g., areca nut chewing) and an outcome (e.g., OSF). The OR indicates the odds of occurring an outcome when people with exposure are compared to those without exposure. When OR is greater than 1 (OR >1 and with confidence intervals greater than one), it means that people who use areca nut would have an increased risk of OSF. When OR of any exposure is less than 1 (OR <1), the chance of occurring OSF would decrease, and the exposure is considered as a protective factor.

## 8.3 Epidemiological Studies Contributing to the Evidence

Epidemiological studies provide the highest level of evidence to study the risk factors associated with a specific disease. Since 1985, when IARC first evaluated the evidence on betel quid-associated disorders [5], several case-control and observational studies have been published. These reports provide updates on the knowledge of the risk of betel quid chewing in OSF from the studies conducted in the recent decades.

### 8.3.1 Risk from Betel Quid and Areca Nut without Added Tobacco

The potential OSF risk from chewing betel quid without added tobacco has been reported from China, India, Pakistan, Sri Lanka, and Taiwan (Table 8.1). There are five community-based studies (three observational and two case-control studies) and one hospital-based clinical study from Taiwan, and all reports support the evidence of developing OSF from chewing betel quid [6–11]. Although in Taiwan most of the betel quid chew-

**Table 8.1** Epidemiologic studies for the association between betel quid and areca nut chewing with oral submucous fibrosis

| Reference (publication year), study location, and period | Characteristic of cases | Characteristic of controls | Exposure categories | Odds ratio (95% confidence interval) | Study design; Reference group; adjustment for potential confounders |
|---|---|---|---|---|---|
| Betel quid and areca nut without added tobacco | | | | | |
| Sinor et al. (1990) [16], India | 60 OSF cases confirmed in a dental clinic | 60 clinic-based without oral disorders | Current chewers | 78.0 (5.7–1062.5) | Design: matched case-control study<br>Reference: occasional chewers<br>Controls matched by age, gender, and SES<br>Adjustment: no, 95% CIs are calculated from Table 2 |
| Maher et al. (1994) [17], Pakistan, 1989–1990 | 157 OSF cases confirmed in a dental clinic | 157 hospital-based without oral disorders | Pan<br>Areca nut only | 32 (6–177)<br>154 (34–693) | Design: matched case-control study<br>Reference: former chewers<br>Controls matched by age, gender, and ethnicity<br>Adjusted by age and gender and computed by unconditional logistic regression |
| Yang et al. (2001) [6], Taiwan | 17.6% OSF cases confirmed by dentists from a community survey of 312 participants (119 men, 193 women) | Rest of survey participants without OSF | Ever chewers | 13.9 (0.8–231.0)[a] | Design: cross-sectional study<br>Reference: never chewers<br>Adjustment: no, calculated from Table 3 |
| Lee et al. (2003) [7], Taiwan, 1994–1995 | 125 histologically confirmed OSF cases (93 men, 1 women) | 876 population controls (844 men, 32 women) | Former chewers<br>Current chewers | 12.1 (2.8–51.9)<br>40.7 (16.0–103.7) | Design: matched case-control study<br>Reference: never chewers<br>Controls matched by age, gender, and area<br>Adjusted by education and occupation in conditional logistic regression |

(continued)

**Table 8.1** (continued)

| Reference (publication year), study location, and period | Characteristic of cases | Characteristic of controls | Exposure categories | Odds ratio (95% confidence interval) | Study design; Reference group; adjustment for potential confounders |
|---|---|---|---|---|---|
| Jacob et al. (2004) [13], India | 170 OSF cases confirmed by dentists and oncologists (31 men, 139 women) | 47,773 controls without oral disorders by health workers | Ever chewers among nonsmokers and nondrinkers | 56.2 (21.8–144.8) | Design: case-control study<br>Reference: never chewers<br>Adjusted by age, gender, education, BMI in nonsmokers and nondrinkers |
| Ranganathan et al. (2004) [14], India, 2000–2003 | 185 histologically confirmed OSF cases (168 men, 17 women) | 185 hospital-based controls without oral disorders | Areca nut<br>Pan masala<br>Betel quid | 3.1 (0.8–11.7)<br>81.5 (5.0–1341.1)<br>29.0 (1.7–492.2)[a] | Design: matched case-control study<br>Reference: no habits<br>Controls matched by age and gender<br>Computed by univariate logistic regression |
| Yang et al. (2005) [8], Taiwan | 62 OSF cases patients detected by screening | 62 controls without oral disorders | Only chewing habit:<br>Both sexes<br>Men<br>Women | 4.5 (1.2–16.9)[a]<br>2.9 (0.3–29.3)[a]<br>5.6 (1.1–28.0)[a] | Design: stratified case-control study<br>Reference: no chewing and no smoking<br>Stratified by age/gender groups and computed by conditional logistic regression |
| Chung et al. (2005) [9], Taiwan, 1998–1999 | 17 OSF cases detected from community survey | 1075 patients examined | Only chewing habit | 65.9 (3.9–999.0) | Design: cross-sectional study<br>Reference: no chewing and no smoking<br>Adjusted by age and smoking |
| Ariyawardana et al. (2006) [18], Sri Lanka | 74 histologically confirmed OSF cases (61 men, 13 women) | 74 hospital-based controls without oral disorders | Areca nut only<br>Betel quid | 11.8 (0.6–217.2)[a]<br>3.1 (0.3–30.4) | Design: matched case-control study<br>Reference: no habits<br>Controls matched by age and gender<br>Adjusted by smoking and drinking and computed by unconditional logistic regression |
| Chen et al. (2006) [10], Taiwan, 1994–2000 | 23 histologically confirmed OSF cases | 23 hospital-based controls without oral disorders | Betel quid | 4.2 (0.5–32.7) | Design: case-control study<br>Reference: no habits<br>Adjusted by age, smoking, and HPV |
| Ahmed et al. (2006) [15], India, 2002–2004 | 157 histologically confirmed OSF cases | 135 hospital-based controls without oral disorders | Pan<br>Pan masala<br>Areca nut only | 41.5 (13.6–127.2)<br>138.2 (37.6–506.7)<br>172.8 (18.0–1662.5) | Design: matched case-control study<br>Reference: never chewers<br>Controls matched by age, gender, religion, and SES<br>Adjustment: no, calculated from Table 7 |

8

**Table 8.1** (continued)

| Reference (publication year), study location, and period | Characteristic of cases | Characteristic of controls | Exposure categories | Odds ratio (95% confidence interval) | Study design; Reference group; adjustment for potential confounders |
|---|---|---|---|---|---|
| Yang et al. (2010) [11], Taiwan, 2005 | 89 OSF cases detected from community screening | 2020 patients examined | Men | | Design: cross-sectional study<br>Reference: never chewers<br>Adjusted by age, smoking, and drinking |
| | | | Former chewers | 13.5 (3.8–46.7) | |
| | | | Current chewers | 22.9 (7.3–71.7) | |
| | | | Women | | |
| | | | Former chewers | 9.3 (3.3–26.0) | |
| | | | Current chewers | 13.0 (5.2–32.6) | |
| Zhang et al. (2012) [12], China | 24 OSF cases detected from community screening | 2356 patients examined | Former chewers<br>Current chewers | 590.3 (33.7–10329.8)[a]<br>202.3 (12.1–3392.4)[a] | Design: cross-sectional study<br>Reference: never chewers<br>Adjustment: no, calculated from Table 6 |
| Betel quid and areca nut with added tobacco | | | | | |
| Sinor et al. (1990) [16], India | 60 OSF cases confirmed in a dental clinic | 60 clinic-based without oral disorders | Current chewers | 106.4 (13.0–870.1) | Design: matched case-control study<br>Reference: occasional areca nut chewer<br>Controls matched by age, gender, and SES<br>Adjustment: no, 95% CIs are calculated from Table 2 |
| Maher et al. (1994) [17], Pakistan, 1989–1990 | 157 OSF cases confirmed in a dental clinic | 157 hospital-based without oral disorders | Pan with tobacco | 64 (15–274) | Design: matched case-control study<br>Reference: former chewers<br>Controls matched by age, gender, and ethnicity<br>Adjusted by age and gender and computed by unconditional logistic regression |
| | | | With and without tobacco combined: | | |
| | | | Both sexes | 94 (23–394) | |
| | | | Men | 136 (7–2477) | |
| | | | Women | 61 (14–262) | |
| Hashibe et al. (2002) [19], India, 1995–1998 | 170 OSF cases confirmed by dentists and oncologists (31 men, 139 women) | 47,773 controls without oral disorders by health workers | With and without tobacco combined: | | Design: case-control study<br>Reference: never chewers<br>Adjusted by age, gender, education, occupation, BMI, drinking, smoking, vegetable intake, and fruit intake |
| | | | Both sexes | 44.1 (22.0–88.2) | |
| | | | Men | 48.6 (6.5–365.4) | |
| | | | Women | 45.1 (21.5–94.8) | |
| Jacob et al. (2004) [13], India | 170 OSF cases confirmed by dentists and oncologists (31 men, 139 women) | 47773 controls without oral disorders by health workers | ever chewers among non-smokers and non-drinkers | 73.0 (32.9–162.2) | Design: case-control study<br>Reference: never chewers<br>Adjusted by age, gender, education, BMI |

(continued)

**Table 8.1** (continued)

| Reference (publication year), study location, and period | Characteristic of cases | Characteristic of controls | Exposure categories | Odds ratio (95% confidence interval) | Study design; Reference group; adjustment for potential confounders |
|---|---|---|---|---|---|
| Ariyawardana et al. (2006) [18], Sri Lanka | 74 histologically confirmed OSF cases (61 men, 13 women) | 74 hospital-based controls without oral disorders | Betel quid | 16.2 (5.9–44.9) | Design: matched case-control study<br>Reference: no habits<br>Controls matched by age and gender<br>Adjusted by smoking and drinking and computed by unconditional logistic regression |
| Ahmed et al. (2006) [15], India, 2002–2004 | 157 histologically confirmed OSF cases | 135 hospital-based controls without oral disorders | Gutka | 234.9 (74.2–743.7) | Design: matched case-control study<br>Reference: never chewers<br>Controls matched by age, gender, religion, and SES<br>Adjustment: no, calculated from Table 7 |
| Mukherjee et al. (2014) [20], India, 2012–2013 | 50 hospital-based OSF cases | 100 hospital-based controls | Gutkha | 145.4 (15.2–1397) | Design: case-control study<br>Reference: not daily users<br>Adjusted by sex, age, alcohol, spicy foods, employment, and education |
| Khan et al. (2020) [21], India, 2013–20147 | 73 hospital OSF cases | 1007 patients with tobacco-related mucosal changes reviewed | Gutkha<br>Betel quid | 17.7 (4.9–64.6)<br>18.6 (5.0–69.0) | Design: cross-sectional study<br>Reference: no smoking<br>Adjusted by smoking habit |

[a]Since the number of OSF patients without lifetime chewing habit is zero, one half is used to replace zero in the computation of odds ratio

ers are also cigarette smokers, tobacco is never added to betel quid [6]. In areca nut-only chewers, without cigarette smoking or alcohol consumption, the OR is 4.5 (95% CI, confidence interval, 1.2–16.9) in Indigenous community and 65.9 times (95% CI, 3.9–999) in Han community for developing OSF as compared to people without any risk factor [8, 9]. In addition, current users are at higher risk than former chewers (OR, 40.7 vs. 12.1 [7]; 22.9 vs. 13.5 in men and 13.0 vs. 9.3 in women [11]).

The betel quid chewing reported in Mainland China is also similar to chewers in Taiwan, in that tobacco is never added to the quid and most of the chewers are also cigarette smokers [12]. The risk of OSF in Hunan province among current chewers was 202.3 (OR, 95% CI, 12.1–3392.4) and among former chewers 590.3 (OR, 95% CI, 33.7–10,329.8). The risk for former chewers in this study is much higher than current chewers. It is possible that former chewers may stop chewing due to symptoms experienced from OSF, which is often referred to as reverse causation.

One community-based and three hospital-based case-control studies conducted in India investigated the OSF risk from betel quid and areca nut without added tobacco [13–16]. From a community-based study with 170 cases and 47,773 controls, ever chewers who were also nonsmokers and nondrinkers, OSF risk was 56.2 (OR, 95% CI, 21.8–144.8) [13]. Sinor et al. [16] reported a risk of 78.0 (OR, 95% CI, 5.7–1062.5) in mawa chewers having investigated 60 OSF cases and 60 matched controls. A matched case-control study with 175 OSF cases shows a risk, among areca nut, pan masala, and betel quid users, of 3.1 (OR, 95% CI, 0.8–11.7), 81.5 (OR, 95% CI, 5.0–1341.1), and 29.0 (OR, 95% CI, 1.7–492.2), respectively [14]. The ORs in another matched case-control study were 41.5 (95% CI, 13.6–127.2) for *pan* users, 138.2 (95% CI, 37.6–506.7) for *pan masala* users, and 172.8 (95% CI, 18.0–1662.5) for users of areca nut only [15]. A similar risk pattern was seen in a matched case-control study from Pakistan [17], with the reported OR for *pan* users being 32 (95% CI, 6–177) and 154 (95% CI, 34–693) for users of areca nut only.

In Sri Lanka, OR of OSF is 3.1 (95% CI, 0.3–30.4) for betel quid users and 11.8 (95% CI, 0.6–217.2) for users of areca nut only [18]. Three studies have ORs for areca nut-only users [14, 15, 18], and only one had significant OR (172.8, 95% CI, 18.0–1662.5 [15]). Users of betel quid without tobacco are reported to have a significant risk of developing OSF.

### 8.3.2 Risk from Betel Quid and Areca Nut with Added Tobacco

Risk from betel quid and areca nut with added tobacco has been reported from India, Pakistan, and Sri Lanka (Table 8.1). There are four hospital-based case-control studies and one community-based case-control study from India that reported risk factors for OSF [13, 15, 16, 19–21]. In the community-based study, areca nut chewers with and without added tobacco have an OSF risk of 44.1 (OR, 95% CI, 22.0–88.2) [19]. Another report from the same study center indicated an OR of 73.0 (95% CI, 32.9–162.2) for ever chewers who were also nonsmokers and nondrinkers [13]. For *gutkha* (which contains both areca nut and tobacco), the OR ranges from 17.7 (95% CI, 4.9–64.6) [21] to 234.9 (95% CI, 74.2–743.7) [15].

The risk of betel quid with added tobacco is 16.2 (OR, 95% CI, 5.9–44.9) reported from Sri Lanka [18] and 18.6 (OR, 95% CI, 5.0–69.0) from India [21].

There are three publications [13, 15, 18], which investigated ORs from both types of quid. To examine whether betel quid with tobacco added has higher risk for OSF than betel quid without tobacco, random effect pooled OR estimates were calculated by the Review Manager 5.4.1 using inverse variance method as shown in Fig. 8.1. The pooled OR estimate from Taiwan is 14.2 (95% CI, 4.1–48.8). The pooled OR estimates from

| Study or Subgroup | Weight | Odds Ratio IV, Random, 95% CI | Year |
|---|---|---|---|
| **2.1.1 Taiwan (quid without added tobacco)** | | | |
| Yang 2001 | 2.6% | 13.90 [0.84, 231.02] | 2001 |
| Lee 2003 | 7.1% | 40.70 [15.97, 103.70] | 2003 |
| Yang 2005 | 5.9% | 4.50 [1.20, 16.90] | 2005 |
| Chung 2005 | 2.7% | 65.90 [4.35, 999.01] | 2005 |
| Chen 2006 | 3.9% | 4.20 [0.54, 32.67] | 2006 |
| **Subtotal (95% CI)** | **22.2%** | **14.21 [4.14, 48.80]** | |
| Heterogeneity: Tau² = 1.08; Chi² = 9.97, df = 4 (P = 0.04); I² = 60% | | | |
| Test for overall effect: Z = 4.21 (P < 0.0001) | | | |
| **2.1.2 India (quid without added tobacco)** | | | |
| Sinor 1990 | 2.9% | 78.00 [5.73, 1062.47] | 1990 |
| Jacob 2004 | 7.1% | 56.20 [21.81, 144.80] | 2004 |
| Ranganathan 2004 (areca nut) | 5.8% | 3.10 [0.82, 11.70] | 2004 |
| Ranganathan 2004 (betel quid) | 2.5% | 29.00 [1.71, 492.19] | 2004 |
| Ranganathan 2004 (pan masala) | 2.6% | 81.50 [4.95, 1341.03] | 2004 |
| Ahmed 2006 (areca nut only) | 3.4% | 172.79 [17.96, 1662.46] | 2006 |
| Ahmed 2006 (pan) | 6.5% | 41.50 [13.54, 127.21] | 2006 |
| Ahmed 2006 (pan masala) | 5.9% | 138.20 [37.69, 506.72] | 2006 |
| **Subtotal (95% CI)** | **36.8%** | **44.28 [16.51, 118.75]** | |
| Heterogeneity: Tau² = 1.18; Chi² = 20.38, df = 7 (P = 0.005); I² = 66% | | | |
| Test for overall effect: Z = 7.53 (P < 0.00001) | | | |
| **2.1.3 India (quid with added tobacco)** | | | |
| Sinor 1990 [wT] | 3.8% | 106.40 [13.01, 870.16] | 1990 |
| Hashibe 2002 [wT] | 7.9% | 44.10 [22.05, 88.21] | 2002 |
| Jacob 2004 [wT] | 7.6% | 73.00 [32.86, 162.19] | 2004 |
| Ahmed 2006 [wT] (Gutka) | 6.4% | 234.91 [74.20, 743.72] | 2006 |
| Mukherjee 2014 [wT] (Gutka) | 3.4% | 145.40 [15.13, 1397.00] | 2014 |
| Khan 2020 [wT] (Gutka) | 5.9% | 17.70 [4.85, 64.60] | 2020 |
| Khan 2020 [wT] | 5.9% | 18.60 [5.01, 69.01] | 2020 |
| **Subtotal (95% CI)** | **41.0%** | **57.54 [29.14, 113.63]** | |
| Heterogeneity: Tau² = 0.43; Chi² = 13.62, df = 6 (P = 0.03); I² = 56% | | | |
| Test for overall effect: Z = 11.67 (P < 0.00001) | | | |
| **Total (95% CI)** | **100.0%** | **38.34 [22.53, 65.26]** | |
| Heterogeneity: Tau² = 0.80; Chi² = 52.38, df = 19 (P < 0.0001); I² = 64% | | | |
| Test for overall effect: Z = 13.44 (P < 0.00001) | | | |
| Test for subgroup differences: Chi² = 3.80, df = 2 (P = 0.15), I² = 47.3% | | | |

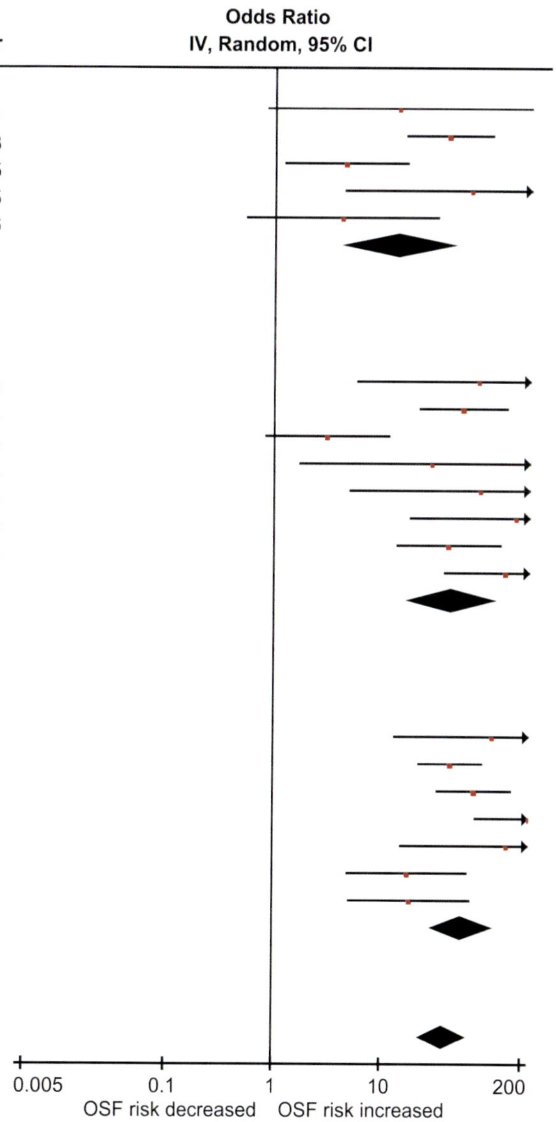


**Fig. 8.1** Pooled estimates for studies from India and Taiwan

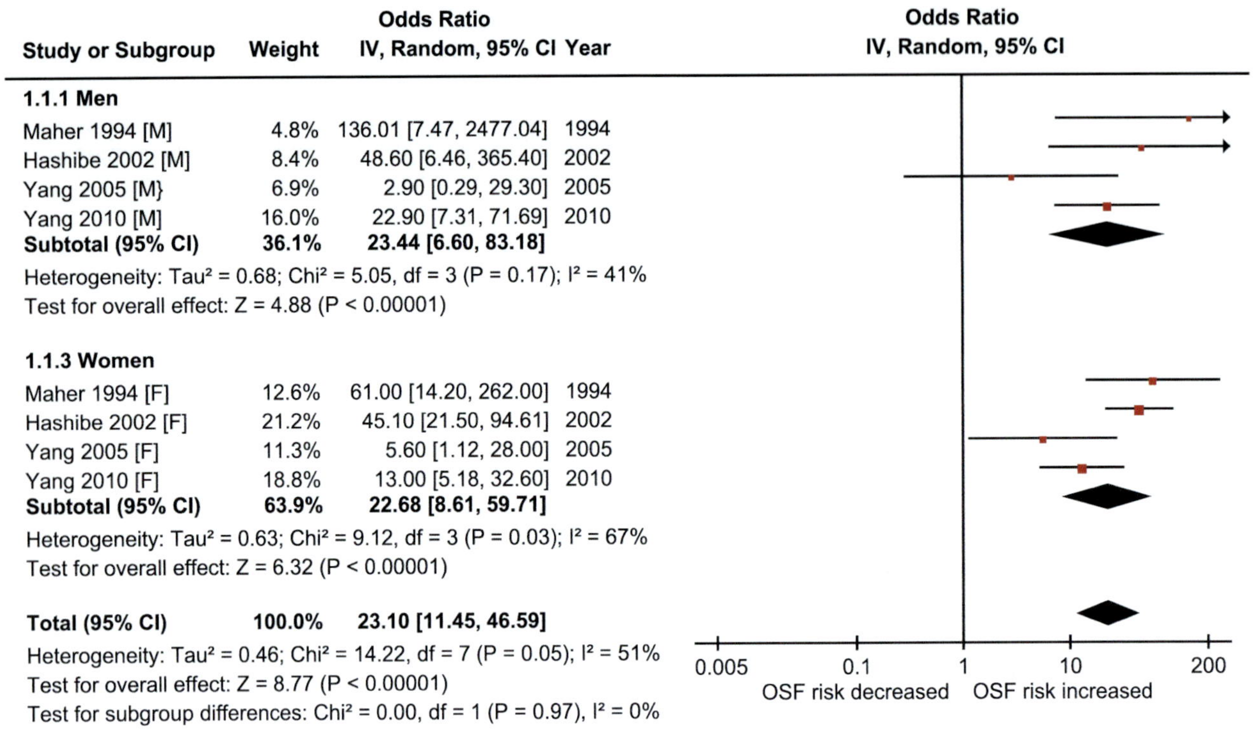


Fig. 8.2 Pooled estimates for men and women comparison



India are 44.3 (95% CI, 16.5–118.8) for nontobacco-added quid and 57.5 (95% CI, 29.1–113.6) for tobacco-added quid. The risks estimated from ORs are higher in betel quid with tobacco than quid without tobacco.

The OSF risk between men and women was also evaluated by random-effect pooled estimates. As shown in Fig. 8.2, the pooled OR was slightly higher in men (23.4; 95% CI, 6.6–83.2) than in women (22.7; 95% CI, 8.6–59.7).

## 8.4 Tobacco, Alcohol, and Synergistic Effect

Users of betel quid and areca nut often simultaneously engage in tobacco smoking or alcohol drinking. The synergistic effects from smoking or drinking alcohol are summarized in Table 8.2. Several studies have investigated the association between tobacco (six reports, [7, 9, 11, 18, 21, 22]) or alcohol (three reports, [7, 18, 21]) and OSF (Table 8.2). The OSF risk in chewers with smoking tobacco ranges from 0.7 (OR, 95% CI, 0.2–3.0) to 29.7 (OR, 95% CI, 3.4–259.9). Among the six studies, only two [7, 9] reported significant ORs for the association between smoking and OSF. The OSF risk in chewers who drank alcohol ranges from 0.9 (OR, 95% CI, 0.2–4.3) to 2.1 (OR, 95% CI, 1.0–4.4). Two studies from Taiwan investigated the synergistic index for the risk of OSF from smoking and alcohol drinking in addition to chewing habit [7, 9]. The synergistic index ranges from 1.2 to 1.6 and was not significant.

There is no strong association between only smoking or alcohol drinking with OSF. This is consistent with the fact that betel quid and areca nut chewing is the etiological factor for OSF.

**Table 8.2** Epidemiologic studies for the association between smoking/drinking and synergistic effects and oral submucous fibrosis

| Reference (publication year), study location, and period | Exposure categories | Odds ratio (95% Confidence Interval) | Synergistic categories | Synergistic index (95% confidence interval) |
|---|---|---|---|---|
| Maher et al. (1994) [17], Pakistan, 1989–1990 | | | Population attributable risk, PAR | 98.6% |
| Lee et al. (2003) [7], Taiwan, 1994–1995 | Smoking | | Synergistic index: | |
| | Past | 6.5 (1.9–22.3) | Cigarette smoking | 1.4 (0.4–4.7) |
| | Current | 7.0 (3.5–14.3) | Alcohol drinking | 1.2 (0.6–2.5) |
| | Drinking | | Population-attributable risk, PAR | 84.5% |
| | Past | 1.4 (0.6–3.4) | | |
| | Current | 1.8 (1.1–3.1) | | |
| Chung et al. (2005) [9], Taiwan, 1998–1999 | Smoking only | 29.7 (3.4–259.9) | Synergistic index | 1.6 |
| Ariyawardana et al. (2006) [18], Sri Lanka | Smoking | 2.8 (0.5–14.1) | | |
| | Alcohol | 0.9 (0.2–4.3) | | |
| Amarasinghe et al. (2010) [22], Sri Lanka, 2006–2007 | Daily smoker | 0.7 (0.2–3.0) | | |
| | Ever smoker | 1.2 (0.3–5.2) | | |
| Yang et al. (2010) [11], Taiwan, 2005 | Smoking | | | |
| | Men | | | |
| | Former | 5.6 (1.6–19.6) | | |
| | Current | 2.2 (0.9–5.3) | | |
| | Women | | | |
| | Current | 1.1 (0.3–3.3) | | |
| | Drinking | | | |
| | Men | | | |
| | Current | 0.7 (0.3–1.6) | | |
| | Women | | | |
| | Current | 1.0 (0.5–1.8) | | |
| Khan et al. (2020) [21], India, 2013–2014 | Smoking | 0.7 (0.4–1.3) | | |
| | Drinking | 2.1 (1.0–4.4) | | |

## 8.5 Dose-Response Effect of Betel Quid and Areca Nut

The dose-response effects from daily frequency and duration of chewing in years are reported in ten studies [7, 8, 11, 13, 16, 17, 19, 20, 23, 24] (**◘** Table 8.3). Increase in daily chewing frequency is associated with increased OSF risk. Majority of these dose-response estimates have strictly increasing trend. Studies that included tests for increasing trend do reveal significant trend effect. In terms of duration of chewing years, four studies report that OR estimates with increasing trend were only seen in women in one study [11]. A reverse trend was observed from two studies [13, 19].

In the investigation of dose-response effects, prespecified intervals of 5 or 10 are commonly used in the literature. Yang et al. [11] used the receiver operating characteristic (ROC) curve with the area under the ROC curve (AUC) to compare the diagnostic accuracy between daily chewing frequency and duration and to



**◘ Table 8.3** Epidemiologic studies for the dose-response relationship of betel quid and areca nut chewing with oral submucous fibrosis

| Reference (publication year), study location, and period | Exposure categories | Odds ratio (95% confidence interval) | *p*-value for trend |
|---|---|---|---|
| Sinor et al. (1990) [16], India | Frequency | | Note: ORs are calculated from Tables 2 and 3 |
| | Times/day | | |
| | 1–5 | 62.4 (7.4–528.5) | |
| | 6–15 | 144.3 (17.6–1183.4) | |
| | 16+ | 234.0 (12.8–4261.3) | |
| | Duration | | |
| | Years | | |
| | 1–5 | 66.3 (7.9–559.6) | |
| | 6–10 | 124.8 (13.5–1154.2) | |
| | 11+ | 169.0 (19.2–1486.7) | |
| Maher et al. (1994) [17], Pakistan, 1989–1990 | Frequency | | |
| | Times/day | | |
| | 1–5 | 84 (20–360) | |
| | 6–10 | 246 (47–1278) | |
| | 11+ | 100 (19–522) | |
| | Duration | | |
| | Years | | |
| | 1–5 | 72 (17–316) | |
| | 6–10 | 137 (29–640) | |
| | 11+ | 109 (25–479) | |
| Hashibe et al. (2002) [19], India, 1995–1998 | Frequency | | |
| | Times/day | | |
| | 1–20 | 28.9 (16.5–50.5) | <0.0001 |
| | 21–40 | 46.8 (24.3–90.2) | |
| | 41+ | 84.3 (32.8–216.8) | |
| | Duration | | |
| | Years | | |

■ **Table 8.3** (continued)

| Reference (publication year), study location, and period | Exposure categories | Odds ratio (95% confidence interval) | *p*-value for trend |
|---|---|---|---|
| | 1–20 | 30.8 (17.6–53.8) | <0.0001 |
| | 21–40 | 34.7 (18.6–64.5) | |
| | 41+ | 22.7 (9.0–57.5) | |
| Lee et al. (2003) [7], Taiwan, 1994–1995 | Frequency | | |
| | Pieces/day | | |
| | 1–10 | 31.4 (11.9–82.5) | <0.05 |
| | 11–20 | 37.4 (12.6–110.4) | |
| | 21+ | 53.5 (16.4–174.8) | |
| | Years | | |
| | 1–10 | 30.9 (11.3–84.7) | <0.05 |
| | 11–20 | 41.9 (14.1–124.9) | |
| | 21+ | 39.3(11.7–131.7) | |
| | Cumulative pack–years | | |
| | 1–10 | 26.5 (10.0–70.3) | <0.05 |
| | 11–20 | 47.0 (15.8–139.8) | |
| | 21+ | 51.4 (16.5–159.7) | |
| Jacob et al. (2004) [13], India | Frequency | | |
| | Times/day | | |
| | 1–10 | 24.6 (9.4–64.3) | <0.0001 |
| | 11+ | 130.9 (35.6–481.5) | |
| | Duration | | |
| | Years | | |
| | 1–10 | 34.4 (13.5–88.1) | <0.0001 |
| | 11+ | 17.6 (4.18–74.3) | |
| Yang et al. (2005) [8], Taiwan | Counts/day | | |
| | 1–9 | 3.7 (0.7–18.9) | |
| | 10–29 | 4.6 (1.2–17.8) | |
| | 30+ | 10.3 (2.4–44.7) | |
| Yen et al. (2007), Taiwan, 1998–1999 | Frequency | | |
| | Pieces/day | | |
| | 1–10 | 1.3 (0.9–1.7) | |
| | 11–20 | 3.9 (2.8–5.6) | |
| | 21+ | 6.9 (5.0–9.6) | |

(continued)

8

**Table 8.3** (continued)

| Reference (publication year), study location, and period | Exposure categories | Odds ratio (95% confidence interval) | *p*-value for trend |
|---|---|---|---|
| Yang et al. (2010) [11], Taiwan, 2005 | Men | | |
| | Counts/day | | |
| | 1–10 | 25.6 (5.5–118.3) | <0.0001 |
| | 11–20 | 27.5 (5.3–144.1) | |
| | 20+ | 33.5 (7.8–143.0) | |
| | Years | | |
| | 0–10 | 42.6 (8.7–207.9) | <0.0001 |
| | 11–20 | 5.0 (0.7–33.2) | |
| | 20+ | 25.5(7.7–84.1) | |
| | Count–years | | |
| | 1st tertile | 40.5 (7.5–218.1) | 0.0114 |
| | 2nd | 37.7 (7.6–187.4) | |
| | 3rd | 22.3 (4.0–123.2) | |
| | Women | | |
| | Counts/day | | |
| | 1–10 | 6.5(1.9–22.9) | 0.0029 |
| | 11–20 | 18.9 (5.6–63.9) | |
| | 20+ | 17.5 (5.6–55.2) | |
| | Years | | |
| | 0–10 | 7.3 (2.0–25.8) | <0.0001 |
| | 11–20 | 8.2 (2.2–30.0) | |
| | 20+ | 13.9 (4.7–40.5) | |
| | Count–years | | |
| | 1st tertile | 5.2 (1.2–23.4) | 0.0143 |
| | 2nd | 19.2 (5.0–73.5) | |
| | 3rd | 16.1 (4.1–63.3) | |
| Mehrotra et al. (2013) [24], India, 2006–2009 | Dose/day | | |
| | Betel quid | | |
| | 1–2 | 0.8 (0.3–1.8) | |
| | 3+ | 2.6 (1.1–6.4) | |
| | Pan masala | | |
| | 1–2 | 14.1 (7.5–26.5) | |
| | 3+ | 17.7 (9.2–34.1) | |
| Mukherjee et al. (2014) [20], India, 2012–2013 | Gutkha | | |
| | 2 packs/day | 3.9 (0.9–18.4) | |
| | 3–4 packs/day | 11.8 (3.5–39.5) | |
| | 5+ packs/day | 89.0 (22.5–352.0) | |

identify the cutoff points in dose-response measures. They found that daily chewing frequency is a better dose-response measure than duration of chewing for predicting the risk of OSF. The cutoff points for higher risk were as low as five for women (sensitivity = 79%, specificity = 83%) and two for men (sensitivity = 82%, specificity = 87%).

## 8.6 Dose-Response of Betel Quid and Areca Nut in Increasing Severity of OSF and Malignant Transformation

The clinical severity of OSF is also associated with the frequency and duration of using betel quid and areca nut. A cross-sectional study of 390 patients with mild (50.5%), moderate (28.2%), or severe (21.3%) OSF [25] found that the severity of OSF increased with frequency, duration, as well as time taken for chewing a quid. Patients who kept the quid in the mouth for longer periods and swallowed the betel juice had a higher risk of severe OSF.

Another cross-sectional study of 765 patients examined the areca nut dose-response effect [26]. The multinomial logistic regression, which simultaneously estimates OR for severe vs. mild and moderate vs. mild, showed that daily frequency is associated with severity (ORs = 1.13 and 1.56, all $p$-value <0.001). However, from the same analysis model, the effect of chewing years was not significantly associated with OSF severity. The cumulative amount of *gutkha* consumption was also found to be positively related to the clinical severity of OSF [27]. A study of 300 OSF patients showed a positive association with the duration of *gutkha* intake but not the daily frequency [28]. Another study of 342 OSF patients also showed positive association between duration and OSF severity [29]. A study of 1000 OSF cases from Central India found that both average daily frequency (1.2 vs. 0.3, $p$-value = 0.001) and chewing years (2.4 vs. 0.74, $p$-value = 0.006) were significant for malignant transformation [30].

A case-control study from China investigated the risk of malignant transformation in OSF patients [31]. The ORs increased as frequency and duration increased for chewing areca nut (alone or with smoking and alcohol drinking).

## 8.7 Conclusions

The consumption of betel quid and areca nut is the primary cause of OSF. Published studies reviewed in this chapter present sufficient evidence to support this conclusion. Although areca nut may be used in various forms around the world, the OSF risk posed by areca nut has been consistently confirmed from epidemiological studies in users of betel quid and areca nut with and without added tobacco. To avoid possible confounding factors, which may jeopardize the actual association, many of the studies are based on case-control design with or without matching. Matching based on age and sex would balance the possible difference from general demographic characteristics. Some studies additionally consider social economic status for matching to account for possible social or cultural differences. In several published studies, the possible confounding effects from tobacco or alcohol consumption have been addressed by multivariate logistic regression with adjustment for tobacco and alcohol use or by stratified groups.

From studies reporting dose-response by examining the daily frequency and duration of use, the effect is clearer for daily frequency, but not duration.

The association between tobacco or alcohol habits with OSF is not conclusive and furthermore does not demonstrate any synergistic effect.

Betel quid and areca nut chewing are the primary lifestyle factors increasing the risk of OSF in humans.

**Summary**

- We conclude that betel quid and areca nut chewing are the primary lifestyle factors for the causation of OSF.
- Daily frequency is the better dose-response measure for predicting the risk of OSF. The cutoff points for higher risk are as low as five times per day for women and two for men.
- Analyzing the current literature, there is no strong association between smoking or alcohol drinking and OSF.

## References

1. Tilakaratne WM, Ekanayaka RP, Warnakulasuriya S. Oral submucous fibrosis: a historical perspective and a review on etiology and pathogenesis. Oral Surg Oral Med Oral Pathol Oral Radiol. 2016;122(2):178–91. https://doi.org/10.1016/j.oooo.2016.04.003.
2. Murti PR, Bhonsle RB, Gupta PC, Daftary DK, Pindborg JJ, Mehta FS. Etiology of oral submucous fibrosis with special reference to the role of areca nut chewing. J Oral Pathol Med. 1995;24(4):145–52.
3. IARC. Betel-quid and areca-nut chewing and some areca-nut derived nitrosamines. IARC Monogr Eval Carcinog Risks Hum. 2004;85:1–334.
4. IARC. Personal habits and indoor combustions. Volume 100 E. A review of human carcinogens. IARC Monogr Eval Carcinog Risks Hum. 2012;100(Pt E):1–538.
5. IARC. Tobacco habits other than smoking, Betel-quid and areca-nut chewing, Some related nitrosamines. IARC Monogr Eval Carcinog Risk Chem Hum. 1985;37:1–268.

6. Yang YH, Lee HY, Tung S, Shieh TY. Epidemiological survey of oral submucous fibrosis and leukoplakia in aborigines of Taiwan. J Oral Pathol Med. 2001;30(4):213–9. https://doi.org/10.1034/j.1600-0714.2001.300404.x.
7. Lee CH, Ko YC, Huang HL, Chao YY, Tsai CC, Shieh TY, et al. The precancer risk of betel quid chewing, tobacco use and alcohol consumption in oral leukoplakia and oral submucous fibrosis in southern Taiwan. Br J Cancer. 2003;88(3):366–72. https://doi.org/10.1038/sj.bjc.6600727.
8. Yang YH, Chen CH, Chang JS, Lin CC, Cheng TC, Shieh TY. Incidence rates of oral cancer and oral pre-cancerous lesions in a 6-year follow-up study of a Taiwanese aboriginal community. J Oral Pathol Med. 2005;34(10):596–601. https://doi.org/10.1111/j.1600-0714.2005.00266.x.
9. Chung CH, Yang YH, Wang TY, Shieh TY, Warnakulasuriya S. Oral precancerous disorders associated with areca quid chewing, smoking, and alcohol drinking in southern Taiwan. J Oral Pathol Med. 2005;34(8):460–6. https://doi.org/10.1111/j.1600-0714.2005.00332.x.
10. Chen PC, Pan CC, Kuo C, Lin CP. Risk of oral nonmalignant lesions associated with human papillomavirus infection, betel quid chewing, and cigarette smoking in Taiwan: an integrated molecular and epidemiologic study. Arch Pathol Lab Med. 2006;130(1):57–61. https://doi.org/10.5858/2006-130-57-ROONLA.
11. Yang YH, Ho PS, Lu HM, Huang IY, Chen CH. Comparing dose-response measurements of oral habits on oral leukoplakia and oral submucous fibrosis from a community screening program. J Oral Pathol Med. 2010;39(4):306–12. https://doi.org/10.1111/j.1600-0714.2009.00820.x.
12. Zhang SS, Li WH, Gao YJ, Liu ZW, Liu L, Tang JQ, et al. Betel-quid and oral submucous fibrosis: a cross-sectional study in Hunan province. China. J Oral Pathol Med. 2012;41(10):748–54. https://doi.org/10.1111/j.1600-0714.2012.01166.x.
13. Jacob BJ, Straif K, Thomas G, Ramadas K, Mathew B, Zhang ZF, et al. Betel quid without tobacco as a risk factor for oral precancers. Oral Oncol. 2004;40(7):697–704. https://doi.org/10.1016/j.oraloncology.2004.01.005.
14. Ranganathan K, Devi MU, Joshua E, Kirankumar K, Saraswathi TR. Oral submucous fibrosis: a case-control study in Chennai, South India. J Oral Pathol Med. 2004;33(5):274–7. https://doi.org/10.1111/j.0904-2512.2004.00116.x.
15. Ahmad MS, Ali SA, Ali AS, Chaubey KK. Epidemiological and etiological study of oral submucous fibrosis among gutkha chewers of Patna, Bihar, India. J Indian Soc Pedod Prev Dent. 2006;24(2):84–9. https://doi.org/10.4103/0970-4388.26022.
16. Sinor PN, Gupta PC, Murti PR, Bhonsle RB, Daftary DK, Mehta FS, et al. A case-control study of oral submucous fibrosis with special reference to the etiologic role of areca nut. J Oral Pathol Med. 1990;19(2):94–8. https://doi.org/10.1111/j.1600-0714.1990.tb00804.x.
17. Maher R, Lee AJ, Warnakulasuriya KA, Lewis JA, Johnson NW. Role of areca nut in the causation of oral submucous fibrosis: a case-control study in Pakistan. J Oral Pathol Med. 1994;23(2):65–9. https://doi.org/10.1111/j.1600-0714.1994.tb00258.x.
18. Ariyawardana A, Athukorala AD, Arulanandam A. Effect of betel chewing, tobacco smoking and alcohol consumption on oral submucous fibrosis: a case-control study in Sri Lanka. J Oral Pathol Med. 2006;35(4):197–201. https://doi.org/10.1111/j.1600-0714.2006.00400.x.
19. Hashibe M, Sankaranarayanan R, Thomas G, Kuruvilla B, Mathew B, Somanathan T, et al. Body mass index, tobacco chewing, alcohol drinking and the risk of oral submucous fibrosis in Kerala, India. Cancer Causes Control. 2002;13(1):55–64. https://doi.org/10.1023/a:1013991025848.
20. Mukherjee D, Oommen AM, Ghom A, George K. Risk factors associated with Oral Sub Mucous Fibrosis (OSMF). Int J Health Sci Res. 2014:4(7).
21. Khan A, Ongole R, Baptist J, Srikant N, Lukmani F. Patterns of tobacco use and its relation to oral precancers and cancers among individuals visiting a tertiary hospital in South India. J Contemp Dent Pract. 2020;21(3):304–9.
22. Amarasinghe HK, Usgodaarachchi US, Johnson NW, Lalloo R, Warnakulasuriya S. Betel-quid chewing with or without tobacco is a major risk factor for oral potentially malignant disorders in Sri Lanka: a case-control study. Oral Oncol. 2010;46(4):297–301. https://doi.org/10.1016/j.oraloncology.2010.01.017.
23. Yen AM, Chen SC, Chen TH. Dose-response relationships of oral habits associated with the risk of oral pre-malignant lesions among men who chew betel quid. Oral Oncol. 2007;43(7):634–8. https://doi.org/10.1016/j.oraloncology.2006.05.001.
24. Mehrotra D, Kumar S, Agarwal GG, Asthana A, Kumar S. Odds ratio of risk factors for oral submucous fibrosis in a case control model. Br J Oral Maxillofac Surg. 2013;51(7):e169–73. https://doi.org/10.1016/j.bjoms.2012.08.001.
25. Reddy V, Wanjari PV, Banda NR, Reddy P. Oral submucous fibrosis correlation of clinical grading to various habit factors. Int J Dent Clin. 2011;3(1):21–4.
26. Hosein M, Mohiuddin S, Fatima N. Association between grading of oral submucous fibrosis with frequency and consumption of areca nut and its derivatives in a wide age group: a multi-centric cross sectional study From Karachi, Pakistan. J Cancer Prev. 2015;20(3):216–22. https://doi.org/10.15430/JCP.2015.20.3.216.
27. Singh A, Lanke RB, Shetty R, Akifuddin S, Sahu M, Singh N, et al. Effect of habits and nutritional status on clinical grading and histopathological staging in patients with oral sub mucous fibrosis. J Clin Diagn Res. 2015;9(10):ZC49–52. https://doi.org/10.7860/JCDR/2015/16013.6648.
28. Siddiqui HK, Khan FR, Sadiq A, Hashmi U, Qaiser Z. Predictors of the severity of oral submucous fibrosis among gutka consumers: a regression analysis. Br J Oral Maxillofac Surg. 2021;59(6):690–4. https://doi.org/10.1016/j.bjoms.2020.09.005.
29. Balsaraf S, Bhambal A, Chole R. Study of oral potentially malignant disorders related to various risk factors amongst the patients attending hospitals in Bhopal, India. Med Pharm Rep. 2019;92(1):66–71. https://doi.org/10.15386/cjmed-906.
30. Hazarey VK, Erlewad DM, Mundhe KA, Ughade SN. Oral submucous fibrosis: study of 1000 cases from central India. J Oral Pathol Med. 2007;36(1):12–7. https://doi.org/10.1111/j.1600-0714.2006.00485.x.
31. Liu B, Shen M, Xiong J, Yuan Y, Wu X, Gao X, et al. Synergistic effects of betel quid chewing, tobacco use (in the form of cigarette smoking), and alcohol consumption on the risk of malignant transformation of oral submucous fibrosis (OSF): a case-control study in Hunan Province, China. Oral Surg Oral Med Oral Pathol Oral Radiol. 2015;120(3):337–45. https://doi.org/10.1016/j.oooo.2015.04.013.


8

# Genetic Aspects of Oral Submucous Fibrosis

*Jay Gopal Ray and Rajiv S. Desai*

## Contents



© The Author(s), under exclusive license to Springer Nature Switzerland AG 2023
S. Warnakulasuriya, K. Ranganathan (eds.), *Oral Submucous Fibrosis*, Textbooks in Contemporary Dentistry,
https://doi.org/10.1007/978-3-031-12855-4_9

## 9.1 Introduction

Oral cancer is a multistep process which may be preceded by oral potentially malignant disorders (OPMDs), such as oral submucous fibrosis (OSF) [1]. The high mortality and morbidity rates associated with oral cancer are because of late diagnosis [2]. Identification of newer techniques to diagnose the disease at the earliest stage is facilitated by advances in research, which include molecular and biochemical markers for early detection. Some of these markers reflect genetic and epigenetic changes [3]. Gene ontology and bioinformatics have been used to identify genes that are mutated, upregulated, or downregulated. However, there are no in silico studies in OSF.

**Learning Goals**

- To understand the genetic alterations in OSF and to examine the biomarkers that may help to identify populations at risk particularly among betel quid/areca nut chewers.

9

## 9.2 Genetic Susceptibility and Gene Expression in Tissue/Organ Fibrosis

In systemic fibrotic conditions involving the liver, kidney, and lung, the association of genetic susceptibility is observed [4–7]. In cirrhosis of the liver, in addition to exogenous factors such as alcohol abuse and viral hepatitis, genetic predisposition significantly contributes to both cirrhosis and liver carcinoma [4]. Besides environmental factors, genetic factors involved in aging/senescence, cell-cell adhesion, and host defense contribute to the increased risk of pulmonary fibrosis [6]. Genetic susceptibility is also important in systemic sclerosis of the skin and internal organs [7].

## 9.3 Genetic Susceptibility in Oral Submucous Fibrosis (OSF)

Genetic susceptibility is important in the development of betel quid (BQ)-induced OSF. The mechanism involved in genetic susceptibility to OSF involves the combined effect of various genes.

### 9.3.1 Collagen 1A1 and Collagen 1A2 (COL1A1 and COL1A2) Gene

The connective tissue extracellular matrix (ECM) forms a three-dimensional scaffold for the cells and is involved in tissue homeostasis by components of ECM such as fibronectin, elastin, collagen, and nonfibrillar protein such as hyaluronan, proteoglycan, and glycoproteins [8]. Cancer progression is intensified by hypoxia and collagen-rich conditions [9]. Impairment of ECM function and ECM-cell interaction play an important role in diseases such as fibrosis, cancer, and osteoarthritis [8].

OSF is a collagen-related disorder having dense collagen deposition in the oral submucosa. Buccal mucosa when exposed to areca alkaloid, due to chewing BQ, accumulate collagen [10].

In OSF, there are alterations in collagen fiber bundle diameter, thickness, and distribution [11]. There is altered expression of type I and type III collagen fibers. In early OSF, and normal mucosa COLI is 85% and COL III 15%. However, as the disease progresses, type III collagen is gradually replaced by type I collagen, thereby leading to collagen I-predominant microenvironment [12].

The stiffness of oral mucosa in OSF is due to loss of procollagen type III, a predominance of collagen type I, and complete loss of collagen type IV [13]. Relative to normal buccal fibroblasts, more type I collagen mRNA and type I collagen trimers are seen in OSF fibroblasts [14].

The genes involved in collagen synthesis (transcription, translation, and posttranslational processing), degradation, and collagen cross-linking include collagen 1A1 and 1A2 (COL1A1 and COL1A2), collagenase-1 (COLase), transforming growth factor-beta (TGF-β), lysyl oxidase, and cystatin C (CST3). These genes are implicated in the pathogenesis of OSF. The constituents of areca nut, mainly arecoline and arecaidine, are found to interact with COL1A1, COL1A2, COLase, and lysyl oxidase (LOX) expressed in fibroblasts. Gene- and gene-environmental interactions explain the differences between individuals having low and high exposure to areca nut (AN). During the development of OSF, the microenvironment around oral fibroblasts can vary between low- and high-exposure groups. This discrepancy may result from fibroblast selection by BQ ingredients or inflammatory factors during the progression of OSF. A high proportion of the OSF risk can be attributed to the genetic component [15].

### 9.3.2 Matrix Metalloproteinases (MMPs)

MMPs constitute a family of neutral proteases which can degrade the ECM [16]. Twenty-eight human MMPs have been identified so far. These enzymes are classified as per their substrate specificity and structural similarities. Among them, a few important examples are collagenases (MMP-1) gelatinases (MMP-2 and MMP-9), stromelysin (MMP-3), and membrane-bound MMPs. MMPs regulate ECM proteolysis and process several biologically active proteins such as cytokines, cell-surface proteins, chemokines, TGF-β 1, and other inflammation-related molecules that contribute to tissue fibrosis [16]. Many MMPs are expressed and activated in OSF patients as well as in head and neck squamous cell carcinoma (HNSCC) [17]. Gene polymorphisms in MMPs are suspected to influence gene expression in OSF.

### 9.3.3 Collagenase-1 (COLase-1, MMP-1)

Interstitial collagenase, also known as collagenase I, or MMP-1 belongs to a subgroup of the MMP family. It is the principal collagenase that cleaves collagen type I, II, III, VII, and X collagen. Collagenase I is important in photocarcinogenesis and photoaging [18]. Collagenase I is produced by various cells such as macrophages, stromal fibroblasts, endothelial cells, epithelial cells, and tumor cells [19]. It is secreted as a pro-collagenase and can be activated by many signaling pathways [20]. In OSF, MMP-1 activity is found to be lower compared to normal oral mucosa indicating a difference in collagen metabolism in patients. However, there is no statistically significant difference among different histological grades of OSF [21, 22]. Elevated expression of MMP-1 in stromal cells of OSF has also been reported [23]. Elevated expressions of MMP-1 have been reported in OSCC patients having BQ-chewing habit [24]. MMP-1 promoter region enhances its transcriptional activity and contributes to carcinogenesis and cancer metastasis. Choudhary et al. reported that single nucleotide polymorphisms (SNPs) in the MMP-1 promoter region are associated with the susceptibility of BQ chewers to HNSCC and OSF in India. Habitual BQ chewing and alcohol consumption enhance the expression of the 2G allele of MMP-1 genes in HNSCC and OSF patients [17]. Moreover, the 2G phenotype of the MMP-1 promoter is found in higher frequency in OSF and OSCC patients in comparison to controls [25].

### 9.3.4 MMP-2 (Gelatinase-A) and MMP-9 (Gelatinase-B)

MMP-2, also known as gelatinase-A, and MMP-9, also known as gelatinase-B, are $Zn^{2+}$-dependent endopeptidases having similar structures. MMP-2 is expressed by a wide variety of cell types in normal conditions, while MMP-9 is expressed in only a few cell types including trophoblasts, osteoclasts, leukocytes, dendritic cells, and precursors [26]. MMP-2 gene is located on chromosome 16q, while MMP-9 is on chromosome 20q. MMP-2 degrades proteins in ECM as well as the basement membrane. It degrades type I, type IV, type V, and type X collagen, elastin, laminin, fibronectin, elastin, and proteoglycans [27]. Mutations in MMP-2 disrupt its transcriptional activity resulting in its increased transcription. Individuals carrying CC genotype are found to express more MMP-2 proteins than individuals carrying TT or CT genotype [28]. Lin et al. assessed the MMP-2 genotype association with the risk of OSF and OSCC in 58 OSF cases, 121 OSCC cases, and 147 control cases. The subjects carrying CC genotype had twofold more risk in the development of OSF [29]. MMP-9 is known to degrade extracellular matrix components such as fibrillin, decorin, elastin type IV, V, XI, and XVI collagen, laminin, and gelatin. It also activates factors such as pro-TNF and pro-TGF [30]. In OSF, expressions of MMP-2, MMP-9, TIMP-1, and TIMP-2 are high compared to healthy oral mucosa [23]. MMP-9 expression has been analyzed in 432 patients and was found to be elevated in saliva, mucosa, and serum of patients in OPMDs compared to control [31]. Arecoline stimulated TIMP-1 expression, but reduced fibroblasts MMP-2 and MMP-9 in buccal mucosa [32].

PCR, RFLP of single nucleotide polymorphisms (SNP) genotyping reveals no significant difference in MMP-2 and MMP-9 polymorphism in OSF patients compared to healthy controls. T allele showed a significant association with increasing clinicopathological grades of HNSCC [17]. Tu et al. studied MMP-9 SNP in BQ-related OSCC, OSF, and non-diseased BQ chewers. Functional association of MMP-9-1562 C/T polymorphism with increased OSCC was seen in young BQ chewers. However, in the elder population, this association was not observed. No association was observed between the joint MMP-9 -1562 C>T and MMP-3 -1171 5A>6A functional polymorphisms and OSCC risk or patient survival [33].

### 9.3.5 MMP-3 (Stromelysin-1)

MMP-3 degrades basal membrane and collagen type II, V, IX, and X. It also induces activation of MMP-1 and MMP-9. MMP-3 gene is located on chromosome 11q22.3. Ye et al. reported 6A allele showing lower promoter activity than the 5A allele in vitro [34]. Tu et al. assessed the association of MMP-3 genotype with OSCC and OSF risk in 71 OSF patients, 150 OSCC patients, and 98 controls. They reported that the frequency of 5A genotype in the MMP-3 promoter was more in the OSF than in the control group; however, no significant differences were observed between the OSCC and control groups. 5A genotype in MMP-3 promoter was found to be associated with OSF risk but not OSCC [35].

In the case-control study of 362 participants (135 HNSCC, 101 OSF, and 126 controls), Choudhary et al. studied the genotype of MMP-3 SNP by PCR-RFLP analysis. The difference in 5A genotype frequency between OSF and control was statistically significant. However, the 5A genotype showed a twofold increased risk for OSF development compared to controls, but this phenomenon was only observed in patients less than 45 years of age. The concluded that MMP-3 genotype expression is associated with 5A alleles, which may play a major role in developing HNSCC and OSF [36].

Zade et al. evaluated the genotype of MMP-3 SNP by PCR analysis of 20 individuals (five OSCC, five OSF, five normal individuals with AN and alcohol habits, and five without the habit). The frequency of 5A genotype in MMP-3 promoter was found to be higher in OSF compared to the control group; however, between OSCC and control group, no significant difference was noted. It was similar to Tu's study where 5A genotype in the MMP-3 promoter is associated with the risk of OSF but not in OSCC in an Indian population [37]. In MMP-3 promoter -1171, 5A>6A, the insertion or deletion of single adenosine could alter the transcription level of the MMP-3 gene. For MMP-3, the frequency of the 5A genotype in the MMP-3 promoter region was higher in the OSF group than in the control group and a greater than twofold risk for developing OSF compared to controls. However, the 5A/5A carrier allele showed an association only in patients less than 45 years of age [37].

9

### 9.3.6 TGF-β and SMAD

A variety of mediators including hormones, cytokines, and growth factors influence the synthesis of collagen TGF-β controls proliferation, differentiation, and function in many cell types. It is known to stimulate collagen production through the regulation of intramembrane proteolysis and CREB3L1 activation [38]. Kale et al. found more adipose tissues and TGF-β expression in early-stage OSF tissues in India [39]. Overexpression of both TGF-β1 and TGF-β2 was reported in OSF tissues, with a higher expression of TGF-β1 than TGF-β2. TGF-β1 is expressed in inflammatory cells, perivascular cells, epithelial cells, muscle and fibroblasts [40–42]. The mRNA level of TGF-β was higher in the early and middle stages of OSF tissues than in healthy patients of Hunan, China [42]. An increased expression of CD105, a TGF-β1 receptor, was associated with hypoxia-induced neoangiogenic activity in OSF. This feature was linked to transformation from normal mucosa to mild and severe epithelial dysplasia [43–45].

A study from Sri Lanka showed that the difference in TGF-β expression was not evident among OSF patients, pan masala (a chewing tobacco and AN product in India) chewers, and healthy oral mucosa. Secretion of TGF-β1 in cultured fibroblasts harvested from the specimens also showed no marked difference [46]. In a recent study, real-time PCR and immunohistochemical staining showed elevated expression of TGF-β1, connective tissue growth factor (CTGF), and decreased expression of bone morphogenetic protein 7 (BMP-7) in OSF. The possible stimulatory effects of areca components on epithelial-mesenchymal transition and expression of smooth muscle actin, CTGF, TGF-β, LIM domain kinase 1 (LIMK1), and p-Smad2 in epithelial cells has also been reported [47–49]. Injection of pan masala extract to buccal mucosa of Sprague Dawley rats on alternate days for 48 weeks induced OSF-like changes with a concomitant elevated expression of TGF-β1 [50].

Chang et al. observed that areca nut extract (ANE) stimulated TGF-β1 and Smad2 in oral keratinocytes and SAS oral cancer cells implicating the involvement of AN in the OSF pathogenesis [51]. Smad2 overexpression has been reported in OSF tissues relative to healthy tissues [52].

The expression of Smad7, an inhibitor of TGF-β, is elevated in OSCC and OSF tissues relative to normal tissues and has been suggested as a diagnostic marker [53]. The association of genotypes of TGF-β1 with the risk of OSF has been investigated. While comparing the frequencies of TC, TT, and CC alleles on the TGF-β1 gene on chromosome 19q, it was found that high OSF risk is associated with CC alleles in both low- and high-exposure groups [15]. An Indian study showed evidence of C-to-T transition (rs13306708) in the 50UTR region of TGF-β1 between OSF patients [27CC, 15CT, 8TT] and control subjects [42CC, 6CT, 2TT]); however, authors could not find polymorphisms in the promoter region and exon 1 of TGF β1 in OSF patients and control subjects [54]. Hsu et al. compared the TGF-β1 codon 10 T/C and codon 25 G/C polymorphisms in patients with oral premalignant lesions and healthy control. They found an association of TGF-β1 codon 10 and 25 polymorphisms with the development of OPMDs [55].

### 9.3.7 Lysyl Oxidase (LOX)

Lysyl oxidase (LOX), also known as protein-lysine 6-oxidase, is a copper-dependent extracellular enzyme that mediates cross-linking of collagen and elastin through posttranslational oxidative deamination of peptidyl lysine residues in their precursors. LOX stabilizes the collagen fibrillar array and contributes to the stiffness and mechanical strength of ECM [56, 57]. LOX and LOX-like proteins participate in tissue fibrosis, tumorigenesis, atherosclerosis, and metastasis by mediating protein expression and regulating signal transduction [56]. LOX overexpression affects tumor desmoplasia (fibrosis) and tumor microenvironment, and stimulates anchorage-independent growth of OSCC cells [56, 58, 59]. LOX expression in blood cells from patients of OSF was found to be similar to, lower than, or higher than age- and sex-matched controls suggesting that changes of LOX in circulating blood cells of OSF were not significant [60]. LOX activity is found to be elevated in fibroblasts cultured from OSF patients when compared with fibroblasts cultured from normal oral mucosa [61]. An epidemiological study showed elevated LOX expression in OSF and oral mucosa adjacent to OSCC tissues [58]. This could be due to the stimulation of LOX expression in oral keratinocytes by ANE. Copper in BQ was found to stimulate LOX expression of fibroblasts, thereby increasing collagen cross-linking and resistance to degradation [62].

LOX, encoded by the LOX gene on chromosome 5q, has been linked with predisposition to OSF. The frequencies of three genotypic variants (AA, AG, and GG) of LOX genes in patients of OSF and controls were investigated. The high OSF risk allele was found to be AA in the low-exposure group, while GG is more prevalent in the high-exposure group [15]. Differences of Arg158Gln SNPs of the LOX genotype between elder BQ chewers and OSF patients were seen in PCR-RFLP and direct sequencing [63]. The Arg158Gln SNP was associated with early clinical stages of OSCC [52]. Thorawat et al. studied LOX G473A SNP in OSF, in BQ chewers without OSF, as well as in healthy controls. LOX G473A SNPs were not present in this Indian cohort [64]. Mukherjee et al. studied the genotype for LOX polymorphism by PCR-RFLP. They observed significantly higher heterozygous G473A genotype in OSF cases, among 26–40-year age group, and in male patients. They also found a higher total soluble collagen level among patients carrying GA or AA genotype [65]. These reports suggest that LOX and LOX-like proteins could be a potential therapeutic target for the treatment of OSF [59].

### 9.3.8 Cystatin C (CST3)

Cystatin C (CST3) is a molecule responsible for the prevention of ECM degradation. The terminal regions of each collagen molecule are composed of terminal peptides, which function in cross-linking and enhancing the strength of collagen fibers. These areas are resistant to attacks by collagenases but are susceptible to serine and cysteine proteinases. These groups of enzymes belong to the cystatin superfamily, namely the type 1 cystatins (stefins A, B), type 2 cystatins, and kininogens. Cystatin C is one of the type 2 cystatins, a class of cysteine proteinase inhibitors found in a variety of human body fluids and secretions. The major function of this enzyme is to provide protection and stabilization of the collagen fibrils [66]. Cystatin plays a crucial role in carcinogenesis and fibrosis of various organs such as the kidney, lung, and liver [67–69]. Cystatin C expression is higher in OSF tissues when compared to normal oral mucosa. It is mainly expressed by fibroblasts, endothelial cells, and inflammatory cells. Fibroblasts from OSF show higher cystatin expression than normal fibroblasts. In addition, arecoline was found to promote cystatin C mRNA and protein expression in a dose-dependent manner [70]. Cystatin C is encoded by the CST3 gene on chromosome 20p. With A being normal allele and B the mutated allele, frequency distribution of AA, AB, and BB on CST3 gene in OSF patients and healthy individuals were showed an increased risk of OSF with high-risk allele AA in those with both low and high exposures to betel quid [15]. There was a consistent relationship between genotype distribution of TGF-β1 and CST3 genes and the risk of OSF in both low- and high-exposure groups [71].

The authors have also investigated the effect of the combination of these six genes for evaluating gene-gene interaction, in both high and low exposures for BQ. Other studies reported that genotypes associated with the highest OSF risk in the lower exposure group were CC of COL1A1, AA of COL1A2, TT of collagenase-1, CC of TGF-β1, AA of LOX, and AA of CST3. On the other hand, TT of COL1A1, BB of COL1A2, AA of collagenase-1, CC of TGF-β1, GG of LOX, and AA of CST3 genes led to the highest risk of OSF in the high-exposure group [71].

An elevated cystatin M was shown to promote the metastasis of OSCC by blocking cathepsin B activity and rescuing tumor cells from TNF-α-induced apoptosis [72]. Salivary cystatin B level was also found to be a valuable prognostic marker for OSCC patients [73]. More studies are needed to clarify the role of various cystatins in OSF and OSCC.

### 9.3.9 Plasminogen Activator Inhibitor (PAI-1)

ECM homeostasis and wound healing are regulated by plasminogen activator inhibitor-1 (PAI-1) by suppression of urokinase plasminogen activator (uPA)/tissue plasminogen activator (tPA)-mediated conversion of plasminogen to plasmin, which activates MMPs and fibrinolysis. Studies on fibrosis models of internal organs such as liver, lung, and kidney have found that PAI-1 deficiency or inhibition of PAI-1 activity attenuates organ fibrosis [74]. TGF-β may stimulate PAI-1 expression through ROS and SMAD-dependent (ALK5/smad2/3) and SMAD-independent (Src/EGFR/MEK/ERK) pathways [75, 76]. When compared to normal buccal fibroblasts, PAI-1 and tPA secretion is increased in fibroblasts derived from OSF. In OSF, the fibroblast ratio of PAI-1/tPA is also increased. Arecoline stimulates PAI and tPA secretion. It also increases the PAI-1/tPA ratio in buccal mucosal fibroblasts [77, 78]. Moreover, when compared to healthy tissue, hypoxia-inducible factor-1α (HIF-1α) showed overexpression in fibroblasts, inflammatory cells, and epithelial cells in OSF tissues. Hypoxia enhanced arecoline-induced ECM and PAI-1 production by buccal mucosal fibroblasts [79]. PAI-1 expression was found to be elevated in OSCC tissues when compared to normal tissues; however, PAI-1 showed little association with the survival rate of OSCC patients [80]. PAI-1 – 675 4G/5G genotypes were reported to be strongly associated with OSCC relative to control subjects in the European population [81, 82]. More studies can clarify PAI-1 polymorphism in the risk and survival of OSF and OSCC patients.

9

### 9.3.10 TIMPs (Tissue Inhibitor Matrix Metalloproteinases)

TIMPs (TIMP-1, TIMP-2, TIMP-3, and TIMP-4) that show differential inhibitory effects on MMPs, a disintegrin, and metalloproteinases (ADAMs) prevent proteolysis of ECM followed by accumulation of ECM/tissue fibrosis [16]. Shrestha and Carnelio reported overexpression of MMP-2 and TIMP-2 in mucosal tissues from early and moderately advanced OSF patients. TIMP-2 was expressed in the deeper connective tissue, lamina propria, and suprabasal layers. MMP-2 found in the basal and suprabasal layers showed differences in expression in these two stages of OSF [83]. Zymography and immunohistochemical staining showed an increase in the expression of MMP-1, MMP-2, MMP-9, TIMP-1, and TIMP-2 in OSF tissues when compared to normal tissues [23]. An in vitro study from Sri Lanka found that fibroblasts from early-stage OSF secrete more TIMP-1 and TIMP-2 compared to fibroblasts from pan masala chewers without OSF and normal buccal mucosal fibroblasts. These differences might be caused by cellular senescence and premature aging of buccal mucosa tissues [46].

Safrole and arecoline stimulate TIMP-1 mRNA and protein expression of buccal fibroblasts [32, 84]. Fibroblasts from OSF tissues were found to secrete more TIMP-1 than fibroblasts from surrounding healthy tissues suggesting that they may have role in the pathogenesis of OSF [32, 84].

Fibroblasts from early-stage OSF were found to have similar levels of TGF-β1, MMP-1, MMP-2, MMP-3, interleukin-6 (IL-6), and IL-8 when compared with fibroblasts from healthy tissues. However, increased TIMP-1 and TIMP-2 secretion from OSF fibroblasts was observed [46].

### 9.3.11 Vascular Endothelial Growth Factor (VEGF)

Transforming growth factor (TGF), vascular endothelial growth factor (VEGF), and basic fibroblast growth factor (bFGF) are tumor growth factors that serve as cancer biomarkers [85]. Adequate blood supply is necessary for the growth of solid tumors, and growth factors responsible for it have been studied extensively in various tumors [86]. Vascular endothelial cells are found to be dormant in adult cells, and they divide less than once in a decade. During the tumor growth phase, hypoxia develops, pro-angiogenic factors increase resulting in angiogenesis and tumor progression. Following upregulation of hypoxia-inducible transcription factor, increased production of VEGF is observed [87]. VEGF is a critical angiogenic cytokine involved in blood supply to neoplastic cells. Also, there is a significant increase in vascularity during the transition from normal oral mucosa to degrees of dysplasia. In addition to its role in angiogenesis in squamous cell carcinoma, VEGF has also been investigated in oral potentially malignant disorders and has been linked to oral cancer metastasis [88]. The polymorphic nature of the VEGF-460/T gene has been assessed in subjects of OSF to identify the progression to malignancy at an early stage [89]. Among subjects, 6.67% showed CT polymorphism and 16.67% of subjects showed TT polymorphism. Thus, VEGF 460 C/T has the potential to be used as a prognostic marker in predicting the malignant transformation of OSF [89].

### 9.3.12 Cytochrome P450 (CYP3A) Gene

Cytochrome P450 3A (CYP3A) gene family has a major role to play in the oxidative metabolism of many xenobiotic substrates and active endogenous substrates. Polymorphisms in the gene for cytochrome P450 enzyme can alter the activation or detoxification of carcinogenic compounds that influence an individual's genetic susceptibility to cancer [90]. Betel chewers having lower CYP3A expression levels are more susceptible to BQ toxicity. Various studies have demonstrated CYP3A gene polymorphism associated with an individual's susceptibility to OSCC and OPMDs among tobacco users [91, 92].

CYP3A polymorphism had also been identified as a genetic marker for OSF susceptibility [93–96]. Choudhari et al. suggested polymorphism in CYP1A1 and CYP2E1 was associated with an increased risk of OSF [94]. Yaming et al. reported a significant association between the gene polymorphism of CYP1A1 at the NcoI site and the risk of OSF when compared to controls. However, no such association was observed for the CYP2E1 gene polymorphism in OSF patients [95]. Identifying CYP polymorphism can be used to screen individuals who are genetically at high risk of developing OSF and cancer, thus helping in guiding treatment regimens for patients.

## 9.3.13 DNA Repair Gene Polymorphism

### 9.3.13.1 X-Ray Cross-Complementing (XRCC) Polymorphism

X-ray cross-complementing (XRCC) genes were discovered mainly through their role in protecting mammalian cells from damage caused by ionizing radiation. They are also important in genetic stability. There are two main pathways in eukaryotic cells for repairing double-strand DNA breakage, namely, nonhomologous end joining and homologous recombination (HR). Nonhomologous end joining provides a mechanism for the repair of double-strand DNA breakage throughout the cell cycle. However, it is particularly important during the G0, G1, and early S phases in mitotic cells and is mediated by the XRCC5, XRCC6, and XRCC7 genes. The DNA repair protein Ku acts as a heterodimer of the two 70 kDa (Ku70) and 80 kDa (Ku80) subunits and binds to DNA ends, nicks, or single- to double-strand transition. It serves as a DNA-binding component of the DNA-dependent protein kinase (DNA-PK) that phosphorylates certain chromatin-bound proteins in vitro. The XRCC5 gene encodes Ku80 and forms a heterodimer with Ku and functions as DNA end binding at the double-strand breakage site. Ku binds to the end of the DNA double-strand breakage and appears to stabilize the binding of the DNA-PKCs to DNA [97–100].

### 9.3.13.2 NADPH Quinone Oxidoreductase 1 (NQ01) C609T

The human NAD(P)H:quinone oxidoreductase 1 gene (NQO1; DT-diaphorase, Enzyme Commission (EC) number 1.6.99.2) occupies 17 kilobase pairs (kb) within a gene-rich region on chromosome 16 at 16q22.1 [101]. This cytosolic flavoenzyme detoxifies quinones (a large class of aromatic compounds found commonly in plants, benzene metabolites, and chemotherapies) to hydroquinones or catechols. The enzyme NAD(P)H:quinone oxidoreductase 1 (NQO1) acts as an antioxidant by catalyzing a 2-electron reduction that bypasses the need for two 1-electron reductions that can result in the production of DNA and protein-damaging reactive oxygen species. In certain conditions (e.g., the presence of

myeloperoxidase or antioxidants), NQO1 can contribute to the formation of reactive oxidation species via oxidative cycling and therefore can act as a prooxidant [102]. NQO1 is constitutively expressed in most tissues including the bone marrow, where expression is thought to be highly inducible by xenobiotics with quinone moieties and is upregulated during times of oxidative or electrophilic stress. Polymorphisms of NQO1 gene have been characterized and known for about two decades [103]. C-to-T substitution at position 609 of NQO1 cDNA codes for a proline-to-serine change at residue 187 is now documented in most cancers.

## 9.3.14 Tumor Necrosis Factor-α (TNF-α)

Tumor necrosis factor-α (TNF-α), situated in the class III region of human leukocyte antigen (HLA), is a mediator with multiple functions, including the regulation of inflammation and transcriptions of collagen and collagenase. Chiu et al. studied a biallelic promoter-region (-308) polymorphism on the TNF-**α** gene and showed a significantly lower TNF-2 allele among OSF subjects than in areca-chewing controls, implying a multifunctional etiological factor of TNF-**α** in OSF pathogenesis [104].

## 9.3.15 p53 Gene Mutations

The p53 gene is a tumor-suppressor gene that is found in the mutated form in common human cancers including OSCC. Characteristics of mutations in the p53 gene of OSCC in betel quid chewers in Sri Lanka have been reported [105].

Trivedy et al. carried out mutation analysis of exons 2–9 for studying p53 mutation in OSF and OSCC by examining the mobility shift in single-strand conformation polymorphism (SSCP). They observed mobility shifts in SSCP indicative of p53 mutation or loss of heterozygosity (detection of the band) in OSF (13/21) and OSCC (15/27), suggesting that p53 mutation/protein stabilization plays a possible role in the pathogenesis of OSF and its malignant transformation [106].

### 9.3.16 Cytotoxic T-lymphocyte-Associated Antigen 4 (CTLA-4); CD 152 (Cluster of Differentiation 152) Gene Polymorphism

CTLA-4 is a negative regulator of T-lymphocyte activation. The particular genotype of the locus encoding the CTLA-4 glycoprotein has been associated with susceptibility to various autoimmune diseases. Shin et al. investigated the possible role of CTLA-4 polymorphism in OSF susceptibility by restriction fragment length polymorphism (RFLP). They found that the G allele at position +49 of exon 1 was significantly associated with OSF, confirming its role in the risk for the development of OSF [107].

### 9.3.17 Major Histocompatibility Complex (MHC) Class I Chain-Related Gene A (MICA) Polymorphism

9

MICA is expressed by keratinocytes and other epithelial cells, and its encoded protein interacts with Υ/δ T-cells localized in the submucosa. Liu et al. analyzed MICA polymorphism in OSF using the ABI prism 377-18 DNA sequencer. The phenotype frequency of allele A6 of MICA in OSF was significantly higher than that of controls, suggesting that allele A6 in MICA might confer risk for OSF [108].

### 9.3.18 Glutathione S-Transferase (GST) Polymorphism

Several allelic variants of polymorphic glutathione S-transferases (GSTs) show impaired enzyme activity and are suspected to increase the host's susceptibility to various cancers. Agrawal et al. showed a higher frequency of both the GSTM1 and GSTT1 null genotype in OSF cases than in controls, suggesting a greater risk associated with the genotype in the development of OSF [109].

### 9.3.19 Apoptosis-Associated Genes FAS and FASL Polymorphism

Wang et al. demonstrated that FAS polymorphism in the form of FAS $A_{-1377}$ $G_{-670}$ versus FAS $G_{-1377}$ $-A_{-670}$ haplotype is significantly correlated with the malignant potential of OSF [110].

### 9.3.20 Loss of Heterozygosity (LOH)

Teh et al. provided evidence of genomic instability in the form of loss of heterozygosity (LOH) in OSF. This acquisition of LOH may subsequently alter gene function and expression. Nearly 50% of OSF cases included in this study demonstrated a small number of discrete hot-spot LOH loci, and the degree of LOH showed a significant positive relationship with OSF grade. Chromosome 13 contains the largest LOH regions from 13q14 to 13q33, in proportion to chromosomal size. Since the chromosome 13q is highly susceptible to genomic instability in HNSCC, it was hypothesized that genes within the 13q14–q33 LOH region found in the OSF may have a crucial part in the initiation of oral carcinogenesis in these patients. Along with this, few other LOH loci with previously identified susceptibility regions in HNSCC: 3p24-p22, 6q26-q27, 9q22.3, 12p11.2, and 20p12-11, were recognized in this study [111].

## 9.4 Conclusion

OSF is an oral potentially malignant condition with a potential for malignant transformation. The pathophysiology of OSF is very complex. Areca nut chewing is the etiological factor in the causation of OSF. Though certain individuals due to their genetic constitution are less prone to develop the disease, susceptible individuals may develop the disease over a short period of exposure to areca nut [112]. The genetic alterations in OSF influence TGF-β pathway and collagen metabolism, inflammatory response, immune response, epithelial-mesenchymal transition, and epithelial differentiation/keratinization. It is, therefore, important to further clarify the molecular mechanisms of BQ-induced OSF and oral cancer to identify high-risk individuals.

**Summary**

BQ components are found to induce extracellular matrix (ECM) deposition via upregulation of TGF-$\beta$1, PAI-1, cystatin, LOX, TIMPs, MMPs, collagenase-1, SMAD, VEGF, cytochrome P450, XRCC, NQO1, TNF-$\alpha$, P53, CTLA-4, CD, MICA, GSTs, FAS, and FASL. The high-risk alleles and genotypes of collagen, TGF-$\beta$1, PAI-1, cystatin, LOX, TIMPs, MMPs, collagenase-1, SMAD, VEGF, cytochrome P450, XRCC, NQO1, TNF-$\alpha$, P53, CTLA-4, CD, MICA, GSTs, FAS, and FASL found in OSF patients with high frequency may change the transcriptional activity and the functions of corresponding proteins and increase the risk of OSF.

**Acknowledgments** Dr. Snehal U. Chavhan B.D.S., Post-Graduate Student,

Department Of Oral Pathology and Microbiology, Nair Hospital Dental College,

Mumbai 400008, Maharashtra, India
Dr. Chetan A. Fukate B.D.S., Post-Graduate Student, Department Of Oral Pathology and Microbiology, Nair Hospital Dental College.
Mumbai 400008, Maharashtra, India

## References

1. Warnakulasuriya S, Johnson NW, van der Waal I. Nomenclature and classification of potentially malignant disorders of the oral mucosa. J Oral Pathol Med. 2007;36(10):575–80. https://doi.org/10.1111/j.1600-0714.2007.00582.x.
2. Rosin MP, Poh CF, Elwood JM, Williams PM, Gallagher R, MacAulay C, Lam WW, Auluck A, Zhang L, Hislop TG. New hope for an oral cancer solution: together we can make a difference. J Can Dent Assoc. 2008;74(3):261–6.
3. Mishra R. Biomarkers of oral premalignant epithelial lesions for clinical application. Oral Oncol. 2012;48(7):578–84. https://doi.org/10.1016/j.oraloncology.2012.01.017.
4. Basyte-Bacevice V, Skieceviciene J, Valantiene I, Sumskiene J, Petrenkiene V, Kondrackiene J, Petrauskas D, Lammert F, Kupcinskas J. *TM6SF2* and *MBOAT7* Gene variants in liver fibrosis and cirrhosis. Int J Mol Sci. 2019;20(6):1277. https://doi.org/10.3390/ijms20061277.
5. Gui Z, Li W, Fei S, Guo M, Chen H, Sun L, Han Z, Tao J, Ju X, Yang H, Wei JF, Tan R, Gu M. Single nucleotide polymorphisms of Ubiquitin-related genes were associated with allograft fibrosis of renal transplant fibrosis. Ann Transplant. 2019;24:553–68. https://doi.org/10.12659/AOT.917767.
6. Mathai SK, Schwartz DA, Warg LA. Genetic susceptibility and pulmonary fibrosis. Curr Opin Pulm Med. 2014;20(5):429–35. https://doi.org/10.1097/MCP.0000000000000074.
7. Angiolilli C, Marut W, van der Kroef M, Chouri E, Reedquist KA, Radstake TRDJ. New insights into the genetics and epigenetics of systemic sclerosis. Nat Rev. Rheumatol. 2018;14(11):657–73. https://doi.org/10.1038/s41584-018-0099-0.
8. Theocharis AD, Manou D, Karamanos NK. The extracellular matrix as a multitasking player in disease. FEBS J. 2019;286(15):2830–69. https://doi.org/10.1111/febs.14818.
9. Xu S, Xu H, Wang W, Li S, Li H, Li T, Zhang W, Yu X, Liu L. The role of collagen in cancer: from bench to bedside. J Transl Med. 2019;17(1):309. https://doi.org/10.1186/s12967-019-2058-1.
10. Harvey W, Scutt A, Meghji S, Canniff JP. Stimulation of human buccal mucosa fibroblasts in vitro by betel-nut alkaloids. Arch Oral Biol. 1986;31(1):45–9. https://doi.org/10.1016/0003-9969(86)90112-3.
11. Tom A, Baghirath V, Krishna B, Ganepalli A, Kumar JV, Mohan SP. Ultrastructural changes of collagen in different histopathological grades of oral submucous fibrosis. J Pharm Bioallied Sci. 2019;11(Suppl. 2):S309–13. https://doi.org/10.4103/JPBS.JPBS_20_19.
12. Kamath VV. The nature of collagen in oral submucous fibrosis: a systematic review of literature. Saudi J Oral Sci. 2014;1:57–64.
13. Reichart PA, van Wyk CW, Becker J, Schuppan D. Distribution of procollagen type III, collagen type VI and tenascin in oral submucous fibrosis (OSF). J Oral Pathol Med. 1994;23(9):394–8. https://doi.org/10.1111/j.1600-0714.1994.tb00083.x.
14. Kuo MY, Chen HM, Hahn LJ, Hsieh CC, Chiang CP. Collagen biosynthesis in human oral submucous fibrosis fibroblast cultures. J Dent Res. 1995;74(11):1783–8. https://doi.org/10.1177/00220345950740111101.
15. Chiu CJ, Chang ML, Chiang CP, Hahn LJ, Hsieh LL, Chen CJ. Interaction of collagen- related genes and susceptibility to betel quid-induced oral submucous fibrosis. Cancer Epidemiol Biomark Prev. 2002;11(7):646–53.
16. Arpino V, Brock M, Gill SE. The role of TIMPs in regulation of extracellular matrix proteolysis. Matrix Biol. 2015;44–46:247–54. https://doi.org/10.1016/j.matbio.2015.03.005.
17. Chaudhary AK, Pandya S, Mehrotra R, Singh M, Singh M. Role of functional polymorphism of matrix metalloproteinase-2 (−1306 C/T and − 168 G/T) and MMP-9 (−1562 C/T) promoter in oral submucous fibrosis and head and neck squamous cell carcinoma in an Indian population. Biomarkers. 2011;16(7):577–86. https://doi.org/10.3109/1354750X.2011.609602.
18. Pittayapruek P, Meephansan J, Prapapan O, Komine M, Ohtsuki M. Role of matrix metalloproteinases in photoaging and photocarcinogenesis. Int J Mol Sci. 2016;17(6):868. https://doi.org/10.3390/ijms17060868.
19. Brinckerhoff CE, Rutter JL, Benbow U. Interstitial collagenases as markers of tumor progression. Clin Cancer Res. 2000;6(12):4823–30.
20. Kumar V, Abbas AK, Fausto N. Robbins and Cortan pathologic basis of disease. seventh ed. Philadelphia, PA: Saunders; 2004. p. 269–342.
21. Shieh TY, Yang JF. Collagenase activity in oral submucous fibrosis. Proc Natl Sci Counc Repub China B. 1992;16(2):106–10.
22. Mishra G, Ranganathan K. Matrix metalloproteinase-1 expression in oral submucous fibrosis: an immunohistochemical study. Indian J Dent Res. 2010;21(3):320–5. https://doi.org/10.4103/0970-9290.70785.
23. Rajendran R, Rajeesh MP, Shaikh S, Shanthi PMR. Expression of matrix metalloproteinases (MMP-1, MMP-2 and MMP-9) and their inhibitors (TIMP-1 and TIMP-2) in oral submucous fibrosis. Indian J Dent Res. 2006;17(4):161–6. https://doi.org/10.4103/0970-9290.29870.
24. Lee CH, Liu SY, Lin MH, Chiang WF, Chen TC, Huang WT, Chou DS, Chiu CT, Liu YC. Upregulation of matrix metalloproteinase-1 (MMP-1) expression in oral carcinomas of betel quid (BQ) users: roles of BQ ingredients in the acceleration of tumour cell motility through MMP-1. Arch Oral Biol. 2008;53(9):810–8. https://doi.org/10.1016/j.archoralbio.2008.05.004.
25. Chaudhary AK, Pandya S, Mehrotra R, Bharti AC, Jain S, Singh M. Functional polymorphism of the MMP-1 promoter (−1607 1G/2G) in potentially malignant and malignant head and neck lesions in an Indian population. Biomarkers. 2010;15(8):684–92. https://doi.org/10.3109/1354750X.2010.511267.
26. Sternlicht MD, Werb Z. How matrix metalloproteinases regulate cell behavior. Annu Rev. Cell Dev Biol. 2001;17:463–516. https://doi.org/10.1146/annurev.cellbio.17.1.463.
27. Nelson AR, Fingleton B, Rothenberg ML, Matrisian LM. Matrix metalloproteinases: biologic activity and clinical implications. J Clin Oncol. 2000;18(5):1135–49. https://doi.org/10.1200/JCO.2000.18.5.1135.
28. Price SJ, Greaves DR, Watkins H. Identification of novel, functional genetic variants in the human matrix metalloproteinase-2 gene: role of Sp1 in allele-specific transcriptional regulation. J Biol Chem. 2001;276(10):7549–58. https://doi.org/10.1074/jbc.M010242200.
29. Lin SC, Lo SS, Liu CJ, Chung MY, Huang JW, Chang KW. Functional genotype in matrix metalloproteinases-2 promoter is a risk factor for oral carcinogenesis. J Oral Pathol Med. 2004;33(7):405–9. https://doi.org/10.1111/j.1600--0714.2004.00231.x.
30. Witty JP, Foster SA, Stricklin GP, Matrisian LM, Stern PH. Parathyroid hormone- induced resorption in fetal rat limb bones is associated with production of the metalloproteinases

collagenase and gelatinase B. J Bone Miner Res. 1996;11(1):72–8. https://doi.org/10.1002/jbmr.5650110111.
31. Venugopal A, Uma Maheswari TN. Expression of matrix metalloproteinase-9 in oral potentially malignant disorders: a systematic review. J Oral Maxillofac Pathol. 2016;20(3):474–9. https://doi.org/10.4103/0973-029X.190951.
32. Chang YC, Yang SF, Tai KW, Chou MY, Hsieh YS. Increased tissue inhibitor of metalloproteinase-1 expression and inhibition of gelatinase A activity in buccal mucosal fibroblasts by arecoline as possible mechanisms for oral submucous fibrosis. Oral Oncol. 2002;38(2):195–200. https://doi.org/10.1016/s1368-8375(01)00045-8.
33. Tu HF, Wu CH, Kao SY, Liu CJ, Liu TY, Lui MT. Functional −1562 C-to-T polymorphism in matrix metalloproteinase-9 (MMP-9) promoter is associated with the risk for oral squamous cell carcinoma in younger male areca users. J Oral Pathol Med. 2007;36(7):409–14. https://doi.org/10.1111/j.1600--0714.2007.00552.x.
34. Ye S. Polymorphism in matrix metalloproteinase gene promoters: implication in regulation of gene expression and susceptibility of various diseases. Matrix Biol. 2000;19(7):623–9. https://doi.org/10.1016/s0945-053x(00)00102-5.
35. Tu HF, Liu CJ, Chang CS, Lui MT, Kao SY, Chang CP, Liu TY. The functional (− 1171 5A-- > 6A) polymorphisms of matrix metalloproteinase 3 gene as a risk factor for oral submucous fibrosis among male areca users. J Oral Pathol Med. 2006;35(2):99–103. https://doi.org/10.1111/j.1600-0714.2006.00370.x.
36. Chaudhary AK, Singh M, Bharti AC, Singh M, Shukla S, Singh AK, Mehrotra R. Synergistic effect of stromelysin-1 (matrix metalloproteinase-3) promoter (−1171 5A-> 6A) polymorphism in oral submucous fibrosis and head and neck lesions. BMC Cancer. 2010;10(369):1–9. https://doi.org/10.1186/1471-2407-10-369.
37. Zade PR, Gosavi SR, Hazarey VK, Ganvir SM. Matrix metalloproteinases-3 gene-promoter polymorphism as a risk factor in oral submucous fibrosis in an Indian population: a pilot study. J Investig Clin Dent. 2017;8(3):e12228. https://doi.org/10.1111/jicd.12228.
38. Chen Q, Lee CE, Denard B, Ye J. Sustained induction of collagen synthesis by TGF-β requires regulated intramembrane proteolysis of CREB3L1. PLoS One. 2014;9(10):e108528. https://doi.org/10.1371/journal.pone.0108528.
39. Kale AD, Mane DR, Shukla D. Expression of transforming growth factor β and its correlation with lipodystrophy in oral submucous fibrosis: an immunohistochemical study. Med Oral Patol Oral Cir Bucal. 2013;18(1):e12–8. https://doi.org/10.4317/medoral.18226.
40. Thangjam GS, Agarwal P, Balapure AK, Rao SG, Kondaiah P. Regulation of extracellular matrix genes by arecoline in primary gingival fibroblasts requires epithelial factors. J Periodontal Res. 2009;44(6):736–43. https://doi.org/10.1111/j.1600-0765.2008.01185.x.
41. Kamath VV, Krishnamurthy S, Satelur KP, Rajkumar K. Transforming growth factor- β1 and TGF-β2 act synergistically in the fibrotic pathway in oral submucous fibrosis: An immunohistochemical observation. Indian J Med Paediatr Oncol. 2015;36(2):111–6. https://doi.org/10.4103/0971-5851.158842.
42. Gao Y, Ling T, Wu H. Expression of transforming growth factor beta 1 in keratinocytes of oral submucous fibrosis tissue. Zhonghua Kou Qiang Yi Xue Za Zhi. 1997;32(4):239–41.
43. Das RK, Pal M, Barui A, Paul RR, Chakraborty C, Ray AK, Sengupta S, Chatterjee J. Assessment of malignant potential of oral submucous fibrosis through evaluation of p63, E-cadherin and CD105 expression. J Clin Pathol. 2010;63(10):894–9. https://doi.org/10.1136/jcp.2010.078964.
44. Anura A, Das RK, Pal M, Paul RR, Ray AK, Chatterjee J. Correlated analysis of semi- quantitative immunohistochemical features of E-cadherin, VEGF and CD105 in assessing malignant potentiality of oral submucous fibrosis. Pathol Res Pract. 2014;210(12):1054–63. https://doi.org/10.1016/j.prp.2014.06.009.
45. Gadbail AR, Chaudhary M, Sarode SC, Gondivkar S, Tekade SA, Zade P, Hande A, Sarode GS, Patil S. Ki67, CD105, and α-SMA expression supports the transformation relevant dysplastic features in the atrophic epithelium of oral submucous fibrosis. PLoS One. 2018;13:e0200171.
46. Pitiyage GN, Lim KP, Gemenitzidis E, Teh MT, Waseem A, Prime SS, Tilakaratne WM, Fortune F, Parkinson EK. Increased secretion of tissue inhibitors of metalloproteinases 1 and 2 (TIMPs-1 and -2) in fibroblasts are early indicators of oral sub-mucous fibrosis and ageing. J Oral Pathol Med. 2012;41(6):454–62. https://doi.org/10.1111/j.1600--0714.2012.01129.x.
47. Khan I, Agarwal P, Thangjam GS, Radhesh R, Rao SG, Kondaiah P. Role of TGF-β and BMP7 in the pathogenesis of oral submucous fibrosis. Growth Factors. 2011;29(4):119–27. https://doi.org/10.3109/08977194.2011.582839.
48. Khan I, Kumar N, Pant I, Narra S, Kondaiah P. Activation of TGF-β pathway by areca nut constituents: a possible cause of oral submucous fibrosis. PLoS One. 2012;7(12):e51806. https://doi.org/10.1371/journal.pone.0051806.
49. Kondaiah P, Pant I, Khan I. Molecular pathways regulated by areca nut in the etiopathogenesis of oral submucous fibrosis. Periodontol. 2000;80(1):213–24. https://doi.org/10.1111/prd.12266.
50. Maria S, Kamath VV, Satelur K, Rajkumar K. Evaluation of transforming growth factor beta1 gene in oral submucous fibrosis induced in Sprague-Dawley rats by injections of areca nut and pan masala (commercial areca nut product) extracts. J Cancer Res Ther. 2016;12(1):379–85. https://doi.org/10.4103/0973-1482.148729.
51. Chang MC, Pan YH, Wu HL, Lu YJ, Liao WC, Yeh CY, Lee JJ, Jeng JH. Stimulation of MMP-9 of oral epithelial cells by areca nut extract is related to TGF-β/Smad2-dependent and -independent pathways and prevented by betel leaf extract, hydroxychavicol and melatonin. Aging (Albany NY). 2019;11(23):11624–39. https://doi.org/10.18632/aging.102565.
52. Zagabathina S, Ramadoss R, Ah HP, Krishnan R. Comparative evaluation of SMAD- 2 expression in oral submucous fibrosis and reactive oral lesions. Asian Pac J Cancer Prev. 2020;21(2):399–403. https://doi.org/10.31557/APJCP.2020.21.2.399.
53. Hu X, Xiong H, Wang W, Huang L, Mao T, Yang L, Wang C, Huang D, Wu J, Xia K, Su T. Study on the expression and function of smad family member 7 in oral submucous fibrosis and oral squamous cell carcinoma. Arch Oral Biol. 2020;112:104687. https://doi.org/10.1016/j.archoralbio.2020.104687.
54. Rajendran R, Harish RK, Anil S, Vidyadharan R, Banerjee M. Transforming growth factor-β-1 polymorphisms are infrequent but exist at selected loci in oral submucous fibrosis. Indian J Dent Res. 2010;21(3):413–9. https://doi.org/10.4103/0970-9290.70815.
55. Hsu HJ, Yang YH, Shieh TY, Chen CH, Kao YH, Yang CF, Ko EC. Role of cytokine gene (interferon-γ, transforming growth factor-β1, tumor necrosis factor-α, interleukin-6, and interleukin-10) polymorphisms in the risk of oral precancerous lesions in Taiwanese. Kaohsiung J Med Sci. 2014;30(11):551–8. https://doi.org/10.1016/j.kjms.2014.09.003.
56. Wang Y, Long J, Wang X, Sun Y. Association of the plasminogen activator inhibitor- 1 (PAI-1) Gene-675 4G/5G and − 844 A/G promoter polymorphism with risk of keloid in a Chinese


9

Han population. Med Sci Monit. 2014;20:2069–73. https://doi.org/10.12659/MSM.892397.
57. Guo DC, Regalado ES, Gong L, Duan X, Santos-Cortez RL, Arnaud P, Ren Z, Cai B, Hostetler EM, Moran R, Liang D, Estrera A, Safi HJ, University of Washington Center for Mendelian Genomics, Leal SM, Bamshad MJ, Shendure J, Nickerson DA, Jondeau G, Boileau C, Milewicz DM. LOX mutations predispose to thoracic aortic aneurysms and dissections. Circ Res. 2016;118(6):928–34. https://doi.org/10.1161/CIRCRESAHA.115.307130.
58. Shieh TM, Lin SC, Liu CJ, Chang SS, Ku TH, Chang KW. Association of expression aberrances and genetic polymorphisms of lysyl oxidase with areca-associated oral tumorigenesis. Clin Cancer Res. 2007;13(15 Pt 1):4378–85. https://doi.org/10.1158/1078-0432.CCR-06-2685.
59. Chitty JL, Setargew YFI, Cox TR. Targeting the lysyl oxidases in tumour desmoplasia. Biochem Soc Trans. 2019;47(6):1661–78. https://doi.org/10.1042/BST20190098.
60. Chaurasia A, Singh N, Sahu D, Mishra A. Comparative evaluation of role of Lysyl oxidase gene (LOXG473A) expression in pathogenesis and malignant transformation of Oral Submucous Fibrosis. J Clin Exp Dent. 2019;11(10):e858–64. https://doi.org/10.4317/jced.55980.
61. Ma RH, Tsai CC, Shieh TY. Increased lysyl oxidase activity in fibroblasts cultured from oral submucous fibrosis associated with betel nut chewing in Taiwan. J Oral Pathol Med. 1995;24(9):407–12. https://doi.org/10.1111/j.1600-0714.1995.tb01210.x.
62. Tilakaratne WM, Klinikowski MF, Saku T, Peters TJ, Warnakulasuriya S. Oral submucous fibrosis: review on aetiology and pathogenesis. Oral Oncol. 2006;42(6):561–8. https://doi.org/10.1016/j.oraloncology.2005.08.005.
63. Shieh TM, Tu HF, Ku TH, Chang SS, Chang KW, Liu CJ. Association between lysyl oxidase polymorphisms and oral submucous fibrosis in older male areca chewers. J Oral Pathol Med. 2009;38(1):109–13. https://doi.org/10.1111/j.1600--0714.2008.00695.x.
64. Thorawat A, Nandimath K, Hiremath S, Naikmasur VG. Molecular screening of lysyl oxidase G473A polymorphism in oral submucous fibrosis. J Oral Maxillofac Pathol. 2014;18(2):207–10. https://doi.org/10.4103/0973-029X.140751.
65. Mukherjee S, Katarkar A, Dhariwal R, Mohanty S, Mahato B, Ray JG, Chaudhuri K. Effect of lysyl oxidase G473 A polymorphism on lysyl oxidase and total soluble collagen expression in oral submucous fibrosis. Asian Pac J Cancer Prev. 2021;22(8):2493–9. https://doi.org/10.31557/APJCP.2021.22.8.2493.
66. Eley BM, Cox SW. Advances in periodontal diagnosis. 6. Proteolytic and hydrolytic enzymes of inflammatory cell origin. Br Dent J. 1998;184(6):268–71. https://doi.org/10.1038/sj.bdj.4809599.
67. Sung SA, Kim DH, Oh KH, Han SY, Han KH. The role of Cathepsin B in peritoneal fibrosis due to peritoneal dialysis. Int J Nephrol. 2019;2019:4150656. https://doi.org/10.1155/2019/4150656.
68. Lalmanach G, Saidi A, Marchand-Adam S, Lecaille F, Kasabova M. Cysteine cathepsins and cystatins: from ancillary tasks to prominent status in lung diseases. Biol Chem. 2015;396(2):111–30. https://doi.org/10.1515/hsz-2014-0210.
69. Breznik B, Mitrović A, Lah TT, Kos J. Cystatins in cancer progression: more than just cathepsin inhibitors. Biochimie. 2019;166:233–50. https://doi.org/10.1016/j.biochi.2019.05.002.
70. Chung-Hung T, Shun-Fa Y, Yu-Chao C. The upregulation of cystatin C in oral submucous fibrosis. Oral Oncol. 2007;43(7):680–5. https://doi.org/10.1016/j.oraloncology.2006.08.009.
71. Cheng RH, Wang YP, Chang JY, Pan YH, Chang MC, Jeng JH. Genetic susceptibility and protein expression of extracellular matrix turnover-related genes in oral submucous fibrosis. Int J Mol Sci. 2020;21(21):8104. https://doi.org/10.3390/ijms21218104.
72. Vigneswaran N, Wu J, Zacharias W. Upregulation of cystatin M during the progression of oropharyngeal squamous cell carcinoma from primary tumor to metastasis. Oral Oncol. 2003;39(6):559–68. https://doi.org/10.1016/s1368-8375(03)00038-1.
73. Carnielli CM, Macedo CCS, De Rossi T, Granato DC, Rivera C, Domingues RR, Pauletti BA, Yokoo S, Heberle H, Busso-Lopes AF, Cervigne NK, Sawazaki-Calone I, Meirelles GV, Marchi FA, Telles GP, Minghim R, Ribeiro ACP, Brandão TB, de Castro G Jr, González-Arriagada WA, Gomes A, Penteado F, Santos-Silva AR, Lopes MA, Rodrigues PC, Sundquist E, Salo T, da Silva SD, Alaoui-Jamali MA, Graner E, Fox JW, Coletta RD, Paes Leme AF. Combining discovery and targeted proteomics reveals a prognostic signature in oral cancer. Nat Commun. 2018;9(1):3598. https://doi.org/10.1038/s41467-018-05696-2.
74. Flevaris P, Vaughan D. The role of plasminogen activator inhibitor type-1 in fibrosis. Semin Thromb Hemost. 2017;43(2):169–77. https://doi.org/10.1055/s-0036-1586228.
75. Samarakoon R, Higgins SP, Higgins CE, Higgins PJ. The TGF-β1/p53/PAI-1 signaling axis in vascular senescence: role of Caveolin-1. Biomol Ther. 2019;9(8):341. https://doi.org/10.3390/biom9080341.
76. Samarakoon R, Higgins PJ. Integration of non-SMAD and SMAD signaling in TGF- beta1-induced plasminogen activator inhibitor type-1 gene expression in vascular smooth muscle cells. ThrombHaemost. 2008;100(6):976–83.
77. Yang SF, Hsieh YS, Tsai CH, Chou MY, Chang YC. The upregulation of type I plasminogen activator inhibitor in oral submucous fibrosis. Oral Oncol. 2003;39(4):367–72. https://doi.org/10.1016/s1368-8375(02)00123-9.
78. Yang SF, Hsieh YS, Tsai CH, Chen YJ, Chang YC. Increased plasminogen activator inhibitor-1/tissue type plasminogen activator ratio in oral submucous fibrosis. Oral Dis. 2007;13(2):234–8. https://doi.org/10.1111/j.1601-0825.2006.01272.x.
79. Tsai CH, Lee SS, Chang YC. Hypoxic regulation of plasminogen activator inhibitor-1 expression in human buccal mucosa fibroblasts stimulated with arecoline. J Oral Pathol Med. 2015;44(9):669–73. https://doi.org/10.1111/jop.12284.
80. Huang CF, Yu GT, Wang WM, Liu B, Sun ZJ. Prognostic and predictive values of SPP1, PAI and caveolin-1 in patients with oral squamous cell carcinoma. Int J Clin Exp Pathol. 2014;7(9):6032–9.
81. Vairaktaris E, Serefoglou Z, Avgoustidis D, Yapijakis C, Critselis E, Vylliotis A, Spyridonidou S, Derka S, Vassiliou S, Nkenke E, Patsouris E. Gene polymorphisms related to angiogenesis, inflammation and thrombosis that influence risk for oral cancer. Oral Oncol. 2009;45(3):247–53. https://doi.org/10.1016/j.oraloncology.2008.05.003.
82. Vylliotis A, Yapijakis C, Nkenke E, Nisyrios T, Avgoustidis D, Adamopoulou M, Ragos V, Vassiliou S, Koronellos N, Vairaktaris E. Effect of thrombosis-related gene polymorphisms upon oral cancer: a regression analysis. Anticancer Res. 2013;33(9):4033–9.
83. Shrestha A, Carnelio S. Evaluation of matrix metalloproteinases-2 (MMP-2) and tissue inhibitors of metalloproteinases-2 (TIMP-2) in oral submucous fibrosis and their correlation with disease severity. Kathmandu Univ Med J (KUMJ). 2013;11(44):274–81. https://doi.org/10.3126/kumj.v11i4.12521.
84. Shieh DH, Chiang LC, Shieh TY. Augmented mRNA expression of tissue inhibitor of metalloproteinase-1 in buccal mucosal fibroblasts by arecoline and safrole as a possible pathogenesis for

oral submucous fibrosis. Oral Oncol. 2003;39(7):728–35. https://doi.org/10.1016/s1368-8375(03)00101-5.
85. Reddy SB, Reddy MB, Shyam NDVN. Tumour markers in oral neoplasia. IJDA. 2010;2:103–14.
86. Johnstone S, Logan RM. The role of vascular endothelial growth factor (VEGF) in oral dysplasia and oral squamous cell carcinoma. Oral Oncol. 2006;42(4):337–42. https://doi.org/10.1016/j.oraloncology.2005.06.020.
87. Roskoski R Jr. Vascular endothelial growth factor (VEGF) signaling in tumor progression. Crit Rev. Oncol Hematol. 2007;62(3):179–213. https://doi.org/10.1016/j.critrevonc.2007.01.006.
88. Shang ZJ, Li JR, Li ZB. Circulating levels of vascular endothelial growth factor in patients with oral squamous cell carcinoma. Int J Oral Maxillofac Surg. 2002;31(5):495–8. https://doi.org/10.1054/ijom.2002.0284.
89. Rai DV, Guttal KS, Kulkarni BB, Hiremath S, Burde KN. Vascular endothelial growth factor (VEGF) gene polymorphism in oral submucous fibrosis subjects: a preliminary study. Asian J Med Sci. 2016;7(5):10–6.
90. Hernando-Rodriguez M, Rey-Barja N, Marichalar-Mendia X, Rodriguez-Tojo MJ, Acha-Sagredo A, Aguirre-Urizar JM. Role of cytochrome P-450 genetic polymorphisms in oral carcinogenesis. J Oral Pathol Med. 2012;41(1):1–8. https://doi.org/10.1111/j.1600-0714.2011.01067.x.
91. Kao SY, Wu CH, Lin SC, Yap SK, Chang CS, Wong YK, Chi LY, Liu TY. Genetic polymorphism of cytochrome P4501A1 and susceptibility to oral squamous cell carcinoma and oral precancer lesions associated with smoking/betel use. J Oral Pathol Med. 2002;31(9):505–11. https://doi.org/10.1034/j.1600--0714.2002.00158.x.
92. Liu S, Park JY, Schantz SP, Stern JC, Lazarus P. Elucidation of CYP2E1 5′ regulatory RsaI/PstI allelic variants and their role in risk for oral cancer. Oral Oncol. 2001;37(5):437–45. https://doi.org/10.1016/s1368-8375(00)00099-3.
93. Li N, Hu Q, Jiang C, Hu Y, Yuan Y, Jian X, Tang Z, Guo F. Novel genetic biomarkers for susceptibility to oral submucous fibrosis: cytochrome P450 3A. Med Hypotheses. 2011;77(5):834–6. https://doi.org/10.1016/j.mehy.2011.07.049.
94. Chaudhuri SR, Mukherjee S, Paul RR, Haldar A, Chaudhuri K. CYP1AI and CYP2E1 gene polymorphisms may increase susceptibility to oral submucous fibrosis among betel quid chewers of eastern India. Gene. 2013;513(2):268–71. https://doi.org/10.1016/j.gene.2012.10.043.
95. Yaming P, Urs AB, Saxena A, Zuberi M. Roles of CYP1A1 and CYP2E1 gene polymorphisms in oral submucous fibrosis. Asian Pac J Cancer Prev. 2016;17(7):3335–40.
96. Villard PH, Seree EM, Re JL, De Meo M, Barra Y, Attolini L, Dumenil G, Catalin J, Durand A, Lacarelle B. Effects of tobacco smoke on the gene expression of the Cyp1a, Cyp2b, Cyp2e, and Cyp3a subfamilies in mouse liver and lung: relation to single strand breaks of DNA. Toxicol Appl Pharmacol. 1998;148(2):195–204. https://doi.org/10.1006/taap.1997.8332.
97. Mimori T, Hardin JA, Steitz JA. Characterization of the DNA-binding protein antigen Ku recognized by autoantibodies from patients with rheumatic disorders. J Biol Chem. 1986;261(5):2274–8.
98. Jackson SP. DNA-dependent protein kinase. Int J Biochem Cell Biol. 1997;29(7):935–8. https://doi.org/10.1016/s1357-2725(97)00006-x.
99. Mukherjee S, Bhowmik AD, Roychoudhury P, Mukhopadhyay K, Ray JG, Chaudhuri K. Association of XRCC1, XRCC3, and NAT2 polymorphisms with the risk of oral submucous fibrosis among eastern Indian population. J Oral Pathol Med. 2012;41(4):292–302. https://doi.org/10.1111/j.1600--0714.2011.01097.x.
100. Liao PH, Yang HW, Huang YF. Genetic expression signatures of oral submucous fibrosis and oral cancer-A preliminary microarray report. J Dent Sci. 2016;11(4):457–62. https://doi.org/10.1016/j.jds.2013.02.017.
101. Warnakulasuriya S, Trivedy C, Peters TJ. Areca nut use: an independent risk factor for oral cancer. BMJ. 2002;324(7341):799–800. https://doi.org/10.1136/bmj.324.7341.799.
102. Jaiswal AK, McBride OW, Adesnik M, Nebert DW. Human dioxin-inducible cytosolic NAD(P)H:menadione oxidoreductase. cDNA sequence and localization of gene to chromosome 16. J Biol Chem. 1988;263(27):13572–8.
103. Ross D, Kepa JK, Winski SL, Beall HD, Anwar A, Siegel D. NAD(P)H:quinone oxidoreductase 1 (NQO1): chemoprotection, bioactivation, gene regulation and genetic polymorphisms. Chem Biol Interact. 2000;129(1–2):77–97. https://doi.org/10.1016/s0009-2797(00)00199-x.
104. Chiu CJ, Chiang CP, Chang ML, Chen HM, Hahn LJ, Hsieh LL, Kuo YS, Chen CJ. Association between genetic polymorphism of tumor necrosis factor-alpha and risk of oral submucous fibrosis, a pre-cancerous condition of oral cancer. J Dent Res. 2001;80(12):2055–9. https://doi.org/10.1177/00220345010800120601.
105. Chiba I, Muthumala M, Yamazaki Y, Uz Zaman A, Iizuka T, Amemiya A, Shibata T, Kashiwazaki H, Sugiura C, Fukuda H. Characteristics of mutations in the p53 gene of oral squamous-cell carcinomas associated with betel-quid chewing in Sri Lanka. Int J Cancer. 1998;77(6):839–42. https://doi.org/10.1002/(sici)1097-0215(19980911)77:6<839::aid-ijc7>3.0.co;2-v. Erratum in: Int J Cancer 1999;80(3):486
106. Trivedy C, Warnakulasuriya KA, Tavassoli M, Steingrimsdottir H, Penhallow J, Maher R, Johnson NW. p53 aberrations in oral submucous fibrosis and oral squamous cell carcinoma detected by immunocytochemistry and PCR-SSCP. J Oral Pathol Med. 1998;27(2):72–7. https://doi.org/10.1111/j.1600-0714.1998.tb02097.x.
107. Shin YN, Liu CJ, Chang KW, Lee YJ, Liu HF. Association of CTLA-4 gene polymorphism with oral submucous fibrosis in Taiwan. J Oral Pathol Med. 2004;33(4):200–3. https://doi.org/10.1111/j.0904-2512.2004.00081.x.
108. Liu CJ, Lee YJ, Chang KW, Shih YN, Liu HF, Dang CW. Polymorphism of the MICA gene and risk for oral submucous fibrosis. J Oral Pathol Med. 2004;33(1):1–6. https://doi.org/10.1111/j.1600-0714.2004.00047.x.
109. Agrawal D, Gupta S, Agarwal D, Gupta OP, Agarwal M. Role of GSTM1 and GSTT1 polymorphism: susceptibility to oral submucous fibrosis in the North Indian population. Oncology. 2010;79(3–4):181–6. https://doi.org/10.1159/000318533.
110. Wang LH, Ting SC, Chen CH, Tsai CC, Lung O, Liu TC, Lee CW, Wang YY, Tsai CL, Lin YC. Polymorphisms in the apoptosis-associated genes FAS and FASL and risk of oral cancer and malignant potential of oral premalignant lesions in a Taiwanese population. J Oral Pathol Med. 2010;39(2):155–61. https://doi.org/10.1111/j.1600-0714.2009.00873.x.
111. Teh MT, Tilakaratne WM, Chaplin T, Young BD, Ariyawardana A, Pitiyage G, Lalli A, Stewart JE, Hagi-Pavli E, Cruchley A, Waseem A, Fortune F. Fingerprinting genomic instability in oral submucous fibrosis. J Oral Pathol Med. 2008;37(7):430–6. https://doi.org/10.1111/j.1600-0714.2008.00643.x.
112. Ray JG, Chatterjee R, Chaudhuri K. Oral submucous fibrosis: a global challenge. Rising incidence, risk factors, management, and research priorities. Periodontol. 2019;80(1):200–12. https://doi.org/10.1111/prd.12277.

# Diet and Micronutrients

*Madhura Murittige Gopalakrishna and Roopa S. Rao*

Contents



© The Author(s), under exclusive license to Springer Nature Switzerland AG 2023
S. Warnakulasuriya, K. Ranganathan (eds.), *Oral Submucous Fibrosis*, Textbooks in Contemporary Dentistry,
https://doi.org/10.1007/978-3-031-12855-4_10

## 10.1 Introduction

Oral submucous fibrosis (OSF) is a potentially malignant disorder, primarily caused by areca nut consumption, and is characterized by fibrotic changes of oral and pharyngeal tissues. The etiopathogenesis of OSF is a complex orchestration involving a multitude of molecules and enzymes [1–6]. In this chapter, we discuss the role of diet, nutrition, and micronutrients as risk or protective factors in the causation of OSF.

> WCRF/AICR defines "**Nutrition** as the set of integrated processes by which cells, tissues, organs, and indeed a whole organism acquire the energy and nutrients needed to function normally and have a normal structure" [7]

10

Nutrition plays a significant role in the growth, development, and functioning of an organism. Finally, all the energy requirements for body metabolism will be met by the nutritional status of the diet consumed. The so-called diet comprises essential nutrients that are to be mandatorily obtained from an external source, and some components will be converted into essential ingredients by the body from the consumed dietary portion. Further, the diet encompasses certain elements that are not essential nutrients but may influence the body's metabolism. Such compounds are phytochemicals, fiber, caffeine, and others [7].

**A healthy diet includes the following: (WHO Recommendation) [8, 9]**

- Fruit, vegetables, legumes (e.g., lentils and beans), nuts, and whole grains (e.g., unprocessed maize, millet, oats, wheat, and brown rice)
- At least 400 g (i.e., five portions) of fruits and vegetables per day, excluding potatoes, sweet potatoes, cassava, and other starchy roots

A healthy diet comprises macro- and micronutrients. The **micronutrients** are needed by the body in smaller amounts, and they represent **vitamins, minerals, trace elements**, and **antioxidants**. These micronutrients have a great impact on the overall health of an individual. The micronutrients empower the body to produce hormones, enzymes, and other substances required for normal growth and development. The deficiency states of micronutrients may result in diseases affecting different parts of the body including oral tissues; further, these deficiency states may also result in fatal and life-threatening conditions [10–13].

The mineral component of the micronutrients could be further typed as macrominerals and microminerals. The microminerals are the trace elements that exist in smaller amounts in natural and perturbed environments and play a significant role in various physiological and metabolic phenomena of the human body [14].

**Learning Goals**

- Epidemiological evidence on diet and nutrition in OSF
- Role of trace elements (Cu, Zn, Fe, Se) in OSF
- Role of vitamins in OSF
- Evidence from interventional studies in OSF

## 10.2 Epidemiological Evidence on Diet and Nutrition

An epidemiological (population-based case-control) study [15], was designed to assess the dietary factors in oral potentially malignant disorders (OPMDs) in Gujarat, India. The primary objective was to check the association of dietary components (antioxidants, vitamins, minerals, and fiber) with OPMDs of the oral cavity. A food frequency questionnaire (FFQ) was developed and tested to collect the dietary information to assess the exposure to various nutrients. Out of 5018 male subjects consuming tobacco, 318 exhibited OPMDs and qualified as cases. Age- and gender-matched healthy individuals without oral lesions were selected as the control group. The common OPMDs observed were OSF and oral leukoplakia. The FFQ was composed of questions on the frequency and quantity of 92 food items consumed, reflecting >95% of exposure to comprehensive energy, fiber, fat, minerals, and vitamins. Of all the dietary elements, the fiber component was observed to be significantly protective for oral submucous fibrosis with a 10% reduction in risk per g day ($P < 0.05$). The study revealed a strong linear protective effect (OR = 0.89) on a continuous scale (g $d^{-1}$), $P < 0.02$.

In another epidemiological study by Gupta et al. [16], the influence of dietary factors on OPMDs in a Kerala population (India) was assessed. A customized food frequency questionnaire (FFQ) was developed and validated for estimating the nutrient exposure in the target population. In a house-to-house survey, 5056 tobacco users were screened. Among this population, 226 people exhibited OPMDs, and were recruited as cases. Equal number of age- and gender-matched controls were selected for the control group. OSF was the second common OPMD (next to oral leukoplakia) observed in the population. The confirmatory diagnosis of OSF was based on the presence of palpable fibrous bands. After adjusting for tobacco use, the intake of fruits, vegetables, and β-carotene showed an inverse relation to risk and an average reduction of about 10% per quartile of exposure. Zinc was shown to have a dose-response gradient and a larger effect in men. This study was undertaken to check the reduced risk of OPMDs in individuals who consume more fruits and vegetables; it confirmed the influence of these dietary factors in the development of OPMDs that had included both oral leukoplakia and oral submucous fibrosis [16].

The next section of this chapter highlights the role of dietary components in the disease process of OSF. Here, we discuss the role of trace elements, e.g., copper, zinc, iron, and selenium, in OSF and the role of vitamins in OSF.

## 10.3 Role of Trace Elements in OSF

### 10.3.1 Role of Copper

Copper (Cu) is the third most ample trace element in humans. Copper accounts for 75–100 mg of the total body. Copper is found almost in every tissue of the body, and the chief storage organs are the liver and brain, heart, kidney, and muscle. Further, copper is transported as ceruloplasmin into the plasma and excreted in the bile. In erythrocytes, 60% of the copper is found as copper-zinc metalloenzyme superoxide dismutase, and the remaining 40% is bound to other amino acids and proteins. Copper is a significant component of various enzymes involved in vital biological functions. Of significance in OSF is the synthesis of collagen and elastin as copper is a cofactor for the enzyme lysyl oxidase. Moreover, copper can act as an antioxidant protecting the tissues from oxidative stress, as well as a prooxidant causing damage to tissues [17–24].

The WHO Collaborating Centre research group based at King's College London first described raised copper levels in areca nut [25]. Copper dissolves in saliva and remains in the oral fluids for 30 min. This facilitates the uptake of copper by oral epithelial cells. The absorption of copper by oral mucosal keratinocytes is by a nonenzyme-dependent diffusion process, bound to metallothionein. With regard to areca nut chewing, there is raised level of copper seen in OSF patients. The higher copper levels upregulate the activity of lysyl oxidase causing more collagen production [26, 27]. In addition, when Cu is found in higher concentrations, there is a release of active oxygen species that further brings about oxidative damage to the cell [28, 29].

Several subsequent studies have shown elevated levels of Cu in the sera of OSF patients [29–34]. This has been attributed to the chewing of areca nut that is rich in Cu (302 nmol/g). The liver releases ceruloplasmin, a copper-carrying protein. The decreased catabolism of ceruloplasmin increases Cu levels in OSF patients. Further, the higher levels of Cu induce oxidative stress by Fenton and Haber-Weiss reaction. The serum copper levels in OSF patients show a gradual increase with advanced stages of the disease [30–35].

The role of Cu has been an interesting subject of investigation in carcinogenesis. High levels of copper within the cells generate hydroxyl radicals that can result in damage to the DNA and proteins. This may activate tumor necrosis factor-alpha and vascular endothelial growth factors. These factors are important for tumor growth and metastasis. During the malignant transformation of OSF, a four- to eightfold increase in the blood level of ceruloplasmin has been observed. Ceruloplasmin acts as a source of Cu ions, initiates LDL oxidation, and plays a role in the malignant transformation of OSF to carcinoma [36–42].

However, two studies have reported low levels of Cu in OSF patients when compared to healthy volunteers providing contradictory evidence. Varghese et al. speculated that the reduced Cu levels observed in the study could be attributed to the difference in laboratory methodologies employed and patient selection. Atomic absorption spectrophotometry was used to measure Cu levels, and the patients recruited for the study were not on any treatment in contrast to earlier studies where colorimeter was used and patients were on some form of treatment for OSF [43]. The study by Anuradha et al. also reported lower levels of Cu in OSF patients. In this study the cohort had poor dietary patterns and loss of appetite, suggesting reverse causation, also, the sample size was low [44]. However, many later studies have shown raised Cu levels in OSF patients, with atomic absorption spectrophotometry analysis [32, 45, 46].

### 10.3.2 Role of Zinc

Zinc (Zn) is the second most abundant transition metal in humans that appears in all enzyme systems. In blood plasma, Zn is transported by albumin and transferrin. Zn exhibits catalytic, regulatory, and structural roles in a biological system. Zn also shows antioxidant and antimicrobial properties.

An animal study (on rodents) has shown that Zn-deficient diet could result in change in the keratinization pattern (parakeratosis from orthokeratinization) of the oral mucosa.

Zn is a cofactor for the superoxide dismutase enzyme, and many studies have shown lower levels of Zn in OSF patients. This could be due to higher Cu levels and oxidative stress. Another interesting finding is lower levels of iron and higher serum levels of Zn in OSF patients. This is due to the common transporter molecule, transferrin, that carries both iron and Zn. Thus, OSF patients exhibiting lower iron levels would exhibit higher serum Zn levels.

The natural antioxidant of humans, superoxide dismutase, is a Cu–Zn protein complex that shows an anticarcinogenic effect in OSF. Additionally, Zn reduces the activity of Cu-coupled lysyl oxidase and thus inhibits collagenic cross-linkage. Further, Zn promotes collagenic degradation via collagenases and matrix metalloproteinases. By interfering with the mucosal absorption of Cu, Zn shows an inverse relation with Cu. Higher Zn levels hamper Cu absorption as both the metals are absorbed through metallothioneins. Thus, the Cu:Zn ratio could be a reliable biomarker for assessing carcinogenesis. There is limited literature suggesting a carcinogenic effect of Zn [47–58].



The Zn level in body fluids (serum/plasma/saliva) of OSF patients has been evaluated in numerous studies. Of these, only four studies have not reported lower Zn levels in OSF patients. In one such study by Khanna et al., higher Zn levels were observed in OSF patients, but it was not statistically significant. The reason for elevated Zn levels was attributed to consumption of gutkha with higher Zn content [31, 33, 35, 44–46, 59–65].

The various effects of reduced Zn levels in OSF patients are the following:

(i) Zn acts as a first-line defense against oxidative stress by forming cofactor Cu/Zn-superoxide dismutase enzyme [66].
(ii) Zn is pivotal for the gene expression of metallothionein, which removes hydroxyl ions and confers protection against oxidative damage [67].
(iii) Zn competes with other transition metals for binding sites, thereby reducing those metals from generating hydroxyl ions [67].
(iv) Excessive cellular uptake of Zn for neutralization of free radicals [68].

Important attributes of Zn in preventing the development of malignancy [67]:

(a) The tumor suppressor protein, p53, is Zn dependent and is involved in the repair of DNA.
(b) The apoptotic regulating transcription factors, AP-1 and NF-kB, show alterations with reduced cellular levels of Zn.

Lower levels of Zn may induce overexpression of COX-2 that promotes cell proliferation, prevents apoptosis, and therefore contributes to the malignant transformation of OSF [67].

### 10.3.3 Role of Iron

Iron (Fe) is the most abundant essential trace element in humans. Iron is an important component of heme and various enzymes in the body [69, 70]. The vital functions carried out by iron are the transport of oxygen, synthesis of DNA, energy metabolism, development and maintenance of oral mucosa. Iron deficiency leads to Plummer-Vinson's syndrome. Patients who have Plummer-Vinson's syndrome (sideropenic dysphagia) exhibit features of anemia; further glossitis, angular cheilitis, and koilonychia are noticed. These patients have greater risk of developing oral, postcricoidal, and esophageal carcinomas.

Further, the investigations on iron levels in OSF patients have revealed lower serum iron concentrations when compared to healthy controls [44, 60, 71–80].

The suggestions for diminished levels of iron in OSF patients could be due to:

(i) Excessive use of iron for the hydroxylation of lysine and proline during collagen synthesis.
(ii) The mechanical injury caused by areca nut chewing hampers intake of a nutritionally balanced diet.
(iii) Vegetarian diet may predispose an individual to greater depletion of iron stores.

Ultimately, chronic iron deficiency in areca nut chewers is a factor that facilitates the development of OSF. Further, features of anemia have been noticed in the advanced stage of OSF [81, 82].

### 10.3.4 Role of Selenium

Selenium is yet another vital trace element that is an important constituent of antioxidant enzymes: glutathione peroxidase and thioredoxin reductase [83]. Lower serum levels of selenium have been reported in OSF patients when compared to normal individuals [84].

## 10.4 Role of Vitamins

In a case-control study (OSF, $n = 40$; control, $n = 25$), deficiency of vitamin B12 and iron was reported in OSF patients when compared to healthy volunteers. Further, the red cell indices such as packed cell volume, mean corpuscular volume, and mean corpuscular Hb were significantly reduced in OSF patients [85].

Another case-control study showed high frequencies of vitamin B12, folic acid deficiencies, and gastric parietal cell antibody positivity in OSF patients when compared to healthy individuals [86].

Shetty et al. in their study observed lower serum and salivary levels of ascorbic acid with progressibe worsening of histopathological grading of OSF. The likely reason for lower levels of ascorbic acid is that it may have been used for the excessive synthesis of collagen during the progression of OSF [87].

Another study evaluated mean serum vitamin A and vitamin E levels in OSF patients. There was no statistically significant difference in these vitamin levels between OSF and control groups. It has been suggested that these vitamins are used by the tissues to combat oxidative stress generated due to the consumption of areca nut [88].

## 10.5 Interventional Studies

In an interventional study on OSF by Maher et al. [89], the beneficial clinical response to multiple micronutrients was evaluated in Karachi, Pakistan. Out of 169 OSF subjects recruited for the study, 117 compliant individuals were given daily oral micronutrient (vitamins and minerals) supplementations for 1–3 years. There was a significant improvement in symptoms, such as burning sensation, intolerance to spicy food, and restricted mouth opening. The interincisor distance increased in 48 (41%) and there was regression of concomitant lesions like oral leukoplakia and/or erythroplakia [89].

**Summary**

**Points of clinical relevance:**

Factors that promote fibrosis in Oral Submucous Fibrosis are as follows:

- Low dietary fibre
- Higher levels of copper
- Lower levels of Zinc, Iron, and Selenium
- Lower levels of Vitamins A, B, C, and E
- Dietary supplementation of the micronutrients has shown improvement in signs and symptoms of OSF

## References

1. Pindborg JJ, Sirsat SM. Oral submucous fibrosis. Oral Surg Oral Med Oral Pathol. 1966;22(6):764–79. https://doi.org/10.1016/0030-4220(66)90367-7.
2. Sinor PN, Gupta PC, Murti PR, Bhonsle RB, Daftary DK, Mehta FS, et al. A case-control study of oral submucous fibrosis with special reference to the etiologic role of areca nut. J Oral Pathol Med. 1990;19(2):94–8.
3. Maher R, Lee AJ, Warnakulasuriya KA, Lewis JA, Johnson NW. Role of areca nut in the causation of oral submucous fibrosis: a case-control study in Pakistan. J Oral Pathol Med. 1994;23(2):65–9. https://doi.org/10.1111/j.1600-0714.1994.tb00258.x.
4. Murti PR, Bhonsle RB, Gupta PC, Daftary DK, Pindborg JJ, Mehta FS. Etiology of oral submucous fibrosis with special reference to the role of areca nut chewing. J Oral Pathol Med. 1995;24(4):145–52. https://doi.org/10.1111/j.1600-0714.1995.tb01156.x.
5. Tilakaratne WM, Klinikowski MF, Saku T, Peters TJ, Warnakulasuriya S. Oral submucous fibrosis: review on etiology and pathogenesis. Oral Oncol. 2006;42(6):561–8. https://doi.org/10.1016/j.oraloncology.2005.08.005.
6. Xu H, Lyu F, Song J, Xu Y, Jiang E, Shang Z, et al. Research achievements of oral submucous fibrosis: progress and prospect. Biomed Res Int. 2021.; Article ID 6631856; https://doi.org/10.1155/2021/6631856.
7. World Cancer Research Fund/American Institute of Cancer Research. Diet, nutrition, physical activity, and cancer: a global perspective. Continuous Update Project Expert Report 2018. www.dietandcancerreport.org
8. World Health Organization—Healthy Diet. https://www.who.int/news-room/fact-sheets/detail/healthy-diet, last accessed 28th Aug 2021
9. Diet, nutrition and the prevention of chronic diseases: report of a Joint WHO/FAO Expert Consultation. WHO Technical Report Series, No. 916. Geneva: World Health Organization; 2003.
10. World Health Organization—Health Topics. https://www.who.int/health-topics/micronutrients#tab=tab_1, last accessed 28th Aug 2021
11. Enwonwu CO, Phillips RS, Falkler WA Jr. Nutrition and oral infectious diseases: state of the science. Compend Contin Educ Dent. 2002;23(5):431–4.
12. Moynihan PJ. The role of diet and nutrition in the etiology and prevention of oral diseases. Bull World Health Organ. 2005;83(9):694–9.
13. Chen M, Andersen R, Barmes M, David E, Leclerq M, Lyttle H, et al. Comparing oral health care systems: a second international collaborative study. World Health Organization; 1997. https://apps.who.int/iris/handle/10665/41976
14. Bhattacharya PT, Misra SR, Hussain M. Nutritional aspects of essential trace elements in oral health and disease: an extensive review. Scientifica (Cairo). 2016;2016:5464373. https://doi.org/10.1155/2016/5464373.
15. Gupta PC, Hebert JR, Bhonsle RB, Sinor PN, Mehta H, Mehta FS. Dietary factors in oral leukoplakia and submucous fibrosis in a population-based case control study in Gujarat, India. Oral Dis. 1998;4:200–6.
16. Gupta PC, Hebert JR, Bhonsle RB, Murti PR, Mehta H, Mehta FS. Influence of dietary factors on oral precancerous lesion in a population-based case-control study in Kerala, India. Cancer. 1999;85(9):1885–93.
17. Adelstein SJ, Vallee BL. Copper metabolism in man. N Engl J Med. 1961;265:892–7. https://doi.org/10.1056/NEJM196111022651806.
18. Harris ED. Copper homeostasis: the role of cellular transporters. Nutr Rev. 2001;59(9):281–5. https://doi.org/10.1111/j.1753-4887.2001.tb07017.x.
19. Araya M, Pizarro F, Olivares M, Arredondo M, Gonzalez M, Mendez M. Understanding copper homeostasis in humans and copper effects on health. Biol Res. 2006;39(1):183–7. https://doi.org/10.4067/S0716-97602006000100020.
20. Bonham M, O'Connor J, Hannigan B, Strain J. The immune system as a physiological indicator of marginal copper status? Brit J Nutr. 2002;87(5):393–403. https://doi.org/10.1079/BJN2002558.
21. Rakel D. Integrative medicine. 2nd ed. Philadelphia, PA: Saunders Elsevier; 2007.
22. Davis CD. Low dietary copper increases fecal free radical production, fecal water alkaline phosphatase activity and cyto-

toxicity in healthy men. J Nutr. 2003;133(2):522–7. https://doi.org/10.1093/jn/133.2.522.
23. Willis MS, Monaghan SA, Miller ML, McKenna RW, Perkins WD, Levinson BS, Bhushan V, Kroft SH. Zinc-induced copper deficiency: a report of three cases initially recognized on bone marrow examination. Am J Clin Pathol. 2005;123(1):125–31. https://doi.org/10.1309/v6gvyw2qtyd5c5pj.
24. Osredkar J, Sustar N. Copper and zinc, biological role and significance of copper/zinc imbalance. J Clinic Toxicol S. 2011;3(2161):0495.
25. Trivedy CR, Warnakulasuriya KA, Peters TJ, Senkus R, Hazarey VK, Johnson NW. Raised tissue copper levels in oral submucous fibrosis. J Oral Pathol Med. 2000;29(6):241–8. https://doi.org/10.1034/j.1600-0714.2000.290601.x.
26. Trivedy C, Baldwin D, Warnakulasuriya S, Johnson N, Peters T. Copper content in Areca catechu (Betel nut) products and oral submucous fibrosis. Lancet. 1997;349(17):1447.
27. Trivedy C, Warnakulasuriya KA, Hazarey VK, Tavassoli M, Sommer P, Johnson NW. The upregulation of lysyl oxidase in oral submucous fibrosis and squamous cell carcinoma. J Oral Pathol Med. 1999;28(6):246–51. https://doi.org/10.1111/j.1600-0714.1999.tb02033.x.
28. Desai VD, Kumar MVS, Bathi RJ, Gaurav I, Sharma R. Molecular analysis of trace elements in oral submucous fibrosis and future perspectives. Universal Res J Dent. 2014;4(1):26–35. https://doi.org/10.4103/2249-9725.127070.
29. Rajalalitha P, Vali S. Molecular pathogenesis of oral submucous fibrosis—a collagen metabolic disorder. J Oral Pathol Med. 2005;34(6):321–8. https://doi.org/10.1111/j.1600--0714.2005.00325.x.
30. Theophanides T, Anastassopoulou J. Copper and carcinogenesis. Crit Rev Oncol Hematol. 2002;42(1):57–64. https://doi.org/10.1016/s1040-8428(02)00007-0.
31. Gaetke LM, Chow CK. Copper toxicity, oxidative stress, and antioxidant nutrients. Toxicology. 2003;189(1–2):147–63. https://doi.org/10.1016/s0300-483x(03)00159-8.
32. Shettar SS. Estimation of serum copper and zinc levels in patients with oral submucous fibrosis. J Indian Acad Oral Med Radiol. 2010;22(4):193–6.
33. Tadakamadla J, Kumar S, Mamatha GP. Evaluation of serum copper and iron levels among oral submucous fibrosis patients. Med Oral Patol Oral Cir Bucal. 2011;16(7):e870–3. https://doi.org/10.4317/medoral.17083.
34. Ayinampudi BK, Narsimhan M. Salivary copper and zinc levels in oral pre-malignant and malignant lesions. J Oral Maxillofac Pathol. 2012;16(2):178–82. https://doi.org/10.4103/0973-029X.98452.
35. Rajendran R, Vasudevan DM, Vijayakumar T. Serum levels of iron and proteins in oral submucous fibrosis (OSMF). Ann Dent 1990;49(2):23-25, 45.
36. Hosthor SS, Mahesh P, Priya SA, Sharada P, Jyotsna M, Chitra S. Quantitative analysis of serum levels of trace elements in patients with oral submucous fibrosis and oral squamous cell carcinoma: a randomized cross-sectional study. J Oral Maxillofac Pathol. 2014;18(1):46–51. https://doi.org/10.4103/0973-029X.131902.
37. Jani YV, Chaudhary AR, Dudhia BB, Bhatia PV, Soni NC, Patel PS. Evaluation of role of trace elements in oral submucous fibrosis patients: a study on Gujarati population. J Oral Maxillofac Pathol. 2017;21(3):455. https://doi.org/10.4103/jomfp.JOMFP_106_14.
38. Sutton HC, Winterbourn CC. On the participation of higher oxidation states of iron and copper in Fenton reactions. Free RadicBiol Med. 1989;6(1):53–60. https://doi.org/10.1016/0891-5849(89)90160-3.
39. Nasulewicz A, Mazur A, Opolski A. Role of copper in tumour angiogenesis—clinical implications. J Trace Elem Med Biol. 2004;18(1):1–8. https://doi.org/10.1016/j.jtemb.2004.02.004.
40. Al-Rawi NH, Talabani NGA. Quantitative analysis of trace elements in saliva of oral cancer patients from Iraq. J Coll Dent. 2005;17(2):32–5.
41. Mukhopadhyay CK, Mazumder B, Lindley PF, Fox PL. Identification of the prooxidant site of human ceruloplasmin: a model for oxidative damage by copper bound to protein surfaces. Proc Natl Acad Sci U S A. 1997;94(21):11546–51. https://doi.org/10.1073/pnas.94.21.11546.
42. Jayadeep A, Raveendran Pillai K, Kannan S, Nalinakumari KR, Mathew B, Krishnan Nair M, Menon VP. Serum levels of copper, zinc, iron and ceruloplasmin in oral leukoplakia and squamous cell carcinoma. J Exp Clin Cancer Res. 1997;16(3):295–300.
43. Varghese I, Sugathan CK, Balasubramoniyan G, Vijayakumar T. Serum copper and zinc levels in premalignant and malignant lesions of the oral cavity. Oncology. 1987;44(4):224–7. https://doi.org/10.1159/000226482.
44. Anuradha CD, Devi CSS. Studies on the hematological profile and trace elements in oral submucous fibrosis. J Clin Biochem Nutr. 1995;19:9–17.
45. Gupta RP, Rai K, Hemani DD, Gupta AK. Study of trace elements (copper & zinc) in oral submucous fibrosis. Indian J Otolaryngol. 1987;39:104–6.
46. Khanna S, Udas AC, Kumar GK, Suvarna S, Karjodkar FR. Trace elements (copper, zinc, selenium and molybdenum) as markers in oral sub mucous fibrosis and oral squamous cell carcinoma. J Trace Elem Med Biol. 2013;27(4):307–11. https://doi.org/10.1016/j.jtemb.2013.04.003.
47. Wapner RA. Protein nutrition and mineral absorption. Boca Raton, FL: CRC Press; 1990.
48. Broadley MR, White PJ, Hammond JP, Zelko I, Lux A. Zinc in plants. New Phytol. 2007;173(4):677–702. https://doi.org/10.1111/j.1469-8137.2007.01996.x.
49. Whitney EN, Rolfes SR. Understanding nutrition. 10th ed. Boston, MA: Thomson Learning; 2010.
50. Sandstead HH. Understanding zinc: recent observations and interpretations. J Lab Clin Med. 1994;124(3):322–7.
51. McCarthy TJ, Zeelie JJ, Krause DJ. The antimicrobial action of zinc ion/antioxidant combinations. J Clin Pharmacy Therap. 1992;17(1):51–4. https://doi.org/10.1111/j.1365-2710.1992.tb01265.x.
52. Fabris N, Mocchegiani E. Zinc, human diseases and aging. Aging Clin Exp Res. 1995;7:77–93.
53. Milbury PE, Richer AC. Understanding the antioxidant controversy: scrutinizing the "Fountain of Youth". Greenwood Publishing Group; 2008.
54. Das M, Das R. Need of education and awareness towards zinc supplementation: a review. Int J Nutr Metab. 2012;4(3):45–50. https://doi.org/10.5897/IJNAM11.043.
55. Jayadeep A, Raveendran KP, Kannan S, Nalinakumari KR, Mathew B, Krishnan NM, et al. Serum levels of copper, zinc, iron, and ceruloplasmin in oral leukoplakia and squamous cell carcinoma. J Exp Clin Can Res. 1997;16(3):295–300.
56. Ray JG, Ghosh R, Mallick D, Swain N, Gandhi P, Ram SS, Selvaraj S, Rathore A, Mathummal S, Chakraborty A. Correlation of trace elemental profiles in blood samples of Indian patients with leukoplakia and oral submucous fibrosis. Biol Trace Elem Res. 2011;144(1–3):295–305. https://doi.org/10.1007/s12011-011-9091-0.
57. Desai V, Kumar M, Bathi R, Gaurav I, Sharma R. Molecular analysis of trace elements in oral submucous fibrosis and future perspectives. Univ Res J Dent. 2014;4(1):26–35. https://doi.org/10.4103/2249-9725.127070.

58. Mulware SJ. Trace elements and carcinogenicity: a subject in review. 3 Biotech. 2013;3(2):85–96. https://doi.org/10.1007/s13205-012-0072-6.
59. Díez M, Arroyo M, Cerdàn FJ, Muñoz M, Martin MA, Balibrea JL. Serum and tissue trace metal levels in lung cancer. Oncology. 1989;46(4):230–4. https://doi.org/10.1159/000226722.
60. Balpande AR, Sathawane RS. Estimation and comparative evaluation of serum iron, copper, zinc, and copper/zinc ratio in oral leukoplakia, submucous fibrosis and squamous cell carcinoma. J Indian Acad Oral Med Radiol. 2010;22(2):73–6.
61. More CB, Patel H. Trace elements in potentially oral malignant disorders and oral malignant lesion-a biochemical study. Int J Oral Maxillofac Dis. 2016;1(2):1–7.
62. Yadav A, Kumar L, Misra N, Deepak U, Shiv Kumar GC. Estimation of serum zinc, copper, and iron in the patients of oral submucous fibrosis. Natl J Maxillofac Surg. 2015;6(2):190–3. https://doi.org/10.4103/0975-5950.183851.
63. Srileka M. Copper and zinc level in oral submucosal fibrosis (OSMF) patients. J Pharm Sci Res. 2015;7(8):573–4.
64. Neethi H, Patil S, Rao RS. Estimation of serum copper and zinc levels in oral submucous fibrosis: an atomic absorption spectroscopic study. J Contemp Dent Pract. 2013;14(5):801–5. https://doi.org/10.5005/jp-journals-10024-1406.
65. Kode MA, Karjodkar FR. Estimation of the serum and the salivary trace elements in OSMF patients. J Clin Diagn Res. 2013;7(6):1215–8. https://doi.org/10.7860/JCDR/2013/5207.3023.
66. Klotz LO, Kröncke KD, Buchczyk DP, Sies H. Role of copper, zinc, selenium and tellurium in the cellular defense against oxidative and nitrosative stress. J Nutr. 2003;133(5 Suppl. 1):1448S–51S. https://doi.org/10.1093/jn/133.5.1448S.
67. Ho E. Zinc deficiency, DNA damage and cancer risk. J Nutr Biochem. 2004;15(10):572–8. https://doi.org/10.1016/j.jnutbio.2004.07.005.
68. Prasad AS. Zinc is an antioxidant and anti-inflammatory agent: its role in human health. Front Nutr. 2014;1:14. https://doi.org/10.3389/fnut.2014.00014.
69. Vasudevan DM, Sreekumari S. Textbook of biochemistry for medical students. 5th ed. New Delhi, India: Jaypee; 2007.
70. Satyanarayana U, Chakrapani U. Essentials of biochemistry, book and allied. 2nd ed. Kolkata, India: Elsevier; 2008.
71. Shetty SR, Babu S, Kumari S, Shetty P, Hegde S, Karikal A. Status of trace elements in saliva of oral precancer and oral cancer patients. J Cancer Res Ther. 2015;11(1):146–9. https://doi.org/10.4103/0973-1482.137973.
72. Okade AR, Hallikeri KS, Trivedi DJ. Salivary estimation of copper, iron, zinc, and manganese in oral submucous fibrosis patients: a case-control study. Clin Can Invest J. 2015;4(3):302–6. https://doi.org/10.4103/2278-0513.156075.
73. Tiwari R, David CM, Mahesh DR, Sambargi U, Rashmi KJ, Benakanal P. Assessment of serum copper, iron and immune complexes in potentially malignant disorders and oral cancer. Braz Oral Res. 2016;30(1):e101. https://doi.org/10.1590/1807-3107BOR-2016.vol30.0101.
74. Khanna SS, Karjodkar FR. Circulating immune complexes and trace elements (Copper, Iron and Selenium) as markers in oral precancer and cancer: a randomised, controlled clinical trial. Head Face Med 2006;2:33. doi: https://doi.org/10.1186/1746-160X-2-33.
75. Shetty SR, Babu S, KumariS SP, Hegde S, Karikal A. Role of serum trace elements in oral precancer and oral cancer: a biochemical study. J Can Res Treat. 2013;1(1):1–3.
76. Guruprasad R, Nair PP, Singh M, Singh M, Singh M, Jain A. Serum vitamin c and iron levels in oral submucous fibrosis. Indian J Dent. 2014;5(2):81–5. https://doi.org/10.4103/0975-962X.135266.
77. Thakur M, Guttikonda VR. Estimation of hemoglobin, serum iron, total iron-binding capacity and serum ferritin levels in oral submucous fibrosis: a clinicopathological study. J Oral Maxillofac Pathol. 2017;21(1):30–5. https://doi.org/10.4103/jomfp.JOMFP_131_15.
78. Ganapathy KS, Gurudath S, Balikai B, Ballal S, Sujatha D. Role of iron deficiency in oral submucous fibrosis: an initiating or accelerating factor. J Indian Acad Oral Med Radiol. 2011;23(1):25–8. Retrieved from https://www.proquest.com/scholarly-journals/role-iron-deficiency-oral-submucous-fibrosis/docview/868927327/se-2
79. Novacek G. Plummer-Vinson syndrome. Orphanet J Rare Dis. 2006;1:36. https://doi.org/10.1186/1750-1172-1-36.
80. Lee J, Cho Y. Effect of ascorbic acid, silicon and iron on collagen synthesis in the human dermal fibroblast cell (HS27). FASEB J. 2008;22(S2):672. https://doi.org/10.1096/fasebj.22.2_supplement.672.
81. Pawlak R, Berger J, Hines I. Iron status of vegetarian adults: a review of literature. Am J Lifestyle Med. 2016;12(6):486–98. https://doi.org/10.1177/1559827616682933.
82. Mohammad H, Hadi NI, Younus S, Ahmed F, Younus N. Potentially significant biomarkers in oral submucous fibrosis. Pakistan J Med Dent. 2015;4(2):51–6.
83. Rayman MP. Selenium and human health. Lancet. 2012;379(9822):1256–68. https://doi.org/10.1016/S0140-6736(11)61452-9.
84. Khanna S, Udas AC, Kumar GK, Suvarna S, Karjodkar FR. Trace elements (copper, zinc, selenium, and molybdenum) as markers in oral submucous fibrosis and oral squamous cell carcinoma. J Trace Elem Med Biol. 2013;27(4):307–11. https://doi.org/10.1016/j.jtemb.2013.04.003.
85. Patil DJ, Joshi M. Evaluation of hematological profile in oral submucous fibrosis: a cross-sectional study. J Oral Maxillofac Pathol. 2020;24:575.
86. Wang YP, Wu YC, Cheng SJ, Chen HM, Sun A, Chang JY. High frequencies of vitamin B12 and folic acid deficiencies and gastric parietal cell antibody positivity in oral submucous fibrosis patients. J Formos Med Assoc. 2015;114(9):813–9. https://doi.org/10.1016/j.jfma.2015.05.011.
87. Shetty SR, Babu S, Kumari S, Shetty P, Vijay R, Karikal A. Evaluation of micronutrient status in serum and saliva of oral submucous fibrosis patients: a clinicopathological study. Indian J Med Paediatr Oncol. 2012;33(4):224–6. https://doi.org/10.4103/0971-5851.107087.
88. Jain A, Kaur G, Ranjan R, Singh D, Porwal D, Shekhawat A. Estimation of serum level of Vitamin A and E in OSMF patients. Int J Appl Dent Sci. 2020;6(2):174–6.
89. Maher R, Aga P, Johnson NW, Sankaranarayanan R, Warnakulasuriya S. Evaluation of multiple micronutrient supplementation in the management of oral submucous fibrosis in Karachi. Pakistan. Nutr Cancer. 1997;27(1):41–7. https://doi.org/10.1080/01635589709514499.

# Aetiopathogenesis of Oral Submucous Fibrosis

Contents

# In Vivo and In Vitro Experimental Evidence

*Primali Jayasooriya and Upul Dissanayake*

**Contents**



© The Author(s), under exclusive license to Springer Nature Switzerland AG 2023
S. Warnakulasuriya, K. Ranganathan (eds.), *Oral Submucous Fibrosis*, Textbooks in Contemporary Dentistry,
https://doi.org/10.1007/978-3-031-12855-4_11

## 11.1 Introduction

Analytical epidemiology studies in humans described in ▶ Chap. 8 provide strong evidence that areca nut is the major risk factor for the development of oral submucous fibrosis (OSF). However, mechanistic evidence is needed when examining the etiological role of a substance or an agent in the development of a specific disease. International Agency for Research in Cancer (IARC-1985, 2004) [1, 2] has examined the mechanistic data in evaluating carcinogenicity of areca nut as well as its role in OSF. The summary article from most recent IARC meeting published in 2020 [3] indicates arecoline as "*possibly carcinogenic to humans*" (*group 2B*) based on *strong* mechanistic evidence.

Constituents of areca nut extract (ANE) include saccharides, polyphenols, fats, alkaloids, minerals, tannins, and crude fiber [4]. Alkaloids in areca nut include arecoline, arecaidine, guvacoline, and guvacine, which comprise 0.15–0.67% of Areca nut extract (ANE) [4]. Analysis of areca nut alkaloids revealed dry areca nut, pan masala, gutkha, and Chinese areca nut to contain total alkaloids ranging from 2.86 to 9.91 (mg/g product dry weight) [5]. Arecoline has been shown to generate its detrimental effects via stimulating the proliferation of fibroblasts with collagen synthesis, reducing collagen degradation and collagen phagocytosis by fibroblasts, and generating inflammation through ROS production [6]. Other components of areca nut that contribute to the pathogenesis include polyphenols and copper, which play a role in abnormal collagen cross-linking leading to reduced collagen degradation [7]. In addition, mechanical irritation by components of betel quid is thought to aid diffusion of alkaloids and flavonoids into the subepithelial connective tissue [8]. Another component of betel quid-slaked lime facilitates conversion of arecoline into arecaidine and aid in its penetration into oral mucosa [9]. This chapter describes the mechanistic evidence on the role of areca nut together with contribution from genetic factors, which ultimately allows to draw conclusions on the initiation and development of OSF.

11

**Learning Goals**

- Understand the experimental evidence supporting the role of areca nut in the pathogenesis of OSF
- Recognize the constituents of areca nut/betel quid that contribute to OSF
- Identify inflammatory and fibrogenic cytokines and prooxidants that are induced by areca nut/ANE
- Identify the contribution of fibroblasts, myofibroblasts, keratinocytes, and lymphocytes in the pathogenesis of OSF
- Know the genetic polymorphisms that make an individual more susceptible to develop OSF

## 11.2 In Vivo Experimental Evidence on OSF

The main objective of this chapter is to discuss the published experimental evidence supporting etiological risk factors of OSF. In vivo animal studies and human studies that deal with the analysis of body fluids serum/plasma and saliva of etiological constituents are presented first followed by in vitro studies giving experimental evidence of how areca nut and its constituents contribute to the pathogenesis of OSF.

### 11.2.1 In Vivo Animal Models of OSF Induced by ANE/Commercial Areca Nut Products

The best in vivo evidence regarding the contribution of areca nut as an etiological factor in OSF is obtained from animal studies [10–17]. Chiang et al. [12] describe a dermal model for OSF, which has the advantage of rapid development of fibrosis within 2–4 weeks; though the site difference could affect the interpretation of pathologic mechanisms of OSF. Other studies describe the developement of OSF within the oral cavity in experimental animals [10, 11, 13–17], and therefore they are more appropriate to interpret the effect of areca nut/commercial areca nut products in the pathogenesis of OSF. The in vivo OSF models have been developed in BALB/C mice [11, 12, 14, 17], Wistar albino rats [10, 16], and Sprague-Dawley rats [13, 15] with ANE [11–13, 17], arecoline with or without mechanical stimulation [14, 15], pan masala extracts [10, 13], and arecoline gel [16]. The mode of administration of the agents varied across studies: local applications of solutions [11], gel [16], and paste [10] in addition to local injections [12, 13, 15, 17] and systemic administration via drinking water [14]. Due to these methodological differences, time taken for the development of OSF shows a wide variation (14 days to 600 days) (◘ Table 11.1).

Khrime et al. in 1991 [10] developed a model for OSF by painting the oral cavities of 21 albino rats with a paste of areca nut (pan masala) preparation on alternative days. Starting from 2 months up to 6 months, gradual increase in submucosal collagen indicative of OSF was observed in a time-dependent manner in 88.2% of

**Table 11.1** Summary of in vivo experimental evidence supporting areca nut/arecoline as an etiological factor contributing to OSF in animal models

| Reference | Methodology | Findings | Strengths (S)/limitations (L) |
|---|---|---|---|
| [10] | Instant betel nut preparation (pan masala) painted on buccal mucosa of 21 albino rats on alternative days for 6 months. Compared with a control group of 14 albino rats | At the end of 6 months, 88.2% of biopsies obtained from test group showed increased submucosal collagen indicative of OSF. A gradual increase in collagen was observed at 2-, 4-, and 6-month time points.<br>Observed mild leukoplakia correlated to mild-to-moderate loss of nuclear polarity and increase in keratoses/parakeratoses<br>Increase in inflammatory cell infiltration and vascularity was noted when compared to the control group | S: First in vivo study to show etiological contribution of betel nut preparation in the development of OSF<br>L: Issues with reproducibility, increase in vascularity observed in test group is unexpected and controversial as with advancement of OSF, submucosal tissue becomes avascular |
| [11] | Aqueous ANE (prepared by dissolving 265 g areca nut in 1L NaCl) was applied on buccal mucosa of 20 female BALB/c strain mice weighing 28–30 g twice daily 6 days per week for 300–600 days. A control group of 20 mice was treated with 50 mM NaCl | By the end of 600 days, ANE-treated group showed significant epithelial atrophy, fibrosis, and muscle atrophy characteristic of OSF compared to the control group<br>Progressive reduction in fibroblast density and vascular density was evident from 300- to 600-day treatment groups | S: First reproducible in vivo model to show the contribution of areca nut in the development of OSF<br>Gradual increase in histopathological evidence supportive of OSF shown at four time points<br>Use of aqueous ANE, to simulate the actual scenario that occurs in betel/areca nut chewers<br>L: Long duration taken for the development of OSF-like features |
| [12] | Two groups of 24 BALB/c mice each were injected with ANE 10 mg/ml and 20 mg/ml on the shaved skin. Third group of 24 mice received 0.5 mg/ml bleomycin injection, while 24 mice in control group received PBS injections. 6 mice in each group were sacrificed on 3rd, 7th, 14th, and 30th days of treatment<br>In addition to routine H&E sections, immunohistochemistry and immune blot techniques had been used to evaluate α-SMA and CTGF levels | Mice that received both concentrations of ANE injections were shown to have increased dermal thickness as well as increased dermal collagen deposition compared to control group<br>ANE-induced fibrosis was shown to be produced in a dose-dependent manner, with mice receiving 20mg/ml ANE showing 2.7-fold increase in collagen compared to the control<br>It was also confirmed that ANE could induce fibrotic marker genes α-SMA and CTGF gene expression | S: Rapid development of fibrosis<br>First study to show that ANE is capable of inducing fibrotic marker gene expression<br>L: Use of ANE injections does not exactly replicate the actual scenario that leads to the development of OSF in humans<br>Site differences may also hinder the interpretation of features expected to occur in OSF naturally |
| [13] | Three groups of Sprague-Dawley rats (10 in each group) received buccal mucosal injections of areca nut (33 mg/ml), pan masala (33 mg/ml), and 0.2 ml of sterile saline, respectively, on alternate days for 48 weeks. Rats were sacrificed at 6-week intervals. TGF-β expression was assessed using RT-PCR | Histopathological changes supportive of OSF such as atrophic epithelium, partial or complete loss of rete ridges, juxta-epithelial hyalinization, inflammation, and accumulation of dense bundles of collagen fibers in the lamina propria were observed in both areca nut- and pan masala-treated groups<br>Epithelial atrophy was reported to occur at an earlier time in mice receiving pan masala injections compared to mice receiving areca nut<br>In contrast, fibrosis started to develop at an earlier time point in the mice receiving areca nut injections compared to pan masala<br>Highest level of TGF-β expression was evident at 18th week in areca nut-treated group while in pan masala-treated group it was at 24th week. This can be correlated with the time when maximum fibrosis was observed histopathologically.<br>Thereafter, a downward trend of TGF-β expression was observed | S: Provides evidence implicating both areca nut and pan masala as the etiological agents in OSF<br>Correlates the histopathological change of fibrosis with fibrogenic cytokine expression pattern, indicating areca nut's ability to stimulate TGF-β expression<br>L: Does not support the observation that commercial areca products have the ability to develop OSF at a faster rate compared to naturally occurring areca nut<br>Use of injection as a mode of delivery is not an exact replication of what takes place in humans |

(continued)

**Table 11.1** (continued)

| Reference | Methodology | Findings | Strengths (S)/limitations (L) |
|---|---|---|---|
| [14] | Arecoline (1000 mg/L) was added to drinking water to develop OSF in 40 BALB/c mice in experimental group, while distilled water was given to 40 mice in the control group. Mice were sacrificed during a period of 20 weeks at 8, 12, 16, and 20 weeks of treatment | By the 8th week, mice started to develop epithelial atrophy and accumulation of collagen in the lamina propria<br>By 20th week, hyaline degeneration of the connective tissues was observed on the tongue and palatal mucosa<br>Collagen I was found to gradually increase, and by 20th week it was the sole constituent of lamina propria. Collagen III was found to decrease over time | S: Arecoline without the other constituents was shown to produce OSF-like changes<br>L: The fact that arecoline was added to drinking water in a higher concentration than that observed in areca nut chewers' saliva is different to the actual scenario that occurs in humans<br>Collagen III expression was found to be increased in a subsequent report (15) |
| [15] | Arecoline (0, 0.5, 2.0, 8.0 mg/ml) was used for 20 weeks to induce OSF in Sprague-Dawley rats. Control group of 8 rats each received mechanical stimulation with or without a brush<br>Expression pattern of TGF-β and collagen III was evaluated | Moderate and high concentrations of arecoline was shown to reduce mouth opening and produce typical OSF pathological features in the buccal mucosae.<br>The expression levels of collagen III and TGF-β1 were significantly increased in the test group compared to the control group. Mechanical stimulation alone did not produce clinical or pathological features supportive of OSF | S: Convincingly shows that mechanical stimulation per se is not capable of inducing clinical/pathological features supportive of OSF<br>L: Collagen III expression was found to be reduced in another report (14) |
| [16] | 1% arecoline hydrobromide mucoadhesive gel was applied with a cotton bud unilaterally on to the buccal mucosa of the experimental animals daily for 4 months. After application of the gel, the animals were fasted for a period of 6 h and then were fed with regular diet | By the 2nd month of treatment, epithelial atrophy and collagen accumulation were observed. A white mucosal patch, thin epithelial lining, and dense collagen at submucosa were observed with biopsy taken at the end of 4th month compared to no changes observed in the oral mucosa of rats in the control group | S: Considering the fact that a gel containing arecoline initiating features of OSF gives a better model more closely resembling the actual situation encountered in the oral cavity in humans<br>This finding also allows us to speculate that arecoline plays a significant role in the pathogenesis of OSF |



the biopsies. In addition, cytological atypia suggestive of leukoplakia was also described, which is a feature that has not been described in any other OSF animal models.

The first reproducible animal model for OSF was developed in 2007 by Perera et al. [11]. They developed the animal model by applying aqueous ANE (prepared by adding 265 g areca nut per liter of 0.9% normal saline) on the buccal mucosa of mice twice a day, 6 days per week. Mice were sacrificed at 300, 350, 450, and 600 days of treatment. Their findings revealed significantly higher scores for epithelial atrophy, connective tissue fibrosis, and muscle atrophy characteristic of OSF, in the test group compared to the control group at 600 days of treatment. These changes were shown to gradually develop by comparing groups that received treatment for 300–450 days.

In order to avoid the long duration for the development of OSF in the model developed by Perera et al. [11], Chiang et al. [12] developed an alternative dermal model by subcutaneously injecting 100 μl of ANE in 10 mg/ml or 20 mg/ml concentrations on the shaved skin of mice. Animals were sacrificed at 3, 7, 14, and 30 days. Their results showed a significant increase in dermal thickness and collagen deposition in the groups receiving ANE compared to the control. ANE was also shown to induce the expression of fibrotic marker genes alpha smooth muscle actin (α-SMA) and connective tissue growth factor (CTGF) in the skin lesions. Chiang et al. [17] went on to successfully induce fibrosis of the buccal mucosa in a mouse model with pathological features similar to OSF in 4 weeks by submucosal injection of ANE at 20 mg/ml concentration once every 2 days.

Maria et al. [13] were also successful in developing OSF animal models by injecting 0.2 ml (33 mg/ml) of areca nut or pan masala extracts for 48 weeks on alternate days. The histopathological findings were presented at 6-week intervals, and in the test group which received ANE, mice showed development of epithelial atrophy by the 24th week while in mice receiving pan masala epithelial atrophy was evident from the 6th week. In contrast, increased collagen deposition was identified by the 6th week in the pan masala group, while in ANE group, by the 12th week. In addition, corresponding to histopathological findings, maximum upregulation of TGF-β1 gene was evident after 18 and 24 weeks of treatment, in mice receiving ANE and pan masala, respectively. However, overall mice injected with pan masala did not show more significant rapid development of OSF compared with those injected with ANE, in contrast to an observational study on humans by Babu et al. [18], where chewing of pan masala/gutkha was associated with earlier presentation of OSF than betel quid use.

Wen et al. [14] developed their OSF model by giving mice in the experimental group arecoline diluted to a concentration of 1000 mg/L in drinking water for a period of 20 weeks. Mice were sacrificed at 8, 12, 16, or 20 weeks. A significant reduction in mouth opening was observed in the experimental group compared to the control from the 16th week onwards, though fibrous bands were not observed. Pathological changes, epithelial atrophy, and accumulation of collagen similar to that in OSF started to appear by the 8th week. With the advancement of the disease, a reduction in angiogenesis and significant increase in m-RNA type I collagen expression was observed. The most significant finding of the study was that pure arecoline in the absence of polyphenols, physical stimulation, or lime was shown to be capable of inducing histopathological changes compatible with OSF in mice.

Yang et al. [15] developed OSF in a rat model by using 0.5, 2, and 8 mg/ml of arecoline. In their study, rats who received moderate-to-high concentrations of arecoline showed features of OSF by 16 weeks, with significant increase in TGF-β and type III collagen. Mechanical stimulation alone failed to develop OSF. Desai et al. (16) induced OSF in the experimental animals by applying 1% arecoline hydrobromide mucoadhesive gel daily for 4 months. In their study, histopathological changes similar to OSF started to appear by the 2nd month.

According to the findings of the in vivo animal studies, ANE, commercial areca nut products such as pan masala, as well as arecoline alone have been shown to induce OSF-like changes confirming the fact that areca nut, especially the alkaloid arecoline, is a significant chemical agent in the pathogenesis of OSF. OSF is a generalized condition that is not restricted only to the site where the etiological agent comes in contact in the oral mucosa. Experimental evidence from Perera et al. [11] supports this observation as they show that when ANE is applied to buccal mucosa, OSF-like features also develop in the ventral surface of the tongue (◘ Figs. 11.1 and

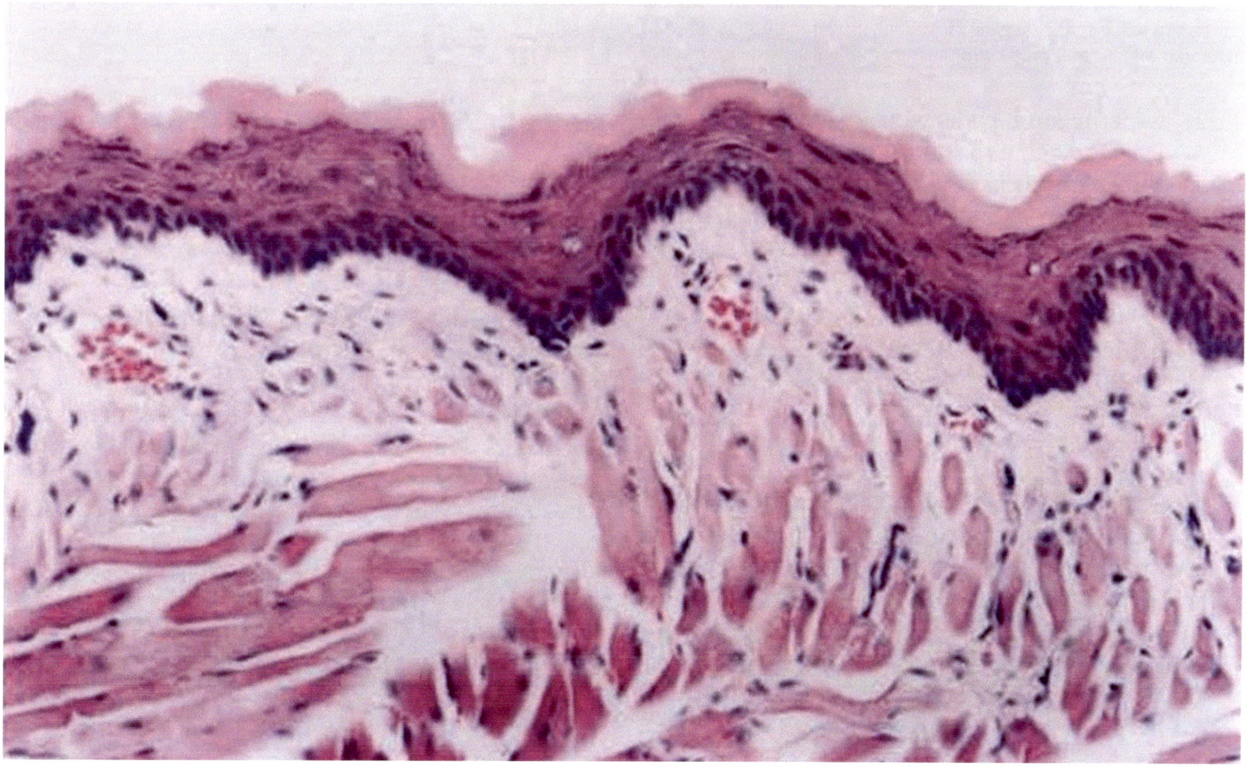

◘ **Fig. 11.1** Photomicrograph taken from the ventral surface of the tongue of a mouse in the control group following NaCl application of buccal mucosa for 600 days. The epithelium, is of normal thickness while connective tissue underneath the epithelium is vascular and contains plump fibroblasts

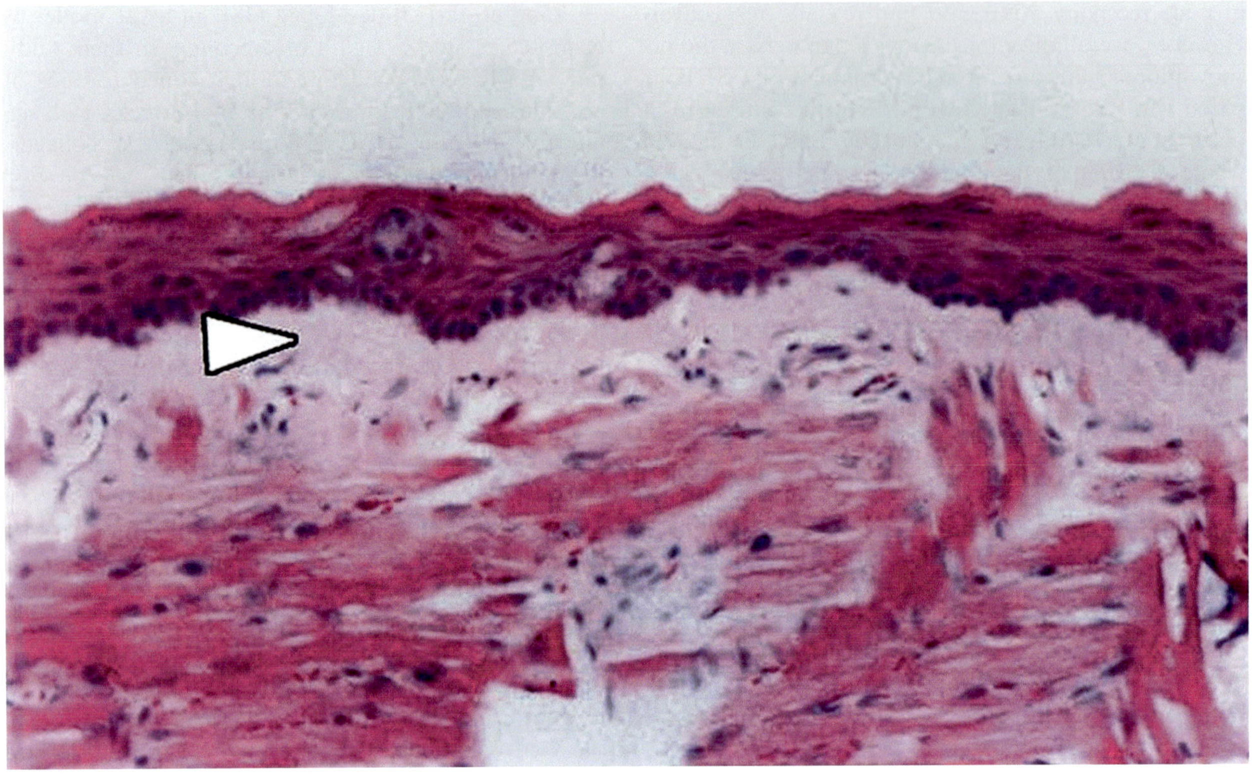

11

**Fig. 11.2** Photomicrograph taken from the ventral surface of the tongue of a mouse in the experimental group following ANE application to the buccal mucosa for 600 days. The epithelium is atrophic and contains a juxta-epithelial zone of hyalinization and fibrosis, which is avascular and acellular indicating histopathological evidence of OSF

Figure credits: Dr Sumeth Perera, Senior Lecturer in Biochemistry, Department of Biochemistry, Faculty of Medicine, University of Sabaragamuwa, Sri Lanka

11.2). Experimental evidence also shows the ability of ANE or arecoline to induce increased expression of TGF-β, a fibrogenic cytokine and type I and III collagen m-RNA leading to increased collagen production and fibrosis. Except for Khrime et al. [10], other investigators do not show if all animals exposed to ANE/arecoline developed OSF. Thus, it is difficult to draw conclusions if any factor other than ANE/arecoline contributes to the disease in animal models.

**Important**

**The role played by areca nut in OSF identified through** in vivo **animal studies**

Experimental evidences show that arecoline is the main constituent of areca nut capable of producing features similar to OSF in mice/rats. Mechanical stimulation in the absence of areca nut constituents has not been able to produce OSF-like lesions in animal models. Fibrosis that occurs has been correlated with increased type I and/or III collagen production by evaluating its m-RNA expression.

### 11.2.2 In Vivo Experimental Evidence of Chili as a Risk Factor of OSF

In the early 1960s, Sirsat and Khanolka attempted to develop an in vivo animal model for OSF using capsaicin, the active ingredient of chili as the etiological agent [19]. Their results showed that capsaicin had some effect on connective tissues, but they were cautious in indicating chili as an etiological factor as any nonspecific irritant could produce similar lesions. Considering the fact that OSF is completely absent in countries that have high chili consumption, there is insufficient experimental evidence at present to implicate chili as an etiological factor in OSF, in spite of some epidemiological evidence [20, 21] and early observational studies [22] to the contrary.

**Tip**

There is insufficient experimental evidence to implicate chili as an etiological factor in OSF.

### 11.2.3 In Vivo Human Experimental Studies Dealing with OSF Patients

#### 11.2.3.1 Inflammatory Cytokine Production by Peripheral Blood Mononuclear Cells

Haque et al. [23] analyzed spontaneous and stimulated production of IL-1β, IL-6, IL-8, TNF-α, and interferon-gamma (IFN-ɣ) in peripheral blood monocytes in patients with OSF, relatives of OSF patients, and control group including both Indians and Caucasians without the habit of betel quid chewing. Results revealed upregulation of pro-inflammatory cytokines in OSF patients, and IFN-ɣ, the anti-fibrotic cytokine, was underexpressed indicating that the imbalance between the two groups of cytokines may play a role in the pathogenesis of OSF.

#### 11.2.3.2 Elevated Levels of Copper from Areca Nut and Drinking Water Reduce Collagen Degradation

Areca nut products are a rich source of copper as shown by Trivedy et al. [24]. Their results showed that mean dry weight of copper in eight areca nut products was 302 (±SD 92) nmol/g. Salivary copper levels were shown to be significantly higher with areca nut chewing than without chewing in normal healthy individuals [24]. Trivedy et al. [25] also showed that both epithelium and connective tissue of OSF patients contained higher levels of copper compared to a control sample. They concluded that substantial amounts of copper released from areca products induce lysyl oxidase activity, upregulate collagen synthesis by fibroblasts, and facilitate its cross-linking, thereby, inhibiting its degradation. Arakeri et al. [26] by comparing three groups, namely OSF patients who chewed gutkha, individuals who chewed gutkha without OSF, and individuals who did not chew gutkha, showed that OSF patients who chewed gutkha had the highest copper concentration in drinking water as well as in plasma and in saliva. Their conclusion was that copper does play a role in the pathogenesis, though it is not the only cause. Though not directly related to OSF, experimental evidence has shown that catechin in the presence of copper stimulates lysyl oxidase activity in chick aorta [27]. Thus, it can be speculated that catechin present in areca nut may also contribute to the pathogenesis of OSF by stimulating lysyl oxidase enzyme activity.

#### 11.2.3.3 Genetic Susceptibility in Individuals with OSF

Considering the fact that increased collagen synthesis and reduced collagen degradation play a role in the pathogenesis of OSF, polymorphisms in collagen-related genes have been investigated. Chiu et al. [28] compared the relationship between OSF and polymorphisms in collagen 1A1 and 1A2 (COL1A1 and COL1A2), collagenase-1 (COLase), transforming growth factor-β1 (TGF-β1), lysyl oxidase (LOX), and cystatin C (CST3), between patients with low and high exposure to betel quid. PCR-based RFLP was performed in 166 OSF patients and 284 betel quid chewers without OSF. In COL1A1 gene, high-OSF-risk allele in low-exposure group was found to be CC, while it was TT in high-exposure group. For COL1A2 gene, high-OSF-risk allele was AA in low-exposure group and BB in high-exposure group. Risk of OSF was shown to increase with increasing number of high-risk alleles in both low and high exposure to betel quid groups. These results suggested that susceptibility to OSF could involve multigenic mechanisms modified by the betel quid-exposure dose.

MMP-1 is the main enzyme that cleaves collagen including type I, the major collagen of OSF. Chaudhary et al. [29] show that single nucleotide polymorphisms (SNPs) in MMP-1 promoter region (−1607) 2G allele are associated with susceptibility of Indian betel quid chewers to OSF, while another study did not show a similar relationship [30]. MMP-3 degrades basement membrane and collagen II, IV, IX, and X and activates MMP-1 and -9. Tu et al. investigated the effect of insertion/deletion (−1171 5A–6A) polymorphisms in MMP-3 promoter region by PCR in 71 OSF patients and revealed that 5A genotype of MMP-3 promoter was associated with the risk of OSF [31]. Chaudhary et al. [32] on the other hand showed that 5A allele was associated with the risk of OSF in Indian patients younger than 45 years while 6A allele was associated with the risk of OSF in all age groups.

TGF-β polymorphisms in OSF patients have been studied by Chiu [28] and Rajendran [33]. Chui et al. showed that high OSF risk was associated with CC alleles in both high- and low-exposure groups [28], while Rajendran et al. [33] showed high frequency of C-to-T transition in the UTR region in OSF patients compared to control. Regarding the LOX gene, Chiu et al. [28] showed that AA and GG were the high-risk allele for low and high exposure to betel chewing groups, respectively. Sheih et al. [34] showed the presence of a G-to-A polymorphism at nucleotide 473, which caused a non-conservative Arg158Gln change in the LOX amino acid sequence in OSF patients older than 50 years. Ray et al. [35] showed that with respect to LOX, G > A (473), a significantly higher number of individuals from Kolkotta were found to carry the heterozygous GA allele in individuals aged <30 years. However, there were significant differences with respect to the carrier status of GA allele among people of different regions of India. Cystatin C (CST3) is a molecule that prevents ECM degradation, by inhibiting the action of cysteine proteinases. High-OSF-risk allele in CST3 gene was found to be AA in both low- and high-exposure groups [28].

MICA (major histocompatibility complex class I chain-related gene A) is expressed by keratinocytes, and its protein has been shown to interact with T cells localized in the submucosa. When MICA polymorphism was analyzed in 80 OSF patients and 351 unrelated controls using DNA sequencing, allele A6 in MICA was found to confer risk for OSF [36]. In a study by Agrawal et al. [37] on allelic variants of polymorphic glutathione S-transferases (GSTs) that show impaired enzyme activity, they found that the frequency of both the GSTM1 and GSTT1 null genotypes was higher in OSF patients than in controls. They concluded that the GSTM1 and GSTT1 null genotypes, separately or in combination, increase the risk of developing OSF in the North Indian population. Mukharjee et al. [38] showed that polymorphisms at N-acetyltransferase 2 locus, XRCC3 Thr 241 Met, and combination of SNPs XRCC3 Thr 241 Met - NAT2 A857G increase the risk of OSF in men exposed to areca nut or smokeless tobacco. The cytochrome P4501A1 (CYP1A1) enzyme is central to the metabolic activation of carcinogens released by betel quid (xenobiotics), whereas CYP2E1 metabolizes the nitrosamines and tannins. Chaudrari et al. [39] investigated the polymorphisms at CYP1A1m1 (T3801C), m2 (A2455G), and CYP2E1 PstI site (nucleotide 21259) in 75 OSF patients and 150 controls from an eastern Indian population by the PCR-RFLP method. Results show that polymorphism in CYP1A1 and CYP2E1 may confer an increased risk for OSF.

11

A significant association of certain human leukocyte antigens (HLA) and haplotypic pairs with OSF has been reported [40, 41]. Chen et al. [40] reported that increased phenotypic frequency of HLA-B76 and higher frequencies in haplotypes HLA-B76-Cw7 and HLA-B62/Cw7 confer higher genetic susceptibility to OSF in Taiwanese smokers. In addition, HLA-DRB1*0301 and HLA-DQB1*0503 were shown to be associated with the susceptibility to OSF and smoking behavior by Prohit et al. [41].

Considering the polymorphisms that have been detected in patients with OSF as well as in betel quid chewers without OSF [28–41], contribution from more than one polymorphism may make a person susceptible to develop OSF, confirming the multigenic nature of the disease.

**Tip**

**The role of genetic polymorphisms in the development of OSF**

Genetic polymorphisms in collagen, MMP, TGF-β, lysyl oxidase, and cystatin genes have been identified in individuals more susceptible to develop OSF. Investigators also identified polymorphisms in MICA, GST, CYP, and HLA genes, which were significantly associated with OSF patients compared to the control population.

### 11.2.4 In Vivo Experimental Evidence of Analysis of Areca Nut Alkaloids in Saliva

When betel quid/commercial areca nut products are chewed, harmful components implicated in the pathogenesis of OSF should be transferred into saliva in order to diffuse into the oral mucosa, to provide evidence that areca nut plays a main etiological role in OSF. However, studies that analyze areca nut alkaloids and their metabolites in saliva are sparse [42–46]. Cox et al. [42] analyzed saliva in 32 habitual areca nut chewers and 6 persons who denied areca nut use as the control group over a period of 50 min at 5-min intervals, after chewing 0.5 g of areca nut by chewers and a rubber-based material by the control group. The results were compared with respect to two critical arecoline concentrations: 0.1 μg/ml for collagen stimulation and more than 10 μg/ml for cytotoxicity [47, 48]. Results revealed that all chewers had salivary arecoline exceeding either one of the critical values during chewing. Critical arecoline concentration, 0.1 μg/ml, was achieved by all subjects in 85% of the time points, while >10 μg/ml arecoline concentration was achieved by approximately one-third of subjects in 30% of the time points studied.

Lee at al. [43] in a similar study analyzed salivary arecoline, arecaidine, and N-methylnipecotic acid over a period of 35 min in five subjects after chewing on 5 g of areca nut. Results show that saliva of all participants reached the critical arecoline concentration of >10 μg/ml during chewing, while the highest levels of arecoline and arecaidine were achieved 5 min after areca nut chewing, and then the alkaloid levels decreased gradually. Maximum N-methylnipecotic acid level (which is the major metabolite of arecoline and arecaidine [49]) was evident 10 min after areca nut chewing.

Venkatesh et al. [44] analyzed salivary arecoline levels in 50 individuals, who used commercially available areca nut for more than 3 years. In contrast to other studies [42, 43], salivary arecoline concentrations during chewing were lower (0.06–0.1 μg/ml) than after chewing (0.1–0.3 μg/ml). The most significant finding of the study [44] was the fact that the group that chewed on the placebo also had high arecoline levels, which was attributed to re-secretion of arecoline that has been previously absorbed by the oral mucosa. In contrast to studies [42–44] that analyzed short-term areca nut alkaloid concentrations in saliva, Franke et al. [45] in their pilot study involving four betel chewers found arecoline, guvacoline, arecaidine, and guvacine for up to 8 h following exposure, both in saliva and urine. Further, they found that arecoline/arecaidine ratio in saliva was 4:1, while in urine it was 1:10 [45], which provides indirect evidence of conversion of arecoline into arecaidine as a requirement for detrimental effects of the areca nut alkaloids to take effect. The fact that the amount of arecaidine secreted by urine is more than the amount found in saliva indicates that arecoline is converted to arecaidine most probably by esterases secreted by fibroblasts. If this conversion takes place solely due to lime (calcium hydroxide) as previously indicated, experimental evidence should show higher salivary concentration of arecaidine.

Irrespective of the differences in methodologies and results, all studies [42–46] confirm that individual variations exist with respect to significant alkaloid concentrations identified in saliva, which can be used to support the fact that not all individuals who chew areca nut develop OSF or malignancy. Lack of experimental evidence regarding salivary areca nut alkaloid concentrations of OSF patients is a limitation that was identified in the published literature.

**Tip**

**How long do harmful concentrations of areca nut alkaloids remain in saliva?**

Experimental evidence shows that areca nut alkaloids at harmful concentrations may remain in saliva as long as 8 h post-exposure to areca nut/betel quid. These alkaloids may also get re-secreted into saliva through oral mucosa; thus, the time which alkaloids remain in saliva may not solely depend on the frequency of chewing.

#### 11.2.4.1 Pro-inflammatory Cytokines in Serum and Saliva in OSF Patients

Several in vivo human studies have confirmed that pro-inflammatory cytokine levels both in serum and saliva are elevated in OSF patients [23, 50, 51]. Kaur et al. [50] analyzed serum and salivary TNF-α, IL-6, and IL-8 levels in 52 OSF patients using enzyme-linked immunoassay (ELISA) and found a progressive increase in all three cytokines when the grade of dysplasia increased (which was correlated with advancement of the OSF). They also showed that the cytokine levels detected in saliva were higher than the levels detected in serum. These findings are similar to those reported by Dineshkumar et al. [51] that, IL-6 was three times higher in saliva compared to serum in 50 OSF patients. In vitro experimental evidence by Wang et al. [52] and Jeng et al. [53] showed that the production of inflammatory cytokines by gingival fibroblasts and keratinocytes in the presence of arecoline support the involvement of arecoline in increased levels of salivary and serum pro-inflammatory cytokines detected in OSF patients [23, 50, 51] which provides further evidence of the role played by arecoline in the pathogenesis of OSF.

#### 11.2.4.2 Oxidative Stress Generated by ANE in OSF Patients

ROS generation by ANE may occur due to autooxidation in the oral cavity or metabolism involving intracellular enzymes such as cytochrome P450. In vivo experimental evidence related to oxidative stress [54–61] have been assessed using lipid peroxidation products, malonaldehyde (MDA) [54, 58, 59] and 8-isoprostane [57]; prooxidants such as lipid peroxide, conjugated dienes, hydroxyl radicals [60], hydrogen peroxide [62] and antioxidant levels [54–57, 59, 61] in the saliva and serum of OSF patients. In all reported studies, a general trend of elevated levels of prooxidants or their metabolites were observed in OSF patients compared to healthy individuals [54–56, 58, 59]. In contrast, a significant reduction in antioxidant levels was observed in OSF patients compared to healthy individuals [54–57, 59, 61]. These findings indicate that oxidative stress generated by ANE is a mechanism that is important in the development of OSF.

Nair et al. [60] designed a series of experiments to assess hydroxyl radical (HO.) formation during chewing of betel quid by evaluating the formation of ortho- and meta-tyrosine from L-phenylalanine. Both forms of tyrosine were generated in vitro in the presence of extracts of areca nut and/or catechu, metal ions such as $Cu^{2+}$ and $Fe^{2+}$, and lime (alkaline pH). Exclusion of any of these ingredients from the reaction mixture significantly reduced the yield of tyrosine. Addition of hydroxyl radical scavengers was shown to inhibit phenylalanine oxidation in a dose-dependent fashion. The in vivo component of the study was done by assessing the saliva of five volunteers who chewed betel quid consisting of betel leaf, areca nut, catechu, slaked lime (without tobacco), and phenylalanine. Their saliva, collected after chewing betel quid with phenylalanine, contained high concentrations of o- and m-tyrosine. These studies demonstrate that the hydroxyl radical is formed during betel quid chewing which may produce DNA damage in oral epithelial cells.

#### 11.2.4.3 Involvement of Autoimmunity in the Etiology of OSF

Although studies that deal with direct identification of auto-antigens are sparse [63], a few studies that deal with the identification of several autoantibodies including antinuclear (ANA), anti-smooth muscle (SMA), anti-gastric parietal cell (GPCA), anti-thyroid microsomal (TMA), and anti-reticulin antibodies are available in literature [64–66]. Immune complexes have also been investigated in order to ascertain an autoimmune basis for OSF [67]. Wang et al. [63], using a proteome microarray and ELISA, validated 8 auto-antigens that were frequently found in the serum of patients with OSF compared to healthy individuals. Out of all validated auto-antigens, they selected PTMA which was found in high frequency in OSF patients for further investigations. PTMA overexpression was associated with TGF-β-induced fibrosis, while PTMA knockdown reversed fibrosis in human fibroblast cultures.

Chiang et al. [64] after analyzing 5 autoantibodies in 109 OSF patients revealed that the presence of serum GPCA and ANA in OSF patients was associated with daily consumption of betel quid. They also speculated higher frequencies of specific HLA-DR antigens in OSF patients as a contributing factor in autoantibody production. Gupta et al. [65] investigated ANA levels in three groups of individuals (OSF patients; control with and without betel quid chewing) and reported that significantly higher ANA levels were identified in OSF patients compared to healthy individuals. In addition, ANA levels were significantly higher in females compared to males, and it correlated with reduced mouth opening. Shah et al. [67] investigated ESR, and serum IgA, IgG, and IgM levels of 113 OSF patients and 25 controls. Their results of elevated serum immunoglobulin levels in OSF patients compared to the control led to the postulation of possible immunological basis for OSF.



Chen et al. [40], among others, have studied alterations in cellular/humoral response and report on HLA antigen and certain phenotypic and haplotypic alterations that make individuals susceptible to develop OSF. In contrast, Van Wyk et al. [68] could not identify HLA antigen phenotypes that make an individual more susceptible to develop the disease.

Although the data on various HLA types, elevated autoantibody levels, and detection of immune complexes tend to support an autoimmune basis for OSF, the number of cases considered in these studies are insufficient to draw definitive conclusions. Further investigations are required to confirm the contribution of auto-antigen/autoantibody generation as an etiological factor responsible for OSF.

#### 11.2.4.4 Involvement of Micronutrients in the Etiology of OSF

Trace elements that have been investigated in the saliva/plasma of OSF patients include Zn, Cu, Fe, and Se [24, 69–72]. Zn is important for the activation of antioxidant enzymes and superoxide dismutase (SOD). In OSF patients, levels of SOD were found to be reduced compared to controls [60]. Together with copper [69], iron acts as a cofactor for prolyl hydroxylase and lysyl hydroxylase, which are enzymes involved in the hydroxylation of collagen [70]. Excessive collagen synthesis in OSF is associated with a decline in the levels of serum and plasma Fe in OSF patients, while copper levels become elevated [70]. Deficiency of iron in OSF reduces levels of cytochrome oxidase, resulting in atrophy of the epithelium. Taken together, reduced and elevated levels of micronutrients in serum/plasma/saliva have been observed in OSF patients. However, there is insufficient evidence to indicate that these micronutrients are the sole cause of OSF.

## 11.3 In Vitro Experimental Evidence Supporting the Role Played by Areca Nut/Betel Quid in OSF

### 11.3.1 Collagen Synthesis

Literature reveals contradictory results on arecoline concentrations required for collagen synthesis by cultured fibroblasts [47, 73–76]. In vitro studies involving human fibroblasts in culture show that arecoline concentrations above 0.1 μg/ml are required for cell stimulation and collagen synthesis while concentrations above 10–50 μg/ml are cytotoxic [47, 48, 73, 77, 78]. Most of the in vitro studies that assess collagen synthesis have measured radioactive collagen by incorporating 3H proline [47, 77–82] or 3H leucine [33], while a single study each used biochemical measurement of hydroxyproline content in lieu of total collagen [73] and photometric method [74]. RT-PCR-based m-RNA expression of collagen genes has been used to assess patterns of collagen synthesis induced by arecoline [75]. In addition, m-RNA levels of heat-shock protein 47 (HSP47), a molecular chaperone involved in the processing and quality type I collagen, have also been investigated [76].

Canniff and Harvey in 1981 [47] used three crude extracts of areca nut to stimulate collagen synthesis in cultures of human fibroblasts, with a pulse of 3H proline. When cultures were analyzed for radioactive collagen, all three extracts at a concentration of 10 μg/ml were found to stimulate collagen synthesis by 150% supporting an etiological role of areca nut in OSF. Harvery et al. [77] also showed that exposure of fibroblasts to arecoline and arecaidine was associated with a concentration-dependent increase in collagen synthesis and cell proliferation. Cell proliferation was evaluated using methylene blue staining assay, and arecoline was found to stimulate fibroblast proliferation up to 10 μg/ml, while it was cytotoxic at 100 μg/ml. However, arecaidine even at 100 μg/ml was capable of maintaining cell proliferation. Based on these results, Harvey et al. [77] concluded that arecaidine was the more potent stimulator of collagen synthesis and cell proliferation. They also used evidence put forward by Nieschultz and Schmersahl [62] to suggest that fibroblasts possess an esterase capable of hydrolyzing arecoline to arecaidine. In contrast to Harvey et al. [77], van Wyk et al. [81] reported that arecoline and arecaidine extracted from raw, baked, and boiled nuts at concentrations of 2.75 μg/ml and 10.6 μg/ml, respectively, inhibit fibroblast growth. Recent study [83] confirms that arecoline at a concentration of <16 μg/ml stimulates proliferation of oral fibroblasts. This process was shown to be mediated via Egr-1, which is a typical immediate early gene by trans-activating Wnt5a.

Kuo et al. [80] compared biosynthesis of collagen in fibroblast cultures established using biopsies of ten OSF patients with tissue from age- and sex-matched controls undergoing third molar extractions. Collagen synthesis was assessed using the same technique described by Canniff and Harvey [47, 77]. Results showed that in four OSF fibroblast strains, there was a 1.5-fold increase in collagen synthesis compared to age-, sex-, and passage-matched controls. It was also found that OSF fibroblasts have higher procollagen m-RNA and produce type I collagen trimer, which is resistant to degradation. However, the fact that 6 out of 10 OSF fibroblast cultures failed to show an increase in collagen synthesis was attributed to the fact that it is not only increased synthesis of collagen that contributes to the pathogenesis of OSF. Though this in vitro study does not directly deal with the effects of areca nut alkaloids, the fact that the experiment was performed using fibroblasts established from OSF patients who used areca nut supports its inclusion.

In contrast to early studies that show increased collagen synthesis [47, 77, 80], several studies [78, 81, 82, 84] show inhibition of collagen or protein synthesis at 0.4–1.0 mM (62 μg/ml and 155 μg/ml) concentrations of arecoline, which are much higher concentrations than generally detected in saliva even in individuals who chew commercial areca products [44]. Xia et al. in 2009 [73] investigated the influence of oral keratinocytes on collagen metabolism by establishing keratinocyte and fibroblast cultures from three healthy individuals. They assessed collagen metabolism in four study groups, namely fibroblast alone without stimulation by arecoline, fibroblasts stimulated with 20 μg/ml arecoline, fibroblasts cocultured with keratinocytes without arecoline pretreatment, and fibroblasts cocultured with keratinocytes pretreated with 20 μg/ml arecoline. The hydroxyproline content was determined after alkaline hydrolysis using a commercial kit, which was considered as the amount of total collagen. According to their results, two study groups with only fibroblasts produced two times more soluble collagen than the fibroblasts that were cocultured with keratinocytes. On the other hand, the group that had fibroblasts cocultured with keratinocytes pretreated with arecoline had higher levels of soluble collagen though it did not reach the amount of collagen secreted by study groups, which only had fibroblasts. This indicates that keratinocytes in the presence of arecoline participate in increasing collagen synthesis. Further, they observed active MMP-9 in the coculture groups but not in groups that contained only fibroblasts. Xia et al. [73] suggested a possible interaction of oral keratinocytes exposed to arecoline in stimulating fibroblasts to increase collagen production in OSF.

Krishnakumar et al. [74] evaluated collagen synthesis by a photometric method in fibroblast and keratinocyte mono- and cocultures exposed to ANE and commercially available smokeless tobacco products at concentrations ranging from 20 to 320 μg/ml. ANE at 20 μg/ml concentrations in fibroblast monocultures had higher amount of collagen compared to fibroblasts exposed to 20 μg/ml of commercial smokeless tobacco products. Cocultures had less amount of secreted collagen similar to that reported in previous studies [73, 75]. However, at higher concentrations, smokeless tobacco induced higher amount of collagen production, though it was less than the amount induced by ANE. Thus, ANE was concluded to be the most potent inducer of collagen synthesis.

Thangjam et al. [75] demonstrated reduced expression of m-RNA of collagen genes 1A1 and 3A1, when gingival fibroblasts were exposed to 50 μg/ml of arecoline. However, when the gingival fibroblasts were cultured with human keratinocytes (Ha CaT) with and without arecoline exposure, both groups showed 6- and 1.9-fold increase in m-RNA expression in 1A1 and 3A1 genes, respectively. This observation was noted in both groups of keratinocytes with and without arecoline exposure. The results confirm the observations of Xia et al. [73], who showed the contribution of keratinocytes in collagen synthesis. The factor secreted by keratinocytes was identified as TGF-β, and it was shown to be activated through muscarinic acetylcholine receptor pathway [75].

Yang et al. [76] investigated the m-RNA expression by RT-PCR of heat-shock protein 47 (HSP47), a molecular chaperone of type I collagen in fibroblast cultures established from 20 OSF patients and tissue obtained during third molar extractions. Results revealed higher expression of HSP47 m-RNA in OSF fibroblasts compared to normal fibroblasts. Exposure of normal fibroblasts to arecoline at 80 μg/ml resulted in threefold increase in HSP47 m-RNA. Thus, Yang et al. [76] concluded that accumulation of collagen in OSF patients may occur due to increased HSP induced by arecoline.

**Important**

**Influence of areca nut on collagen synthesis by fibroblasts**

In vitro studies have shown the ability of areca nut alkaloids to stimulate fibroblast proliferation and increase collagen synthesis in the presence of keratinocytes. However, not all fibroblast cultures established from OSF patients show significant increase in collagen synthesis, which points towards the contribution of events other than increased collagen synthesis in the pathogenesis of OSF.

11

## 11.3.2 In Vitro Experimental Evidence Supportive of Inflammation Induced by Arecoline/ANE

### 11.3.2.1 Contribution of Pro-inflammatory Cytokines

Inflammatory cytokines secreted by fibroblasts are capable of inducing chronic inflammation and have been shown to play a role in the initiation and progression of fibrosis elsewhere in the body [85]. Wang et al. [52] using buccal mucosal fibroblast cultures established from healthy individuals show that exposure to arecoline at 80 μg/ml concentration for four days increased IL-2, IL-6, and IL-21 production but decreased TGF-β production. When fibroblasts continued to grow further for three days without arecoline, a significant increase in cytokine expression was still seen in the experimental group compared to fibroblasts that were not exposed to arecoline. It shows that even in the absence of stimulation by ANE, cells that have been primed are capable of maintaining the inflammatory process. In addition, the cytokine supernatant in the presence of peripheral blood mononuclear cells shows increase in T helper 17 cells (Th17), which induce inflammation and reduction in regulatory T cells (Treg) which suppress the immune response. It was confirmed using Q-PCR that there was a high level of RORγt expression characteristic of Th17, while Foxp3 expression which is characteristic of Treg was lower in the experimental group. Authors [52] showed that arecoline-induced IL-6 stimulated CD4+ T cells to differentiate into Th17 via STAT3 pathway, which has a pro-inflammatory effeact. However, as Th17 cells promote autoimmune response in tissues, whether autoimmunity has any influence in the pathogenesis of OSF is yet to be confirmed with strong evidence.

In addition to gingival fibroblasts [52], gingival keratinocytes were also found to be capable of producing IL-6 and TNF-α [53]. Jeng et al. [53] have shown that ANE (100–400 μg/ml) induced IL-6 and TNF-α production by gingival keratinocytes. It was also shown that IL-6 (5–100 ng/ml) suppressed gingival keratinocyte growth while enhancing oral fibroblast growth. In order to identify the interplay between epithelial cells and immune cells, PGE2, IL-6, and TNF-α secreted by epithelial cells were incubated with peripheral blood monocytes. Jeng et al. [53] showed that the cytokine-rich supernatant secreted by epithelial cells was incapable of not only activating CD4+ and CD8+ cells but also suppressing T cell activation. In addition to the observation of suppressing T cell activation being inconsistent with the findings by Wang et al. [52], it is also difficult to explain the role played by T cells in inducing chronic inflammation, which is a well-described phenomenon, on the basis of results presented by Jeng et al. [53].

### 11.3.2.2 Contribution of Pro-inflammatory Enzymes and Molecules

Tsai et al. [86] exposed buccal mucosal fibroblasts to arecoline at 20–160 μg/ml concentrations and evaluated cyclooxygenase 2 (COX-2) enzyme levels by RT-PCR. Results revealed that resting fibroblasts did not produce COX-2 m-RNA, while the highest amount of COX-2 m-RNA was observed at 2 h following exposure to arecoline at 80 μg/ml concentration. Tsai et al. [86] by showing the presence of COX-2 in both in vivo and in vitro experiments support the involvement of COX-2-mediated inflammatory process in the pathogenesis of OSF and the importance of arecoline as an etiological factor. Jeng et al. [87] in a similar study showed that gingival keratinocytes exposed to ANE (200–800 μg/ml) for 24 hours exhibited prostaglandin E (PGE) production. It was attributed to the induction of cyclooxygenase-2 (COX-2) mRNA expression and protein production. They also confirmed that ANE at 800–1200 μg/ml induced cell death, which could not be inhibited by indomethacin. It led Jeng et al. [87] to confirm that ANE-induced cytotoxicity was not mediated by PGE2. These results suggest that areca nut alkaloids are capable of inducing inflammation via its stimulatory effects on the PGEs, COX-2 production, and associated tissue inflammatory responses. Chang et al. [88] also confirm the ability of ANE to induce the secretion of pro-inflammatory mediators by epithelial cells. They showed that auto-oxidation or metabolic activation of ANE components by cytochrome P450 1A1 may generate ROS. ANE was shown to upregulate the expression of cyclooxygenase-2 (COX-2), CYP1A1, and hemeoxygenase-1 (HO-1), but inhibit the expression of keratin 5/14, cyclin B1, and cdc25C in keratinocytes. Their conclusion was that ROS could activate multiple signaling pathways such as EGFR, Src, and Ras to affect cdc25C, cyclin B1, and keratin 14 expression to mediate MEK/ERK signaling, COX-2 expression, and PGE production. Interestingly, *Piper betle* leaf extract was found to inhibit the ANE-induced $PGE_2$ production and COX 2 m-RNA production.

These experimental evidences show that persistent inflammation of the oral mucosa which could be initiated by chemical mediators of areca nut as well as by mechanical trauma from coarse fibers of areca nut induces chronic inflammation by activation of T lymphocytes. Some of the T lymphocytes which may differentiate into Th17 cells exhibit significant pro-inflammatory response through IL-17. Stimulation of these pro-inflammatory cytokines produced by epithelial cells, fibroblasts, and lymphocytes contributes to a critical step in the pathogenesis of OSF. Another important observation was that once primed by arecoline, fibroblasts retain the ability to secrete cytokines for a few days, even without arecoline in the culture medium. Therefore, inflammation induced by arecoline may persist for several days in areca nut chewers even when they are not chewing areca nut.

**Tip**

**Areca nut-induced inflammation in OSF**

Experimental evidence confirms the ability of areca nut alkaloids to induce inflammation through stimulating keratinocytes, fibroblasts, and lymphocytes to produce inflammatory cytokines (IL-2, IL-6, IL-21, and TNF-α). The cytokines in turn increase the T helper cells, which play a role in maintaining persistent inflammation together with inflammatory mediators COX and PGE. In vivo evidence confirms the presence of high levels of inflammatory cytokines in the saliva of OSF patients compared to individuals without disease.

### 11.3.3 Experimental Evidence Supporting Arecoline/ANE in Stimulating Fibrogenic Cytokines

Experimental evidence supporting ANE in the induction and activation of TGF-β, CTGF, and early growth response-1 (Egr-1) molecules responsible for fibrosis has been established by several studies [89–91]. Khan et al. [89] exposed primary gingival fibroblasts (hGF) and human keratinocytes (HaCaT) to the water extract of areca nut, different alkaloids (arecoline 400 μM, arecaidine 1000 μM, guvacine 1000 μM), and polyphenols (catechin 170 μM, tannin 6 μM). Their results showed that in addition to arecoline, arecaidine, guvacine, and polyphenols, catechin and tannin were also potent inducers of pro-fibrogenic TGF-β signaling in keratinocytes. The spent medium of the epithelial cultures exposed to areca nut extract revealed TGF-β by ELISA. Gene expression profiling of both water and alcohol extracts of areca nut revealed that 1331 genes were differently expressed, which involved genes contributing to pathways in cancer, cell cycle, cytokine-cytokine receptor interaction, and Wnt signaling pathway. They showed that both water and alcohol extracts of areca nut induced p-SMAD2 and TGF-β downstream targets in HaCaT cells but not in hGF, suggesting that epithelial cells could be the source of TGF-β in the development of OSF. However, it was also shown that TGF-β induced in the epithelium by areca nut acts on the fibroblasts in a pro-fibrogenic manner for the induction of matrix components such as collagens.

Pant et al. [90] designed a series of experiments to identify how areca nut-induced TGF-β in epithelial cells acts on fibroblasts. Human gingival fibroblasts were treated with areca nut and/or TGF-β followed by transcriptome profiling. The expressions of 413 genes in fibroblasts were increased by areca nut and TGF-β together. They also found that differentially expressed genes of OSF tissues compared to normal tissues overlapped significantly with areca nut- and TGF-β-induced genes in epithelial cells and fibroblasts. Several pathways were found to be common between OSF tissues and areca nut +TGF-β-treated gingival fibroblasts. Areca nut together with TGF-β enhanced fibroblast activation as demonstrated by increased αSMA, γSMA, and collagen gel contraction by hGF cells. Furthermore, TGF-β secreted by areca nut-treated epithelial cells influenced fibroblast activation and other genes implicated in fibrosis. These data establish a role for areca nut through epithelial-mesenchymal interaction in OSF. According to the results, Pant et al. [90] proposed a model on the role of areca nut and TGF-β in OSF progression as follows: areca nut exposure induces and activates TGF-β in epithelial cells. Both areca nut and TGF-β act on fibroblasts to induce endothelin and CTGF, which are also pro-fibrogenic cytokines. These cytokines (including TGF-β through αvβ6) induce fibroblasts to convert into myofibroblasts expressing γSMA and αSMA markers with resultant overall increase in collagen production. Collagen maturation and stabilizing enzymes (BMP1 and PLOD2, respectively) can also be induced by areca nut along with TGF-β, which increase the collagen, resulting in excessive deposition of extracellular matrix characteristic of OSF.

Early growth response-1 (Egr-1) is a zinc finger transcription factor that is expressed in fibrotic diseases and is essential for the fibrotic response to TGF-β. Heish et al. [91] showed that fibroblasts treated with 0.1 mM arecoline for 2 h have fourfold increase in Egr-1 protein levels and sevenfold increase in Egr-1 m-RNA levels. With further investigations, ROS, JNK, and ERK were shown to be involved in the arecoline-induced Egr-1 protein expression. In addition to Egr-1, arecoline has been shown to induce human buccal mucosal fibroblasts to produce CTGF, both of which are important mediators of fibrotic response [91]. Heish et al. [91] also showed that TGF-β-neutralizing antibody inhibits Egr-1 and CTGF production, which meant that arecoline induced Egr-1 and CTGF that was mediated through TGF-β signaling pathway.



Several mechanisms have been shown to activate TGF-β including αvβ6 integrin [92, 93], ROS [92], and c-Jun N-terminal kinase (JNK) via M receptor [93]. Moutasim et al. [94] investigated the functional role of αvβ6 using oral keratinocyte with high αvβ6 (VB6) expression. In the presence of arecoline, integrin avβ6 expression was found to be upregulated resulting in significant αvβ6-dependent activation of TGF-β1 through M4 muscarinic acetylcholine receptor. In addition, experimental evidence indicates that alkaloids and polyphenols present in ANE activate THBS1 (activator of latent TGF-β) in HeCaT [93, 94]. It has also been shown by Heish et al. [92] that arecoline-induced mitochondrial ROS activates latent TGF-β1 to its active form, which in turn stimulates the synthesis of other fibrogenic cytokines such as CTGF. Pant et al. [93] have shown that arecoline activates JNK through M receptor and ROS, and after JNK phosphorylation, it activates activating transcription factor 2 (ATF2) and TGF-β. On the other hand, treatment of keratinocytes and oral fibroblasts with TGF-β resulted in downregulation of BMP7, which is a known negative modulator of fibrosis [89–95]. In addition, Chang et al. [95] report that thrombin-induced CTGF synthesis is mediated through TGF-β signaling.

TGF-β stimulates procollagen gene expression, which ultimately results in the increase in collagen synthesis and fibrosis. Taken together, upregulation of fibrogenic TGF-β induced by areca nut and downregulation of anti-fibrotic BMP7 have been experimentally shown to contribute to the pathogenesis of OSF.

**Important**

**What components of areca nut induce TGF-β?**

Experimental evidence reveals that in addition to the constituents of areca nut—arecoline, arecaidine, guvacine, and polyphenols—catechin and tannin are also potent inducers of pro-fibrogenic TGF-β signaling in keratinocytes.

**What is the role of TGF-β in OSF?**

Once activated, TGF-β stimulates

1. Increase collagen production through
   Differentiation of fibroblasts to myofibroblasts expressing SMA phenotype
   Inducing production of collagen maturation and stabilizing enzymes
   Stimulating the expression of other fibrotic genes such as Egr-1 and CTGF
2. Inhibit collagen degradation through
   Activation of TIMP, TMG-2, and PAI genes

### 11.3.4 Experimental Evidence of Areca Nut Extract/Arecoline Contributing to Myofibroblast Activation

Persistent activation of myofibroblasts leads to pathological fibrosis through its contraction [96, 97] and dysregulation of ECM synthesis (type 1 collagen and fibronectin). Myofibroblasts are also considered to produce more ECM than fibroblasts. In addition to the role played by TGF-β through SMAD signaling [94], transdifferentiation of myofibroblasts in the presence of arecoline has been shown to be maintained by ZEB1 and 2, Snail, IL-6, and LINC00312 [98–101].

Twist is an epithelial-mesenchymal transcription factor implicated in the differentiation of myofibroblasts. Lee et al. [96] showed that arecoline could increase Twist m-RNA and protein in a dose-dependent manner in buccal mucosal fibroblasts. Myofibroblast activity including collagen gel contraction and migration was shown to be dependent on Twist. These experiments show that arecoline-induced upregulation of Twist is one factor that produces dysregulation of myofibroblastic activity. A study by Chang et al. [97] also revealed that ANE induced collagen gel contraction in buccal mucosal fibroblasts. With further series of experiments, it was shown that contraction was related to PLC/IP3/Ca (2+)/calmodulin and Rho signaling pathway as well as actin filament polymerization and was not purely dependent on ROS production. Chang et al. and Liao et al. [98, 99] showed that trans-differentiation of buccal mucosal fibroblast to myofibroblast with α-SMA and ZEB1 expression was induced by arecoline. Knockdown of ZEB1 was shown to inhibit arecoline-induced α-SMA promoter activity, protein expression, and collagen gel contraction in buccal mucosal fibroblasts. In addition, Liao et al. [99] showed arecoline-induced downregulation of miR-200b as a mechanism that induced increased ZEB2 expression. Their results suggested that downregulation of miR-200b may contribute to the pathogenesis of areca quid-associated OSF through the expression of ZEB2 and myofibroblast hallmarks. Peng et al. [100] showed that arecoline activated Snail-triggered myofibroblast trans-differentiation through increased expression of α-SMA, collagen I, and IL-6. Moreover, IL-6 in buccal mucosal fibroblasts was found to further increase the expression of Snail and mediate Snail-induced myofibroblast activation. These findings suggested that Snail and IL-6 regulate the areca nut-associated myofibroblast trans-differentiation. Yu et al. [101] showed that long noncoding RNA, LINC00312, was associated with fibrosis factors, such as α-SMA, type I collagen, and fibronectin. They showed that the inhibition of LINC00312 downregulated the myofibroblast activities, including collagen gel contractility and gene expression of myofibroblast markers.

Taking all the experimental evidence into consideration, persistent activation of myofibroblasts by ANE/arecoline results in pathological fibrosis due to dysregulation of extracellular matrix (ECM) synthesis and degradation.

### 11.3.5 Experimental Evidence of Decreased Collagen Degradation and Clearance by Areca Nut

A reduction in collagen degradation and clearance may occur due to changes in collagen stabilization, defective ECM dynamics, and defects in collagen phagocytosis. Studies that deal with the effect of areca nut products on TGF-β, TIMPs, PAI, lysyl oxidase/copper, cystatin, and KGF will be discussed, with respect to ECM turnover. TGF-β decreases the collagen degradation by activation of TIMPs, TMG-2, and PAI genes. Significance of tissue inhibitor of metalloproteinase (TIMP) 1 and 2 in collagen turnover has been shown in several studies [102–104]. Chang et al. [102] evaluated the levels of TIMP-1 and -2 in fibroblasts established from OSF patients and healthy individuals. Their results indicated that OSF fibroblasts have higher TIMP expression than fibroblasts obtained from healthy individuals. Using Western blots and gelatin zymography, arecoline was shown to elevate TIMP-1 expression at concentration levels under 20 mg/ml in a dose-dependent manner. In addition, arecoline was found to inhibit MMP-2 secretion and production at the concentration level of 40 mg/ml. Therefore, it was concluded that arecoline acts as an inhibitor of MMP-2 while stimulating TIMP-1 activity, leading to the accumulation of ECM components in areca quid-associated OSF. Similar results were observed by Sheih et al. [103] who showed that on exposure to arecoline and safrole, OSF fibroblasts produced more TIMP-1 protein and expressed higher levels of TIMP-1 m-RNA compared to normal buccal mucosal fibroblasts. Xia et al. [73] showed that the coculture group with arecoline-treated keratinocytes produced the highest amount of TIMP compared to other groups and concluded that TIMP together with keratinocytes plays a pivotal role in the pathogenesis of OSF. Pitiyage et al. [104] also demonstrated elevated TIMP-1 and -2 levels in OSF fibroblasts compared to normal fibroblasts, while TIMP levels were seen to increase in normal fibroblasts with the introduction of DNA double-strand breaks. Flavonoids in areca nut have been shown to inhibit the MMP activity [2].

S100A4, a calcium-binding protein, initiates the onset and progression of fibrosis in many organs [105]. Influence of S100A4 protein on the expression of TIMP-1/MMP was evaluated using S100A4 knockdown buccal mucosal fibroblasts in the presence of arecoline. Results indicate that there is significant downregulation of TIMP-1/MMP in the absence of S100A4, and thus it can be concluded that S100A4 regulates TIMP activity in OSF [105].

In addition to the action of TIMP, experimental evidence by Scutt et al. [106] showed that reconstituted collagen fibrils on rat dermis when treated by crude ANE or purified tannins/catechin are resistant to both human and bacterial collagenase. They concluded that tannin, which is a major component of areca nut, induces fibrosis in OSF patients which is resistant to degradation by collagenases. Transglutaminase-2 (TGM-2) is a Ca2+-dependent enzyme that produces cross-linking to stabilize proteins. Arecoline was shown to induce TGM-2 mRNA and protein expression in human gingival fibroblast cells [107, 108]. The TGM-2 expression was hypothesised to be induced by ROS initiated by arecoline or through TGF-β. These studies provide evidence to support the role played by arecoline in stabilizing collagen through TGM-2 overexpression in OSF. The role of plasminogen activator inhibitor-1 (PAI-1) is to inhibit plasmin-dependent ECM degradation leading to its accumulation in various organs. Yang and Tsai [109, 110] show that OSF fibroblasts express significantly higher PAI-1 m-RNA compared to normal buccal mucosal fibroblasts. In addition, when normal fibroblasts were exposed to arecoline (0–160 μg/ml), it increased PAI-1 expression in a dose-dependent manner. Tsai et al. [110] showed that PAI-1 expression depends on the activation of HIF1α and TGF-β, which are also dependent on activation by arecoline. It can be concluded that PAI-1 may play a role in promoting fibrogenesis in OSF patients by inhibiting the conversion of procollagenase to collagenase.

Lysyl oxidase is an extracellular enzyme that is secreted by fibroblasts. It requires copper as a cofactor and it initiates the cross-linking of collagen and elastin which is more resistant to digestion by mammalian collagenase. Ma et al. [69] compared the lysyl oxidase activity of fibroblasts obtained from normal oral mucosa and OSF patients associated with areca nut chewing. The results revealed that lysyl oxidase activity in OSF fibroblasts was greater than that in normal fibroblasts. They postulated that an increased lysyl oxidase level seen in OSF fibroblasts may give rise to collagen resistant to digestion by collagenase. Trivedy *et al.* confirmed the importance of copper in collagen synthesis by showing that the addition of copper to normal fibroblasts causes a significant increase in the synthesis of collagen, with a peak production observed at a concentration of 50 mM copper chloride [111].

11

Cystatin C is a protein that inhibits cysteine proteinases and has been shown to be upregulated in fibrotic diseases elsewhere in the body. It has been shown to play a role in inhibiting the degradation of collagen. On evaluation of cystatin C by RT-PCR and ELISA, OSF fibroblasts demonstrated significantly higher cystatin C expression than normal buccal mucosal fibroblasts. In addition, arecoline was found to elevate cystatin C m-RNA and protein expression in a dose-dependent manner, leading to the stabilization of collagen fibrils in OSF [112].

Keratinocyte growth factor-1 (KGF-1) is a potent inhibitor of collagenase secreted by epithelial cells. Tsai et al. [113] showed that KGF-1 m-RNA was upregulated in fibroblasts obtained from OSF patients and buccal mucosal fibroblasts subjected to arecoline (0–80 μg/ml) in a dose-dependent manner compared to buccal mucosal fibroblasts without exposure to arecoline.

Experimental evidences on collagen phagocytosis of OSF fibroblasts and normal buccal mucosal fibroblasts with or without exposure to areca nut alkaloids have been presented by Tsai and Sheih [114, 115]. Tsai et al. [114] evaluated the degradation of collagen by fibroblast phagocytosis with collagen and fibronectin-coated fluorescent latex beads in OSF and normal buccal mucosal fibroblast cultures. When fluorescence associated with internalized beads was measured by flow cytometry, results revealed that normal fibroblast cultures contained 70 and 75% of fibronectin and collagen phagocytic cells in contrast to 10% and 15% of phagocytic cells in OSF cultures. In addition, when normal fibroblasts were incubated with areca nut alkaloids (arecoline, arecaidine), dose-dependent reduction in phagocytic cells was observed, which confirmed the negative influence of areca nut alkaloids on collagen and fibronectin phagocytosis. Consistent with Tsai et al. [114], Sheih et al. [115] showed that in addition to arecoline, safrole (which is a component of betel quid in some countries such as Taiwan and Papua New Guinea) and nicotine, which are released in saliva during betel quid chewing and smoking, can also inhibit collagen phagocytosis by fibroblasts in a dose-dependent manner contributing to the pathogenesis of OSF.

**Important**

**The role of areca nut and copper in decreasing collagen degradation**

Experimental evidence shows that reduced extracellular matrix degradation could be achieved in the following ways:

1. Arecoline stimulates TIMP-1 expression in fibroblasts while reducing MMP-2 expression with the net effect of reduced collagen degradation.
2. TMG-2 (which is activated through TGF-β or ROS) produces cross-linking to stabilize collagen, which prevents its degradation.
3. Arecoline stimulates PAI-1, which inhibits plasmin-dependent ECM degradation.
4. Arecoline elevates cystatin C m-RNA and protein expression in a dose-dependent manner, leading to stabilization of collagen fibrils in OSF.
5. Lysyl oxidase secreted by fibroblasts produces cross-linking in collagen in the presence of copper, which reduces its degradation. Areca nut is a rich source of copper, while it was also shown that fibroblasts harvested from OSF patients secrete a higher amount of lysyl oxidase.
6. Arecoline stimulates TGF-β expression in keratinocytes, which in turn activates TIMP-1, TMG-2, and PAI.

### 11.3.6 In Vitro Evidence of Oxidative Stress and ROS Generation by Betel Quid

Areca nut, lime, heavy metals (copper and ferrous ions), and inflorescence of *Piper betle* and betel leaves have been identified as components of betel quid contributing to ROS generation [116, 117]. Direct in vitro evidence of arecoline-induced ROS generation in human keratinocytes and fibroblasts was shown in studies by Heish et al. [92] and Lee et al. [108], where ROS was shown to activate TGF-β from the latent complex [92] and upregulate transglutaminase-2 [108]. Heish et al. [92] showed that mitochondria-targeted antioxidant completely suppressed arecoline-induced latent TGF-β1 activation and both mitochondrial and total cellular ROS. Lee et al. [108] showed that arecoline concentrations greater than 20 μg/ml significantly upregulated intracellular ROS generation in buccal mucosal fibroblasts in a dose-dependent manner. Similarly, arecoline was found to increase transglutaminase-2 protein in a dose-dependent manner in buccal mucosal fibroblasts by Western blot analysis. Also, the production of both ROS and transglutaminase-2 was shown to be inhibited or reduced by antioxidants glutathione precursor N-acetyl-L-cysteine (NAC) and epigallocatechin-3-gallate (EGCG). Therefore, Lee et al. [108] proposed that increased production of transglutaminase-2 by arecoline stimulation in fibroblasts may be mediated by intracellular ROS.

Illeperuma et al. [118] designed a study to see whether the cytokines released from ANE-exposed fibroblasts were induced by ROS. Their results revealed that ROS induced IL-6 and IL-8 secretion in fibroblasts exposed to areca nut. Similarly, Chang et al. [119] showed that ANE increased the expression of cyclooxygenase-2, prostaglandin E2, and IL-1α in human immune cells through oxidative stress. Indirect evidence of the involvement of oxidative stress/ROS as a pathological mechanism in OSF can be found in studies by Yang [76], Tsai [51], Heish [91], and Deng [120], where antioxidant NAC was found to inhibit or reduce arecoline-induced HSP47, COX-2, Erg-1, and CTGF expression by fibroblasts/epithelial cells in culture.

Cytotoxicity induced by arecoline has been shown to be mediated by ROS, which leads to suppression of catalase activity in the epithelium. Therefore, Khan et al. [121] designed a study to identify the mechanisms that contribute to epithelial atrophy in OSF by exposing human gingival fibroblasts and keratinocytes to areca nut water extract (ANW) and ANE. ANE was shown to generate more ROS in epithelial cells compared to ANW in a dose-dependent manner. On the other hand, both AWE and ANE did not induce fibroblast to generate ROS. Thus surprisingly, AWE was shown to be cytotoxic to keratinocytes, while it induced proliferation of fibroblasts through IGF. Their results showed that arecoline enhances the oxidative reduction potential of copper resulting in the cleavage of DNA, which generates an apoptotic response in epithelium. Khan et al. [121] theorized ROS-induced apoptosis as the mechanism responsible for the atrophy of OSF epithelium.

In contrast to previous studies which showed generation of oxidative stress by ANE/arecoline, Paranagama et al. [122] and Sazwi et al. [123] among others have shown antioxidant activity of traditional betel quid (TBQ) which contained areca nut [122] and betel quid which contained areca nut with *Uncaria gambir* with or without calcium hydroxide [123], within the scope of their study design. Ethyl acetate extract of TBQ was shown to contain a high amount of polyphenols and demonstrated DPPH and ABTS radical scavenging activity and ability to reduce ferric, which conferred antioxidant ability. TBQ was also shown to protect human gingival fibroblasts from $H_2O_2$-induced oxidative stress. Sazwi et al. [123] revealed that *Uncaria gambir* demonstrated the highest antioxidant activity (DPPH, FRAP, and Fe). It was also shown that betel quid without calcium hydroxide had higher antioxidant activity. The molecule responsible for antioxidant activity was identified as quinic acid by Sazwi et al. [123]. In contrast to previous studies [122, 123] where antioxidant properties were attributed to polyphenols and quinic acid, Tsai et al. [124] assessed the m-RNA levels of HO-1 (hemo-oxygenase-1), which is a stress-inducible protein that acts as an antioxidant in fibroblast cultures in the presence of arecoline. They demonstrated that OSF fibroblasts expressed significantly higher HO-1 mRNA expression than normal buccal mucosal fibroblasts, while arecoline was also found to elevate HO-1 mRNA and protein expression in a dose-dependent manner. From these studies, it can be concluded that betel quid as well as areca nut have both antioxidant and prooxidant properties.

Experimental evidence shows that areca nut, lime, heavy metals (copper and ferrous ions), and inflorescence of *Piper betle* and betel leaves are components of betel quid contributing to ROS generation. Prooxidant properties/ROS has been shown to maintain inflammation, activate TGF-β, and increase the expression of other fibrogenic genes Egr-1 and CTGF, which promote fibrosis, while paradoxically also reducing collagen degradation through activation of TMG-2. On the other hand, experimental evidence supporting betel quid's antioxidant properties also exists [122, 123]. However, at present, there is insufficient evidence to indicate whether harmful effects of ROS get diminished by the antioxidant properties of betel quid during the development of OSF.

### 11.3.7 The Role of Arecoline-Induced Autophagy in OSF

Autophagy is a process of self-digestion where damaged cell components are metabolized and released back into the cytoplasm. Three main categories of autophagy are micro-autophagy, macro-autophagy, and chaperone-mediated autophagy. HIF-1α has been implicated as a major regulator of autophagy under hypoxic conditions, which led investigators to explore the role of autophagy in OSF [125]. Li et al. [125] investigated the effect of TGF-β signaling on autophagy and revealed that TGF-β stimulated the expression of light chain 3(LC) m-RNA (commonly used as a marker of autophagy) as well as its protein in fibroblasts. On incubation of fibroblast with a known autophagy inhibitor, chloroquine leads to reduced expression of Col 1A2 gene. Though areca nut constituents have not been directly investigated in relation to autophagy by Li et al. [125], the fact that ANE has been shown to produce and activate TGF-β [89] signifies the importance of areca nut in the induction of autophagy.

Dai et al. [126] investigated whether arecoline could induce autophagy to affect angiogenesis of human umbilical vein endothelial cells (HUVECs). Results revealed that HUVECs treated with arecoline exhibited increased autophagosomes and LC3 expression with reduced expression of p62. Incorporation of chloroquine had the opposite effect with a reduction in LC3 expression and increased expression of p62. Authors theorized that high levels of autophagy induced by arecoline could inhibit angiogenesis and thereby contribute to the pathogenesis of OSF.



Zhu et al. [127] treated human oral keratinocytes with 15 μg/ml of arecoline and found a greater number of autophagic vacuoles after 6–24 h of arecoline treatment compared to 0–3 h, by transmission electron microscopy. They also showed that with chloroquine, apoptosis and caspase-3 was reduced when compared to arecoline used alone. These findings confirmed autophagy and apoptosis as mechanisms that produce epithelial atrophy, which was shown to be directly mediated by arecoline. In addition, Tseng et al. [128] have shown that arecoline at 0.4 and 0.8 mM concentrations induces apoptosis of endothelial cells. This increase in apoptosis was correlated to an increase in the subpopulation of G0/G1 endothelial cells, which is a hallmark of apoptosis. Thus, it can be concluded that arecoline-induced apoptosis of endothelial cells and induction of autophagy are the mechanisms by which reduced vascularity occurs in OSF.

## 11.4 Experimental Evidence-Based Outline of Mechanisms by Which Etiological Agents Contribute to the Development of OSF

Considering significant number of experimental evidence related to etiology of OSF that exists in the literature, etiological contribution from areca nut, betel quid, micronutrients, and genetic polymorphisms is outlined by correlating the hallmarks of OSF: aberrant ECM metabolism - initiating both increased synthesis and reduction in degradation of ECM, epithelial atrophy, and reduced vascularity. Betel quid/areca nut chewing releases alkaloids arecoline, arecaidine, guvacoline, and guvacine into saliva. The most significant alkaloids arecoline and arecaidine in saliva reach a concentration that can stimulate collagen synthesis within 5 min and continue to induce collagen synthesis for approximately 8 h. Both chemical trauma from areca nut alkaloids/flavonoids and mechanical trauma from coarse fibers of areca nut allow the diffusion of detrimental substances into the oral mucosa.

Areca nut extract contributes to deranged ECM metabolism by initiating both increased synthesis and reduction in degradation of ECM including collagen and fibronectin. In the epithelium, arecoline has been shown to induce keratinocytes to produce TGF-β, which is activated by ROS, muscarinic acetylcholine and αvβ6 receptors. TGF-β, through SMAD/non-SMAD pathways, induces Egr-1, CTGF, as well as myofibroblastic phenotype with α-SMA and vimentin expression, which ultimately leads to increase in collagen synthesis. Experimental evidences supporting persistent inflammation are shown by increased levels of inflammatory cytokines in the saliva of OSF patients. The ability of arecoline to induce inflammatory mediators supports the chronic inflammatory nature of OSF. Experimental evidence shows that arecoline plays a main role in inducing TGF-β, TIMPs, PAI, lysyl oxidase, cystatin, and KGF expression, which ultimately results in reduced collagen degradation. Tannins and catechins present in ANE have been shown to contribute to cross-linking and creating collagen that is resistant to collagenase (MMP), while safrole present in the inflorescence of *Piper betle* has been shown to increase TIMP-1 production and reduce collagen phagocytosis. Experimental evidence indicates that arecoline-induced apoptosis of endothelial cells and induction of autophagy are the mechanisms by which reduced vascularity occurs in OSF. Arecoline has been shown to enhance the oxidative reduction potential of copper resulting in cleavage of DNA, which generates an apoptotic response in epithelium, leading to epithelial atrophy (Table 11.2).

Ca $(OH)_2$ or lime, a component present in betel quid and commercial areca nut products, and/or an esterase that is present in fibroblasts has been speculated to convert arecoline to arecaidine, which is identified as the active alkaloid which initiates a cascade of events resulting in OSF. Evidence indicating increased excretion of arecaidine in urine is the main observation that can be found to support its involvement in the pathogenesis of OSF.

The major etiological role played by areca nut in the development of OSF is confirmed by the ability of ANE to induce OSF-like lesions in mouse models. Highlighting the importance of arecoline in inducing OSF, arecoline

**Table 11.2** In vitro experimental evidence supporting etiological contribution of areca nut/betel quid and commercial smokeless tobacco products

| Reference | Cell type/dose of constituents of areca nut/betel quid or commercial smokeless tobacco product | Effect |
|---|---|---|
| [47] | Fibroblasts subjected to ANE at 10 μg/ml | Stimulated and increased collagen synthesis by 150% |
| [77] | Human fibroblasts subjected to arecoline and arecaidine at 0–100 μg/ml | In fibroblasts exposed to arecoline or arecaidine for 24 h, there was concentration-dependent stimulation of collagen synthesis; arecaidine consistently produced greater stimulation than arecoline<br>Arecoline and arecaidine stimulated the rate of proliferation of fibroblasts over a 5-day culture period in a concentration-dependent manner |
| [73] | Human fibroblasts monocultures and fibroblasts and keratinocyte cocultures were stimulated with arecoline at 20 μg/ml | Fibroblasts cocultured with keratinocytes pretreated with arecoline had higher levels of soluble collagen though it did not reach the amount of collagen secreted by study groups which only had fibroblasts<br>Active MMP-9 was observed in the coculture groups but not in groups that contained only fibroblasts<br>Coculture group produced higher amounts of TIMP |
| [74] | Human fibroblasts monocultures and fibroblasts and keratinocyte cocultures were stimulated with ANE, commercial smokeless tobacco products (gutkha and Hans) at concentrations ranging from 20 to 320 μg/ml and time intervals of 12, 24, 48, and 72 h | ANE at 20 μg/ml showed increased collagen production compared to commercial tobacco products. Gutkha and Hans showed higher collagen synthesis at 160 and 80–320 μg/ml, respectively<br>Monocultures showed increased collagen synthesis than cocultures |
| [75] | HaCaT keratinocytes, were exposed to 0–50 μg/ml arecoline | It induced expression of TGF-β, through muscarinic acetylcholine receptor-intracellular $Ca^{2+}$-PKC pathway<br>Gingival fibroblasts were induced to produce collagens 1A1 and 3A1 by arecoline in the presence of spent medium of cultured human keratinocytes, which was shown to contain TGF-β |
| [76] | Buccal mucosal fibroblasts were exposed to 0–160 μg/ml arecoline | Arecoline upregulated HSP47 expression via P13K, Cox-2, MEK pathways |
| [52] | Fibroblasts were stimulated by arecoline at 0–80 μg/ml concentrations | Arecoline at 80 μg/ml concentration for four days increased IL-2, IL-6, and IL-21 production but decreased TGF-β production<br>When cytokine-containing medium was cocultured with PBMC, it increased T helper cells, which are also potent stimulators of inflammation |
| [53] | Gingival keratinocytes were exposed to ANE at 100–400 μg/ml | ANE induced IL-6 and TNF-α production by gingival keratinocytes<br>IL-6 was found to stimulate gingival fibroblast growth |
| [86] | Buccal mucosal fibroblasts were exposed to arecoline at 0–160 μg/ml | Arecoline at 80 μg/ml induced cyclooxygenase-2 expression within half an hour, but subsequently expression subsided. COX expression was concluded to be an early response. Decreased thiol content was involved in the induction of COX |
| [87] | Gingival keratinocytes exposed to 200–800 μg/ml ANE for 24 h | ANE induced threefold increase of PGE and 1.7-fold increase of PGF. At higher concentration of 800–1200 μg/ml, cell death occurred |
| [89] | Primary human gingival fibroblasts and HaCaT keratinocytes were exposed to water ANE and different alkaloids (arecoline 400 μM, arecaidine 1000 μM, guvacine 1000 μM), polyphenols (catechin 170 μM, tannin 6 μM) | Both water and alcohol extracts of ANE induced TGF-β signaling in epithelial cells by increased levels of p-SMAD2. It was also established that arecoline, arecaidine, guvacine, and polyphenols were capable of inducing TGF-β expression in HaCaT cells<br>Both polyphenols and alkaloids induced TGF-β2 and THBS1 (activator of latent TGF-β) in HaCaT cells suggesting that areca nut-mediated activation of p-SMAD2 involves upregulation and activation of TGF-β |
| [91] | Buccal mucosal fibroblasts were exposed to arecoline at 0–0.4 mM concentration | Arecoline-induced upregulation of Egr-1 with the involvement of JNK and ERK pathways |
| [94] | Keratinocytes were exposed to arecoline at 5–10 μg/ml | Arecoline-induced upregulation of αvβ6 integrin expression with the involvement of muscarinic acetylcholine receptors |

(continued)

**Table 11.2** (continued)

| Reference | Cell type/dose of constituents of areca nut/betel quid or commercial smokeless tobacco product | Effect |
|---|---|---|
| [93] | HaCaT cells were subjected to areca nut treatment (5 μg/ml) at 0.5-, 1-, 2-, 4-, 6-, 12-, and 24-h time points | Increase in TGF-β2 mRNA and protein was induced by areca nut after 2-h treatment with the activation of downstream effectors, SMAD2 and 3 |
| [96] | Buccal mucosal fibroblasts were exposed to arecoline at 0–20 μg/ml | Arecoline treatment was found to increase Twist protein expression in a dose-dependent manner. Twist protein played a significant role in myofibroblast trans-differentiation |
| [98] | Buccal mucosal fibroblast cultures were exposed to 0–20 μg/ml concentration of arecoline | Arecoline induced ZEB1, α SMA, and vimentin expression, indicating myofibroblast phenotype |
| [103] | Buccal mucosal fibroblasts were exposed to 0–50 μg/ml concentrations of betel quid ingredients arecoline, arecaidine, and safrole. OSF fibroblasts were assessed for TIMP in the presence of betel quid ingredients | OSF fibroblasts secreted more TIMP compared to normal fibroblasts, with and without betel quid components<br>Both arecoline and safrole showed dose-dependent increase in TIMP-1 expression as well as protein synthesis |
| [105] | Buccal mucosal fibroblasts were exposed to 0–20 μg/ml of arecoline | Arecoline upregulated S100A4 expression with NF-ĸB, ERK, and mTOR pathways being involved. It is involved in upregulating TIMP/MMP |
| [108] | Buccal mucosal fibroblasts were exposed to 0–160 μg/ml of arecoline | Arecoline induced upregulation of transglutaminase-2 expression, which was induced by ROS |
| [109] | Buccal mucosal fibroblasts were exposed to 0–160 μg/ml of arecoline | Arecoline induced plasminogen activator inhibitor-1 |
| [110] | Buccal mucosal fibroblasts were exposed to 0–160 μg/ml of arecoline | Arecoline was found to upregulate HIF1α protein expression in a dose-dependent manner. It was also found to upregulate PAI-1 protein expression in a dose-dependent manner under environmental hypoxia and normoxic conditions |
| [108] | Normal oral fibroblasts and OSF fibroblasts were assessed for lysyl oxidase activity and proliferation rates | OSF fibroblasts showed a faster proliferative activity, increased protein content, and increased lysyl oxidase than normal fibroblasts |
| [111] | Human oral fibroblasts were incubated with copper chloride at concentrations ranging from 0.01 to 500 μM for 24 h, and in vitro cell proliferation was evaluated | Copper chloride increased collagen synthesis by oral fibroblasts compared with growth without copper |
| [112] | Buccal mucosal fibroblasts were subjected to 0–80 μg/ml of arecoline | Arecoline induced upregulation of cystatin C expression |
| [113] | Buccal mucosal fibroblasts were subjected to 0–80 μg/ml of arecoline | Arecoline induced keratinocyte growth factor-1 expression |
| [115] | Fibroblasts obtained from normal and diseased (OSF) were compared with respect to phagocytic activity. Normal fibroblast cultures were then exposed to 10–50 μg/ml of arecoline, nicotine, and safrole | Collagen phagocytosis of fibroblast from normal region was higher than fibroblast obtained from diseased region<br>In the presence of arecoline, safrole, and nicotine, phagocytic activity of normal fibroblasts was significantly reduced |
| [120] | Buccal mucosal fibroblasts were subjected to 0–0.4 mM of arecoline | Arecoline induced upregulation of CTGF expression via NF-ĸB, JNK, and p38. Decreased thiol content was involved in induction |
| [124] | Buccal mucosal fibroblasts were subjected to 0–80 μg/ml of arecoline | Arecoline induced upregulation of hemo-oxygenase-1 expression |
| [126] | Human umbilical vein endothelial cells were subjected to 30 μg/ml of arecoline at 0-, 3-, 6-, 12-, and 24-h time points | Arecoline was shown to induce autophagy in HUVEC, which results in reduced angiogenesis |

alone without the other constituents of areca nut has been shown to be capable of producing OSF-like lesions in mice. However, in humans, the fact that not all betel/areca nut chewers develop OSF supports the involvement of genetic polymorphisms in the pathogenesis of OSF. Taken together, experimental evidence ultimately supports a polygenic nature, which involves both environmental (areca nut) and genetic components in the development of OSF.

## 11.5 Experimental Evidence That Is Required to Complete the Etiological Picture of OSF

1. Is it arecoline or arecaidine which plays the main etiological role in OSF?
2. How do areca nut alkaloids and polyphenol concentrations differ in areca nut chewers with and without OSF?
3. Does T helper cell-induced autoimmunity play a role in OSF?
4. Do the concentrations of areca nut alkaloids producing increased collagen synthesis and reduced degradation differ geographically among humans or depending on the type of areca nut?
5. Would other constituents of areca nut in the absence of arecoline produce OSF?
6. Why do all mice subjected to ANE develop OSF while only a portion of humans who use areca nut develop OSF?
7. Do antioxidant properties of betel quid play a protective role among areca nut chewers who do not develop OSF?
8. Which genetic polymorphism combination/s makes an individual more susceptible to OSF?

**Summary**

In summary, experimental evidence supports the major role played by areca nut alkaloids arecoline and/or arecaidine in producing inflammation, increased collagen synthesis, collagen cross-linking, decreased collagen degradation, and autophagy, which ultimately leads to the development of OSF. Experimental evidence also shows that the genetic makeup or polymorphisms could make an individual more susceptible to develop OSF. Collectively, all evidence supports an essential contribution from environmental risk factors (areca nut use) and genetic polymorphisms, which confirms the multifactorial nature of OSF.

## References

1. Betel-quid and areca-nut chewing. IARC Monogr Eval Carcinog Risk Chem Hum. 1985;37:137–202.
2. IARC Working Group on the Evaluation of Carcinogenic Risks to Humans. Betel-quid and areca-nut chewing and some areca-nut derived nitrosamines. IARC Monogr Eval Carcinog Risks Hum. 2004;85:1–334.
3. IARC Monographs Vol 128 Group. Carcinogenicity of acrolein, crotonaldehyde, and arecoline. Lancet Oncol. 2021;22(1):19–20. https://doi.org/10.1016/S1470-2045(20)30727-0.
4. Sharan RN, Mehrotra R, Choudhury Y, Asotra K. Association of betel nut with carcinogenesis: revisit with a clinical perspective. PLoS One. 2012;7(8):e42759. https://doi.org/10.1371/journal.pone.0042759.
5. Jain V, Garg A, Parascandola M, Chaturvedi P, Khariwala SS, Stepanov I. Analysis of alkaloids in areca nut-containing products by liquid chromatography-tandem mass spectrometry. J Agric Food Chem. 2017;65(9):1977–83. https://doi.org/10.1021/acs.jafc.6b05140.
6. Tilakaratne WM, Klinikowski MF, Saku T, Peters TJ, Warnakulasuriya S. Oral submucous fibrosis: review on aetiology and pathogenesis. Oral Oncol. 2006;42(6):561–8.
7. Rai A, Siddiqui M, Paraveen S, Rasheed A, Ali S. Molecular pathogenesis of oral submucous fibrosis: a critical appraisal. Biomed Pharmacol J. 2019;12:4.
8. Prabhu RV, Prabhu V, Chatra L, Shenai P, Suvarna N, Dandekeri S. Areca nut and its role in oral submucous fibrosis. J Clin Exp Dent. 2014;6(5):e569–75. https://doi.org/10.4317/jced.51318.
9. Sarode SC, Mahuli A, Sarode GS, Mahuli S. Why only areca nut chewing cannot cause oral submucous fibrosis? Med Hypotheses. 2013;81(1):47–9. https://doi.org/10.1016/j.mehy.2013.02.025.
10. Khrime RD, Mehra YN, Mann SB, Mehta SK, Chakraborti RN. Effect of instant preparation of betel nut (pan masala) on the oral mucosa of albino rats. Indian J Med Res. 1991;94:119–24.
11. Sumeth Perera MW, Gunasinghe D, Perera PA, Ranasinghe A, Amaratunga P, Warnakulasuriya S, Kaluarachchi K. Development of an in vivo mouse model to study oral submucous fibrosis. J Oral Pathol Med. 2007;36:273–80.
12. Chiang MH, Chen PH, Chen YK, Chen CH, Ho ML, Wang YH. Characterization of a Novel dermal fibrosis, model induced by areca nut extract that mimics oral submucous fibrosis. PLoS ONE. 2016;11:e0166454.
13. Maria S, Kamath VV, Satelur K, Rajkumar K. Evaluation of transforming growth factor beta1 gene in oral submucous fibrosis induced in Sprague-Dawley rats by injections of areca nut and pan masala (commercial areca nut product) extracts. J Cancer Res. 2016;12:379–85.
14. Wen QT, Wang T, Yu DH, Wang ZR, Sun Y, Liang CW. Development of a mouse model of arecoline-induced oral mucosal fibrosis. Asian Pac J Trop Med. 2017;10:1177–84.
15. Yang B, Fu MF, Tang ZG. Rat model with oral submucous fibrosis induced by arecoline and mechanical stimulation. Hua Xi Kou Qiang Yi Xue Za Zhi. 2019;37:260–4.
16. Desai VC, Shirsand SB, Malpani A, Hiremath S. Evaluation of mucoadhesive dexamethasone sodium phosphate gel in the treatment of arecoline-induced oral submucous fibrosis in Wistar albino rats: a cross-sectional study. Indian J Dent Res. 2020;31(5):685–93. https://doi.org/10.4103/ijdr.IJDR_685_19.

17. Chiang MH, Lee KT, Chen CH, Chen KK, Wang YH. Photobiomodulation therapy inhibits oral submucous fibrosis in mice. Oral Dis. 2020;26(7):1474–82. https://doi.org/10.1111/odi.13409.
18. Babu S, Bhat RV, Kumar PU, Sesikaran B, Rao KV, Aruna P, Reddy PR. A comparative clinico-pathological study of oral submucous fibrosis in habitual chewers of pan masala and betelquid. J Toxicol Clin Toxicol. 1996;34(3):317–22. https://doi.org/10.3109/15563659609013796.
19. Sirsat SM, Khanolkar VR. Submucous fibrosis of the palate in diet-preconditioned Wistar rats. Induction by local painting of capsaicin--an optical and electron microscopic study. Arch Pathol. 1960;70:171–9.
20. Tang JG, Jian XF, Gao ML, Ling TY, Zhang KH. Epidemiological survey of oral submucous fibrosis in Xiangtan City, Hunan Province. China. Commun Dent Oral Epidemiol. 1997;25(2):177–80. https://doi.org/10.1111/j.1600-0528.1997.tb00918.x.
21. Ahmad MS, Ali SA, Ali AS, Chaubey KK. Epidemiological and etiological study of oral submucous fibrosis among gutkha chewers of Patna, Bihar, India. J Indian Soc Pedod Prev Dent. 2006;24(2):84–9. https://doi.org/10.4103/0970-4388.26022.
22. Seedat HA, Van Wyk CW. Submucous fibrosis in non-betel nut chewing subjects. J Biol Buccale. 1988;16:3–6.
23. Haque MF, Meghji S, Khitab U, Harris M. Oral submucous fibrosis patients have altered levels of cytokine production. J Oral Pathol Med. 2000;29(3):123–8. https://doi.org/10.1034/j.1600-0714.2000.290304.x.
24. Trivedy C, Baldwin D, Warnakulasuriya S, et al. Copper content in Areca catechu (betel nut) products and oral submucous fibrosis. Lancet. 1997;349:1447.
25. Trivedy CR, Warnakulasuriya KA, Peters TJ, Senkus R, Hazarey VK, Johnson NW. Raised tissue copper levels in oral submucous fibrosis. J Oral Pathol Med. 2000;29(6):241–8. https://doi.org/10.1034/j.1600-0714.2000.290601.x.
26. Arakeri G, Hunasgi S, Colbert S, Merkx MA, Brennan PA. Role of drinking water copper in pathogenesis of oral submucous fibrosis: a prospective case control study. Br J Oral Maxillofac Surg. 2014;52(6):507–12. https://doi.org/10.1016/j.bjoms.2014.03.023.
27. DiSilvestro RA, Harris ED. Evaluation of (+)-catechin action on lysyl oxidase activity in aortic tissue. Biochem Pharmacol. 1983;32(2):343–6. https://doi.org/10.1016/0006-2952(83)90565-8.
28. Chiu CJ, Chang ML, Chiang CP, Hahn LJ, Hsieh LL, Chen CJ. Interaction of collagen-related genes and susceptibility to betel quid-induced oral submucous fibrosis. Cancer Epidemiol Biomark Prev. 2002;11(7):646–53.
29. Chaudhary AK, Pandya S, Mehrotra R, Bharti AC, Jain S, Singh M. Functional polymorphism of the MMP-1 promoter (-1607 1G/2G) in potentially malignant and malignant head and neck lesions in an Indian population. Biomarkers. 2010;15(8):684–92.
30. Lin SC, Chung MY, Huang JW, Shieh TM, Liu CJ, Chang KW. Correlation between functional genotypes in the matrix metalloproteinases-1 promoter and risk of oral squamous cell carcinomas. J Oral Pathol Med. 2004;33(6):323–6. https://doi.org/10.1111/j.1600-0714.2004.00214.x.
31. Tu HF, Liu CJ, Chang CS, et al. The functional (-1171 5A–>6A) polymorphisms of matrix metalloproteinase 3 gene as a risk factor for oral submucous fibrosis among male areca users. J Oral Pathol Med. 2006;35(2):99–103.
32. Chaudhary AK, Singh M, Bharti AC, et al. Synergistic effect of stromelysin-1 (matrix metalloproteinase-3) promoter (-1171 5A-> 6A) polymorphism in oral submucous fibrosis and head and neck lesions. BMC Cancer. 2010;10:369.
33. Rajendran R, Harish RK, Anil S, Vidyadharan R, Banerjee M. Transforming growth factor-β-1 polymorphisms are infrequent but exist at selected loci in oral submucous fibrosis. Indian J Dent Res. 2010;21(3):413–9. https://doi.org/10.4103/0970-9290.70815.
34. Shieh TM, Tu HF, Ku TH, Chang SS, Chang KW, Liu CJ. Association between lysyl oxidase polymorphisms and oral submucous fibrosis in older male areca chewers. J Oral Pathol Med. 2009;38(1):109–13.
35. Ray JG, Mukherjee S, Mahato B, Sripathi Rao BH, Chaudhuri K. Comparative distribution of lysyl oxidase (G473A) and NQO1 (C609T) polymorphism among tea-garden workers (habitual chewers of betel quid) of Darjeeling district and Kolkata city of West Bengal. Contemp Clin Dent. 2013;4(4):476–81.
36. Liu CJ, Lee YJ, Chang KW, Shih YN, Liu HF, Dang CW. Polymorphism of the MICA gene and risk for oral submucous fibrosis. J Oral Pathol Med. 2004;33(1):1–6.
37. Agrawal D, Gupta S, Agarwal D, Gupta OP, Agarwal M. Role of GSTM1 and GSTT1 polymorphism: susceptibility to oral submucous fibrosis in the North Indian population. Oncology. 2009;79(3-4):181–6.
38. Mukherjee S, Bhowmik AD, Roychoudhury P, Mukhopadhyay K, Ray JG, Chaudhuri K. Association of XRCC1, XRCC3, and NAT2 polymorphisms with the risk of oral submucous fibrosis among eastern Indian population. J Oral Pathol Med. 2012;41(4):292–302.
39. Chaudhuri SR, Mukherjee S, Paul RR, Haldar A, Chaudhuri K. CYP1AI and CYP2E1 gene polymorphisms may increase susceptibility to oral submucous fibrosis among betel quid chewers of Eastern India. Gene. 2013;513(2):268–71.
40. Chen HM, Hsieh RP, Yang H, Kuo YS, Kuo MY, Chiang CP. HLA typing in Taiwanese patients with oral submucous fibrosis. J Oral Pathol Med. 2004;33(4):191–9. https://doi.org/10.1111/j.0904-2512.2004.00195.x.
41. Purohit A, Purohit BM, Mani A, Bhambal A. Genetic implications of HLA-DR and HLA-DQ genotype on tobacco smoking and oral submucous fibrosis. Oral Health Prev Dent. 2020;18(1):455–60. https://doi.org/10.3290/j.ohpd.a44683.
42. Cox S, Vickers ER, Ghu S, Zoellner H. Salivary arecoline levels during areca nut chewing in human volunteers. J Oral Pathol Med. 2010;39(6):465–9. https://doi.org/10.1111/j.1600--0714.2009.00881.x.
43. Lee HH, Chen LY, Wang HL, Chen BH. Quantification of salivary arecoline, arecaidine and N-methylnipecotic acid levels in volunteers by liquid chromatography-tandem mass spectrometry. J Anal Toxicol. 2015;39(9):714–9. https://doi.org/10.1093/jat/bkv077.
44. Venkatesh D, Puranik RS, Vanaki SS, Puranik SR. Study of salivary arecoline in areca nut chewers. J Oral Maxillofac Pathol. 2018;22(3):446. https://doi.org/10.4103/jomfp.JOMFP_143_18.
45. Franke AA, Li X, Lai JF. Pilot study of the pharmacokinetics of betel nut and betel quid biomarkers in saliva, urine, and hair of betel consumers. Drug Test Anal. 2016;8(10):1095–9. https://doi.org/10.1002/dta.1912.
46. Khokhar A, GVR R, Deswal BS, Mohapatra S. Study of salivary arecoline in areca nut chewers. Int J Scientific Res. 2017;6(12)
47. Canniff JP, Harvey W. The aetiology of oral submucous fibrosis: the stimulation of collagen synthesis by extracts of areca nut. Int J Oral Surg. 1981;10(Suppl. 1):163–7.


11

48. Chang YC, Tai KW, Cheng MH, Chou LS, Chou MY. Cytotoxic and non-genotoxic effects of arecoline on human buccal fibroblasts in vitro. J Oral Pathol Med. 1998;27:68–71.
49. Giri S, Idle JR, Chen C, Zabriskie TM, Krausz KW, Gonzalez FJ. A metabolomic approach to the metabolism of the areca nut alkaloids arecoline and arecaidine in the mouse. Chem Res Toxicol. 2006;19:818–27.
50. Kaur J, Jacobs R. Proinflammatory cytokine levels in oral lichen planus, oral leukoplakia, and oral submucous fibrosis. J Korean Assoc Oral Maxillofac Surg. 2015;41(4):171–5. https://doi.org/10.5125/jkaoms.2015.41.4.171.
51. Dineshkumar T, Ashwini BK, Rameshkumar A, Rajashree P, Ramya R, Rajkumar K. Salivary and serum interleukin-6 levels in oral premalignant disorders and squamous cell carcinoma: diagnostic value and clinicopathologic correlations. Asian Pac J Cancer Prev. 2016;17(11):4899–906. https://doi.org/10.22034/APJCP.2016.17.11.4899.
52. Wang L, Gu L, Tang Z. Cytokines secreted by arecoline activate fibroblasts that affect the balance of TH17 and Treg. J Oral Pathol Med. 2020;49(2):156–63. https://doi.org/10.1111/jop.12965.
53. Jeng JH, Wang YJ, Chiang BL, Lee PH, Chan CP, Ho YS, Wang TM, Lee JJ, Hahn LJ, Chang MC. Roles of keratinocyte inflammation in oral cancer: regulating the prostaglandin E2, interleukin-6 and TNF-alpha production of oral epithelial cells by areca nut extract and arecoline. Carcinogenesis. 2003;8:1301–15. https://doi.org/10.1093/carcin/bgg083.
54. Gupta S, Reddy MV, Harinath BC. Role of oxidative stress and antioxidants in aetiopathogenesis and management of oral submucous fibrosis. Indian J Clin Biochem. 2004;19(1):138–41. https://doi.org/10.1007/BF02872409.
55. Chitra S, Balasubramaniam M, Hazra J. Effect of α-tocopherol on salivary reactive oxygen species and trace elements in oral submucous fibrosis. Ann Clin Biochem. 2012;49(3):262–5. https://doi.org/10.1258/acb.2011.011050.
56. Bose KS, Vyas P, Singh M. Plasma non-enzymatic antioxidants-vitamin C, E, beta-carotenes, reduced glutathione levels and total antioxidant activity in oral sub mucous fibrosis. Eur Rev Med Pharmacol Sci. 2012;16(4):530–2.
57. Meera S, Sarangarajan R, Rajkumar K. 8-Isoprostane: a salivary oxidative stress biomarker for oral submucous fibrosis and oral squamous cell carcinoma. J Oral Maxillofac Pathol. 2020;24(2):279–84. https://doi.org/10.4103/jomfp.JOMFP_235_19.
58. Ganta SR, Chittemsetti S, Sravya T, Guttikonda VR. Salivary malondialdehyde in oral submucous fibrosis—a marker for oxidative damage. J Oral Maxillofac Pathol. 2021;25(1):82–7. https://doi.org/10.4103/jomfp.JOMFP_279_18.
59. Shakunthala GK, Annigeri RG, Arunkumar S. Role of oxidative stress in the pathogenesis of oral submucous fibrosis: a preliminary prospective study. Contemp Clin Dent. 2015;6(Suppl. 1):S172–4. https://doi.org/10.4103/0976-237X.166823.
60. Nair UJ, Nair J, Friesen MD, Bartsch H, Ohshima H. Ortho- and meta-tyrosine formation from phenylalanine in human saliva as a marker of hydroxyl radical generation during betel quid chewing. Carcinogenesis. 1995;16(5):1195–8. https://doi.org/10.1093/carcin/16.5.1195.
61. Uikey AK, Hazarey VK, Vidya SM. Estimation of antioxidant dismutase and glutathione peroxidase in oral submucous fibrosis. J Oral Maxillofac Pathol. 2003;7(2):44–5.
62. Nieschultz V, Schmersahl P. Zur Phamakologie der Wirkstoffe des Betels Umwenlung des arecolin in arecadin. Arzneimitrel-Forsch. 1968;18:222–5.
63. Wang J, You J, Wang L, Wang H, Tian T, Wang W, Jia L, Jiang C. PTMA, a new identified autoantigen for oral submucous fibrosis, regulates oral submucous fibroblast proliferation and extracellular matrix. Oncotarget. 2017;8(43):74806–19. https://doi.org/10.18632/oncotarget.20419.
64. Chiang CP, Hsieh RP, Chen TH, Chang YF, Liu BY, Wang JT, Sun A, Kuo MY. High incidence of autoantibodies in Taiwanese patients with oral submucous fibrosis. J Oral Pathol Med. 2002;31(7):402–9. https://doi.org/10.1034/j.1600--0714.2002.00117.x.
65. Wang YP, Wu YC, Cheng SJ, Chen HM, Sun A, Chang JY. High frequencies of vitamin B12 and folic acid deficiencies and gastric parietal cell antibody positivity in oral submucous fibrosis patients. J Formos Med Assoc. 2015;114(9):813–9. https://doi.org/10.1016/j.jfma.2015.05.011.
66. Gupta A, Das SN, Das BK, Bhuyan L. Characterization of anti-nuclear antibodies in patients with oral submucous fibrosis and its clinicopathologic implications—an immunofluorescence study. J Oral Maxillofac Pathol. 2021;25(1):201. https://doi.org/10.4103/jomfp.jomfp_376_20.
67. Shah N, Kumar R, Shah MK. Immunological studies in oral submucous fibrosis. Indian J Dent Res. 1994;5(3):81–7.
68. Van Wyk CW, Grobler Rabie AF, Martel RW, Hammond MG. HLA antigens in oral submucous fibrosis. J Oral Pathol Med. 1994;23:23–7.
69. Ma RH, Tsai CC, Shieh TY. Increased lysyl oxidase activity in fibroblasts cultured from oral submucous fibrosis associated with betel nut chewing in Taiwan. J Oral Pathol Med. 1995;24(9):407–12. https://doi.org/10.1111/j.1600-0714.1995.tb01210.x.
70. Sachdev PK, Freeland-Graves J, Beretvas SN, Sanjeevi N. Zinc, copper, and iron in oral submucous fibrosis: a meta-analysis. Int J Dent. 2018;2018:3472087. https://doi.org/10.1155/2018/3472087.
71. Anuradha CD, Devi CS. Serum protein, ascorbic acid and iron and tissue collagen in oral submucous fibrosis—a preliminary study. Indian J Med Res. 1993;98:147–51.
72. Khanna SS, Karjodkar FR. Circulating immune complexes and trace elements (copper, iron and selenium) as markers in oral precancer and cancer: a randomised, controlled clinical trial. Head Face Med. 2006;2:33.
73. Xia L, Tian-You L, Yi-Jun G, Dong-Sheng T, Wen-Hui L. Arecoline and oral keratinocytes may affect the collagen metabolism of fibroblasts. J Oral Pathol Med. 2009;38(5):422–6. https://doi.org/10.1111/j.1600-0714.2009.00758.x.
74. Krishnakumar K, Ramadoss R, Krishnan R, Sukhija H. In vitro quantification of collagen and Snail1 gene expression in experimentally induced fibrosis by arecoline and commercial smokeless tobacco products. Asian Pac J Cancer Prev. 2020;21(4):1143–8. https://doi.org/10.31557/APJCP.2020.21.4.1143.
75. Thangjam GS, Agarwal P, Balapure AK, Rao SG, Kondaiah P. Regulation of extracellular matrix genes by arecoline in primary gingival fibroblasts requires epithelial factors. J Periodontal Res. 2009;44(6):736–43. https://doi.org/10.1111/j.1600-0765.2008.01185.x.
76. Yang SF, Tsai CH, Chang YC. The upregulation of heat shock protein 47 expression in human buccal fibroblasts stimulated with arecoline. J Oral Pathol Med. 2008;37(4):206–10. https://doi.org/10.1111/j.1600-0714.2007.00633.x.
77. Harvey W, Scutt A, Meghji S, Canniff JP. Stimulation of human buccal mucosa fibroblasts in vitro by betel-nut alkaloids. Arch Oral Biol. 1986;31(1):45–9. https://doi.org/10.1016/0003-9969(86)90112-3.

78. Chang YC, Tai KW, Lii CK, Chou MY. Cytopathologic effects of arecoline on human gingival fibroblasts in vitro. Clin Oral Investig. 1999;3:25–9.
79. Van Wyk CW, Olivier A, de Miranda CM, van der Bijl P, Grobler-Rabie AF. Observations on the effect of areca nut extracts on oral fibroblast proliferation. J Oral Pathol Med. 1994;23(4):145–8. https://doi.org/10.1111/j.1600-0714.1994.tb01103.x.
80. Kuo MY, Chen HM, Hahn LJ, Hsieh CC, Chiang CP. Collagen biosynthesis in human oral submucous fibrosis fibroblast cultures. J Dent Res. 1995;74(11):1783–8. https://doi.org/10.1177/00220345950740111101.
81. Jeng JH, Lan WH, Hahn LJ, Hsieh CC, Kuo MYP. Inhibition of the migration, attachment, spreading, growth and collagen synthesis of human gingival fibroblasts by arecoline, a major areca alkaloid, in vitro. J Oral Pathol Med. 1996;25:371–5.
82. Chang MC, Kuo MYP, Hahn LJ, Hsieh CC, Lin SK, Jeng JH. Areca nut extract inhibits the growth, attachment, and matrix protein synthesis of cultured human gingival fibroblasts. J Periodontol. 1998;69:1092–7.
83. Chen Q, Jiao J, Wang Y, Mai Z, Ren J, He S, Li X, Chen Z. Egr-1 mediates low-dose arecoline induced human oral mucosa fibroblast proliferation via transactivation of Wnt5a expression. BMC Mol Cell Biol. 2020;21(1):80. https://doi.org/10.1186/s12860-020-00325-7.
84. Chang YC, Lii CK, Tai KW, Chou MY. Adverse effects of arecoline and nicotine on human periodontal ligament fibroblasts in vitro. J Clin Periodontol. 2001;28(3):277–82. https://doi.org/10.1034/j.1600-051x.2001.028003277.x.
85. Jimenez SA, Hitraya E, Varga J. Pathogenesis of scleroderma. Collagen. Rheum Dis Clin North Am. 1996;22(4):647–74. https://doi.org/10.1016/s0889-857x(05)70294-5.
86. Tsai CH, Chou MY, Chang YC. The up-regulation of cyclooxygenase-2 expression in human buccal mucosal fibroblasts by arecoline: a possible role in the pathogenesis of oral submucous fibrosis. J Oral Pathol Med. 2003;32(3):146–53. https://doi.org/10.1034/j.1600-0714.2003.00004.x.
87. Jeng JH, Ho YS, Chan CP, Wang YJ, Hahn LJ, Lei D. Areca nut extract up-regulates prostaglandin production, cyclooxygenase-2 mRNA and protein expression of human oral keratinocytes. Carcinogenesis. 2000;21:1365–70.
88. Chang MC, Chen YJ, Chang HH, Chan CP, Yeh CY, Wang YL, et al. Areca nut components affect COX-2, cyclin B1/cdc25C and keratin expression, PGE2 production in keratinocyte is related to reactive oxygen species, CYP1A1, Src, EGFR and Ras signaling. PLOS One. 2014;9:e101959.
89. Khan I, Kumar N, Pant I, Narra S, Kondaiah P. Activation of TGF-beta pathway by areca nut constituents: a possible cause of oral submucous fibrosis. PLoS One. 2012;7(12):e51806. https://doi.org/10.1371/journal.pone.0051806.
90. Pant I, Kumar N, Khan I, Rao SG, Kondaiah P. Role of areca nut induced TGF-β and epithelial-mesenchymal interaction in the pathogenesis of oral submucous fibrosis. PLoS One. 2015;10(6):e0129252. https://doi.org/10.1371/journal.pone.0129252.
91. Hsieh YP, Chen HM, Chang JZ, Chiang CP, Deng YT, Kuo MY. Arecoline stimulated early growth response-1 production in human buccal fibroblasts: suppression by epigallocatechin-3-gallate. Head Neck. 2015;37(4):493–7. https://doi.org/10.1002/hed.23614.
92. Hsieh YP, Wu KJ, Chen HM, Deng YT. Arecoline activates latent transforming growth factor β1 via mitochondrial reactive oxygen species in buccal fibroblasts: suppression by epigallocatechin-3-gallate. J Formos Med Assoc. 2018;117(6):527–34. https://doi.org/10.1016/j.jfma.2017.07.003.
93. Pant I, Rao SG, Kondaiah P. Role of areca nut induced JNK/ATF2/Jun axis in the activation of TGF-beta pathway in precancerous oral submucous fibrosis. Sci Rep. 2016;6:34314.
94. Moutasim KA, Jenei V, Sapienza K, Marsh D, Weinreb PH, Violette SM, Lewis MP, Marshall JF, Fortune F, Tilakaratne WM, Hart IR, Thomas GJ. Betel-derived alkaloid up-regulates keratinocyte alphavbeta6 integrin expression and promotes oral submucous fibrosis. J Pathol. 2011;223(3):366–77. https://doi.org/10.1002/path.2786.
95. Chang JZ, Hsieh YP, Lin WH, Chen HM, Kuo MY. Activation of transforming growth factor-β1 by thrombin via integrins αvβ1, αvβ3, and αvβ5 in buccal fibroblasts: suppression by epigallocatechin-3-gallate. Head Neck. 2017;39(7):1436–45. https://doi.org/10.1002/hed.24791.
96. Lee YH, Yang LC, Hu FW, Peng CY, Yu CH, Yu CC. Elevation of Twist expression by arecoline contributes to the pathogenesis of oral submucous fibrosis. J Formos Med Assoc. 2016;115(5):311–7. https://doi.org/10.1016/j.jfma.2015.05.009.
97. Chang MC, Lin LD, Wu HL, Ho YS, Hsien HC, Wang TM, Jeng PY, Cheng RH, Hahn LJ, Jeng JH. Areca nut-induced buccal mucosa fibroblast contraction and its signaling: a potential role in oral submucous fibrosis—a precancer condition. Carcinogenesis. 2013;34(5):1096–104. https://doi.org/10.1093/carcin/bgt012.
98. Chang YC, Tsai CH, Lai YL, et al. Arecoline-induced myofibroblast transdifferentiation from human buccal mucosal fibroblasts is mediated by ZEB1. J Cell Mol Med. 2014;18(4):698–708. https://doi.org/10.1111/jcmm.12219.
99. Liao YW, Yu CC, Hsieh PL, Chang YC. miR-200b ameliorates myofibroblast transdifferentiation in precancerous oral submucous fibrosis through targeting ZEB2. J Cell Mol Med. 2018;22(9):4130–8. https://doi.org/10.1111/jcmm.13690.
100. Peng CY, Liao YW, Lu MY, Yang CM, Hsieh PL, Yu CC. Positive feedback loop of SNAIL-IL-6 mediates myofibroblastic differentiation activity in precancerous oral submucous fibrosis. Cancers (Basel). 2020;12(6):1611. https://doi.org/10.3390/cancers12061611.
101. Yu CH, Fang CY, Yu CC, Hsieh PL, Liao YW, Tsai LL, Chu PM. LINC00312/YBX1 axis regulates myofibroblast activities in oral submucous fibrosis. Int J Mol Sci. 2020;21(8):2979. https://doi.org/10.3390/ijms21082979.
102. Chang YC, Yang SF, Tai KW, Chou MY, Hsieh YS. Increased tissue inhibitor of metalloproteinase-1 expression and inhibition of gelatinase A activity in buccal mucosal fibroblasts by arecoline as possible mechanisms for oral submucous fibrosis. Oral Oncol. 2002;38(2):195–200. https://doi.org/10.1016/s1368-8375(01)00045-8.
103. Shieh DH, Chiang LC, Shieh TY. Augmented mRNA expression of tissue inhibitor of metalloproteinase-1 in buccal mucosal fibroblasts by arecoline and safrole as a possible pathogenesis for oral submucous fibrosis. Oral Oncol. 2003;39(7):728–35. https://doi.org/10.1016/s1368-8375(03)00101-5.
104. Pitiyage GN, Lim KP, Gemenitzidis E, Teh MT, Waseem A, Prime SS, Tilakaratne WM, Fortune F, Parkinson EK. Increased secretion of tissue inhibitors of metalloproteinases 1 and 2 (TIMPs-1 and -2) in fibroblasts are early indicators of oral sub-mucous fibrosis and ageing. J Oral Pathol Med. 2012;41(6):454–62. https://doi.org/10.1111/j.1600--0714.2012.01129.x.
105. Yu CC, Tsai CH, Hsu HI, Chang YC. Elevation of S100A4 expression in buccal mucosal fibroblasts by arecoline: involve-

ment in the pathogenesis of oral submucous fibrosis. PLoS One. 2013;8(1):e55122. https://doi.org/10.1371/journal.pone.0055122.

106. Scutt A, Meghji S, Canniff JP, Harvey W. Stabilization of collagen by betel nut polyphenols as a mechanism in oral submucous fibrosis. Experimentia. 1987;43:391–3.

107. Thangjam GS, Agarwal P, Khan I, Verma UP, Balapure AK, Rao SG, et al. Transglutaminase-2 regulation by arecoline in gingival fibroblasts. J Dent Res. 2009;88(2):170–7.

108. Lee SS, Chen YJ, Tsai CH, Huang FM, Chang YC. Elevated transglutaminase-2 expression mediates fibrosis in areca quid chewing-associated oral submucosal fibrosis via reactive oxygen species generation. Clin Oral Investig. 2016;20(5):1029–34.

109. Yang SF, Hsieh YS, Tsai CH, Chou MY, Chang YC. The upregulation of type I plasminogen activator inhibitor in oral submucous fibrosis. Oral Oncol. 2003;39(4):367–72. https://doi.org/10.1016/s1368-8375(02)00123-9.

110. Tsai CH, Lee SS, Chang YC. Hypoxic regulation of plasminogen activator inhibitor-1 expression in human buccal mucosa fibroblasts stimulated with arecoline. J Oral Pathol Med. 2015;44(9):669–73. https://doi.org/10.1111/jop.12284.

111. Trivedy C, Meghji S, Warnakulasuriya KA, et al. Copper stimulates human oral fibroblasts in vitro: a role in the pathogenesis of oral sub-mucous fibrosis. J Oral Pathol Med. 2001;30:465–70.13.

112. Chung-Hung T, Shun-Fa Y, Yu-Chao C. The upregulation of cystatin C in oral submucous fibrosis. Oral Oncol. 2007;43(7):680–5. https://doi.org/10.1016/j.oraloncology.2006.08.009.

113. Tsai CH, Yang SF, Chen YJ, Chou MY, Chang YC. Raised keratinocyte growth factor-1 expression in oral submucous fibrosis in vivo and upregulated by arecoline in human buccal mucosal fibroblasts in vitro. J Oral Pathol Med. 2005;34(2):100–5. https://doi.org/10.1111/j.1600-0714.2004.00288.x.

114. Tsai CC, Ma RH, Shieh TY. Deficiency in collagen and fibronectin phagocytosis by human buccal mucosa fibroblasts in vitro as a possible mechanism for oral submucous fibrosis. J Oral Pathol Med. 1999;28(2):59–63. https://doi.org/10.1111/j.1600-0714.1999.tb01997.x.

115. Shieh DH, Chiang LC, Lee CH, Yang YH, Shieh TY. Effects of arecoline, safrole, and nicotine on collagen phagocytosis by human buccal mucosal fibroblasts as a possible mechanism for oral submucous fibrosis in Taiwan. J Oral Pathol Med. 2004;33(9):581–7. https://doi.org/10.1111/j.1600--0714.2004.00229.x.

116. Nair UJ, Obe G, Friesen M, Goldberg MT, Bartsch H. Role of lime in the generation of reactive oxygen species from betel-quid ingredients. Environ Health Perspect. 1992;98:203–5.

117. Chen PH, Tsai CC, Lin YC, Ko YC, Yang YH, Shieh TY, et al. Ingredients contribute to variation in production of reactive oxygen species by areca quid. J Toxicol Environ Health A. 2006;69:1055–69.

118. Illeperuma RP, Kim DK, Park YJ, Son HK, Kim JY, Kim J, et al. Areca nut exposure increases secretion of tumor-promoting cytokines in gingival fibroblasts that trigger DNA damage in oral keratinocytes. Int J Cancer. 2015;137:2545–57.

119. Chang LY, Wan HC, Lai YL, Chou IC, Chen YT, Hung SL. Areca nut extracts increased the expression of cyclooxygenase-2, prostaglandin E2 and interleukin-1alpha in human immune cells via oxidative stress. Arch Oral Biol. 2013;58:1523–31.

120. Deng YT, Chen HM, Cheng SJ, Chiang CP, Kuo MY. Arecoline-stimulated connective tissue growth factor production in human buccal mucosal fibroblasts: modulation by curcumin. Oral Oncol. 2009;45(9):e99–e105. https://doi.org/10.1016/j.oraloncology.2009.04.004.

121. Khan I, Pant I, Narra S, Radhesh R, Ranganathan K, Rao SG, Kondaiah P. Epithelial atrophy in oral submucous fibrosis is mediated by copper (II) and arecoline of areca nut. J Cell Mol Med. 2015;19(10):2397–412. https://doi.org/10.1111/jcmm.12622.

122. Paranagama MP, Piyarathne NS, Nandasena TL, Jayatilake S, Navaratne A, Galhena BP, Williams S, Rajapakse J, Kita K. The Porphyromonas gingivalis inhibitory effects, antioxidant effects and the safety of a Sri Lankan traditional betel quid—an in vitro study. BMC Complement Med Ther. 2020;20(1):259. https://doi.org/10.1186/s12906-020-03048-6.

123. Sazwi NN, Nalina T, Abdul Rahim ZH. Antioxidant and cytoprotective activities of Piper betle, Areca catechu, Uncaria gambir and betel quid with and without calcium hydroxide. BMC Complement Altern Med. 2013;13:351. https://doi.org/10.1186/1472-6882-13-351.

124. Tsai CH, Yang SF, Lee SS, Chang YC. Augmented heme oxygenase-1 expression in areca quid chewing-associated oral submucous fibrosis. Oral Dis. 2009;15(4):281–6. https://doi.org/10.1111/j.1601-0825.2009.01523.x.

125. Li J, Zhao TT, Zhang P, Xu CJ, Rong ZX, Yan ZY, Fang CY. Autophagy mediates oral submucous fibrosis. Exp Ther Med. 2016;11(5):1859–64. https://doi.org/10.3892/etm.2016.3145.

126. Dai Z, Zhu B, Yu H, Jian X, Peng J, Fang C, Wu Y. Role of autophagy induced by arecoline in angiogenesis of oral submucous fibrosis. Arch Oral Biol. 2019;102:7–15. https://doi.org/10.1016/j.archoralbio.2019.03.021.

127. Zhu B, Jiang Q, Que G, Dai Z, Wu Y. Role of autophagy and apoptosis in atrophic epithelium in oral submucous fibrosis. J Oral Sci. 2020;62(2):184–8. https://doi.org/10.2334/josnusd.19-0170.

128. Tseng SK, Chang MC, Su CY, Chi LY, Chang JZ, Tseng WY, Yeung SY, Hsu ML, Jeng JH. Arecoline induced cell cycle arrest, apoptosis, and cytotoxicity to human endothelial cells. Clin Oral Investig. 2012;16(4):1267–73. https://doi.org/10.1007/s00784-011-0604-1.

# Fibrogenic Factors and Molecular Mechanisms

*Paturu Kondaiah*

## Contents



© The Author(s), under exclusive license to Springer Nature Switzerland AG 2023
S. Warnakulasuriya, K. Ranganathan (eds.), *Oral Submucous Fibrosis*, Textbooks in Contemporary Dentistry,
https://doi.org/10.1007/978-3-031-12855-4_12

## 12.1 Introduction

Fibrosis is defined as the progressive replacement of healthy parenchymal tissue with collagen-rich extracellular matrix (ECM) that is deposited by activated fibroblasts, resulting in loss of tissue function [1]. Fibrosis is characterized by excess deposition of extracellular matrix components such as collagen and fibronectin, resulting in overgrowth, hardening, and/or scarring of various tissues. Fibrosis occurs in response to a variety of stimuli including persistent infections, carcinogens (areca nut, alcohol), autoimmune reactions, allergic responses, chemical insults, radiation, and mechanical injury [2].

Most chronic fibrotic disorders are caused by a persistent irritant that sustains the production of growth factors, proteolytic enzymes, angiogenic factors, and fibrogenic cytokines, which stimulate the deposition of connective tissue elements that progressively remodel and destroy normal tissue architecture. Chronic inflammation and prolonged damage to the tissue without repair culminate in fibrosis. The tissue repair process typically involves two distinct phases: a regenerative phase, in which injured cells are replaced by cells of the same type without any tissue damage, and a phase known as fibroplasia or fibrosis, in which connective tissues replace normal parenchymal tissue [2].

Under chronic and persistent pathologic circumstances, such as fibrotic diseases, an uncontrolled fibrotic process results in excessive accumulation of extracellular matrix (ECM), including collagen, fibronectin, hyaluronic acid, and proteoglycans, that leads to fibrosis and ultimately organ failure. These fibrotic diseases may occur in multisystem diseases, such as systemic sclerosis (SSc), nephrogenic systemic fibrosis (NSF), and in specific organs like idiopathic pulmonary fibrosis (IPF), renal fibrosis, hepatic cirrhosis, cardiac fibrosis, oral submucous fibrosis, and glaucoma.

Oral submucous fibrosis (OSF) is a chronic debilitating disease of the oral cavity characterized by inflammation and progressive fibrosis of the submucosal tissues (lamina propria and deeper connective tissues). Microscopically, it is characterized by a juxta-epithelial inflammatory reaction followed by fibroelastic change of the lamina propria and epithelial atrophy that leads to stiffness of the oral mucosa, resulting in trismus and inability to eat [3]. This chapter discusses the cellular and molecular mechanisms involved in the pathogenesis of oral submucous fibrosis.

**Learning Goals**

- Understand the role of areca nut in fibrosis
- Learn the mechanisms and how areca nut induces fibrosis
- Discuss the biological factors involved in fibrosis
- Outline the inflammatory mediators involved during fibrosis
- Explore the mechanisms of carcinogenesis in OSF

## 12.2 Areca Nut in the Molecular Pathogenesis of OSF

Areca nut has been classified as a Class I carcinogen by IARC [4]. The chemical composition of areca nut comprises alkaloids, flavonoids, and tannins, along with carbohydrates, proteins, fats, crude fiber, and elements. Of these, an important constituent is the alkaloid arecoline [4, 5]. Tissue inflammation and reactive oxygen species produced by areca nut and its components cause the epithelial cells to activate the transforming growth factor-beta (TGF-β) signaling pathways. TGF-β and its downstream target proteins promote the fibroblast-mediated production of extracellular matrix deposition.

Oral submucous fibrosis (OSF) is a potentially malignant condition that develops under continuous exposure to the components of the areca nut [6]. Arecoline causes inhibition of elements involved in the degradation of extracellular matrix (ECM) and synthesis of matrix components that disturbs the homeostasis of ECM. Arecoline activates the oral tissue to express TNF-α, which stimulates cell inflammation. Cell inflammation will activate "the wound-healing reaction," which decreases MMP and increases TIMP expression. This TIMP and MMP expression profile is also found in the oral tissue of OSF patients. The function of MMP is to degrade the extracellular matrix protein, and TIMP inhibits this process. This contributes to the abnormal collagen deposition in the lamina propria of the oral mucosa. Inflammation also stimulates the cell to express basic fibroblast growth factor (bFGF) and TGF-β1. The bFGF in oral cells contributes to the collagen deposition disorder in OSF. TGF-β1 stimulates fibroblasts to transform to myofibroblasts, which are mainly responsible for collagen production and tissue contraction. The physiological process of myofibroblasts undergoing apoptosis after wound healing is disrupted in OSF.

The TGF-β signaling is responsible for ceasing the cell cycle and promoting apoptosis in the unrepaired damaged cells while the cells are damaged by stimulants. TGF-β also activates the downstream gene and connective tissue growth factor (CTGF) expression to promote the fibroblast-mediated production of extracellular matrix deposition [7]. It enhances the expression of several inhibitors of proteinases, including tissue inhibitors of metalloproteinases (TIMPs), plasminogen activator inhibitors (PAI-1), and cysteine proteinase inhibitor cystatin C in fibroblasts [8–10] along with the induction of factors that enhance the stability of ECM, such as heat-shock protein-47 (Hsp-47) and transglutaminase-2 (TGM-2) [11, 12]. Arecoline also decreases the phagocytosis of collagen by fibroblasts [13].

Arecoline increases the level of reactive oxygen species (ROS) in OSF patients' serum. Serum ROS attacks the structure of the blood vessels in endothelial cells and induces cell senescence and DNA double-strand breaks.

The decrease in blood flow around the oral mucosa causes epithelial atrophy. The cell inflammation reaction and ROS stimulate the cell to activate the TGF-β signaling pathways. The imbalance, between the synthesis of reactive oxygen species and cellular ability to detoxify the reactive intermediates, leads to oxidative stress. Such stress can result in the production of peroxides and free radicals that can damage cellular components, including proteins, lipids, and DNA. Areca nut extract induces oxidative damage to isolated and cellular DNA, by the generation of hydrogen peroxide. Areca nut at concentrations in the range of 800–1200 μg/mL cause cytotoxicity to oral epithelial cells by deregulation of cell cycle control specifically through G2/M cell cycle arrest, by reducing glutathione levels, and by intracellular production of hydrogen peroxide. Areca nut extract at a concentration of 100 μg/mL was cytotoxic to normal human buccal fibroblast cultures, and the addition of reduced glutathione to these cultures produced a significant reduction in cytotoxicity. Various studies are conducted in vitro to assess the effect of arecoline on the expression of proteins whose expression profile is perturbed in oral submucous fibrosis (OSF) [14] (◘ Table 12.1).

In addition, copper in the areca nut participates in the cross-linking of collagen. It enhances the stiffness of the oral submucous tissue and exacerbates the limitation of mouth opening and trismus. Commercial areca nut contains a significantly higher level of copper than the raw areca nut. Higher serum copper found among OSF patients is considered to be one of the factors that induce OSF [7].

The majority of areca nut-regulated genes are compromised by transforming growth factor-β pathway inhibitors, indicating the regulation of this pathway and its significance in the pathogenesis of oral submucous fibrosis [15]. The transforming growth factor-β is the major factor that influences fibroblast activation, extracellular matrix production, and other aspects important in fibrosis [16]. The other genes regulated by areca nut during myofibroblast transdifferentiation include S100A4, Zeb1, and Twist [17–19]. The reactive oxygen species (ROS), transforming growth factor-β1 (TGF-β1), and hypoxia-inducible factor-1α (HIF-1α) are the three key mediators of the effects induced by arecoline in the pathogenesis of OSF [20] (◘ Figs. 12.1 and 12.2).

◘ **Table 12.1** A collective representation of various studies conducted in vitro to assess the effect of arecoline on the expression of proteins whose expression profile is perturbed in oral submucous fibrosis (OSF) cases

| Serial no. | Cell type and dose of arecoline | Effects | ROS/receptor/pathways involved | Expression in OSF specimen (compared to normal mucosal specimen) | Reference |
|---|---|---|---|---|---|
| 1. | Buccal mucosal fibroblasts (0–200 μg/mL) | Arecoline induced upregulation of vimentin expression | – | Moderately advanced/advanced OSF specimen showed higher expression of intermediate filament vimentin in the cytoplasm of fibroblasts in the connective tissue | Chang et al. (2002b) |
| 2. | Buccal mucosal fibroblasts (0–160 μg/mL) | Arecoline induced cyclooxygenase-2 expression, the induction subsided after some time | Decreased thiol content involved in induction | Moderate cases of OSF showed higher expression of cyclooxygenase-2 in epithelial cells, fibroblasts, and inflammatory cells, whereas advanced cases showed weak expression | Tsai et al. (2003) |
| 3. | Buccal mucosal fibroblasts (0–160 μg/mL) | Arecoline induced upregulation of plasminogen activator inhibitor-1 (PAI-1) expression | – | Moderately advanced/advanced OSF specimens showed higher expression of plasminogen activator inhibitor-1 in fibroblasts, endothelial cells, and inflammatory cells | Yang et al. (2003) |
| 4. | Buccal mucosal fibroblasts (0–80 μg/mL) | Arecoline induced upregulation of insulin-like growth factor-1 expression | – | Moderately advanced/advanced OSF specimens showed higher expression of insulin-like growth factor-1 in fibroblasts, endothelial cells, and inflammatory cells of connective tissue | Tsai et al. (2005a) |

(continued)

**Table 12.1** (continued)

| Serial no. | Cell type and dose of arecoline | Effects | ROS/receptor/pathways involved | Expression in OSF specimen (compared to normal mucosal specimen) | Reference |
|---|---|---|---|---|---|
| 5. | Buccal mucosal fibroblasts (0–80 μg/mL) | Arecoline induced upregulation of keratinocyte growth factor-1 expression | – | Moderately advanced/advanced OSF specimen showed higher expression of keratinocyte growth factor-1 in the epithelial cells and to a lesser degree in fibroblast and endothelial and inflammatory cells | Tsai et al. (2005b) |
| 6. | Buccal mucosal fibroblasts (0–80 μg/mL) | Arecoline induced upregulation of cystatin C expression | – | The connective tissue of moderately advanced/advanced OSF specimen showed higher expression of cystatin C in fibroblasts, endothelial cells, and inflammatory cells | Tsai et al. (2007) |
| 7. | Buccal mucosal fibroblasts (0–160 μg/mL) | Arecoline induced upregulation of heat-shock protein 47 (Hsp-47) expression | PI3K, Cox-2, and MEK pathways are involved. Decreased intracellular thiol content involved in induction | OSF specimen showed higher expression of heat-shock protein 47 mRNA | Yang et al. (2008) |
| 8. | Buccal mucosal fibroblasts (0–160 μg/mL) | Arecoline induced upregulation of heme-oxygenase-1 (HO-1) expression | – | OSF specimen showed higher expression of heme-oxygenase-1 in fibroblasts, epithelial cells, and inflammatory cells | Tsai et al. (2009) |
| 9. | Buccal mucosal fibroblasts (0–0.4 mM) | Arecoline induced upregulation of connective tissue growth factor (CTGF) expression | NF-κB, JNK, p38 pathways involved. Decreased intracellular thiol content involved in induction | OSF specimen showed higher expression of connective tissue growth factor in fibroblasts, endothelial cells, and epithelial cells (in some cases) | Deng et al. (2009) |
| 10. | HaCaT keratinocyte (0–50 μg/mL) | Arecoline induced expression of transforming growth factor-β2 | Muscarinic acetylcholine receptor-intracellular [$Ca^{2+}$] rise-PKC activation pathway involved. Decreased intracellular thiol content involved in induction | OSF specimen showed higher expression of transforming growth factor β2 mRNA | Thangjam et al. (2009) |
| 11. | Keratinocyte (5 10 μg/mL) | Arecoline induced upregulation of αvβ6 integrin expression | Muscarinic acetylcholine receptor involved | OSF specimen showed higher expression of αvβ6 integrin | Moutasim et al. (2011) |
| 12. | Buccal mucosal fibroblasts (0–20 μg/mL) | Arecoline induced upregulation of S100A4 expression | NF-κB, ERK, mTOR pathways are involved | OSF specimen showed higher expression of S100A4 | Yu et al. (2013) |
| 13. | Buccal mucosal fibroblasts (0–160 μg/mL) | Arecoline induced upregulation of protease-activated receptor-1 (PAR-1) expression | ERK, PI3K, Cox-2, TK pathways involved. Decreased intracellular thiol content involved in induction | Moderately advanced/advanced OSF specimen showed higher expression of protease-activated receptor-1 in fibroblasts and inflammatory cells | Tsai et al. (2013) |
| 14. | Buccal mucosal fibroblasts (0–20 μg/mL) | Arecoline induced ZEB1, α-smooth muscle actin (α-SMA), and vimentin expression | – | OSF specimen showed higher expression of ZEB1 localized in the nucleus of fibroblast and α-SMA in fibroblast and blood vessel | Chang et al. (2014) |

**Table 12.1** (continued)

| Serial no. | Cell type and dose of arecoline | Effects | ROS/receptor/pathways involved | Expression in OSF specimen (compared to normal mucosal specimen) | Reference |
|---|---|---|---|---|---|
| 15. | Buccal mucosal fibroblasts (0–160 μg/mL) | Arecoline induced upregulation of hypoxia-inducible factor-1α expression | – | Moderately advanced/advanced OSF specimen showed higher expression of hypoxia-inducible factor-1α in fibroblasts, epithelial cells, and inflammatory cells | Tsai et al. (2015) |
| 16. | Buccal mucosal fibroblasts (0–0.4 mM) | Arecoline induced upregulation of early growth response-1 (Egr-1) expression | JNK, ERK pathways involved. Decreased intracellular thiol content involved in induction | OSF specimen showed higher expression of early growth response-1 in epithelial cells, fibroblasts, inflammatory cells | Hsieh et al. (2015) |
| 17. | HaCaT keratinocytes (0–0.16 mM) | Arecoline induced downregulation of miR-203, downregulation of cytokeratin CK 19 and E-cadherin, upregulation of N-cadherin and vimentin, increased expression of SFRP4, and decreased expression of TM4SF1 | – | OSF specimen showed lower expression of miR-203 and transmembrane 4 L six family member 1 (TM4SF1) and higher expression of secreted frizzled related protein 4 (SPRP4) | Zheng et al. (2015) |
| 18. | Buccal mucosal fibroblasts (0–20 μg/mL) | Arecoline induced upregulation of Twist | – | OSF specimen showed higher expression of Twist mRNA and protein | Lee et al. (2016) |
| 19. | Buccal mucosal fibroblasts (0–160 μg/mL) | Arecoline induced upregulation of transglutaminase-2 (TGM-2) expression | | | |

*ROS* reactive oxygen species, *PI3K* phosphatidylinositol 3-kinase, *Cox-2* cyclooxygenase-2, *MEK* mitogen-activated protein kinase, *JNK* c-Jun NH2-terminal kinase

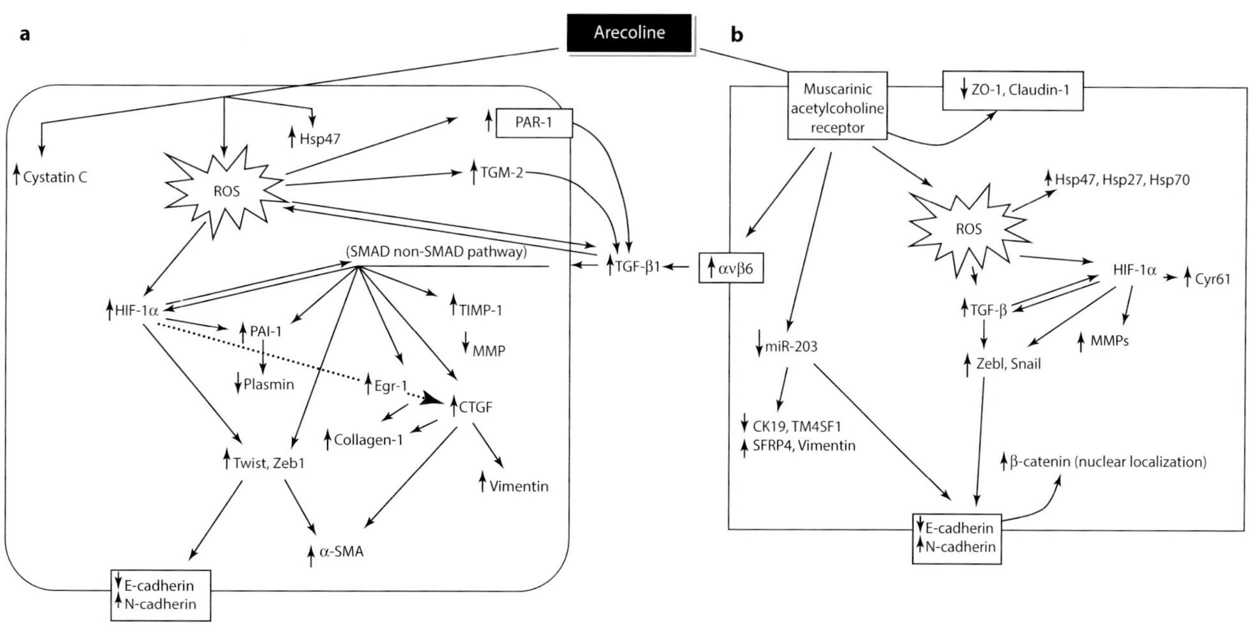


**Fig. 12.1** Induction cascade induced by arecoline in fibroblasts **a** and epithelial cells **b** facilitating the development of OSF

All abbreviations have been elaborated in text except: *N-cadherin* neural cadherin, *CK 19* cytokeratin 19, *TM4SF1* transmembrane 4 L six family member 1, *SFRP4* secreted frizzled related protein 4. Both hard dashed arrows and dotted arrow indicate the same

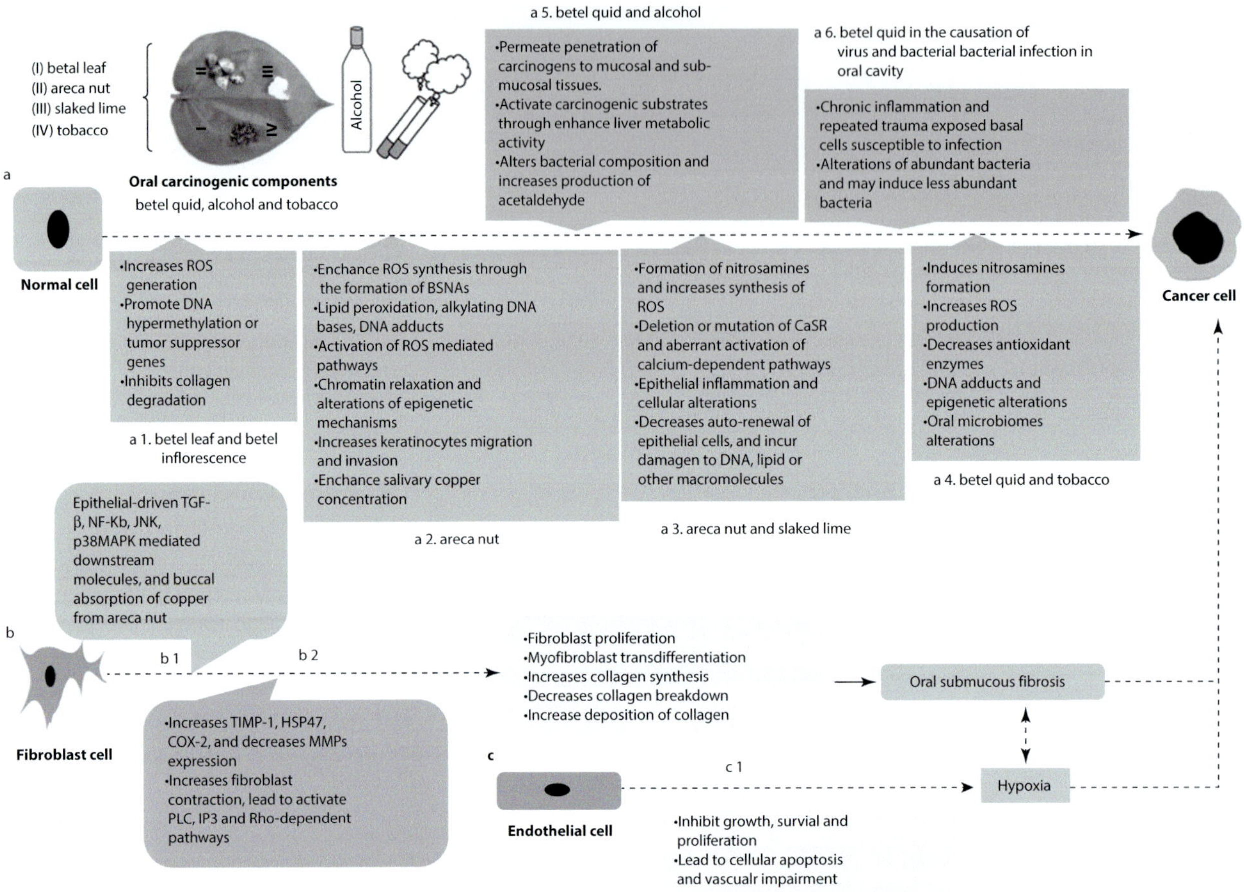


**Fig. 12.2** Possible mechanisms involved in the role of betel quid in oral squamous cell carcinoma and its malignant transformation [21]

(a, 1) Betel leaf and betel inflorescence increase ROS generation and contribute to DNA adducts

(a, 2) Areca nut alkaloids increase ROS generation, alkylate the DNA bases, and form DNA adducts. ROS can apparently activate TGF-β, NF-kB, JNK, and p38MAPK pathways. Areca nut induces αvβ6 integrin and mediates the migration and invasion of keratinocytes

(a, 3) Areca nut and slaked lime induce the generation of ROS through formation of nitrosamines, leading to epithelial inflammation. Excess calcium can alter macromolecules and contribute to oral mucosal inflammation

(a, 4) Tobacco and betel quid can form BSNAs and TSNAs, resulting in the induction of epigenetic silencing of tumor suppressor genes. Tobacco may alter oral bacterial microbiomes involved in carcinogenesis

(a, 5) Alcohol may damage epithelial cells and facilitate the penetration of carcinogens by increasing the epithelial permeability of cell membranes. Additionally, alcohol might activate carcinogenic substrates by increasing its metabolism. It can also induce the production of acetaldehyde, an oral carcinogen involved in oral cancer

(a, 6) Chronic inflammation and repeated trauma might be associated with immune suppression, which may facilitate viral infection at the buccal mucosa and induce changes in bacterial communities. These effects may be involved in carcinogenesis in the oral mucosa of betel quid chewers

(b, 1) TGF-β-, NF-kB-, JNK-, and p38MAPK-mediated downstream targets act on fibroblasts and lead to its proliferation, inducing collagen synthesis

(b, 2) Areca nut chemicals increase collagen synthesis, decrease its breakdown, and activate proliferative cascades in fibroblasts; these factors may be involved in the pathogenesis of OSF

(c, 1) Areca nut contents act on endothelial cells and inhibit their growth, survival, and proliferation. These effects may induce vascular impairment and lead to hypoxia. Hypoxia may further influence oral carcinogenesis by inducing hypoxia-mediated pathways

12

> **Important**
> **Biological factors involved in fibrosis and extracellular matrix (ECM) remodeling:**

| | |
|---|---|
| • Transforming growth factor-β (TGF-β) | • Matrix metalloproteinases (MMPs) |
| • Epidermal growth factor (EGF) | • Tissue inhibitors of matrix metalloproteinases (TIMPs) |
| • Fibroblast growth factor (bFGF) | • Nuclear factor-κB (NF-κB) |
| • Connective tissue growth factor (CTGF) | • JNK pathway |
| • Platelet-derived growth factor (PDGF) | • p38 |
| • Insulin-like growth factor (IGF)-1/2 | • MAPK pathway |
| • NOTCH | • αv integrins (β1, β3, β5, β8) |

## 12.3 Inflammation in Oral Submucous Fibrosis

Fibrosis is initiated by cellular injury that is presumably sensed through impaired cell-cell or cell-ECM interactions (◘ Fig. 12.1). This damage at the cellular level promotes localized fibrin clot formation. The pro-inflammatory factors released by damaged cells activate the innate immune response. The molecules, collectively known as "damage-associated molecular patterns" (DAMPs), either of intracellular origin or released from the ECM, promote an inflammatory response that results in the recruitment of neutrophils and macrophages to phagocytose necrotic cells and cell debris. During this acute inflammatory response, cells release cytokines, chemokines, and growth factors, including transforming growth factor-β (TGF-β), that facilitate the recruitment and proliferation of fibroblasts. Activated fibroblasts and myofibroblasts that provide cell and tissue contractility show an enhanced deposition of ECM proteins and stabilize the fibrotic tissue architecture [22].

The inflammation in submucous fibrosis decreases matrix metalloproteinases (MMPs) and increases tissue inhibitors of matrix metalloproteinase (TIMP) expression similar to wound healing. This contributes to the abnormal collagen deposition in OSF. Inflammation also stimulates the cells to express basic fibroblast growth factor (bFGF) and transforming growth factor β-1 (TGF-β1), contributing to the collagen deposition disorder in OSF. Unlike in wound healing, where myofibroblasts undergo apoptosis, in OSF, TGF-β1 stimulates fibroblasts to transform into myofibroblasts, which results in collagen production and wound contraction [1, 2] (◘ Fig. 12.3).

> **Important**
> Inflammatory mediators involved in OSF pathogenesis are:
> - Interleukins (IL-1β, IL-6, IL-8, IL-15)
> - Interferon-γ (IFN-γ)
> - Monocyte chemoattractant protein-1 (chemokine (C-C motif) ligand 2 [CCL2])
> - Tumor necrosis factor-α (TNF-α)
> - Heat-shock proteins 70 (Hsp 70)
> - Cyclooxygenase-2 (COX-2)

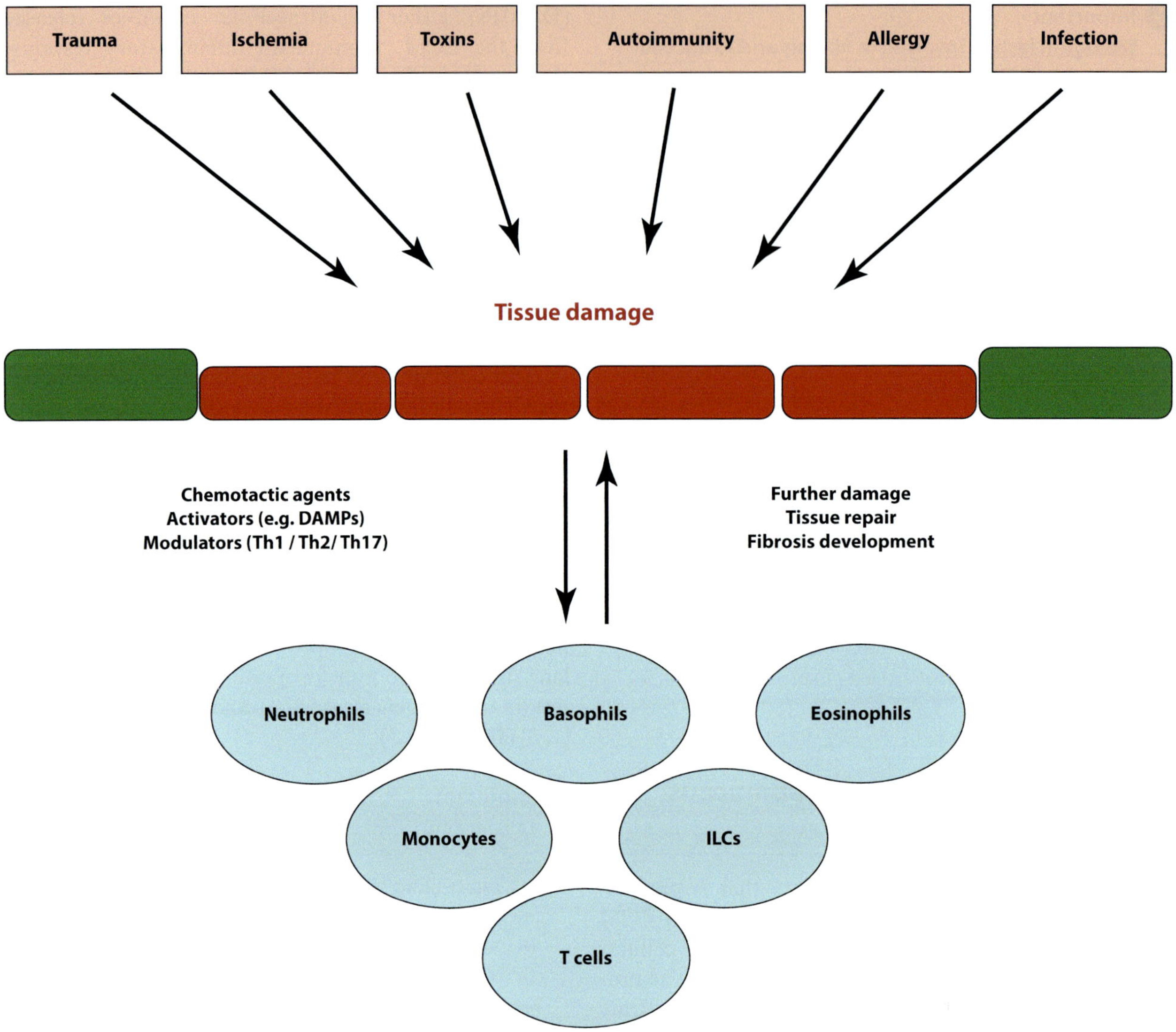


**Fig. 12.3** Interdependence of tissue damage and inflammation. Various types of tissue damage lead to recruitment, activation, and polarization of immune cells. Inflammation can induce further tissue damage or trigger tissue repair and fibrosis



## 12.4 Regulation of Inflammatory Mediators in Oral Submucous Fibrosis

**Cyclooxygenase-2 (COX-2):** Prostaglandin-endoperoxide synthase, commonly called as cyclooxygenase (COX), is the key regulatory enzyme in tissue inflammation and is present in two isoforms COX-1 and COX-2. COX-2 is an inducible form of COX, and its overexpression has been shown to promote tumorigenesis by activation of carcinogens, cytokines, neoangiogenesis, stimulating progression and inhibiting apoptosis. There is a significant increase in COX-2 expression in OSF tissues compared to normal subjects [23].

**Heat-shock protein-70 (Hsp-70):** Heat-shock proteins are a highly conserved group of protective cellular proteins whose synthesis is increased in response to a variety of environmental or pathophysiological stresses, including anoxia, ischemia, heavy metal ions, ethanol, nicotine, surgical stress, viral agents, starvation, inflammation, water deprivation, and nitrogen deficiency. These proteins play an important role in the maintenance of cellular homeostasis, both under normal conditions and during stress. Heat-shock proteins are overexpressed in a wide range of human cancers and are implicated in tumor cell proliferation, differentiation, invasion, metastasis, death, and recognition by the immune system. They are useful biomarkers for carcinogenesis in tissues and signal the degree of differentiation and the aggressiveness of cancers. Thubashini et al. report a significant increase in the expression of Hsp-70 ($p < 0.001$) as the tissue progressed from OSF towards OSCC [24].

In a study by Das et al., differentially expressed proteins between oral submucous fibrosis tissue and normal tissues were recorded by proteomic analysis using two-dimensional electrophoresis (2DE) and MALDI-TOF mass spectrometry. By proteomic analysis, 15 proteins were found to be upregulated and 10 proteins were downregulated in the OSF tissues compared to the control tissues. Among these identified proteins, Hsp-70 1B, calreticulin, and lumican variant exhibited higher expression in OSF tissues compared to the control tissues. Immunohistochemical analysis also showed elevated expression of these proteins in OSF tissues. Gene expression analysis by real-time quantitative RT-PCR showed that Hsp-70 1B, calreticulin, and lumican variant significantly increased (6.2-, 3.3-, 2.8- fold, respectively), whereas enolase 1 decreased by 0.5-fold in the OSF tissues, which was consistent with proteomic results [25, 26].

**Chemokine (C-C motif) ligand 2 [CCL2]:** Chemokines are leukocyte chemoattractants that act with pro-fibrotic cytokines in the development of fibrosis by recruiting myofibroblasts, macrophages, and other cells in OSF. Among all the chemokines, monocyte chemoattractant protein-1 (chemokine (C-C motif) ligand 2 [CCL2]) is a major pro-fibrotic mediator with an established role in the fibrosis of different organs of the body. CCL2 expression has been identified in different inflammatory and fibrotic diseases such as atherosclerosis, hepatic cirrhosis, pulmonary fibrosis, or glomerulosclerosis. It is expressed by a wide variety of cell types, including leukocytes and resident cells.

Sarode et al. designed a study to investigate the expression of CCL2 in OSF and its correlation with myofibroblasts. CCL2 expression in basal cells (CCL2-B) and connective tissue (CCL2-CT), and α-SMA, showed significantly increased expression in advanced OSF as compared with early OSF and controls. Significant differences were observed in the expression of CCL2-B between control and OSF ($p = 0.002$), control and advanced OSF ($p = 0.005$), and early and advanced OSF ($p = 0.0377$). In OSF group, a significant correlation was observed between CCL2-B and CCL2-CT ($p < 0.00001$), CCL2-B and α-SMA ($p < 0.00001$), and CCL2-CT and α-SMA ($p < 0.00001$) [27].

**Mast cell tryptase and mast cell chymase:** Mast cells may be activated by a number of stimuli. Following activation by immunological or non-immunological stimuli, mast cells release a wide range of preformed mediators from their granules. Mast cell products degrade connective tissue matrix to provide space for neovascular sprouts. Mast cells frequently accumulate at the site of fibrosis, such as the skin involved in scleroderma and fibrotic lung tissue, suggesting its contribution to the pathogenesis of various fibrotic conditions [28].

Betel quid components induce the production of various inflammatory mediators such as prostanoids, interleukin (IL)-6, tumor necrosis factor (TNF)-α, IL-8, and granulocyte-macrophage colony-stimulating factor (GMCSF), which stimulate the infiltration of inflammatory cells like mast cells and facilitate their differentiation and activation in the oral mucosa. The inflammatory cells releasing cytokines may act as the stimulant for the increase in the number of mast cells in OSF [28].

Mast cells promote angiogenesis by secreting angiogenic factors or enzymes that degrade extracellular matrix. Mast cell products, including histamine, basic fibroblast growth factor (bFGF), and heparin, directly affect endothelial cells by stimulating their migration or proliferation or indirectly affect them by degrading the connective tissue matrix, thereby providing space for the development of neovascular sprouts. Angiogenic factors like vascular endothelial growth factor (VEGF), bFGF, and platelet-derived growth factor-AB stimulate mast cell migration. In the hypoxic areas, they produce angiogenic products that stimulate the infiltration of more mast cells. Mast cell-derived heparin and TGF-β have shown to display chemotactic activity for endothelial cells and stimulate the growth of fibrotic tissue.

Sabarinath et al. observed statistically significant increase of intact mast cells from normal mucosa to different grades of OSF, but degranulated mast cells were significantly increased only in the very early and early stages of OSF. On the contrary, they were decreased in moderately advanced stage in which the functional contribution of fibroblasts supersedes the demand for nutritional supply [28].

Mast cells (MCs) produce and store various pro-fibrotic cytokines including transforming growth factor-β (TGF-β), fibroblast growth factor (FGF), platelet-derived growth factor (PDGF), interleukin-1 and -6 (IL-1 and IL-6), and tumor necrosis factor-α (TNF-α). Human MCs also contain two types of serine protease, tryptase and chymase. Tryptase is a trypsin-like enzyme, and chymase is a chymotrypsin-like enzyme. Based on their protease content, human MCs are divided into two phenotypes: mast cells secreting both tryptase and chymase are termed MCTC, while mast cells secreting only tryptase are termed MCT. All human tissues contain both the mast cell phenotypes. However, the ratio is different in each anatomical site. MCTC predominates in the skin, heart, synovial fluid, and small intestinal submucosa, and MCT predominates in the lungs and the small intestinal mucosa. MC tryptase and chymase, the most abundant pro-fibrotic cytokines of human MC, have been studied in various fibrotic disorders.

Yadav demonstrated the immunohistochemical expression of MC tryptase and chymase in 20 cases of OSF, 10 cases of oral squamous cell carcinoma (OSCC), and 10 cases of healthy controls. Subepithelial zone of stage 1 and 2 and deep zone of stage 3 and 4 OSF demonstrated increased tryptase-positive MCs. OSCC revealed a proportionate increase in tryptase- and chymase-positive MCs irrespective of the areas of distribution [29].

### 12.4.1 Pro-inflammatory Cytokines

Cytokines are low-molecular-weight polypeptides or glycoproteins which are secreted by immune cells (lymphocytes, macrophages, natural killer (NK) cells, mast cells, and stromal cells). They are ubiquitous, perform multiple biological activities, and are involved in many physiological processes. Cytokines are important for the normal functioning of the immune system, regulation of growth, and development and activation of the inflammatory response. Cytokines have a pleiotropic effect on many different cell types. Cytokines usually act as intercellular (paracrine) and/or intracellular (autocrine) signals within local tissues. They can also serve as endocrine mediators. Many inflammatory mediators, such as interleukin-1 (IL-1), interleukin-6 (IL-6), interleukin-15 (IL-15), and tumor necrosis factor-α (TNF-α), are involved in the pathogenesis of inflammatory fibrotic diseases. Levels of cortisol and inflammatory cytokines, including IL-1β, IL-15, and TNF-α in inflammation, are induced by the foreign materials, and therefore it is important to understand the changes in cortisol and cytokine levels among betel-chewing individuals [30, 31].

Haque et al. have shown a higher expression of interleukin-1 (IL-1) α and IL-1β, IL-6, basic fibroblast growth factor (bFGF), platelet-derived growth factor (PDGF), and transforming growth factor-β (TGF-β) and a lower expression of interferon (IFN)-β and IFN-γ in both the epithelium and underlying connective tissue of OSF specimens compared to normal oral mucosa specimens [32].

In addition, the peripheral blood mononuclear cells from OSF patients have been found to secrete an increased level of stimulated IL-1β, tumor necrosis factor-α (TNF-α), IL-6, and IL-8 and a decreased level of stimulated interferon-gamma (IFN-γ) compared to Caucasian and Indian controls. These two studies by Haque et al. suggest that a local and systemic upregulation of fibrogenic cytokines together with systematic downregulation of anti-fibrotic cytokines underlies the pathogenesis of OSF [33, 34]. Chiu et al. have observed a link between TNF-α allelic polymorphism and occurrence of OSF [35].

Studies have suggested that the nuclear factor-κB (NF-κB) signaling pathway plays a critical role in carcinogenesis, protection from apoptosis, and chemoresistance in a number of cancer types, including head and neck cancer, breast cancer, hepatocellular carcinoma, and gastric cancer 8–12. The NF-κB-dependent cytokine levels are elevated in saliva and tissue specimens of patients with oral potentially malignant disorders [36].

Different cytokines are expressed by cancerous cells, the most common of which include tumor necrosis factor alpha (TNF-α), IL-1, IL-6, and IL-8. TNF-α, IL-6, and IL-8 are potent angiogenic meditators with significant effects on tumor growth and are associated with increased tumor vessel density and a poor clinical outcome. Thus, these cytokines might act as surrogate biomarkers of angiogenesis and prognosis. The excessive cell proliferation and activation of cellular actions can be instigated by chronic inflammation, which leads to the induction of irreversible DNA damage. TNF-α, IL-6, and IL-8 released through the inflammatory response promote tumor growth, which further stimulates the inflammatory response, resulting in cyclic progression. Kaur et al. observed that serum and salivary TNF-α, IL-6, and IL-8 levels were upregulated in precancerous lesions and conditions. Pro-inflammatory cytokine levels are elevated in submucous fibrosis due to immunoregulatory activity. Increased levels of NF-κB mediators might be associated with the development of oral precancerous and cancerous lesions. In the normal cell, stimulation of cytokines causes growth inhibition, while in oral cancer cells, stimulation of cytokines leads to upregulation of positive cell cycle regulators including NF-κB, signal transducers, and activators of transcription and the mitogen-activated protein kinase/extracellular signal-regulated pathway [37].

Upregulation of TNF-α, IL-6, and IL-8 might be protective in action. NF-κB activation leads to the upregulation of anti-apoptotic genes as a cell survival mechanism, by inducing physiological stress, which triggers an inflammatory response. In addition, NF-κB induces cytokines that regulate TNF-α, IL-6, and IL-8, which leads to the recruitment of leukocytes to the sites of inflammation. The levels of serum and salivary TNF-α, IL-6, and IL-8 were also statistically significantly increased in oral leukoplakia, submucous fibrosis, and lichen-planus in contrast to normal healthy subjects ($p < 0.05$) [37].

Interleukin-8 (IL-8) is a prototypical member of the CXC chemokine family, the chemokines in which

12

the first two amino-terminal cysteine residues are separated by an intervening amino acid. The amino terminus of the majority of the CXC chemokines contains three amino acid residues, glutamic acid–leucine–arginine, the ELR motif. Members that contain the ELR motif (ELR+) are potent promoters of angiogenesis, and those that lack the ELR motif (ELR−) are potent inhibitors of angiogenesis. IL-8 is an ELR+ pluripotent cytokine that promotes angiogenesis in OSCC. Punyani et al. reported that the levels of salivary IL-8 were found to be significantly elevated in patients with OSCC as compared to the precancer group ($p < 0.0001$). However, the difference in salivary IL-8 concentrations among the precancer group and controls was statistically nonsignificant ($p = 0.738$) [38].

The continuous contact of the alkaloids in the quid on the oral mucosa causes chronic inflammation leading to activation of macrophages and T cells and an increase in the level of cytokines such as interleukin 6 (IL-6), tumor necrosis factor (TNF), interferon-α (IFN-α), and transforming growth factor-beta. Further, microtrauma produced by the friction of coarse fibers of areca nut also facilitates diffusion of the alkaloids into the subepithelial connective tissue resulting in juxta-epithelial inflammatory cell infiltration. Fibrogenic cytokines secreted by activated macrophages or T lymphocytes are very important in the development of fibrotic disorders. Circulating monocytes are attracted to tissues by chemotactic factors and become macrophages under the influence of their microenvironment. Several studies suggest that local and systemic upregulation of fibrogenic cytokines and downregulation of anti-fibrotic cytokines are central to the pathogenesis of OSF [38].

Macrophages have also been implicated in the pathogenesis of OSF. Pereira et al. evaluated the presence of macrophages in various histological stages of OSMF using CD68 antigen, which has been suggested as the most reliable marker for macrophage differentiation. They found a significant increase in macrophage densities in the subepithelial connective tissue of OSF specimens compared to those in control specimens suggesting that the cellular immune response plays an important role in the pathogenesis of OSF [39].

Haque et al. characterized the inflammatory cell infiltrates in the biopsies of oral mucosa from OSF patients demonstrated by IHC. They found activated T lymphocytes as the major cell population and macrophages as the minor cell population [33].

In a Taiwanese study, IL-1β and TNF-α have been demonstrated to upregulate mRNA expression of collagen types I and III. Intradermal injections of TNF-α stimulate the accumulation of fibroblasts and collagen. TNF-α is reported to inhibit adherence and phagocytosis of collagen. On the contrary, IFN-γ is an anti-fibrotic cytokine that can inhibit collagen synthesis. Improvement of keloids and hypertrophic scars by the intralesional IFN-γ treatment has been reported. Furthermore, local injections of IFN-γ reduce the contracture formation and facilitate the mouth opening in OSF patients [40].

Haque et al. investigated the presence and distribution of inflammatory cells and MHC class II antigen expression by epithelial and immunocompetent cells using a three-stage immunoperoxidase method on 30 frozen sections of OSMF. All tissues were investigated using antibodies to T cells (CD3), T helper/inducer cells (CD4), T suppressor/cytotoxic cells (CD8), B cells (CD20), naive T cells and monocytes (CD45RA), macrophages, Langerhans cells (CD68), and human leukocyte antigen-DR (HLA-DR)-positive cells (HLA-DR alpha). The predominant cell populations detected in normal tissues were CD3, CD4, and HLA-DR-positive cells. The cell population detected in OSF showed higher numbers of CD3- and HLADR-positive cells compared with those of the normal tissues. The pattern of staining for CD4-positive cells in OSF tissues was similar to that of CD3-positive cells both in the epithelium and connective tissue and was higher than that in normal tissues. A few scattered CD8-positive cells and only occasional CD20- and CD68-positive cells were seen in OSF sections. The presence of these immunocompetent cells and high ratio of CD4 to CD8 in OSF tissues suggest an ongoing cellular immune response leading to a possible imbalance of immunoregulation and alteration in local tissue architecture [41].

Bôas et al. compared the microvascular density (MVD) and infiltrating macrophage density (IMD) in oral OSCCs with different histological grades using antibodies such as von Willebrand factor and CD68. However, a significant correlation between MVD and IMD could not be obtained, suggesting that angiogenesis does not depend on the number of macrophages present in OSCC, but their predominant phenotype [42].

El-Rouby studied the association between tumor-associated macrophages (TAMs) and angiogenesis in formalin-fixed, paraffin-embedded archival material of OSCC and oral verrucous carcinoma. TAMs shown by IHC for CD68 and microvessels demonstrated by IHC for CD31 were quantified using an image analyzer computer system. He observed an increased TAM density associated with angiogenesis in higher histopathological grades in oral cancer [43].

Wehrhan et al. analyzed the macrophage polarization in cervical lymph nodes of OSCC patients. The study revealed an influence of OSCC on macrophage polarization in regional lymph nodes. Markers of malignant behavior in the primary tumor were associated with a shift of macrophage polarization in lymph nodes from the anti-tumoral M1 type to the tumor-promoting M2 type [44].

Pettersen et al. studied the activation state of TAMs in cutaneous SCC where CD163 was identified as a more abundant, sensitive, and accurate marker of TAMs when compared with CD68 [45].

### 12.4.2 Cortisol and Steroids

Arecoline is an alkaloid that can be purified from areca nut. Arecoline is a muscarinic cholinergic agonist that can cause cortisol escape from dexamethasone suppression among normal males and stimulate corticosterone release in rats [46, 47].

Risch et al. found that there was an elevation of plasma cortisol and β-endorphin in human subjects who had majorly been treated with arecoline [48]. Hu et al. found that there was a significant increase in plasma cortisol levels and a significant decrease in plasma IL-1β, IL-15, and TNF-α levels among males who chew areca nut and oral cancer patients compared to mid-aged and young control males. These elevations in plasma cortisol concentrations among areca nut chewers could be due to an increased oxygen consumption response by the adrenal gland or stimulation of the hypothalamic-pituitary-adrenal axis [34].



Furthermore, Hu et al. demonstrated a significant reduction in plasma testosterone levels among areca nut-chewing subjects compared to young control male subjects. This result could be due to these areca nut chewers having consumed the nut for more than 8 years or might be an effect of their older age. On the contrary, increased testosterone secretion by dispersed mouse interstitial cells treated with arecoline (the major component in betel quid) or areca nut extract has been investigated. Yang et al. showed that arecoline stimulates testosterone secretion from mouse interstitial cells that have been treated with ovine LH and that this is independent of the cyclic adenosine monophosphate (cAMP) pathway [49]. Stimulated testosterone production by purified Leydig cells treated with arecoline has also been observed [50].

This stimulatory effect exerted by arecoline would seem to be enhanced by adding human chorionic 15 gonadotropin (hCG), forskolin (cAMP stimulator), or 8-Br-cAMP (cAMP analogue). Calcium channel blockers such as nifedipine, nimodipine, or tetrandrine have been shown to decrease testosterone secretion that has been induced by arecoline. Moreover, enhanced expressions of steroidogenic acute regulatory (StAR) protein and 17β-hydroxysteroid dehydrogenase (17β-HSD) have been observed in Leydig cells treated with arecoline [49, 50].

## 12.5 Fibrogenic Factors and Signaling Pathways

### 12.5.1 Transforming Growth Factor-Beta (TGF-β Family)

The TGF-β superfamily is composed of a large group of proteins, including the activin/inhibin family, bone morphogenetic proteins (BMPs), growth differentiation factors (GDFs), TGF-β subfamily, and glial cell line-derived neurotrophic factor (GDNF) family. TGF-β is a multifunctional peptide that controls various cellular processes, including differentiation, proliferation, migration, extracellular matrix (ECM) remodeling, and apoptosis, all of which influence embryogenesis, wound healing, fibrosis, inflammation, and tumor progression.

Beta-type subfamily growth factors are homodimeric or heterodimeric polypeptides with multiple regulatory properties depending on cell type, growth conditions, and presence of other polypeptide growth factors. Since their expression is also controlled by distinct promoters, their secretion is temporal and tissue specific [51, 52].

***TGF-β isoforms***: There are three known isoforms of TGF-β (TGF-β1, TGF-β2, and TGF-β3) expressed in mammalian tissues; they contain highly conserved regions but diverge in several amino acid regions. All of them function through the same receptor signaling pathways. TGF-β1, the most abundant and ubiquitously expressed isoform, was cloned from human term placenta mRNA. TGF-β2 was first described in human glioblastoma cells. It was found that TGF-β2 is capable of suppressing interleukin-2-dependent growth of T lymphocytes. Hence, it is also called glioblastoma-derived T cell suppressor factor (G-TsF). The third isoform, TGF-β3, was isolated from a cDNA library of human rhabdomyosarcoma cell line. It shares 80% of amino acid sequence with TGF-β1 and TGF-β2 [1, 51, 53].

#### 12.5.1.1 TGF-β Synthesis and Activation

Mature dimeric form of TGF-β, composed of two monomers stabilized by hydrophobic interactions and disulfide bridge, initiates intracellular signaling. The three TGF-βs are synthesized as pro-proteins (pro-TGF-βs) with large amino-terminal pro-domains (called latency-associated proteins—LAPs), which are required for proper folding and dimerization of carboxy-terminal growth factor domain (mature peptide). This complex is called "small latent complex" (SLC) [51].

#### 12.5.1.2 TGF-β Receptors

TβRI and TβRII mediate signal transduction. Both receptors are transmembrane serine/threonine kinases, which associate in a homo- or heteromeric complex and act as tetramers. They are organized sequentially into an N-terminal extracellular ligand-binding domain, a transmembrane region, and a C-terminal serine/threonine kinase domain.

Bioactive forms of TGF-βs are dimers held together by hydrophobic interactions and, in most cases, by an inter-subunit disulfide bond as well. The dimeric structure of these ligands suggests that they function by bringing together pairs of type I and II receptors, forming hetero-tetrameric receptor complexes. Binding of TGF-β to extracellular domains of both receptors also induces proper conformation of the intracellular kinase domains. These receptors are subject to reversible posttranslational modifications (phosphorylation, ubiquitylation, and sumoylation) that regulate stability and availability of receptors as well as SMAD and non-SMAD pathway activation [51].

***TGF-β signaling pathways***: In the canonical signaling, after ligand binding, TGF-β receptors dimerize and phosphorylate intracellular SMAD proteins. Complex of SMAD2 and/or SMAD3 becomes phosphorylated by TβRI and forms a complex with SMAD4, which is subsequently transported into the nucleus where it binds with specific transcription factors (TF) and induces transcription of TGF-β-dependent genes.

Interestingly, in addition to the activation of SMAD transcription factors, several different branching signaling pathways can be activated in many cell types, such as Notch signaling, MAP kinases, AKT/PKB pathway, GTP-binding protein pathway, PTK pathway, NF-κB, and Wnt/β-catenin pathway. The noncanonical mechanisms are not clearly elucidated [1, 51].

#### 12.5.1.3 TGF-β Signaling and Fibrotic Diseases

Several signaling pathways are involved in fibrosis, but TGF-β signaling is the master regulator of fibrosis. TGF-β activation induces fibroblasts to produce excessive ECM, causing fibrosis. Additionally, TGF-β signaling in non-fibroblast cells can also induce fibrosis through the production of fibrotic factors, such as endothelin 1 (ET-1), connective tissue growth factor (CTGF), interleukin (IL)-13, platelet-derived growth factor (PDGF), fibroblast growth factor (FGF-2), and insulin-like growth factor (IGF)-1/2.

TGF-β1 isoform is most implicated in fibrosis. This peptide plays a critical role not only in the synthesis and degradation of ECM but also in the response of cells to ECM mediated through integrin receptors; moreover, specific components of the ECM, in turn, can both deliver TGF-β and regulate its activity. Isoforms of TGF-β, β1, and β2 have been linked to variations of protein expression or function. TGF-β1 is a key regulator of ECM assembly and remodeling. The cytokine TGF-β1 is considered to have a central role in inducing myofibroblastic phenotype, and its expression is increased under numerous fibrotic conditions. Thus, TGF-β signaling pathway might be critical for the pathogenesis of OSF. That TGF-β stimulates fibroblast proliferation and EM elaboration suggests the importance of these cytokines in fibroelastic diseases.

TGF-β is increased in the microenvironment of chronic injury/inflammation and cancer. Once activated by TGF-β ligands, epithelial cells can secrete more fibrotic factors, such as CTGF, to increase fibroblast proliferation. Fibroblasts become activated and turn into myofibroblasts, FAFs, or CAFs, and these cells are important effector cells that can produce excessive ECM, leading to fibrosis and ultimately fibrotic diseases when organ function is hampered. Cytokine paracrine interaction results in the production of connective tissue growth factor (CTGF), interleukin-1β (IL-1β), interleukin-6 (IL-6), interferon-γ (IFN-γ), tumor necrosis factor-α (TNF-α), fibrosis-associated fibroblast (FAF), cancer-associated fibroblast (CAF), and extracellular matrix (ECM) [1, 51] (◘ Fig. 12.4).

> TGF-β signaling is the master regulator of fibrosis. Of the three isoforms, TGF-β1 isoform is most implicated in fibrosis.

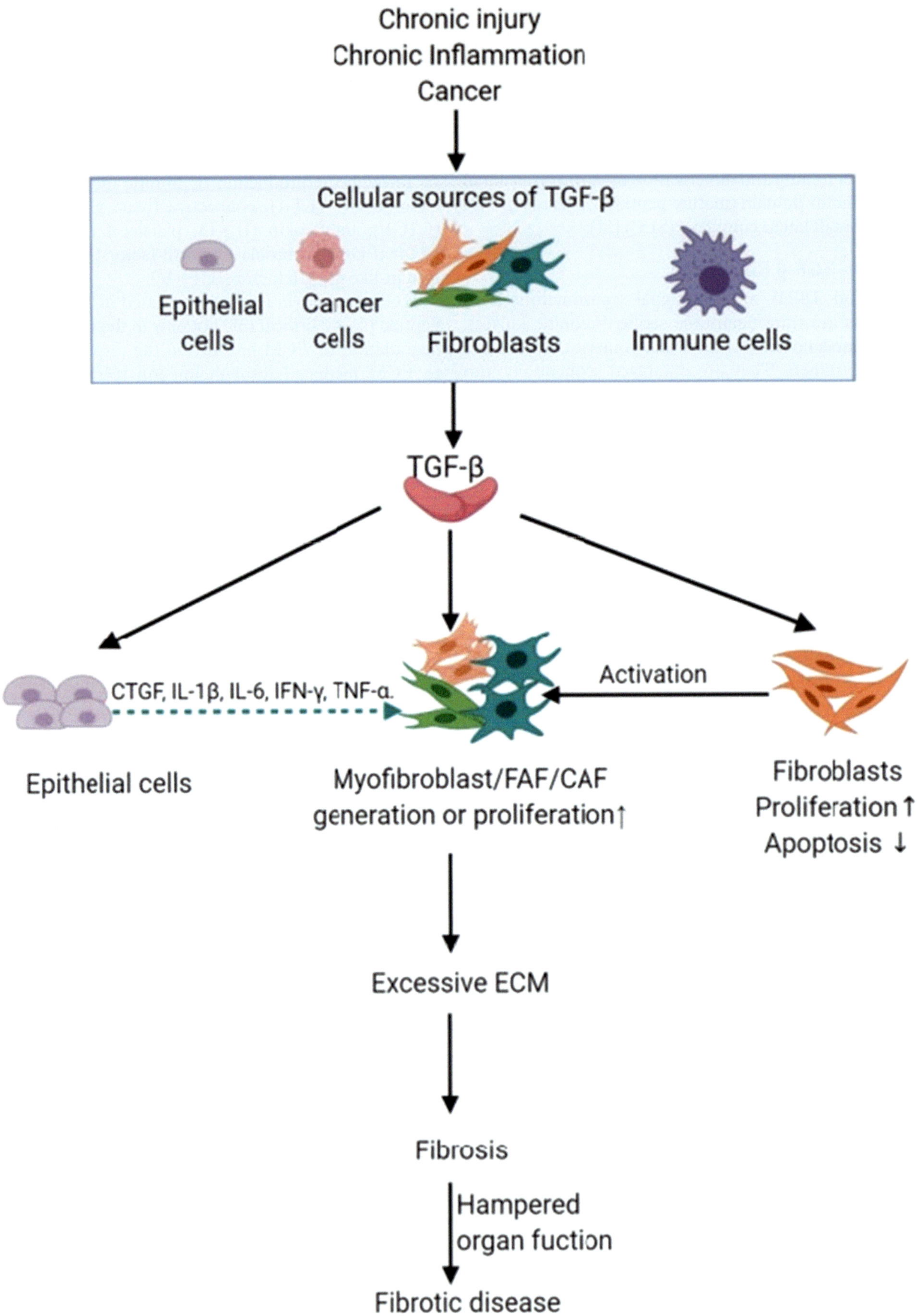


**Fig. 12.4** TGF-β pathway leading to tissue fibrosis

### 12.5.2 Contribution of SMAD and Non-SMAD Signaling Pathways to Fibrosis at the Cellular Level

TGF-β-induced activation of TβRI by TβRII leads to the recruitment and C-terminal phosphorylation of SMAD2 and SMAD3, which then associate with a SMAD4. These activated heterotrimeric SMAD complexes translocate into the nucleus, where they associate with high-affinity DNA-binding transcription factors and transcription cofactors to activate or repress gene transcription. For example, SMAD3/SMAD4 complexes can cooperate with AP1 transcription complexes (Jun–Fos dimers) to promote pro-fibrotic gene transcription. TGF-β also activates non-SMAD signaling, notably the MAPK pathways and Akt–mTOR signaling that also contribute to fibrogenic gene and cell differentiation responses. COL1A2, CCN2 (CTGF), SERPINE1 (PAI-1), FN1, and IL11 encode collagen Iα2, connective tissue growth factor (CTGF), plasminogen activator inhibitor-1 (PAI-1), fibronectin, and interleukin-11, respectively. mTORC1 activation promotes protein translation and contributes to increased collagen synthesis by transcription factor (TF) [1].

#### 12.5.2.1 The Role of Areca Nut and Transforming Growth Factor-β in Oral Submucous Fibrosis Progression

Areca nut can induce and activate transforming growth factor-β in epithelial cells, which can act together on the fibroblast cells and induce the expression of other pro-fibrotic cytokines (endothelin and CTGF). These cytokines can further enhance the fibroid response and aid in the conversion of fibroblasts to myofibroblasts expressing γSMA and αSMA markers. Areca nut and transforming growth factor-β can influence the expression of cytoskeletal reorganizing protein LIMK1. The overall collagen production also increases. Collagen maturation and stabilizing enzymes (BMP1 and PLOD2, respectively) can also be induced by areca nut along with transforming growth factor-β. All these changes may lead to excessive deposition of extracellular matrix characteristic of OSF [54, 55].

#### 12.5.2.2 Transforming Growth Factor-β Regulation by Areca Nut

Areca nut acts on muscarinic acid receptors to release calcium and activate Ca2+/calmodulin-activated kinase II (CAMKII). It also induces intracellular reactive oxygen species (ROS). CAMKII and ROS together activate c-Jun N-terminal kinase (JNK), which subsequently phosphorylates activating transcription factor 2 (ATF2) and c-Jun transcription factors. The two transcription factors induce TGF-β promoter. The translated TGF-β protein can now activate the canonical SMAD signaling pathway and autoinduce TGF-β and other targets in epithelial cells [54, 55].

#### 12.5.2.3 TGF-β in Oral Submucous Fibrosis

Wang et al. report a stronger immunohistochemical expression of TGF-β1 in OSF compared to normal mucosal tissue. There was a strong localized TGF-β1 staining in chronic inflammatory cells. TGF-β1 was highly expressed in OSF tissues compared with normal oral mucosa. The protein expression of TGF-β1 was significantly lower in OSF tissues in the early/intermediate (OSF1) stage than in those in the advanced (OSF2) stage. They also demonstrated that arecoline and TGF-β1 increased the level of CD147 in human oral keratinocytes (HOKs). Transforming growth factor-β1 and β2 showed intense positivity for OSF and scar tissue, whereas mild-to-moderate reactivity was seen in normal oral mucosal tissue. OSF stimulates keratinocytes to produce TGF-β1 and β2. The subsequent passage of the cytokines to the connective tissue initiates changes that result in the pathognomonic fibrosis of the disorder [54–59].

#### 12.5.2.4 Epidermal Growth Factor Receptor

Epidermal growth factor receptor (EGFR), one of the best studied biomarkers, plays an important role in the control of cellular proliferation, apoptosis, invasion, angiogenesis, and metastasis as it works through the tyrosine kinase cascade [60].

EGFR gene is located on chromosome 7p11.2. EGFR gene codes for 11 transcripts, which are splice variants—8 exons and 3 introns.

EGF receptor and its activation: EGFR is the first member of the RTK superfamily to be identified as the epidermal growth factor receptor (EGFR). EGFR (also known as ErbB1 or HER1) is a member of the ErbB/HER family of receptors, which are all single-pass RTKs that derive their name from the discovery that the erythroblastosis tumor virus encodes an aberrant form of the human EGF receptor (ErbB) and that they are a family of human EGF receptors (HER) [60, 61].

The epidermal growth factor receptor (EGFR) belongs to a family of receptor tyrosine kinases that includes three other members (erbB2/HER-2, erbB3/HER-3, and erbB4/HER-4). These receptors are anchored in the cytoplasmic membrane and share a similar structure that is composed of an extracellular ligand-binding domain, a short hydrophobic transmembrane region, and an intracytoplasmic tyrosine kinase domain. EGFR becomes activated by receptor overexpression (frequent in cancer) as well as ligand-dependent and ligand-independent mechanisms [60].

There are six known ligands that bind to the EGFR, including EGF itself and transforming growth factor-α.

Ligand binding to the receptor induces a conformational change of the receptor ectodomain that allows for receptor dimerization and autophosphorylation of several tyrosine residues within the COOH-terminal tail of the receptors. Ligand-independent receptor activation occurs in some tumors that display forms of the EGFR and HER that have a deletion of the extracellular domain that results in constitutive receptor activation. Overexpression of the urokinase-type plasminogen activator receptor also results in ligand-independent activation of the EFGR via the association of a5h1 integrin. Finally, ligand-independent receptor activation occurs as a result of cellular stresses, such as radiation, which silence phosphatases that antagonize the receptor kinase activity, thereby shifting the equilibrium of basal phosphorylation towards the activated state. Activation of the receptor leads to the phosphorylation of key tyrosine residues within the COOH-terminal portion of EGFR and, as a result, provides specific docking sites for cytoplasmic proteins containing Src homology 2 and phosphor-tyrosine-binding domains. Once phosphorylated, the receptor initiates signal transduction through various signaling pathways—MAPK, Akt, ERK, and Jak/STAT pathways [60, 62].

***EGFR signaling***: In canonical EGFR signaling pathway, activation with ligand binding is a well-characterized function of EGFR. With ligand binding, trans-autophosphorylation takes place between tyrosine residues, which triggers the downstream signaling cascades. Conformational changes of C-terminal tail also trigger the components of endocytosis pathway and lead to EGFR internalization. EGFR, without ligand, can also be endocytosed with a rate tenfold lower than the ligand-induced ones. When EGFR is induced with ligand binding on plasma membrane, it is not only phosphorylated, but also ubiquitinated at lysine residues on the cytoplasmic kinase domain by E3 ubiquitin ligase Cbl complex including GRB2 adaptor protein. Concentration of EGF is the regulator of EGFR ubiquitination. At the beginning of internalization of EGFR, ubiquitination drives the non-clathrin endocytosis pathway; at later stages, it steers EGFR to lysosomal degradation. The fate of EGFR depends also on the type of ligand. After internalization, some of its ligands, like TGFA and epiregulin (EREG), dissociate from EGFR in the milder acidic environment of endosome and drive recycling of EGFR to plasma membrane. In contrast, ligands (like EGF) which are not affected by the acidity of endosome, favor the passage of majority of EGFR from early to late endosomes to be degraded by the lysosome. Additionally, heparin-binding EGF-like growth factor (HBEGF) and betacellulin (BTC) drive all EGF receptors to lysosomal degradation.



Ligand-induced EGFR activation in turn activates downstream signaling pathways, including RAS/MAPK pathway, PI3K/AKT pathway, and PLC/protein kinase C cascade. Activation of these pathways with canonical EGFR signaling controls the crucial functions of cells such as survival, proliferation, differentiation, and migration. In addition, activation of EGFR regulates other important metabolic functions such as autophagy in response to cellular or environmental stress via noncanonical signaling. Dealing with stress conditions with the action of noncanonical EGFR signal is preferred in cancer cells to provide advantage for survival and drug resistance (◘ Fig. 12.5).

Following binding, a number of cytoplasmic tyrosine residues are autophosphorylated by the intrinsic receptor kinase. Major pathways mediating EGFR actions include Ras/Raf/MAPK, Stat-1/Stat-3, PI3K/Akt, and Shc/ Grb2/Sos1/Rsk2, although other signaling molecules have also been reported to mediate EGFR's actions [61–69].

#### 12.5.2.5 EGFR Role in Fibrosis

While increased expression of EGFR was noted in the stratum spinosum of the epithelium, TGF-α was restricted to stratum germinativum, indicating an upregulation of TGF-α initially and then exerting a paracrine effect of the non-proliferative cells to increase the expression of cell surface receptor. There was an upregulation of both the TGF-α and EGF in oral submucous fibrosis, implying the activation of RTK pathways and activation of oncogenes such as c-fos and c-myc subsequently. Areca nut extract (ANE) induces activation of RTK signaling by activating the upstream epidermal growth factor receptor (EGFR), Src, and Ras signaling pathways. Increased expression of EGFR has been reported in OSCC and is usually associated with poor prognosis and outcome [70–74]. Meka et al. studied the expression of EGFR in 30 subjects, which included 10 oral leukoplakia (OL), 10 oral submucous fibrosis, and 10 normal oral mucosa as the control group. 40% of oral submucous fibrosis cases showed strong expression (3+), 40% of OL and 30% of OSF cases showed weak expression (2+), and 40% of OL and 30% of OSF cases showed poor expression (1+) compared to controls ($p = 0.012$) [75].

#### 12.5.2.6 Fibroblast Growth Factor Receptor (FGF)

Fibroblast growth factors (FGFs) are broad-spectrum mitogens and regulate a wide range of cellular functions, including migration, proliferation, differentiation, and survival. It is well documented that FGF signaling plays essential roles in the development, metabolism, and tissue homeostasis [76].

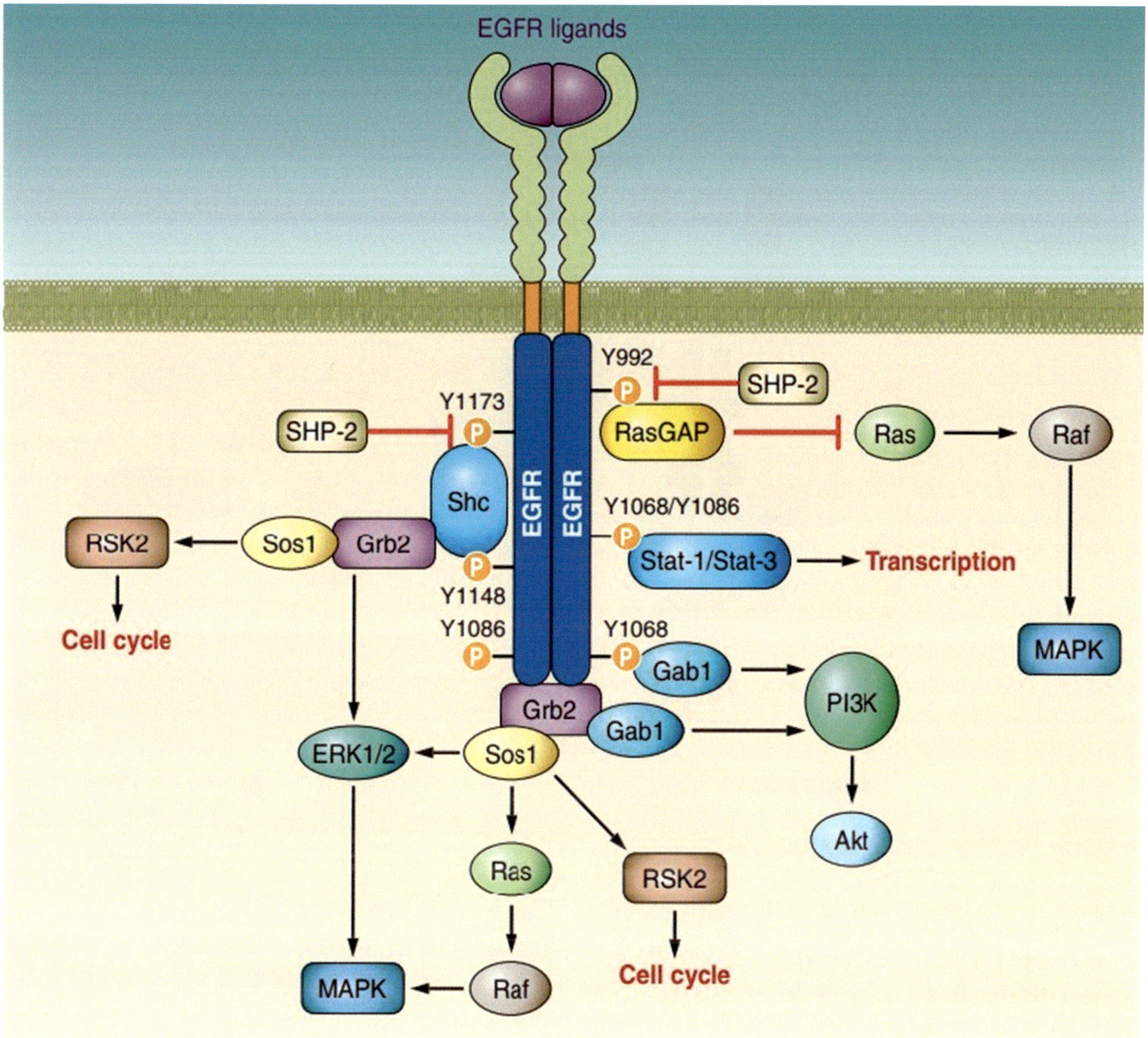


**Fig. 12.5** Potential EGFR signaling pathways activated by ligand binding

FGFR receptors and types: FGF family is one of the most diverse growth factor groups in vertebrates. In mice and humans, 22 FGF ligands have been identified. Based on sequence homology and phylogeny, 18 canonical mammalian FGFs are divided into six subfamilies, including five paracrine subfamilies and one endocrine subfamily. Five paracrine subfamilies contain the FGF1 subfamily (FGF1 and FGF2), the FGF4 subfamily (FGF4, FGF5, and FGF6), the FGF7 subfamily (FGF3, FGF7, FGF10, and FGF22), the FGF8 subfamily (FGF8, FGF17, and FGF18), and the FGF9 subfamily (FGF9, FGF16, and FGF20). The FGF19 subfamily (FGF19, FGF21, and FGF23) signals in an endocrine manner [77].

FGFR gene and signaling: FGFR1 and FGFR2 genes are located at chromosomes 8p11.23 and 10q26.13, respectively, and code for 24 exons. FGFs exert their pleiotropic effects by binding and activating high-affinity tyrosine kinase receptors that are coded by four genes (FGFR1, FGFR2, FGFR3, and FGFR4) and FGFRL1, a truncated FGFR without intracellular domain 2 in mammals. FGFRs are single-pass transmembrane proteins containing an extracellular domain, a transmembrane domain (TMD), and an intracellular tyrosine kinase domain. Among them, the extracellular domain is composed of three immunoglobulin (Ig)-like domains (D1–D3), an acidic region, a heparin-binding motif for FGFs, heparan cofactors, and partner proteins. The TMD anchors the receptors in cell membrane and facilitate its dimerization. In the cytosol, the juxtamembrane region of FGFRs is involved in receptor dimerization, while the split kinase domains are

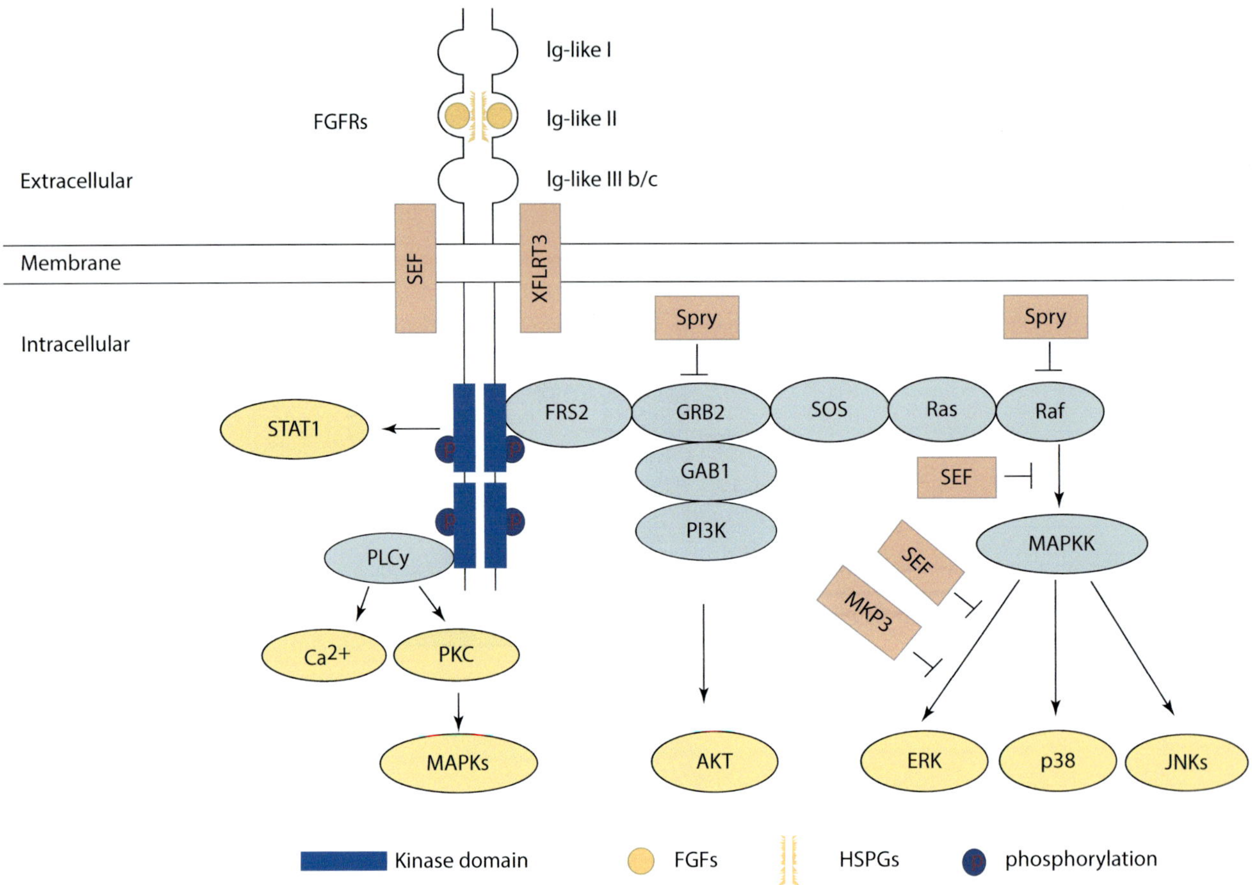


**Fig. 12.6** The classical FGF/FGFR pathways

12

required for the transmitting of FGF-related signaling [78] (Fig. 12.6).

Binding of appropriate growth factors to receptors triggers the conformational changes of FGFRs, resulting in dimerization and activation of FGFRs. Activated FGFRs phosphorylate FRS2a and FRS2a that bind to SH2 domain-containing adaptor Grb2. Grb2 will subsequently bind to SOS, GAB1, and Cbl through its SH3 domain to activate Ras/Raf/MAPKs, including ERK MAPK, p38 MAPK, and JNK MAPK. The activated FGFRs also activate phosphatidylinositol (PI)-3 kinase and STAT. FGFRs recruit and phosphorylate PLCγ. Among the members of the FGF synexpression group, SEF and XFLRT3 are transmembrane proteins and can interact directly with FGFRs. SEF functions as a negative regulator by affecting the phosphorylation of the MAPK ERK cascade. XFLRT3 forms a complex with FGF receptors and enhances FGF/FGFR signaling. Spry acts at the level of Grb2 and/or the level of Raf to attenuate FGF/FGFR signaling. MKP3 negatively regulates FGF/FGFR signaling by dephosphorylating the activated ERK, FGFR substrate 2α (FRS2α), GRB2-associated binding protein 1 (GAB1), growth factor receptor-bound 2 (GRB2), protein kinase C (PKC), and Son of Sevenless (SOS) [78].

#### 12.5.2.7 Role of FGF in Fibrosis

Basic fibroblast growth factor-2 (bFGF2) induces EMT by decreasing the expression of cytokeratin and E-cadherin and inducing the expression of vimentin, FSP-1, and α-SMA. bFGF is upregulated in the early stages of OSF, with increased expression in fibroblasts and endothelial cells. The expression in fibroblasts may be due to the heparan sulfate, which shows enrichment of bFGF-binding domains in fibrotic lesions, and these regions may play an important role in the fibrogenesis through their interaction with endogenous bFGF [79–86]. Pandiar et al. reported a decrease in bFGF expression in OSF compared to normal subjects [74, 87].

FGF2 induces angiogenesis, and its receptors may play a role in the synthesis of collagen. It is involved in the transmission of signals between the epithelium and connective tissue, and influences growth and differentiation of a wide variety of tissues including epithelia. Studies have reported FGF2 overexpression in high-grade malignant tumors and malignant transformation of normal cells transfected with FGF2 gene. FGF2 is involved in the invasion of cancer cells and the proliferation of fibroblasts around cancer cells in an autocrine or paracrine fashion [88, 89].

FGF2 is involved in the induction of angiogenesis in several cancers, pheochromocytoma, renal cell carcinoma, astrocytoma, bladder carcinoma, hepatocellular carcinoma, and prostate cancer, and also in the signals between the epithelium and connective tissue, influencing growth and differentiation. Raimondi et al. have reported FGF2 immunostaining in the cytoplasm of the basal layers of the epithelium in hamster cheek pouch model of oral cancer. Nayak et al. observed a decrease in the expression of FGF2, FGFR2, and FGFR3 in OSF compared to normal subjects [90].

#### 12.5.2.8 Notch

Notch signaling is a highly conserved, ubiquitous, cell-cell communication pathway involved in cell fate, proliferation, and tissue homeostasis both in embryonic development and in adult life. Notch gene is located on chromosome 9q34.3, and its transcript includes 34 exons.

Notch activation requires binding between the Notch receptor exposed on the surface of a "signal-receiving cell" and the Notch ligand on a juxtaposed "signal-sending cell." Receptor-ligand interactions commit Notch receptor to a two-step proteolytic cascade generating a transcriptionally active intracellular fragment.

Notch signaling network is an evolutionarily conserved intercellular signaling pathway that regulates interactions between physically adjacent cells. Five ligands, namely Delta-like 1, Delta-like 3, Delta-like 4, Jagged-1, and Jagged-2, were identified for the four notch receptor members Notch 1, Notch 2, Notch 3, and Notch 4 in mammals. The Notch receptors are single transmembrane polypeptides synthesized in the endoplasmic reticulum and transported to the cell surface through the trans-Golgi network. They share structural elements containing an extracellular domain with multiple epidermal growth factor-like (EGF) repeats, transmembrane domain, and an intracellular domain with multiple subdomains [91, 92].

The Notch proteins are cleaved in the trans-Golgi network and presented on the cell surface as a heterodimer. Binding of ligands from the surface of neighboring cells to the receptor on the adjacent cell induces the conformational change of Notch, leading to the exposure of S2 site, and triggers sequentially proteolytic cleavage by A disintegrin and metalloprotease (ADAM) and the γ-secretase complex. Cleavage by ADAM produces a substrate for the second cleavage by the presenilin-containing γ-secretase complex, releasing the Notch intracellular domain (NICD). The cleaved NICD is then translocated to the nucleus where it binds with the transcription factor CBF1/suppressor of hairless/Lag1 (CSL) and modulates gene expression. Without NICD, CBF1 (also known as RBPJ) protein binds to the consensus DNA sequence in association with SMART/HDAC complex, acting as a transcriptional repressor. Interaction between NICD and CBF1 displaces the SMART/HDAC corepressor complex, which is replaced with a co-activator complex (MAML1–3, EP300, and SNW1). This results in the transcriptional activation of the target genes primarily involving two families of helix-loop-helix transcription factors Hes (hairy/enhancer of split) and Hey (hairy/enhancer of spit related with YRPW motif). In addition to this canonical signaling pathway, noncanonical Notch signaling independent of either CBF1 or γ-secretase cleavage or both has been identified.

Posttranslational modifications including O-fucosylation and O-glycosylation via fringe proteins (lunatic, radical, and manic) regulate the specificity of Notch receptor-ligand binding and are also critical for its function. Termination of Notch signaling in the cell can occur naturally at or downstream of the Notch receptor. The Notch receptor can undergo lysosomal degradation involving the ubiquitin ligase Itch/AIP4 or Nedd4, which acts together with Numb and Itch/AIP4. GSK3 controls NICD1 ubiquitination and proteasome-mediated degradation by phosphorylation of the NICD and regulates the NICD interaction with the E3 ubiquitin ligase CDC4/FBW7 [91, 93] (◘ Fig. 12.7).

Before integration into the plasma membrane, Notch receptor is decorated with different glycans by a complex series of enzymatic reactions occurring within the endoplasmic reticulum (ER) or the Golgi network. Posttranslational adducts determine a differential responsiveness of Notch-expressing cells to the ligands. Thereafter, Notch receptor is cleaved at the level of the S1 cleavage site (S1) by a furin-like convertase residing in the trans-Golgi network. The cleavage results in the formation of a heterodimeric receptor, consisting of a Notch extracellular domain (NECD) and a Notch transmembrane domain (NTMD) held together by $Ca^{2+}$-dependent ionic bonds. Similarly, also Notch ligand undergoes a "maturation process" consisting of its endocytosis, ubiquitination by the Neuralized and Mindbomb E3 ubiquitin ligases, and "recycling" to the plasma membrane. Notch ligands belong to the Delta/Serrate/LAG2 (DSL) protein family. After ligand binding, the mature Notch receptor is subjected to two successive proteolytic cleavages (S2 and S3 cleavage). The first cleavage is exerted by an ADAM metalloprotease (e.g., ADAM17) close to the transmembrane domain to generate the Notch extracellular truncation (NEXT) fragment (S2 cleavage). The second is operated by the γ-secretase complex within the transmembrane domain of the NEXT fragment (S3 cleavage) or in endosomes, to dump into the cytoplasm the biologically active Notch intracellular domain (NICD). In the cell nucleus, NICD

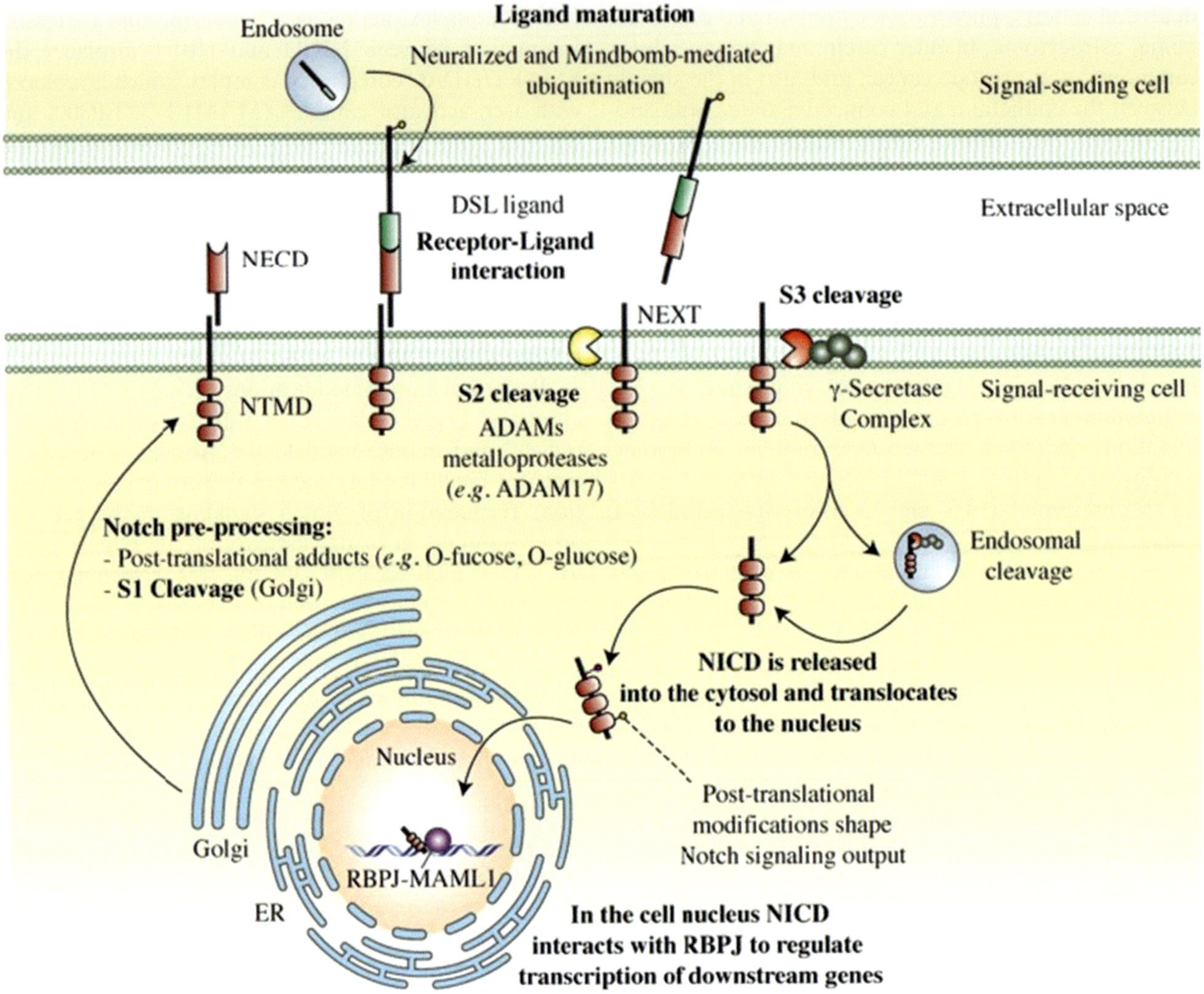


**Fig. 12.7** An overview of Notch maturation, activation, and processing

forms a trimeric complex with RBPJ and MAML1, which initiates transcription of Notch downstream target genes [91].

### 12.5.2.9 Notch and Myofibroblast Differentiation

Myofibroblasts are the major extracellular matrix-producing cells. They are enriched in injured tissue undergoing repair/remodeling and are thought to promote repair by contracting the edges of the wound. Additionally, myofibroblasts produce matrix to facilitate the repair process. If they do not undergo apoptosis upon successful repair, excessive matrix production by persistent myofibroblasts can result in exuberant scar formation and fibrosis. Thus, chronic fibrotic lesions in diverse tissues are characterized by the persistence of these myofibroblasts. Recent evidence further indicates that the Notch signaling pathway is also involved in the regulation of myofibroblast differentiation in chronic fibrosis in the lung, kidney, liver, heart, and skin [94, 95].

### 12.5.2.10 Notch and Epithelial-Mesenchymal Transition (EMT)

The role of Notch signaling in the regulation of EMT is suggested by indirect and direct studies. Notch signaling molecules are reported to activate TGF-β in rat mesangial cells under hyperglycemic conditions. Since EMT is associated with chronic fibrosis in the kidney, lung, liver, and heart, evidence for Notch signaling in EMT focused on epithelial cells derived in these tissues. In rat alveolar epithelial cell line, ectopic expression of the NICD or by co-culture with Jagged1 expression cells induced the expression of mesenchymal marker genes including ACTA2, collagen I, and vimentin with concomitant reduction in the expression of epithelial marker genes such as E-cadherin, occludin, and zonula occludens-1. In addition to these direct effects mediated by its intracellular domain, Notch can indirectly regulate EMT through other signaling pathways, including TGF-β, NF-κB, and β-catenin, and through the action of various regulatory miRNAs [94].

Lunde et al. explored the genome-wide profiles of chromosomal aberrations in samples of oral cancer (OC), oral submucous fibrosis (OSF), and their corresponding normal oral mucosa and found that Notch 4 was one among the 30 genes that showed significant amplifications in their genetic profile [96].

#### 12.5.2.11 Integrins

Integrins, a family of transmembrane cell adhesion molecules, play a key role in mediating intercellular and cell-matrix interactions. Thus, integrins provide a major node of communication between the extracellular matrix, inflammatory cells, fibroblasts, and parenchymal cells and, as such, are intimately involved in the initiation, maintenance, and resolution of tissue fibrosis. Integrins are composed of non-covalent α/β heterodimers of which there are 24 known members in humans and comprise 18 different α subunits and 8 β subunits. They can translate extracellular signals, resulting in a wide range of downstream effects on cell adhesion, migration, proliferation, differentiation, and apoptosis. Of particular note is the αv subunit, which forms heterodimers with the β1, β3, β5, β6, or β8 subunits [97, 98].

#### 12.5.2.12 Role of Integrins in Fibrosis

αv integrins (β1, β3, β5, β8) expressed on fibroblasts and αvβ6 expressed on epithelia activate transforming growth factor-beta (TGF-β) through their interaction with a linear arginine-glycine-aspartic acid (RGD)-binding motif present on the latency-associated peptide (LAP) in the extracellular matrix (ECM). TGF-β released from the ECM by injured epithelia might directly signal to the myofibroblast to promote further ECM production. Furthermore, αv integrins on myofibroblasts can release active TGF-β from the ECM, which further drives the production by myofibroblasts [99, 100] (◘ Fig. 12.8).

One cell type intrinsically involved in organ scarring is the myofibroblast that provides a major source of ECM proteins during fibrogenesis. Being highly contractile cells, myofibroblasts express several αv integrins that transmit the force generated by the actin cytoskeleton to the ECM. αv integrins (β1, β3, β5, β8) expressed on fibroblasts and αvβ6 expressed on epithelia activate transforming growth factor-beta (TGF-β) through their interaction with a linear arginine-glycine-aspartic acid (RGD)-binding motif present on the latency-associ-

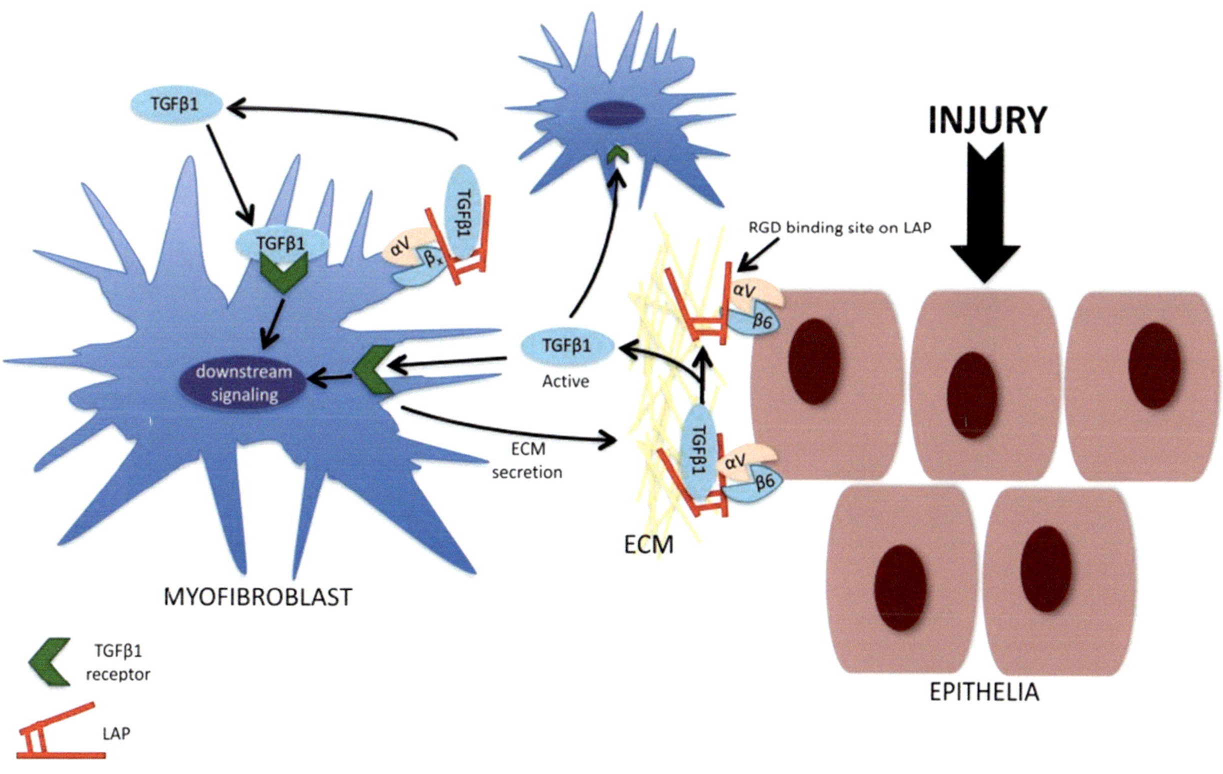


◘ **Fig. 12.8** Complex interplay of αv integrin-mediated regulation of tissue fibrosis ated peptide (LAP) in the extracellular matrix (ECM). TGF-β released from the ECM by injured epithelia might directly signal to the myofibroblast to promote further ECM production. Furthermore, αv integrins on myofibroblasts can release active TGF-β from the ECM; this TGF-β then signals in an autocrine manner to drive further ECM production by myofibroblasts [97].

Myofibroblast αv integrins are able to liberate and thereby activate TGF-β1 deposits in the ECM via mechanical force. Further insights into this process have been provided by Klingberg et al. (2014) who demonstrated, through a series of in vitro experiments, that latent ECM-bound TGF-β1 is primed by the stiffening of the surrounding ECM, such that greater amounts are released compared with a relaxed ECM. Therefore, prior to force-mediated activation of TGF-β1, myofibroblasts actively reorganize the ECM, increasing the bioavailability of the bound latent TGF-β1 complex.

Myofibroblasts express αvβ1 integrin, which can activate (release) TGF-β1 (and presumably TGF-β3) by virtue of αvβ1 interaction with the RGD sequence in the LAP component of the small and large latent TGF-β complexes (SLC and LLC, respectively). Such activation may involve mechanical traction exerted by connections between αvβ1 integrin and contractile cytoskeleton and between latent TGF-β (LTBP) component of the LLC and matrix proteins such as fibrillins and fibronectin. Free TGF-β induces collagen gene transcription and translation by myofibroblasts in a SMAD-dependent fashion and also induces the differentiation of myofibroblasts from a variety of potential progenitors [99] (◘ Fig. 12.9).

A subset of the integrin family (αv integrins) plays a key role in the activation of latent TGF-β1. Specifically, the integrins αvβ3, αvβ5, αvβ6, and αvβ8 have been shown to bind the RGD sequence in the latency-associated peptide (LAP) of TGF-β1 and -β3 and have the potential to activate latent TGF-β6, 7, 8, 9, and 10.

There is evidence to prove that the cells with increased β1 integrin expression are stem cell populations of the epithelium. β1 integrin regulates keratinocyte proliferation, and it is also responsible for the maintenance of skin stem cells. Loss of β1 integrin reduces the proliferation of keratinocytes. Depending on the environmental cues, integrins take part both in the survival as well as in the apoptosis mechanisms. Ligated integrin relays survival signals, whereas unligated integrins can promote pro-apoptotic cascades. The epithelial atrophy in moderate and advanced OSF without epithelial dysplasia may be attributed to the lower percentage of β1 integrin-



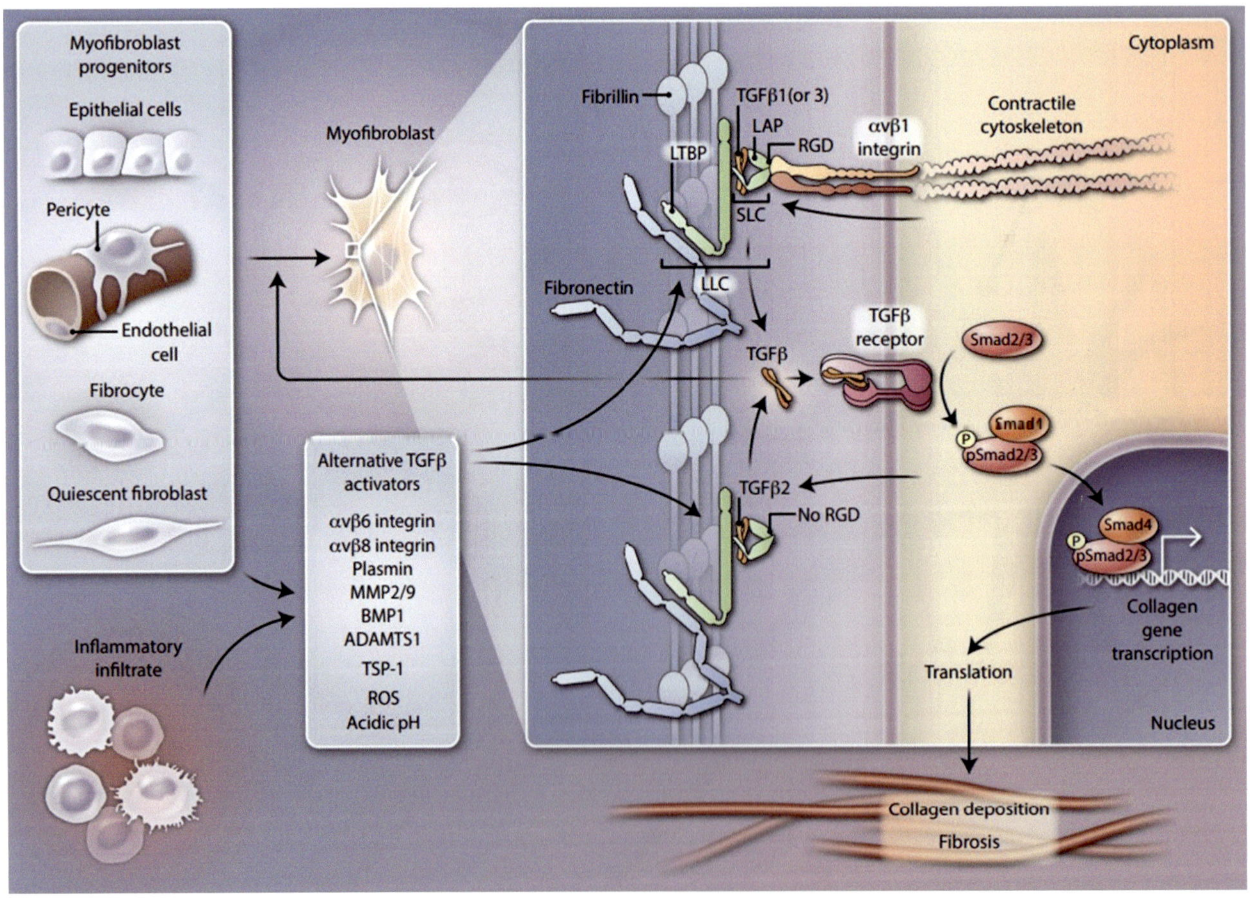


◘ **Fig. 12.9** Integrin-activated TGF-β inducing fibrosis

positive cells, which indicates the decrease in the stem cell population in the basal layer. The OSF with pronounced atrophy showed marked reduction in the thickness of the spinous layer. The reduction in the number of stem cells and its influence on proliferation could be considered as one major event involved in such alteration [101–103]. Veeravarmal et al. have demonstrated that the non-dysplastic epithelium of OSF with severe atrophy showed lowest percentage of β-integrin expression. It is inferred that the absence of stem cells and proliferation may attribute to the atrophy [104].

> Upregulated expression of αvβ6 integrin of keratinocytes under arecoline's effect supports the activation of latent TGF-β1 present in ECM that in turn triggers the myofibroblastic transformation of fibroblasts.

## 12.6 Extracellular Matrix, and Epithelial-to-Mesenchymal Transition

### 12.6.1 Molecular Characterization/Molecular Pathogenesis of Oral Submucous Fibrosis

Oral submucous fibrosis pathogenesis is characterized by an imbalance between collagen deposition and degradation, leading to fibrosis, and both these processes have been postulated to contribute to pathogenesis. Type I collagen, which has been found to be the predominant isoform, is composed of two α1 (I) and one α2 (I) polypeptide chains, produced by the COL1A1 and COL1A2 genes. One other important observation relates to the expression of pro-fibrotic cytokines in oral submucous fibrosis tissues. Earlier reports suggested increased expression of transforming growth factor-β by immunohistochemical staining of oral submucous fibrosis tissues. The importance of transforming growth factor-β in the regulation of extracellular matrix synthesis has been known for several decades. Since then, several fibrotic conditions that affect mankind have been found to involve transforming growth factor-β, and the mechanisms involved in tissue fibrosis are increasingly understood. Fibroblasts in oral submucous fibrosis tissues have been shown to synthesize higher levels of collagen than normal fibroblasts do. This could be due to an irreversible transformation of these into activated fibroblasts similar to those described in the stroma of epithelial malignancies: so-called cancer-associated fibroblasts. Immunohistochemical analysis shows a significant association between the increased expression of type I collagen and its chaperone colligin/heat-shock protein 47 in oral submucous fibrosis lesions. As colligin plays a vital role in the folding and assembling of collagen, it could be possible that the increased level of collagen in oral submucous fibrosis tissues is because of its overstabilization by colligin. The other major mechanism that can promote fibrosis is by reducing collagen degradation, leading to stabilization of collagen bundles. Collagenases are zinc endopeptidases and are considered as the major matrix-degrading enzymes in collagen homeostasis. There are three mammalian collagenases: matrix metalloproteinases, 1, 8, and 13, belonging to the family of matrix metalloproteinases, which are the principal secreted endopeptidases capable of cleaving collagenous extracellular matrix. Collagenase activity in oral submucous fibrosis tissue fibroblast cells was found to be lower than that in normal fibroblasts. Also, areca nut polyphenols (catechin and tannin) are known to reduce collagenase activity and increase cross-linking of collagen fibrils, making them less susceptible to collagenase degradation. This imbalance between collagen synthesis and degradation may lead to excessive pro-collagen 1α1 chains, relative to 1α2, resulting in the alteration of the tri-helical structure of collagen molecules, from 2:1 to 3:1. Although the biological significance of this changed composition of collagen 1 is not clear, this form of collagen is more resistant to degradation by proteases than the normal collagen molecule is. Collagen production and degradation are also finely controlled by the balance of the pro-fibrogenic and anti-fibrogenic cytokines. A change in the expression of pro-fibrogenic and anti-fibrogenic cytokines can change the homeostasis of collagen production, leading to pathological conditions like the various forms of fibrotic disease [54].

#### 12.6.1.1 Factors Regulating Extracellular Matrix (ECM) Remodeling

Equilibrium between two enzyme groups, matrix metalloproteinases (MMPs) and TIMPs, is mandatory to achieve accurate and balanced collagen metabolism and thereby maintain the normal integrity of connective tissue. In OSF, the equilibrium between MMPs and TIMPs is disturbed in such a manner that it ultimately results in increased deposition of ECM. Arecoline influences the deposition of extracellular matrix (ECM) by increasing the production of tissue inhibitor of metalloproteinase-1 (TIMP-1) and decreasing matrix metalloproteinases (MMPs).

Involvement of the connective tissue growth factor (CTGF) in fibrosis in many human tissues is well established. CTGF is only produced by hepatic stellate and kidney mesangial cells in adults under normal conditions. Deng et al. showed the expression of CTGF in OSF fibroblasts and endothelial cells in all of the OSF cases included in their study. In vitro, arecoline stimulated CTGF production in buccal mucosal fibroblasts through the generation of reactive oxygen species (ROS) and by the activation of NFekB, JNK, and p38 MAPK pathways. It is also known that NFekB, JNK, and p38 are strongly activated by ROS.

In the early stages of OSF, overexpression of tenascin, perlecan, fibronectin, and collagen type III may be found in the lamina propria and submucosa, and extensive and irregular deposits of elastin have been found around muscle fibers in the intermediate stage, together with these molecules. In the advanced stage of OSF, collagen type I appears to dominate the ECM. The gene expression levels of the molecules varied with the progression of fibrosis. This pattern of ECM remodeling steps in OSF is similar to the normal granulation tissue formation and maturation process. Difficulty in opening the mouth may be related to loss of various ECM molecules, such as elastin, and replacement of muscle by collagen type I [105, 106].

#### 12.6.1.2 Matrix Metalloproteinases and Tissue Inhibitors of Matrix Metalloproteinases (MMPs and TIMPs)

Matrix metalloproteinases (MMPs) are zinc-dependent endopeptidases that are capable of degrading extracellular matrix proteins. MMPs are a family of zinc- and calcium-dependent proteolytic enzymes, which are involved in a wide variety of biological processes ranging from physiological role such as cell proliferation and differentiation, normal development, and wound healing to pathological states associated with inflammation, degeneration, tumor metastasis, and growth. MMPs and TIMPs play a pivotal role in maintaining the balance in remodeling of the ECM, and disruption of this balance may result in diseases associated with uncontrolled turnover of matrix. The major subgroups are interstitial collagenases, gelatinases, stromelysin, and membrane-bound MMPs. They are produced by several cell types, including fibroblasts, macrophages, neutrophils, and some epithelial cells. Their secretion is induced by certain stimuli, including growth factors, cytokines, and physical stress.

12

Collagenase, a member of the MMP family, is secreted as a latent precursor (procollagenase) and is activated by chemicals such as free radicals produced during the oxidative burst of leukocytes and proteinases. Members of the collagenase subgroup of MMPs, that is, collagenase 1 (MMP-1), collagenase 2 (MMP-8), and collagenase 3 (MMP-13), are the principal neutral proteinases capable of degrading native fibrillar collagens in the extracellular space. Collagenase-1 (MMP-1) is produced by a wide variety of normal cells such as stromal fibroblasts, macrophages, endothelial cells, and epithelial cells, as well as by numerous tumors, suggesting a broad-based role for this collagenase in biology.

MMP-13 is a member of the collagenase family, which degrades fibrillar collagens of types I, II, III, IV, X, and XIV, tenascin, fibronectin, aggrecan, vesicant, and fibrillin-I. It also plays a key role in the activation cascade, both activating and being activated by several MMPs. Elevated MMP-13 levels have been reported in a number of malignancies and have also been associated with tumor behavior and prognosis. The imbalance between the activities of MMPs and TIMPs is associated with pathological conditions, namely proliferative scarring, keloid, submucosal fibrosis, gingival overgrowth, and plantar fibromatosis [107].

Mishra et al. and Shrestha et al. report an increase in MMP-1 and MMP-2 expression, respectively, by immunohistochemical analysis in OSF, whereas Illeperuma et al. demonstrate a decrease in MMP-1 expression [108].

Illeperuma et al. showed that MMP-1 expression was attenuated in OSF, while TGF-β1 expression was upregulated compared to normal oral mucosa. No significant relationship was found between epithelial dysplasia and expressions of TGF-β1, MMP-1, and TIMP-1 in OSF. This study provides further evidence that the fibrotic process in OSF is not only due to excessive collagen deposition but also due to disequilibrium in the ECM remodeling process. Neither the ECM remodeling process nor the tissue fibrosis of OSF directly shows any significant effect on epithelial dysplasia. TIMP-1 expression was reduced, and TIMP-2 expression was increased in the studies done by Illeperuma et al. and Shrestha et al., respectively [59].

#### 12.6.1.3 Alpha-Smooth Muscle Actin (α-SMA)

α-SMA is involved in wound healing and tissue repair. Less generally appreciated is the notion that the transformation of fibroblast to myofibroblasts is a key, perhaps essential, event for the cells to perform these functions. α-SMA is significantly increased in oral submucous fibrosis.

Myofibroblasts are a unique group of cells phenotypically intermediate between smooth muscle cells and fibroblasts. They can be identified by certain characteristic features of the cytoskeleton, particularly by the expression of α smooth muscle actin, and are believed to be primary producers of extracellular matrix. Myofibroblasts appear to be major effector cells in many fibrotic disorders like scleroderma, hepatic and pancreatic fibrosis, and pulmonary fibrosis. Myofibroblasts may stimulate tumor progression by increasing the growth of cancer cells, inducing blood vessel formation and lymphangiogenesis, after injury. In addition to their normal role in tissue homeostasis and repair, altered number and function of myofibroblasts have been implicated in diseases with increased extracellular matrix (ECM) deposition and resultant fibrosis. These cells attenuate cancer cell death and stimulate invasion and metastasis by activating proteolysis. The arrangement of myofibroblasts is confined to the stroma immediately adjacent to the tumor islands, and tumor-free stroma is devoid of myofibroblasts. The presence of myofibroblasts in close proximity to tumor cells is supported by two hypotheses: Myofibroblasts can possibly be derived from the epithelial mesenchymal transition of the tumor cells, and myofibroblasts form tunnels that lead the invasive tumor cells in vitro. Therefore, myofibroblasts act as key players in collective tumor invasion as they are capable of remodeling the extracellular matrix and providing the mechanical propulsive force that facilitates invasion [109–112].

#### 12.6.1.4 Epithelial-Mesenchymal Transition in Oral Submucous Fibrosis

An alarming complication associated with OSF is the higher risk of transforming to oral squamous cell carcinoma (OSCC). It has been described that the pathological changes in the connective tissue of OSF are likely to affect the overlying epithelium and induce EMT. Epithelial-to-mesenchymal transition (EMT) is a biological process involving the transition of a polarized epithelial cell into a cell that has the characteristics of a mesenchymal phenotype. EMT is crucial for developmental milestones such as gastrulation of the metazoans, neural crest formation, and heart morphogenesis. EMT is shown to be elicited following chronic inflammation and during wound healing. The role of EMT has increasingly gained significance as an essential process in fibrosis and carcinogenesis.

EMT is a process in which there is a reduced expression of epithelial genes (E-cadherin) and an increase in the expression of mesenchymal genes (N-cadherin) and EMT transcription factors. Together with an altered localization of the β-catenin, the epithelial cells lose their phenotype and intercellular adhesions. Besides, there is an increased expression of vimentin, signifying a mesenchymal change in the cytoskeleton. An increase in tenascin implies that the matrix deposition enables the migration of cells. Significantly, the matrix metalloproteinase 9 (MMP-9) overexpression demonstrates the disruption of the basement membrane and the proneness of cells to infiltrate the underlying stroma [113–115].

The inflammatory reaction antecedent to fibrosis and the role of EMT in fibrogenesis and malignant transformation in other organs point to the involvement of EMT in the pathogenesis of OSF and its malignant transformation. The inflammatory cytokines produced in response to the inflammation may mediate the progression of OSF via various EMT pathways. The membranous loss of E-cadherin, β-catenin, cytokeratin 5 (CK 5), and cytokeratin 14 (CK 14) with an overwhelming expression of vimentin, N-cadherin, and α-smooth muscle actin (α-SMA) seen in OSF further confirms the role of EMT in OSF [116–119].

## 12.7 Epithelial Factors

### 12.7.1 E-cadherin

The cell adhesion molecule, E-cadherin (E-cad), is a tumor suppressor that is expressed in epithelial tissues. E-cad, 120 kDa glycoprotein, is a calcium-dependent cell-surface adhesion molecule that works as an intercellular adhesion molecule between epithelial cells and is also involved in the transduction of signals controlling various cellular events, including polarity, differentiation, growth, and cell migration. In addition, E-cad has the ability to inhibit cell proliferation by upregulating the p27 via epidermal growth factor receptor. Therefore, E-cad is described as a major growth or proliferation suppressor biomarker. The loss in E-cad expression has been correlated with cancer progression. E-cadherin is also known to express in various carcinomas of head and neck, esophagus, prostrate, pancreas, stomach, and uterine cervix, and its reduced expression has been correlated with aggressive behavior, high proliferation, invasion, metastasis, and poor prognosis of cancer [120, 121].

A decrease in E-cadherin levels in OSF compared to normal has been reported. E-cad was decreased in OSF compared to normal and habit group without OSF. E-cad expression was similar in OSF without dysplasia and with mild dysplasia. A significant loss of membranous E-cadherin was observed in OSF with moderate and severe dysplasia. Increased cytoplasmic E-cad with marked loss of membranous E-cad was seen in OSF with severe dysplasia. E-cadherin expression was reduced with increasing grades of OSCC [120, 121].

**DCs CD303, CD1a, and CD207**—Distribution of immature dendritic cells (DCs), Langerhans cells, and plasmacytoid cells.

Dendritic cells (DCs) are antigen-presenting cells responsible for starting the immune response mediated by B and T lymphocytes. An adequate immune response protects the mucosa from malignant transformation.

CD303 is used to identify plasmacytoid DCs, which are resident in lymphoid or nonlymphoid organs and are responsible for the production of type I interferon. CD303 or blood dendritic cell antigen (BDCA) is a type II lectin used to identify plasmacytoid DC. Plasmacytoid DCs reside in lymphoid and nonlymphoid organs and produce large amounts of type I interferon (IFN). CD303+ cells have been associated with organism defense [122, 123].

CD207/Langerin are effective in identifying immature DCs and Langerhans cells. The expression of the CD207 receptor in DCs evidences that the antigen is effectively coupled with MHC-I and MHC-II, a condition that activates the CD8+ and CD4+ T cells; therefore, the downregulation of this receptor in DCs might indicate a suppression of the T-cell response [122, 124].

CD1a is effective in identifying immature DCs and Langerhans cells. Langerhans cells (LCs), dendritic, non-keratinocytic clear cells of the oral epithelium present in the suprabasal layer, are derived from myeloid stem cells of bone marrow. They are antigen-presenting cells (APCs) that aid to provoke a specific T cell reaction by the interaction of the MHC class II with the CD4+ cells They belong to the family of dendritic cell system (DCS), among which LCs can be differentiated from others by the presence of Birbeck granules [125].

CD1a and CD207 is effective in identifying immature DCs and Langerhans cells. Silva et al. reported an increase in CD303-positive cells and decrease in CD207 and CD1a cells in oral submucous fibrosis compared to the normal subjects [122, 124–126].

### 12.7.2 CD147

CD147, a highly glycosylated transmembrane protein and a member of the immunoglobulin (Ig) superfamily, is extensively expressed on the surface of a myriad of cells, including tumor, epithelial, endothelial, and immune cells. CD147 plays a prominent role in organ fibrosis, which includes liver, renal interstitium, and lung. Upregulation of CD147 is stimulated by TGF-β1, a crucial pro-fibrogenic cytokine, and contributes to pathological angiogenesis by inducing the VEGF-A/VEGFR2 signaling pathway in the liver, which aggravates liver fibrosis.

12

CD147/Emmprin, a highly glycosylated transmembrane protein and a member of the immunoglobulin (Ig) superfamily, is extensively expressed on the surface of a myriad of cells, including tumor, epithelial, endothelial, and immune cells. Wang et al. observed that CD147 was highly expressed in both human oral keratinocytes (HOKs) and fibrotic oral mucosa and that this expression was correlated with TGF-β1 expression. Additionally, CD147 levels were significantly associated with the fibrosis stage. The TGF-β1 signaling pathway was found to be mainly responsible for CD147 upregulation after arecoline treatment, whereas inhibition of TGF-β1 downregulated CD147 expression [56, 127].

### 12.7.3 Cytokeratin

Cytokeratins (CKs) are major intermediate filaments in squamous epithelium and are critical in cell stabilization, shape, intracellular signaling, and transport. They contribute to the maintenance of the cytoskeletal framework of these cells and are specifically expressed by epithelial tissues. Cytokeratin intermediate filaments are present in essentially all epithelial cells and in neoplasms derived from them. Cytokeratins are divided into more than 20 subtypes. This subdivision is based on their isoelective pH as well as their molecular weight. Type I is acidic group with low molecular weight (40–64 kDa), CKs 9–23, and tends to be of lower molecular weight. The basic group (1–8) is of higher molecular weight. Type II is basic or neutral with high molecular weight (52–68 kDa), CKs 1–8 [128, 129].

CK 5/6 is present at the level of the basal layer of the keratinized and non-keratinized stratified squamous epithelia. CK5 expression is decreased at the level of the spinosum stratum of the normal oral mucosa, and in the dysplastic epithelium, CK5 is positive in the basal, parabasal, and stratum spinosum cells [130].

CK 10 expression in keratinized epithelium is a marker for terminal differentiation and maturation of epithelial cells. CK 8 and CK 18 are the most common and characteristic members of the large intermediate filament gene family and are expressed in "simple" or single-layer epithelial tissues, associated with dysplasia grades of tumor precursor lesions and an unfavorable prognosis for patients with SCCs. Loss of CK 8 phosphorylation initiated an increased cell migration and tumor spread in SCCs, whereas loss of CKs 8 and 18 led to alterations in CK 8 and 18 α6β4 integrin-mediated signaling and decreased neoplastic progression [131].

The combined overexpression of CK5 and CK14 was demonstrated in tumors of the oral cavity, in the oropharyngeal, hypopharyngeal, and laryngeal areas, and in the basal actively mitotic cells of the squamous stratified epithelium. The expression of CK5 and CK14 remains high even if the malignant grading decreases. Bag et al. and Nanda et al. have shown an increase in CK 5/6, CK 10, CK 8, and CK 18 in OSF tissue. However, Malik et al. observed a decrease in CK 14 in OSF tissues [129, 132].

### 12.7.4 Annexin and Filamin

The annexins, a multigene family of calcium-dependent phospholipid-binding proteins, have some special functions that include the aggregation of vesicles and regulation of ion channels as well as roles in the regulation of cell cycle, cell signal, and cell differentiation. ANXA4 is related to the loss of cell adhesion and plays important roles in apoptosis, carcinogenesis, chemoresistance, migration, and invasion of cancer cells.

Filamin (FLNA) is a type of actin filament cross-linking protein that participates in cytoskeletal rearrangement. By its scaffolding function, FLNA can interact with more than 90 functionally diverse binding partners to regulate cellular functions and processes. FLNA could be regarded as a novel biomarker for the diagnosis and outcome prediction of cancer because of its ability to control cell mobility, cell-ECM interactions, cell signaling, and DNA damage response. Annexin and filamin are significantly increased in oral submucous fibrosis [133].

### 12.7.5 Loricrin

Loricrin is a major component of the cornified cell envelope (CE) keratins. These keratins are structural proteins and constitute about 85% of a fully differentiated keratinocyte. They belong to a multigene family coded by more than 30 intermediate filament genes and form the cytoskeleton of the vertebrate epithelial cells. It is introduced into the scaffold of the cornified envelope because of its cross-linking and binding property. Interaction of loricrin with the keratin intermediate filaments provides flexibility to the CE. Loricrin also protects against mechanical stress by its association with nectin and calcium induction levels [134].

Chewing hard areca causes both mechanical and chemical stress and creates an environment similar to that of a dry epithelium, leading to expression of loricrin and formation of a CE. Areca nut is usually taken along with lime (calcium hydroxide), and increased calcium concentration aids the barrier recovery process with loricrin being expressed. Variation in the different stages of oral submucous fibrosis could be due to the adapting capacity of the epithelia towards a new stimulus as shown by altered loricrin expression and can be useful in early identification of any transformation potential [134].

Nithya et al. demonstrated significant increase in loricrin expression in OSF in the stratum granulosum and also reported significant association of the marker expression with habits (chewing, alcohol, and smoking) in OSF patients [135].

## 12.8 Receptor Tyrosine Kinase Pathway

RTK signaling pathway can be activated by various growth factors such as epidermal growth factor (EGF), vascular endothelial growth factor (VEGF), platelet-derived growth factor (PDGF), fibroblast growth factor (FGF), and insulin-like growth factor (IGF). These growth factors bind to the external domain of RTK, inducing the dimerization and subsequent autophosphorylation of the tyrosine residue in the receptor, hence activating the downstream signaling pathways such as PI3K/Akt/mTOR and ERK/MAPK pathways [136, 137].

## 12.9 Transcription Factors

The transcription factors bind to the promoter region of the CDH1 gene encoding E-cadherin and thus initiate EMT. An important attribute of EMT is the loss of expression of cell-cell adhesion molecule, E-cadherin. Among the transcription factors directly contributing to this process include snail superfamily of zinc-finger transcription factors, Snail1 and Snail2 (also known as Slug) and zinc-finger E-box-binding homeobox (ZEB) family with the ZF (zinc finger) class of homeodomain transcription factors ZEB1, ZEB2, and TWIST1 gene, which encodes a basic helix-loop-helix (bHLH) transcription factor [4] and lymphoid enhancer-binding factor-1 (LEF-1) [74, 138].

## 12.10 Wnt Signaling Pathway

Wnt signals are transduced through the binding of Wnt proteins to the extracellular domain of frizzled (Fz) protein, in the presence of cofactors such as low-density lipoprotein-related protein5/6 (LRP5/6), which is required to mediate the canonical Wnt signal. In the absence of signaling, β-catenin is degraded by the β-catenin destruction complex, which includes Axin, tumor suppressor adenomatosis polyposis coli (APC), glycogen synthase kinase 3β (GSK-3β), and casein kinase 1α (CK1α). Phosphorylation of β-catenin by this complex drives it for ubiquitination and subsequent proteolytic degradation. In case of Wnt signaling, the binding of Wnt protein to the receptor complex will result in the phosphorylation of LRP5/6 by glycogen synthase kinase 3β and recruitment of cytoplasmic phosphoprotein Dishevelled (Dsh/Dvl) and Axin, which prevents the formation of destruction complex unable to phosphorylate β-catenin, thereby leading to its accumulation in the cytoplasm and translocation into the nucleus. The nuclear β-catenin interacts with transcription factors T cell factor/lymphocyte enhancer factor (TCF/LEF) and inhibits the transcription of E-cadherin to bring about EMT.

A group of secreted Wnt antagonists have been implicated in the regulation of the Wnt/β-catenin-signaling pathway, including Wnt inhibitory factor 1, secreted frizzled-related protein (SFRP), and the dickkopf families. The expression of SERP1 and SERP5 was seen to reduce in OSF undergoing malignant change and was associated with the loss of membranous β-catenin expression. The loss of SERP1 and SERP5 expression was due to promoter methylation. Dickkopf Wnt signaling pathway inhibitor 3 (DKK3) showed upregulation in OSF progressing to OSCC, and a rare mutation of DKK3 was observed in OSCC, along with increased copy numbers. However, in OSF, there was decrease in DKK3 expression seen with further decline with progression in disease. The expression of Wnt inhibitory factor (WIF1), an antagonist of the Wnt signaling, is downregulated in OSF and OSCC due to methylation [139, 140].

## 12.11 Tissue Injury in Oral Submucous Fibrosis

The pathogenesis in OSF is often explained as an overhealing wound because of chronic physical, chemical, and mechanical injury to the oral mucosa. The abrasive character of areca nut inflicts localized microtrauma to the oral mucosa. Betel quid (BQ) constituents released during chewing cause chemical trauma to the oral mucosa. Slaked lime or aqueous calcium hydroxide, one of the BQ constituents, due to its strong alkaline nature (pH = 11) cause chemical irritation to the oral mucosa. The mechanical stress is a direct result of BQ chewing, while the slaked lime component of BQ supplies $Ca^{2+}$ ions. Loricrin, a component of cornified cell envelope, is upregulated by mechanical stress, and there is increased exposure to $Ca^{2+}$ in OSF. The stages of progression of OSF correspond to the stages of maturation of granulation tissue. Immunolocalization patterns of matricellular proteins perlecan and fibronectin explain their role in the maturation of this granulation tissue into fibrosis. Additionally, monocyte chemoattractant protein-1 (MCP-1)/chemokine (C-C motif) ligand 2 (CCL-2)-based recruitment of myofibroblast to the site of epithelial injury in OSF adds credibility to this hypothesis. The upregulation of CCL-2 consequent to chronic epithelial microtrauma neutralizes epithelially derived anti-fibrotic prostaglandin E-2 (PGE-2) through C-C chemokine receptor type 2 (CCR2) or cluster of differentiation 192 (CD192), promoting fibrosis. Filamin-A (FLNA) is one of the two most consistently upregulated biomarkers of squamous cell carcinoma arising in the background of OSF. FLNA is known to shield cells from shear stress, and its upregulation indicates the protective response of oral mucosa towards areca nut chewing-induced mechanical shear stresses [141].

12

**Wound healing versus fibrosis following tissue injury:** In normal wound healing, the activation of myofibroblast is transient, and these cells then undergo apoptosis or quiescence as the provisional ECM degrades and is replaced by parenchymal tissue architecture. However, in fibrosis, chronic injury prevents such resolution of the wound healing cascade, leaving a mixed cell population with pro-inflammatory and pro-fibrotic properties, largely consisting of perpetually activated fibroblasts and myofibroblasts that excessively deposit ECM proteins, including collagens. The fibrotic microenvironment further amplifies the fibrotic response by inducing additional cell damage and oxidative stress due to hypoxia and mechano-transductive signaling in response to dysregulated and enhanced tissue stiffness (◘ Fig. 12.9).

Normal wound healing includes a series of ordered processes: injury, immune cell recruitment and acute inflammation, myofibroblasts' limited activation, and proliferation and ECM homeostasis, leading to wound closure after injury. In pro-fibrotic conditions as observed in OSF, pathological processes including chronic inflammation, myofibroblasts' persistent activation, proliferation, and ECM deposition lead to fibrosis. Fibrosis itself could result in a secondary assault. Extracellular and intracellular factors interact with each other. Their abnormalities contribute to the fibrosis progression and in return are affected by pathological changes [142] (◘ Fig. 12.10).

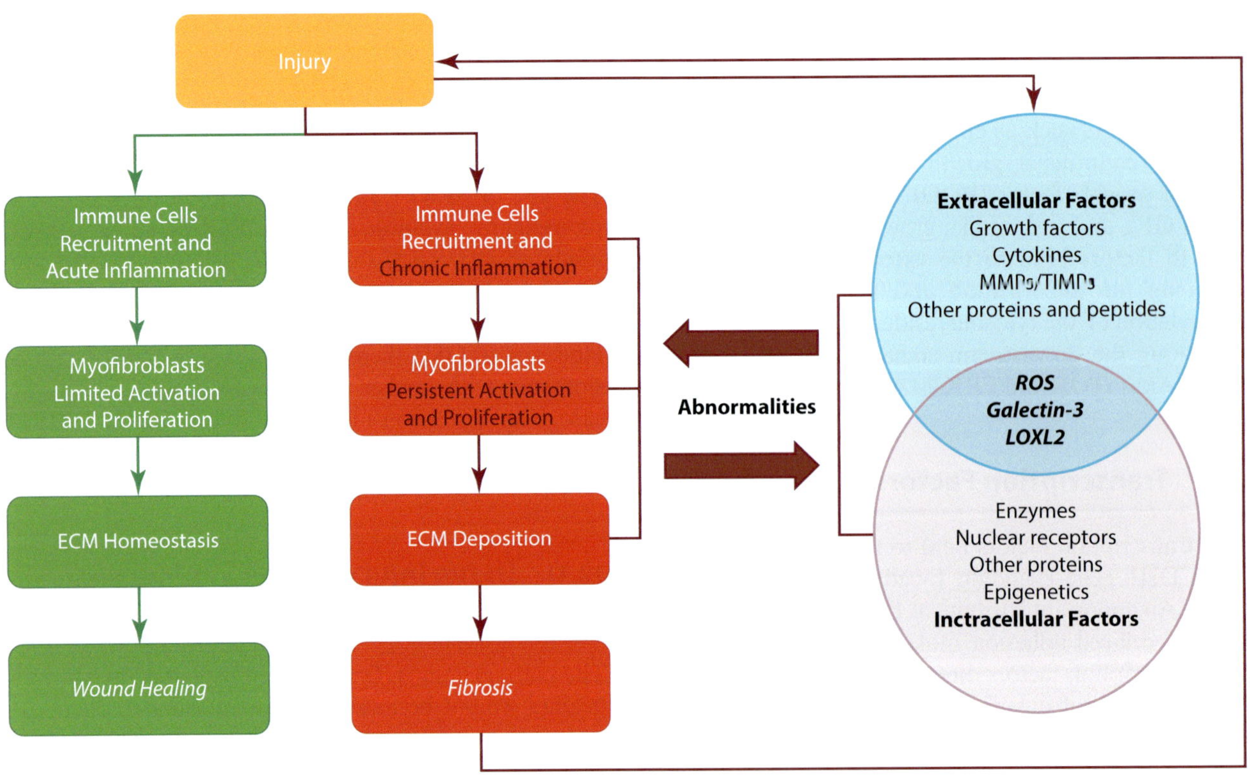


◘ **Fig. 12.10** The cascade of events leading to fibrosis following tissue injury

## 12.12 Anti-fibrotic Factors: Therapeutic Targets for Oral Submucous Fibrosis

**Imatinib:** Imatinib interferes with TGF-β signaling pathways and exerts its anti-fibrotic action. It has shown successful results as an anti-fibrotic drug in preclinical models for treatment of scleroderma. Therefore, it can play an effective role in OSF treatment [143–145].

**Pirfenidone (PFD):** Pirfenidone (5(1H)-pyridone) is a novel anti-fibrotic agent with anti-inflammatory properties used in treating idiopathic lung fibrosis (ILF). ILF is also an inflammatory condition mediated through transforming growth factor-beta (TGF-β). PFD is hypothesized as a novel anti-fibrotic agent beneficial in treating early stages of OSF as both the conditions are mediated through TGF-β. PFD decreases the levels of mRNA encoding type I and III collagen and also inhibits TGF-β1-induced collagen production from fibroblasts. PFD acts by inhibiting tissue inhibitor of metalloproteinase-1 (TIMP-1), pro-inflammatory cytokines TNF-α and fibroblast growth factor (bFGF), and plasminogen activator inhibitor-1 (PAI-1), which are upregulated in OSF. Future randomized clinical trials should be conducted on PFD to understand its efficacy in OSF [143, 146] (◘ Fig. 12.11).

**Nintedanib:** It is used as a second-line drug for lung cancer of the adenocarcinoma subtype. It prevents the phosphorylation of TGF-β1 receptor and reduces excessive ECM production, which is a hallmark of OSF. By inhibiting the platelet-derived growth factor (PDGF) receptor-α and -β, it reduces the level of PDGF, which is upregulated in OSF. It also targets the fibroblast growth factor receptor (FGFR)-1, -2, and -3 and reduces the level of FGF, which is considered a potential biomarker for malignant transformation of OSF. Therefore, nintedanib can be a potential targeted therapy for OSF [147].

**Collagenases:** *Clostridium histolyticum* collagenases (Xiapex) has recently been approved in the management of Dupuytren's contracture, which is characterized by fibrosis. Xiapex contains collagenase which is obtained from the bacterium "*Clostridium histolyticum.*" Collagenase is highly potent and efficaciously digests collagen and its triple helix. Hurst et al. have proven the efficacy of collagenase in the treatment of Dupuytren's contracture in their clinical trial. However, it is not cost effective [147, 148].

**Simtuzumab:** Lysyl oxidase-like 2 (LOXL2) catalyzes collagen cross-linking and is upregulated in OSF. Simtuzumab is a humanized monoclonal antibody targeting the human LOXL2. A phase 2 trial was conducted in idiopathic pulmonary fibrosis (IPF) with simtuzumab, but it was not efficacious in its treatment [149].

**Hyperbaric oxygen therapy (HBO)**: HBO acts by decreasing TNF-α and IL-1, -6, and -8 and enhances wound healing and reduces fibrosis. In vitro studies have demonstrated increased fibroblast proliferation and collagenase synthesis by IL-1 and TNF-α. TNF-α may aggravate fibrosis by inhibition of the collagen phagocytes. The vascular function is impaired in OSF. HBO facilitates angiogenesis through a two-way process:

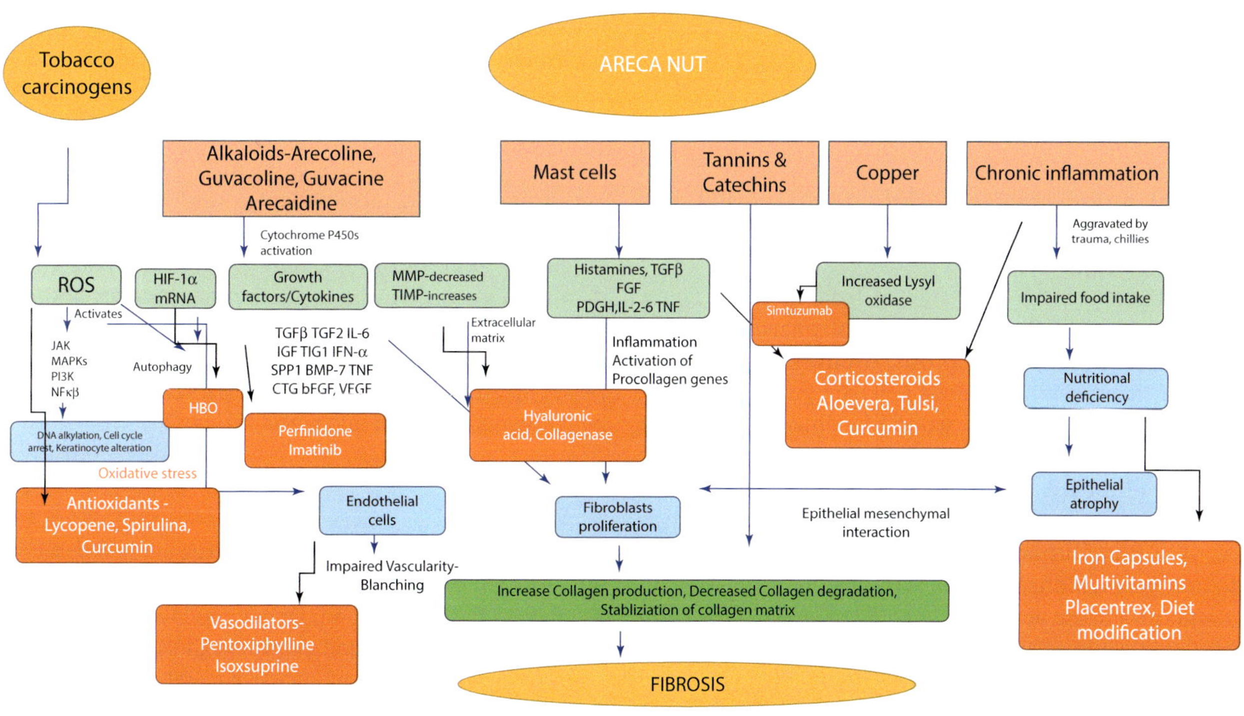


◘ **Fig. 12.11** Targeted drug therapies

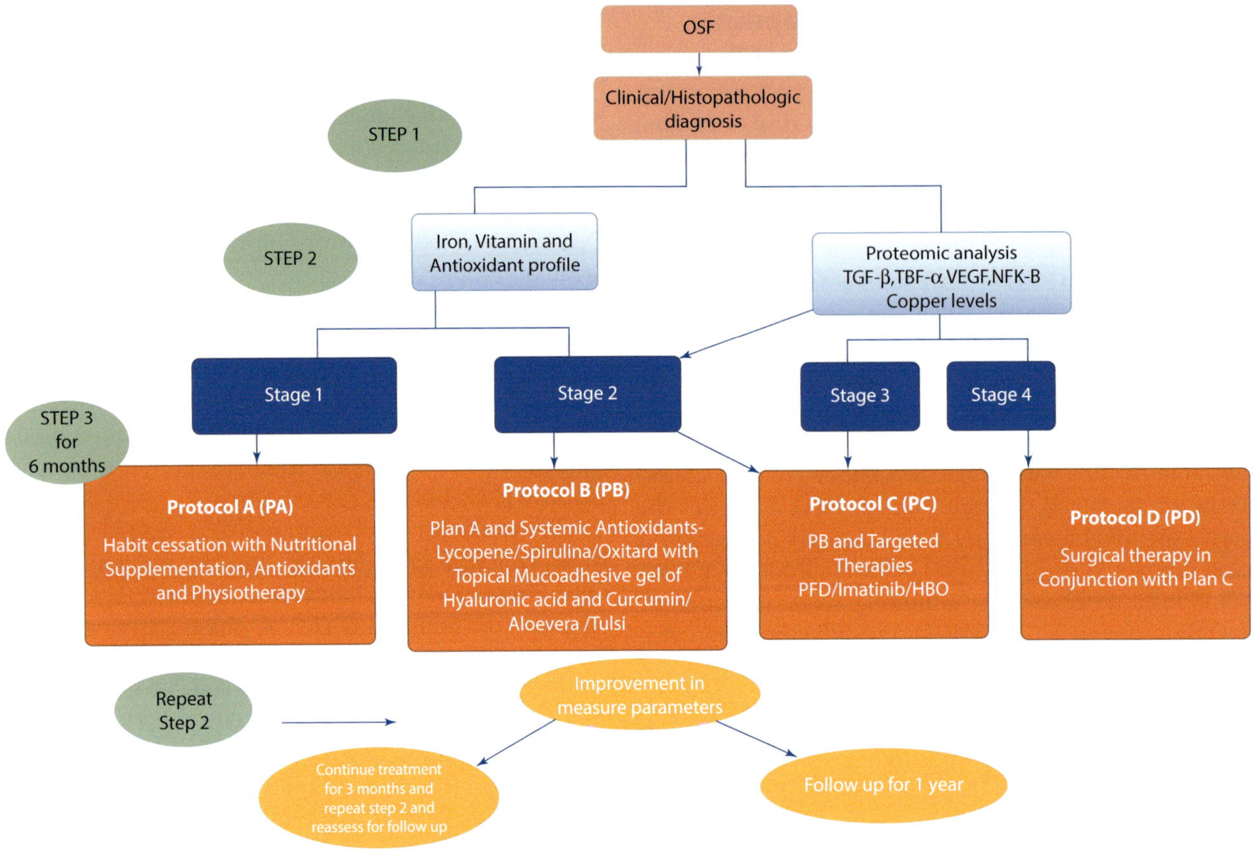




**Fig. 12.12** Stepwise protocol for the management of OSF

by reducing the levels of hypoxia-inducible factor-1α (HIF-1α) and concurrently amplifying the expression of VEGF. These findings suggest that HBO can be used in the management of OSF [150].

**Personalized precision medicine (PPM):** PPM is an upcoming strategy in immunotherapy where the metabolic, proteomic, and genomic analysis is done. Based on PPM, targeted therapies with a systematic and stepwise protocol are tailored for the treatment of OSF [143] (Fig. 12.12).

**Arctigenin**, a lignan extracted from *Arctium lappa*, has been reported to have a variety of pharmacological activities, including anti-fibrosis. Arctigenin was able to abolish the arecoline-induced collagen gel contractility, migration, invasion, and wound-healing capacities of buccal mucosal fibroblasts (BMFs) and downregulate the myofibroblast characteristics of BMFs in a dose-dependent manner. Most importantly, the production of TGF-β in fibrotic BMFs was reduced after exposure to arctigenin, along with the suppression of p-SMAD2, α-smooth muscle actin, and type I collagen A1. In addition, arctigenin was shown to diminish the expression of LINC00974, which has been proven to activate TGF-β/SMAD signaling for oral fibrogenesis. These findings suggest that arctigenin may act as a suitable adjunct therapy for OSF [151].

**Curcumin** is a yellow substance extracted from the roots of the plant *Curcuma longa* (commonly known as turmeric), which belongs to ginger family. Curcumin has been widely used for the management of several medical conditions, such as inflammatory bowel syndrome, rheumatoid arthritis, and pancreatitis. The medicinal benefits of curcumin are attributed to its analgesic, anti-inflammatory, antioxidant, antifibrinolytic, and anticancer properties. An experimental study found that curcumin inhibits the proliferation of fibroblasts and myofibroblasts, disturbs the cell cycle, induces apoptosis by downregulating the Bcl-2/Bax ratio, and decreases the generation of collagen type I and III in myofibroblasts, substantiating its potential preventive and therapeutic benefits in patients with OSF [152, 153].

**Summary**

This chapter describes the role of areca nut in fibrosis. Constituents of areca nut involved in fibrosis are polyphenols (flavonoids and tannins), alkaloids (arecoline, arecaidine, guvacine, and guvacoline), macromolecules (carbohydrates, fats, proteins), mineral matter, and crude fiber. Areca nut induces fibrosis by the activation of reactive oxygen species, fibroblast proliferation, myofibroblast transdifferentiation, increased collagen synthesis, decreased collagen breakdown, and increased deposition of collagen. Biomolecules involved in fibrogenesis are transforming growth factor-β (TGF-β), epidermal growth factor (EGF), fibroblast growth factor (bFGF), connective tissue growth factor (CTGF), platelet-derived growth factor (PDGF), insulin-like growth factor (IGF)-1/2, and Notch. The inflammatory mediators participating in disease evolution are interleukins (IL-1β, IL-6, IL-8, IL-15), interferon-γ (IFN-γ), monocyte chemoattractant protein-1 (chemokine (C-C motif) ligand 2 [CCL2]), tumor necrosis factor-α (TNF-α), heat-shock proteins 70 (Hsp-70), and cyclooxygenase-2 (COX-2). During malignant transformation, carcinogenic agents in areca nut increase reactive oxygen species generation, promote DNA hypermethylation of tumor suppressor genes, induce nitrosamine formation, form DNA adducts, and cause epigenetic alterations. Alterations in oral microbiome may also promote oral carcinogenesis.

## References

1. Budi EH, Schaub JR, Decaris M, Turner S, Derynck R. TGF-β as a driver of fibrosis: physiological roles and therapeutic opportunities. J Pathol. 2021;254(4):358–73. https://doi.org/10.1002/path.5680.
2. Wynn TA. Cellular and molecular mechanisms of fibrosis. J Pathol. 2008;214(2):199–210. https://doi.org/10.1002/path.2277.
3. Pindborg JJ, Sirsat SM. Oral submucous fibrosis. Oral Surg Oral Med Oral Pathol. 1966;22(6):764–79.
4. IARC Working Group on the Evaluation of Carcinogenic Risks to Humans. Betel-quid and areca-nut chewing and some areca-nut-derived nitrosamines. IARC Monogr Eval Carcinog Risks Hum. 2004;85:1–334.
5. Peng W, Liu YJ, Wu N, Sun T, He XY, Gao YX, Wu CJ. Areca catechu L. (Arecaceae): a review of its traditional uses, botany, phytochemistry, pharmacology and toxicology. J Ethnopharmacol. 2015;164:340–56.
6. Angadi PV, Kale AD, Hallikerimath S. Evaluation of myofibroblasts in oral submucous fibrosis: correlation with disease severity. J Oral Pathol Med. 2011;40:208–13.
7. Shen YW, Shih YH, Fuh LJ, Shieh TM. Oral submucous fibrosis: a review on biomarkers, pathogenic mechanisms, and treatments. Int J Mol Sci. 2020;21(19):7231. https://doi.org/10.3390/ijms21197231.
8. Chang YC, Yang SF, Tai KW, Chou MY, Hsieh YS. Increased tissue inhibitor of metalloproteinase-1 expression and inhibition of gelatinase A activity in buccal mucosal fibroblasts by arecoline as possible mechanisms for oral submucous fibrosis. Oral Oncol. 2002a;38:195–200.
9. Tsai CH, Yang SF, Chang YC. The upregulation of cystatin C in oral submucous fibrosis. Oral Oncol. 2007;43:680–5.
10. Yang SF, Hsieh YS, Tsai CH, Chou MY, Chang YC. The upregulation of type I plasminogen activator inhibitor in oral submucous fibrosis. Oral Oncol. 2003;39:367–72.
11. Kondaiah P, Pant I, Khan I. Molecular pathways regulated by areca nut in the etiopathogenesis of oral submucous fibrosis. Periodontol 2000. 2019;80(1):213–24. https://doi.org/10.1111/prd.12266.
12. Yang SF, Tsai CH, Chang YC. The upregulation of heat shock protein 47 expression in human buccal fibroblasts stimulated with arecoline. J Oral Pathol Med. 2008;37:206–10.
13. Lee SS, Chen YJ, Tsai CH, Huang FM, Chang YC. Elevated transglutaminase-2 expression mediates fibrosis in areca quid chewing-associated oral submucocal fibrosis via reactive oxygen species generation. Clin Oral Investig. 2015;20:1029–34.
14. Shieh DH, Chiang LC, Lee CH, Yang YH, Shieh TY. Effects of arecoline, safrole, and nicotine on collagen phagocytosis by human buccal mucosal fibroblasts as a possible mechanism for oral submucous fibrosis in Taiwan. J Oral Pathol Med. 2004;33:581–7.
15. Khan I, Kumar N, Pant I, Narra S, Kondaiah P. Activation of TGF-β pathway by areca nut constituents: a possible cause of oral submucous fibrosis. PLoS One. 2012;7:e51806.
16. Pant I, Kumar N, Khan I, Rao SG, Kondaiah P. Role of areca nut induced TGF-β and epithelial-mesenchymal interaction in the pathogenesis of oral submucous fibrosis. PLoS One. 2015;10:e0129252.
17. Chang YC, Tsai CH, Lai YL, et al. Arecoline-induced myofibroblast transdifferentiation from human buccal mucosal fibroblasts is mediated by ZEB1. J Cell Mol Med. 2014;18:698–708.
18. Lee YH, Yang LC, Hu FW, Peng CY, Yu CH, Yu CC. Elevation of Twist expression by arecoline contributes to the pathogenesis of oral submucous fibrosis. J Formos Med Assoc. 2016;115:311–7.
19. Yu CC, Tsai CH, Hsu HI, Chang YC. Elevation of S100A4 expression in buccal mucosal fibroblasts by arecoline: involvement in the pathogenesis of oral submucous fibrosis. PLoS One. 2013;8:e55122.
20. Das A, Giri S. A review on role of arecoline and its metabolites in the molecular pathogenesis of oral lesions with an insight into current status of its metabolomics. Prague Med Rep. 2020;121(4):209–35. https://doi.org/10.14712/23362936.2020.19.
21. Islam S, Muthumala M, Matsuoka H, Uehara O, Kuramitsu Y, Chiba I, Abiko Y. How each component of Betel Quid is involved in oral carcinogenesis: mutual interactions and synergistic effects with other carcinogens-a review article. Curr Oncol Rep. 2019;21(6):53. https://doi.org/10.1007/s11912-019-0800-8.
22. Mack M. Inflammation and fibrosis. Matrix Biol. 2018;68–69:106–21. https://doi.org/10.1016/j.matbio.2017.11.010.
23. Rangaswamy S, Chikkalingaiah RG, Sharada P, Kumar VK. Expression of cyclooxygenase 2 in oral submucous fibrosis: an immunohistochemical pilot study. J Oral Maxillofac Pathol. 2019;23(2):301.
24. Thubashini M, Malathi N, Kannan L. Expression of heat shock protein70 in oral submucous fibrosis and oral squamous cell carcinoma: an immunohistochemical study. Indian J Dent Res. 2011;22(2):256–9. https://doi.org/10.4103/0970-9290.84299.
25. Das T, Prodhan C, Patsa S, Ray JG, Chaudhuri K. Identification of over expressed proteins in oral submucous fibrosis by proteomic analysis. J Cell Biochem. 2018;119(6):4361–71.
26. Chu HW, Chang KP, Hsu CW, Chang IY, Liu HP, Chen YT, Wu CC. Identification of salivary biomarkers for oral cancer detection with untargeted and targeted quantitative proteomics approaches. Mol Cell Proteomics. 2019;18(9):1796–806. https://doi.org/10.1074/mcp.RA119.001530.
27. Sarode G, Sarode SC, Deshmukh R, Raktade P, Patil S. Myofibroblasts could be recruited in a chemokine (C-C motif) ligand 2-dependent manner in pathogenesis of oral submucous fibrosis. J Oral Maxillofac Pathol. 2016;20(3):445–52.
28. Sabarinath B, Sriram G, Saraswathi TR, Sivapathasundharam B. Immunohistochemical evaluation of mast cells and vascular endothelial proliferation in oral submucous fibrosis. Indian J

Dent Res. 2011;22(1):116–21. https://doi.org/10.4103/0970-9290.80009.
29. Yadav A, Desai RS, Bhuta BA, Singh JS, Mehta R, Nehete AP. Altered immunohistochemical expression of mast cell tryptase and chymase in the pathogenesis of oral submucous fibrosis and malignant transformation of the overlying epithelium. J Investig Clin Dent. 2014;5(3):214–9.
30. Kany S, Vollrath JT, Relja B. Cytokines in inflammatory disease. Int J Mol Sci. 2019;20(23):6008. https://doi.org/10.3390/ijms20236008.
31. Liu C, Chu D, Kalantar-Zadeh K, George J, Young HA, Liu G. Cytokines: from clinical significance to quantification. Adv Sci (Weinh). 2021;8(15):e2004433. https://doi.org/10.1002/advs.202004433.
32. Haque MF, Meghji S, Khitab U, Harris M. Oral submucous fibrosis patients have altered levels of cytokine production. J Oral Pathol Med. 2000;29:123–8.
33. Haque MF, Harris M, Meghji S, Barrett AW. Immunolocalization of cytokines and growth factors in oral submucous fibrosis. Cytokine. 1998;10:713–9.
34. Hu S, Chen W-C, Hwang G-S, Chen S-T, Kuo S-B, Chen Y, Idova G, Wang SW. Changes in plasma steroids and cytokines levels in Betel chewing patients in Taiwan. Steroids. 2016; https://doi.org/10.1016/j.steroids.2016.03.011.
35. Chiu CJ, Chiang CP, Chang ML, Chen HM, Hahn LJ, Hsieh LL, Kuo YS, Chen CJ. Association between genetic polymorphism of tumor necrosis factor-alpha and risk of oral submucous fibrosis, a precancerous condition of oral cancer. J Dent Res. 2001;80:2055–9.
36. Rhodus NL, Ho V, Miller CS, Myers S, Ondrey F. NF-kappaB dependent cytokine levels in saliva of patients with oral preneoplastic lesions and oral squamous cell carcinoma. Cancer Detect Prev. 2005;29:42–5.
37. Kaur J, Jacobs R. Proinflammatory cytokine levels in oral lichen planus, oral leukoplakia, and oral submucous fibrosis. J Korean Assoc Oral Maxillofac Surg. 2015;41(4):171–5. https://doi.org/10.5125/jkaoms.2015.41.4.171.
38. Punyani SR, Sathawane RS. Salivary level of interleukin-8 in oral precancer and oral squamous cell carcinoma. Clin Oral Investig. 2013;17(2):517–24. https://doi.org/10.1007/s00784--012-0723-3.
39. Pereira T, Naik S, Tamgadge A. Quantitative evaluation of macrophage expression using CD68 in oral submucous fibrosis: an immunohistochemical study. Ann Med Health Sci Res. 2015;5(6):435–41. https://doi.org/10.4103/2141-9248.177983.
40. Chiang CP, Wu HY, Liu BY, Wang JT, Kuo MY. Quantitative analysis of immunocompetent cells in oral submucous fibrosis in Taiwan. Oral Oncol. 2002;38:56–63.
41. Haque MF, Harris M, Meghji S, Speight PM. An immunohistochemical study of oral submucous fibrosis. J Oral Pathol Med. 1997;26:75–82.
42. Bôas DS, Takiya CM, Gurgel CA, Cabral MG, Santos JN. Tumor-infiltrating macrophage and microvessel density in oral squamous cell carcinoma. Braz Dent J. 2013;24:194–9.
43. El-Rouby DH. Association of macrophages with angiogenesis in oral verrucous and squamous cell carcinomas. J Oral Pathol Med. 2010;39:559–64.
44. Wehrhan F, Büttner-Herold M, Hyckel P, Moebius P, Preidl R, Distel L, et al. Increased malignancy of oral squamous cell carcinomas (OSCC) is associated with macrophage polarization in regional lymph nodes—an immunohistochemical study. BMC Cancer. 2014;14:522.
45. Pettersen JS, Fuentes-Duculan J, Suárez-Fariñas M, Pierson KC, Pitts-Kiefer A, Fan L, et al. Tumor-associated macrophages in the cutaneous SCC microenvironment are heterogeneously activated. J Invest Dermatol. 2011;131:1322–30.
46. Charles GA, Orsulak PJ, Rush AJ, Fulton CL. Arecoline reverses dexamethasone suppression of cortisol in normal males: a pilot study. Biol Psychiatry. 1995;37:811–6.
47. Overstreet DH, Booth RA, Dana R, Risch SC, Janowsky DS. Enhanced elevation of corticosterone following arecoline administration to rats selectively bred for increased cholinergic function. Psychopharmacology. 1986;88:129–30.
48. Risch SC, Kalin NH, Cohen RM, Weker JL, Insel TR, Cohen ML, Murphy DL. Muscarinic cholinergic influences on ACTH and beta-endorphin release mechanisms in human subjects. Peptides. 1981;2(Suppl. 1):95–7.
49. Yang NY, Kaphle K, Wang PH, Jong DS, Wu LS, Lin JH. Effects of aqueous extracts of "Betel quid" and its constituents on testosterone production by dispersed mouse interstitial cells. Am J Chin Med. 2004;32:705–15.
50. Wang SW, Hwang GS, Chen TJ, Wang PS. Effects of arecoline on testosterone release in rats. Am J Physiol Endocrinol Metab. 2008;295:E497–504.
51. Kubiczkova L, Sedlarikova L, Hajek R, Sevcikova S. TGF-β—an excellent servant but a bad master. J Transl Med. 2012;10:183. https://doi.org/10.1186/1479-5876-10-183.
52. Shi X, Young CD, Zhou H, Wang X. Transforming growth factor-β signaling in fibrotic diseases and cancer-associated fibroblasts. Biomol Ther. 2020;10(12):1666. https://doi.org/10.3390/biom10121666.
53. Garcia-Fernandez N, Marco Molina ML. TGF-β made easy. Open Urol Nephrol J 3b. https://www.ncbi.nlm.nih.gov/gene/7042
54. Kondaiah P, Pant I, Khan I. Molecular pathways regulated by areca nut in the etiopathogenesis of oral submucous fibrosis. Periodontol. 2000;2019(80):213–24. https://doi.org/10.1111/prd.1226.
55. Pant I, Rao SG, Kondaiah P. Role of areca nut induced JNK/ATF2/Jun axis in the activation of TGF-β pathway in precancerous oral submucous fibrosis. Sci Rep. 2016;6:34314.
56. Wang W, Xiong H, Hu Z, Zhao R, Hu Y, Chen W, Han Y, Yang L, Hu X, Wang C, Mao T, Xia K, Su T. Experimental study on TGF-β1-mediated CD147 expression in oral submucous fibrosis. Oral Dis. 2018;24(6):993–1000.
57. Khan I, Agarwal P, Thangjam GS, Radhesh R, Rao SG, Kondaiah P. Role of TGF-β and BMP7 in the pathogenesis of oral submucous fibrosis. Growth Factors. 2011;29(4):119–27. https://doi.org/10.3109/08977194.2011.582839.
58. Kamath VV, Krishnamurthy S, Satelur KP, Rajkumar K. Transforming growth factor-β1 and TGF-β2 act synergistically in the fibrotic pathway in oral submucous fibrosis: an immunohistochemical observation. Indian J Med Paediatr Oncol. 2015;36:111–6.
59. Illeperuma RP, Ryu MH, Kim KY, Tilakaratne WM, Kim J. Relationship of fibrosis and the expression of TGF-β1, MMP-1, and TIMP-1 with epithelial dysplasia in oral submucous fibrosis. Oral Med Pathol. 2010;15:21–8.
60. Chen J, Zeng F, Forrester SJ, Eguchi S, Zhang MZ, Harris RC. Expression and function of the epidermal growth factor receptor in physiology and disease. Physiol Rev. 2016;96(3):1025–69. https://doi.org/10.1152/physrev.00030.2015.
61. Scaltriti M, Baselga J. The epidermal growth factor receptor pathway: a model for targeted therapy. Clin Cancer Res. 2006;12(18):5268–72. https://doi.org/10.1158/1078-0432.CCR-05-1554.
62. http://atlasgeneticsoncology.org/Genes/GC_EGFR.html
63. Porebska I, Harlozinska A, Bojarowski T. Expression of the tyrosine kinase activity growth factor receptors (EGFR, ERB B2,

ERB B3) in colorectal adenocarcinomas and adenomas. Tumor Biol. 2000;21:105–15. https://doi.org/10.1159/000030116.
64. Baekelandt M, Kristensen GB, Tropé CG, Nesland JM, Holm R. Epidermal growth factor receptor expression has no independent prognostic significance in advanced ovarian cancer. Anticancer Res. 1999;19:4469–74.
65. Nankivell P, Williams H, McConkey C, Webster K, High A, MacLennan K, et al. Tetraspanins CD9 and CD151, epidermal growth factor receptor and cyclooxygenase-2 expression predict malignant progression in oral epithelial dysplasia. Br J Cancer. 2013;109:2864–74. https://doi.org/10.1038/bjc.2013.600.
66. Grandis JR, Melhem MF, Gooding WE, Day R, Holst VA, Wagener MM, et al. Levels of TGF-alpha and EGFR protein in head and neck squamous cell carcinoma and patient survival. J Natl Cancer Inst. 1998;90:824–32.
67. Weinstein S, Nuamah I, Tucker J, Montone K. Evaluation of HER-2/ neu (c-erb B-2) oncogene expression in whole organ sections of supraglottic squamous cell carcinoma. Ann Otol Rhinol Laryngol. 1996;105:275–9. https://doi.org/10.1177/000348949610500406.
68. Beckhardt RN, Kiyokawa N, Xi L, Liu TJ, Hung MC, elNaggar AK, et al. HER-2/neu oncogene characterization in head and neck squamous cell carcinoma. Arch Otolaryngol Head Neck Surg. 1995;121:1265–70. https://doi.org/10.1001/archotol.1995.01890110041008.
69. Craven JM, Pavelic ZP, Stambrook PJ, Pavelic L, Gapany M, Kelley DJ, et al. Expression of cerb B-2 gene in human head and neck carcinoma. Anticancer Res. 1992;12:2273–6.
70. Srinivasan M, Jewell SD. Quantitative estimation of PCNA, c-myc, EGFR and TGF- in oral submucous fibrosis—an immunohistochemical study. Oral Oncol. 2001;37:461–7. https://doi.org/10.1016/S1368-8375(00)00115-9.
71. Chang MC, Chen YJ, Chang HH, Chan CP, Yeh CY, Wang YL, et al. Areca nut components affect COX-2, cyclin B1/cdc25C and keratin expression, PGE2 production in keratinocyte is related to reactive oxygen species, CYP1A1, Src, EGFR and Ras signaling. PLoS One. 2014;9:1–12. https://doi.org/10.1371/journal.pone.0101959.
72. Bernardes VF, Gleber-Netto FO, Sousa SF, Silva TA, Aguiar MCF. Clinical significance of EGFR, Her-2 and EGF in oral squamous cell carcinoma: a case control study. J Exp Clin Cancer Res. 2010;29:1–7. https://doi.org/10.1186/1756-9966-29-40.
73. Temam S, Kawaguchi H, El-Naggar AK, Jelinek J, Tang H, Liu DD, et al. Epidermal growth factor receptor copy number alterations correlate with poor clinical outcome in patients with head and neck squamous cancer. J Clin Oncol. 2007;25:2164–70. https://doi.org/10.1200/JCO.2006.06.6605.
74. Shetty SS, Sharma M, Fonseca FP, Jayaram P, Tanwar AS, Kabekkodu SP, Kapaettu S, Radhakrishnan R. Signaling pathways promoting epithelial mesenchymal transition in oral submucous fibrosis and oral squamous cell carcinoma. Jpn Dent Sci Rev. 2020;56(1):97–108. https://doi.org/10.1016/j.jdsr.2020.07.002.
75. Jyothi Meka N, Ugrappa S, Velpula N, Kumar S, Naik Maloth K, Kodangal S, Goyal S. Quantitative immunoexpression of EGFR in oral potentially malignant disorders: oral leukoplakia and oral submucous fibrosis. J Dent Res Dent Clin Dent Prospects. 2015;9(3):166–74. https://doi.org/10.15171/joddd.2015.031.
76. Brooks AN, Kilgour E, Smith PD. Molecular pathways: fibroblast growth factor signaling: a new therapeutic opportunity in cancer. Clin Cancer Res. 2012;18(7):1855–62. https://doi.org/10.1158/1078-0432.CCR-11-0699.
77. https://www.ncbi.nlm.nih.gov/gene/2263.
78. Xie Y, Su N, Yang J, Tan Q, Huang S, Jin M, Ni Z, Zhang B, Zhang D, Luo F, Chen H, Sun X, Feng JQ, Qi H, Chen L. FGF/FGFR signaling in health and disease. Signal Transduct Target Ther. 2020;5(1):181. https://doi.org/10.1038/s41392-020-00222-7.
79. Bishen KA, Radhakrishnan R, Satyamoorthy K. The role of basic fibroblast growth factor in oral submucous fibrosis pathogenesis. J Oral Pathol Med. 2008;37:402–11.
80. Strutz F, Zeisberg M, Ziyadeh FN, Yang C-Q, Kalluri R, Muller GA, et al. Role of basic fibroblast growth factor-2 in epithelial-mesenchymal transformation. Kidney Int. 2002;61:1714–28. https://doi.org/10.1046/j.1523-1755.2002.00333.x.
81. Baird A, Schubert D, Ling N, Guillemin R. Receptor- and heparin-binding domains of basic fibroblast growth factor. Proct Natl Acad Sci U S A. 1988;85:2324–8.
82. Zittermann SI, Issekutz AC. Basic fibroblast growth factor (bFGF, FGF-2) potentiates leukocyte recruitment to inflammation by enhancing endothelial adhesion molecule expression. Am J Pathol. 2006;168:835–46.
83. Hase T, Kawashiri S, Tanaka A, Nozaki S, Noguchi N, Kato K, et al. Correlation of basic fibroblast growth factor expression with the invasion and the prognosis of oral squamous cell carcinoma. J Oral Pathol Med. 2006;35:136–9.
84. Bikfalvi A, Klein S, Pintucci G, Rifkin DB. Biological roles of fibroblast growth factor-2. Endocr Rev. 1997;18:26–45.
85. Jaye M, Lyall RM, Mudd R, Schlessinger J, Sarver N. Expression of acidic fibroblast growth factor cDNA confers growth advantage and tumorigenesis to Swiss 3T3 cells. EMBO J. 1988;7:963–9.
86. Sasda R, Kurokawa T, Iwane M, Igarashi K. Transformation of mouse BALB/c 3T3 cells with human basic fibroblast growth factor cDNA. Mol Cell Biol. 1988;8:588–94.
87. Pandiar D, Shameena PM. Immunohistochemical expression of CD34 and basic fibroblast growth factor (bFGF) in oral submucous fibrosis. J Oral Maxillofac Pathol. 2014;18:155–61.
88. Giri D, Ropiquet F, Ittmann M. Alterations in expression of basic fibroblast growth factor (FGF-2) and its receptor FGFR-1 in human prostate cancer. Clin Cancer Res. 1999;5:1063–71.
89. Raimondi AR, Molinolo AA, Itoiz ME. Fibroblast growth factor-2 expression during experimental oral carcinogenesis. Its possible role in the induction of pre-malignant fibrosis. J Oral Pathol Med. 2006;35:212–7.
90. Nayak S, Goel MM, Makker A, Bhatia V, Chandra S, Kumar S, Agarwal SP. Fibroblast Growth Factor (FGF-2) and its receptors FGFR-2 and FGFR-3 may be putative biomarkers of malignant transformation of potentially malignant oral lesions into oral squamous cell carcinoma. PLoS One. 2015;10(10):e0138801. https://doi.org/10.1371/journal.pone.0138801.
91. Condorelli AG, El Hachem M, Zambruno G, et al. Notch-ing up knowledge on molecular mechanisms of skin fibrosis: focus on the multifaceted Notch signalling pathway. J Biomed Sci. 2021;28:36. https://doi.org/10.1186/s12929-021-00732-8.
92. https://www.ncbi.nlm.nih.gov/gene/4851
93. Liu L, Gao C, Chen G, Li X, Li J, Wan Q, Xu Y. Notch signaling molecules activate TGF-beta in Rat mesangial cells under high glucose conditions. J Diabetes Res. 2013;2013:979702.
94. Hu B, Phan SH. Notch in fibrosis and as a target of anti-fibrotic therapy. Pharmacol Res. 2016;108:57–64. https://doi.org/10.1016/j.phrs.2016.04.010.
95. Aoyagi-Ikeda K, Maeno T, Matsui H, Ueno M, Hara K, Aoki Y, Aoki F, Shimizu T, Doi H, Kawai-Kowase K, Iso T, Suga T, Arai M, Kurabayashi M. Notch induces myofibroblast differentiation of alveolar epithelial cells via transforming growth factor-{beta}-Smad3 pathway. Am J Respir Cell Mol Biol. 2011;45(1):136–44.

96. Lunde ML, Roman E, Warnakulasuriya S, Mehrotra R, Laranne J, Vasstrand EN, Ibrahim SO. Profiling of chromosomal changes in potentially malignant and malignant oral mucosal lesions from South and South-East Asia using array-comparative genomic hybridization. Cancer Genomics Proteomics. 2014;11(3):127–40.
97. Conroy KP, Kitto LJ, Henderson NC. αv integrins: key regulators of tissue fibrosis. Cell Tissue Res. 2016;365(3):511–9. https://doi.org/10.1007/s00441-016-2407-9.
98. Klingberg F, Chow ML, Koehler A, Boo S, Buscemi L, Quinn TM, Costell M, Alman BA, Genot E, Hinz B. Prestress in the extracellular matrix sensitizes latent TGF-1 for activation. J Cell Biol. 2014;207:283–97. https://doi.org/10.1002/jcp.24094.
99. Dietz HC. One integrin to rule them all? Sci Transl Med. 2015;7(288):288fs21. https://doi.org/10.1126/scitranslmed.aab0044.
100. Henderson NC, Sheppard D. Integrin-mediated regulation of TGFβ in fibrosis. Biochim Biophys Acta. 2013;1832(7):891–6. https://doi.org/10.1016/j.bbadis.2012.10.005.
101. Brakebusch C, Fassler R. β1 integrin function in vivo: adhesion, migration and more. Cancer Metastasis Rev. 2005;24(3):403–11.
102. Desgrosellier JS, Cheresh DA. Integrins in cancer: biological implications and therapeutic opportunities. Nat Rev Cancer. 2010;10(1):9–22.
103. Moutasim KA, Jenei V, Sapienza K, Marsh D, Weinreb PH, Violette SM, Lewis MP, Marshall JF, Fortune F, Tilakratne WM, Hart IR, Thomas GJ. Betel-derived alkaloid up-regulates keratinocyte alphavbeta6 integrin expression and promotes oral submucous fibrosis. J Pathol. 2011;223:366–77.
104. Veeravarmal V, Austin RD, Nagini S, Nassar MHM. Expression of β1integrin in normal epithelium, oral submucous fibrosis and oral squamous cell carcinoma. Pathol Res Pract. 2018;214(2):273–80. https://doi.org/10.1016/j.prp.2017.10.013.
105. Tilakaratne WM, Ekanayaka RP, Warnakulasuriya S. Oral submucous fibrosis: a historical perspective and a review on etiology and pathogenesis. Oral Surg Oral Med Oral Pathol Oral Radiol. 2016;122(2):178–91. https://doi.org/10.1016/j.oooo.2016.04.003.
106. Utsunomiya H, Tilakaratne WM, Oshiro K, et al. Extracellular matrix remodeling in oral submucous fibrosis: its stage-specific modes revealed by immunohistochemistry and in situ hybridization. J Oral Pathol Med. 2005;34:498–507.
107. Shrestha A, Carnelio S. Evaluation of Matrix Metalloproteinases-2 (MMP-2) and tissue inhibitors of Metalloproteinases-2 (TIMP-2) in oral submucous fibrosis and their correlation with disease severity. Kathmandu Univ Med J. 2013;44(4):274–81.
108. Mishra G, Ranganathan K. Matrix metalloproteinase-1 expression in oral submucous fibrosis: an immunohistochemical study. Indian J Dent Res. 2010;21:320–5.
109. Gadbail AR, Chaudhary MS, Sarode SC, Gondivkar SM, Belekar L, Mankar-Gadbail MP, Dande R, Tekade SA, Yuwanati MB, Patil S. Ki67, CD105 and α-smooth muscle actin expression in disease progression model of oral submucous fibrosis. J Investig Clin Dent. 2019;10(4):e12443.
110. Gupta K, Metgud R, Gupta J. Evaluation of stromal myofibroblasts in oral leukoplakia, oral submucous fibrosis, and oral squamous cell carcinoma—an immunohistochemical study. Indian J Cancer 2015;52(1):87–92.
111. Jayaraj G, Sherlin HJ, Ramani P, Premkumar P, Natesan A. Stromal myofibroblasts in oral squamous cell carcinoma and potentially malignant disorders. J Oral Biol Craniofac Res. 2015;5(3):165–72.
112. Gandhi P, Prasad UC. Evaluation of myofibroblasts in oral submucous fibrosis and oral squamous cell carcinoma: the pathogenesis and correlation. Dent Res J (Isfahan). 2017;14(5):314–20.
113. Das RK, Anura A, Pal M, Bag S, Majumdar S, Barui A. Epithelio-mesenchymal transitional attributes in oral submucous fibrosis. Exp Mol Pathol. 2013;95:259–69.
114. Lee K, Nelson CM. New insights into the regulation of epithelial—mesenchymal transition and tissue fibrosis, vol. 294. 1st ed. Elsevier Inc.; 2012.
115. Shetty SS, Sharma M, Fonseca FP, et al. Signaling pathways promoting epithelial mesenchymal transition in oral submucous fibrosis and oral squamous cell carcinoma. Jpn Dent Sci Rev. 2020;56(1):97–108. https://doi.org/10.1016/j.jdsr.2020.07.002.
116. Scanlon CS, Van Tubergen EA, Inglehart RC, D'Silva NJ. Biomarkers of epithelial-mesenchymal transition in squamous cell carcinoma. J Dent Res. 2013;92:114–21. https://doi.org/10.1177/0022034512467352.
117. Kriz W, Kaissling B, Le Hir M. Epithelial-mesenchymal transition (EMT) in kidney fibrosis: fact or fantasy? J Clin Invest. 2011;121:468–74. https://doi.org/10.1172/JCI44595.468.
118. Hyun K, Koo G, Han H, Sohn J, Choi W. Epithelial-to-mesenchymal transition leads to loss of EpCAM and different physical properties in circulating tumor cells from metastatic breast cancer. Oncotarget. 2016;7:24677–87.
119. Horowitz JC, Thannickal VJ. Epithelial-mesenchymal interactions in pulmonary fibrosis. Semin Respir Crit Care Med. 2006;27:600–12. https://doi.org/10.1055/s-2006-957332.
120. Prasad RS, Pai A, Shyamala K, Bhadranna A, Shenoy S, Yaji A. Assessment of epithelial-mesenchymal transition signatures in oral submucous fibrosis. J Oral Maxillofac Pathol. 2019;23(2):308.
121. Sharada P, Swaminathan U, Nagamalini BR, Kumar KV, Ashwini BK, Lavanya V. Coalition of E-cadherin and vascular endothelial growth factor expression in predicting malignant transformation in common oral potentially malignant disorders. J Oral Maxillofac Pathol. 2018;22(1):40–7. https://doi.org/10.4103/jomfp.JOMFP_13_18.
122. da Silva LC, Fonseca FP, de Almeida OP, de Almeida Mariz BAL, Lopes MA, Radhakrishnan R, Sharma M, Kowalski LP, Vargas PA. CD1A+ and CD207+ cells are reduced in oral submucous fibrosis and oral squamous cell carcinoma. Med Oral Patol Oral Cir Bucal. 2020;25(1):e49–55.
123. Pellicioli ACA, Bingle L, Farthing P, Lopes MA, Martins MD, Vargas PA. Immunosurveillance profile of oral squamous cell carcinoma and oral epithelial dysplasia through dendritic and T-cell analysis. J Oral Pathol Med. 2017;46(10):928–33. https://doi.org/10.1111/jop.12597.
124. De Monte A, Olivieri CV, Vitale S, Bailleux S, Castillo L, Giordanengo V, Maryanski JL, Segura E, Doglio A. CD1c-related DCs that express CD207/Langerin, but Are Distinguishable from Langerhans cells, are consistently present in human tonsils. Front Immunol. 2016;7:197. https://doi.org/10.3389/fimmu.2016.00197.
125. Narayanan B, Narasimhan M. Langerhans cell expression in oral submucous fibrosis: an immunohistochemical analysis. J Clin Diagn Res. 2015;9(7):ZC39–41.
126. Nyachhyon R, Nagraj SK, Ongole R. Expression of CD1a by Langerhans cells in oral mucosa of submucous fibrosis patients and Arecanut/gutkha chewers. J Nepal Dental Assoc. 2014;14(2):1.
127. Sahaf R, Naseem N, Rehman A-u, Anjum R, Nagi AH. EMMPRIN (CD147) as a potential predictor of oral squamous cell carcinoma progression: a study from Pakistan.


12

J Histol Histopathol. 2017;4(8) https://doi.org/10.7243/2055--091X-4-8.
128. Belaldavar C, Mane DR, Hallikerimath S, Kale AD. Cytokeratins: its role and expression profile in oral health and disease. J Oral Maxillofac Surg Med Pathol. 2016;28: 77–84.
129. Ranganathan K, Kavitha R, Sawant SS, Vaidya MM. Cytokeratin expression in oral submucous fibrosis--an immunohistochemical study. J Oral Pathol Med. 2006;35(1):25–32. https://doi.org/10.1111/j.1600-0714.2005.00366.x.
130. Vasca V, Vasca E, Freiman P, et al. Keratin 5 expression in squamocellular carcinoma of the head and neck. Oncol Lett. 2014;8(6):2501–4. https://doi.org/10.3892/ol.2014.2591.
131. Jacques CM, Pereira AL, Maia V, Cuzzi T, Ramos-e-Silva M. Expression of cytokeratins 10, 13, 14 and 19 in oral lichen planus. J Oral Sci. 2009;51(3):355–65. https://doi.org/10.2334/josnusd.51.355.
132. Frohwitter G, Buerger H, Van Diest PJ, Korsching E, Kleinheinz J, Fillies T. Cytokeratin and protein expression patterns in squamous cell carcinoma of the oral cavity provide evidence for two distinct pathogenetic pathways. Oncol Lett. 2016;12(1):107–13. https://doi.org/10.3892/ol.2016.4588.
133. Liu W, Zeng L, Li N, Wang F, Jiang C, Guo F, Chen X, Su T, Xu C, Zhang S, Fang C. Quantitative proteomic analysis for novel biomarkers of buccal squamous cell carcinoma arising in background of oral submucous fibrosis. BMC Cancer. 2016;16:584.
134. Nithya S, Radhika T, Jeddy N. Loricrin—an overview. J Oral Maxillofac Pathol. 2015;19(1):64–8. https://doi.org/10.4103/0973-029X.157204.
135. Nithya S, Joshua E, Ranganathan K, Thavarajah R, Rao UK. Loricrin expression and its implication in oral submucous fibrosis, hyperkeratosis and normal mucosa with association to habits—an immunohistochemical study. J Oral Biol Craniofac Res. 2019;9(3):226–31. https://doi.org/10.1016/j.jobcr.2019.05.004.
136. Gonzalez DM, Medici D. Signaling mechanisms of the epithelial-mesenchymal transition. Sci Signal. 2014;7:re8. https://doi.org/10.1126/scisignal.2005189.Signaling.
137. Lamouille S, Xu J, Derynck R. Molecular mechanisms of epithelial–mesenchymal transition. Nat Rev Mol Cell Biol. 2014;15:178–96. https://doi.org/10.1038/nrm3758.Molecular.
138. Chang YC, Tsai CH, Lai YL, Yu CC, Chi WY, Li JJ, Chang WW. Arecoline-induced myofibroblast transdifferentiation from human buccal mucosal fibroblasts is mediated by ZEB1. J Cell Mol Med. 2014;18(4):698–708. https://doi.org/10.1111/jcmm.12219.
139. Zhou S, Zhu Y, Mashrah M, Zhang X, He Z, Yao Z, Zhang C, Guo F, Hu Y, Zhang C. Expression pattern of DKK3, dickkopf WNT signaling pathway inhibitor 3, in the malignant progression of oral submucous fibrosis. Oncol Rep. 2017;37(2):979–85.
140. Zhou S, Chen L, Mashrah M, Zhu Y, Liu J, Yang X, He Z, Wang L, Xiang T, Yao Z, Guo F, Yang W, Zhang C. Deregulation of secreted frizzled-related proteins is associated with aberrant β-catenin activation in the carcinogenesis of oral submucous fibrosis. Onco Targets Ther. 2015;8:2923–31.
141. Sharma M, Shetty SS, Radhakrishnan R. Oral submucous fibrosis as an overhealing wound: implications in malignant transformation. Recent Pat Anticancer Drug Discov. 2018;13(3):272–91. https://doi.org/10.2174/1574892813666180227103147.
142. Li X, Zhu L, Wang B, Yuan M, Zhu R. Drugs and targets in fibrosis. Front Pharmacol. 2017;8:855. https://doi.org/10.3389/fphar.2017.00855.
143. More CB, Jatti Patil D, Rao NR. Medicinal management of oral submucous fibrosis in the past decade: a systematic review. J Oral Biol Craniofac Res. 2020;10(4):552–68. https://doi.org/10.1016/j.jobcr.2020.08.004.
144. Moinzadeh P, Hunzelmann N, Krieg T. Pharmacology and rationale for imatinib in the treatment of scleroderma. J Exp Pharmacol. 2013;5:15–22.
145. Akhmetshina A, Venalis P, Dees C, et al. Treatment with imatinib prevents fibrosis in different preclinical models of systemic sclerosis and induces regression of established fibrosis. Arthritis Rheum. 2009;60(1):219–24.
146. Sheshaprasad R, Pai A. Oral sub mucous fibrosis: exploring therapeutic strategies using -anti TGF β drugs. Asian Pac J Cancer Care. 2018;3(2):21–7.
147. Warnakulasuriya S, Kerr AR. Oral submucous fibrosis: a review of the current management and possible directions for novel therapies. Oral Surg Oral Med Oral Pathol Oral Radiol. 2016;122(2):232–41.
148. Hurst LC, Badalamente MA, Hentz VR, et al. Injectable collagenase clostridium histolyticum for Dupuytren's contracture. N Engl J Med. 2009;361(10):968–77.
149. Trivedy C, Warnakulasuriya KA, Hazarey VK, Tavassoli M, Sommer P, Johnson NW. The upregulation of lysyl oxidase in oral submucous fibrosis and squamous cell carcinoma. J Oral Pathol Med. 1999;28(6):246–51.
150. Ye X, Zhang J, Lu R, Zhou G. HBO: a possible supplementary therapy for oral potentially malignant disorders. Med Hypotheses. 2014;83(2):131–6.
151. Lin CY, Hsieh PL, Liao YW, Peng CY, Yu CC, Lu MY. Arctigenin reduces myofibroblast activities in oral submucous fibrosis by LINC00974 inhibition. Int J Mol Sci. 2019;20(6):1328. https://doi.org/10.3390/ijms20061328.
152. Ali A-MS. Efficacy of curcumin for management of oral submucous fibrosis: a systematic review of randomized clinical trials. Oral Surg Oral Med Oral Pathol Oral Radiol. 2019;127:300–8.
153. Zhang SS, Gong ZJ, Li WH, Wang X, Ling TY. Antifibrotic effect of curcumin in TGF-β 1-induced myofibroblasts from human oral mucosa. Asian Pac J Cancer Prev. 2012;13(1):289–94. https://doi.org/10.7314/apjcp.2012.13.1.289.

# Investigative Techniques for Oral Submucous Fibrosis

Contents

# Noninvasive Diagnostic Techniques in Oral Submucous Fibrosis

*Toru Nagao and Alexander Ross Kerr*

## Contents



© The Author(s), under exclusive license to Springer Nature Switzerland AG 2023
S. Warnakulasuriya, K. Ranganathan (eds.), *Oral Submucous Fibrosis*, Textbooks in Contemporary Dentistry,
https://doi.org/10.1007/978-3-031-12855-4_13

## 13.1 Introduction

The clinical diagnosis of oral submucous fibrosis (OSF) is relatively simple and based on presenting signs and symptoms. The potential utility of noninvasive diagnostic techniques in OSF includes early detection of OSF, assessment and monitoring of OSF severity (and response to treatment), and risk stratification or monitoring of OSF patients for malignant transformation (i.e., to oral squamous cell carcinoma (OSCC)). The detection of early-stage OSF before irreversible fibrosis or malignant transformation has occurred may provide opportunities to intervene (such as areca nut cessation) and prevent worsening of the disease and associated morbidity and mortality. Noninvasive diagnostic techniques that offer frontline clinicians in primary care settings more efficient ways to identify patients with early OSF may facilitate earlier interventions. In secondary care settings, such techniques might help expert clinicians to assess disease severity or monitor patients during treatment. The most important parameter is the OSF patient's propensity for malignant transformation necessitating long-term surveillance. OSF patients are reluctant to undergo serial invasive tissue biopsies, and therefore the use of noninvasive diagnostic adjunctive techniques to facilitate the risk stratification for malignant progression would seem reasonable.

This chapter will report on the utility of several noninvasive diagnostic adjunctive techniques and their utility in patients with OSF.



**Learning Goals**

Readers will be able to:

- Appreciate the different noninvasive diagnostic aids that have been tested on patients with oral submucous fibrosis (OSF)
- Identify the utility and limitations of such aids for screening (primary care setting), determination of disease severity, or assessment of risk for malignant transformation of OSF

## 13.2 Measurement of Mouth Opening

The interincisal distance, measured from the maxillary central incisor to the corresponding mandibular central incisor, is simple, reproduceable, and widely employed to assess disease severity in patients with OSF. The mean value of the interincisal distance in normal Nepalese population was 46.8 mm for males and 47.3 mm for females [1], and for Indian population, it was 47.5 mm for males and 44.6 mm for females [2]. A study investigated the maximal mouth opening (MMO) measured by paraclinical workers in patients with OSF compared with normal subjects in Nepal [1]. In this study, the minimum limit for a normal oral opening was determined to be 34 mm among healthy Nepalese adults, and 10 of 13 patients with OSF (histologically confirmed) had a maximum oral opening of less than 34 mm. The authors concluded that reduction of the oral opening as a single screening test for OSF has a sensitivity of 77% and detected only advanced cases. In Taiwan, a study was conducted to develop a scoring system for the early detection of OSF (betel quid users) based on clinical symptoms collected by a self-administered questionnaire [3]. The results showed that a scoring system that included MMO measurement (>35 mm of cutoff value) achieved 82% sensitivity and 85.8% specificity to detect OSF (histologically confirmed).

Measurements of MMO are correlated to the degree of fibrosis, but it is an indirect procedure. Therefore, it does not provide information about the actual condition of oral mucosa [4]. However, measuring MMO may be useful as a screening method in countries where the prevalence of OSF is high, medical resources are scarce, access to care is limited, and a detailed visual and tactile oral examination is not otherwise performed. In such situations, a community worker could simply measure mouth opening with the exclusion of other oral and maxillofacial diseases associated with trismus (i.e., temporomandibular joint disorders, injury to the masticatory muscle, arthritis, and chronic dental infections).

## 13.3 Optical Instruments

### 13.3.1 Tissue Autofluorescence

Evaluating tissue autofluorescence (AF) of oral mucosal sites can inform architectural and metabolic perturbations associated with the presence of oral dysplasia and neoplasia [5]. In vivo adjunctive techniques, both fiber-optic spectroscopic systems measuring the specific spectral signatures of fluorophores and direct visualization devices revealing changes in AF (i.e., retained versus loss of fluorescence visualization (FVR: fluorescence visualization retention vs. FVL: fluorescence visualization loss)), have been tested in patients with OSF. Spectroscopy using a 330 nm light wavelength for excitation demonstrated an AF pattern with two distinct spectral emission bands in patients with OSF compared to those with normal mucosa: at 380 nm (an increased fluorescence compared to normal oral mucosa) dictated by the increased collagen deposition associated with OSF, and at 460 nm (a reduced fluorescence) related to lower epithelial NADH content associated with an atrophic mucosa [6, 7]. This pattern was not deemed sensitive enough to predict the severity of OSF and was attenuated in OSF patients with both concomitant leukoplakia (with or without dysplasia) and benign keratoses. 76% of 88 OSF patients were correctly diagnosed using this pattern from a mixed patient cohort with OSF, leukoplakia, lichen planus, OSCC, and otherwise normal mucosa [8]. However, AF spectroscopy alone has not convincingly been demonstrated to help distinguish between OSF with and without dysplasia or malignancy. Low-level evidence from one study on 40 patients with OSF undergoing AF spectroscopy, coupled with a pre-rinsing with 5-aminolevulinic acid (ALA) to harness PpIX fluorescence, showed that OSF patients with epithelial hyperplasia or dysplasia may be discriminated from OSF patients without epithelial changes [9]. AF spectroscopy requires expensive equipment and therefore has limited applicability in a primary care setting. There is only one study reporting the use of a direct visualization device (VELscope, LED Inc., Vancouver, Canada) in 12 patients with OSF, 11 testing "positive" (i.e., loss of fluorescence) of which 10 demonstrated mild dysplasia, and one OSF patient without dysplasia tested "negative" [10]. Overall, the utility of AF as a noninvasive diagnostic adjunctive technique is limited.

### 13.3.2 Ultrasonography

#### 13.3.2.1 Colored Doppler Ultrasonography

Ultrasonography (USG) is a noninvasive, reproducible, and time-saving examination test method that offers high cost-benefit in medical diagnosis. Ultrasound, a sound energy, is in the form of waves with frequencies of >20 KHz. In medical diagnostics, ultrasound uses frequencies of 2–10 MHz and only the longitudinal mode of ultrasonic vibration. Colored Doppler, combining USG and the Doppler system, is a color-coded representation of blood flow velocity of the reflecting tissue. USG quantitatively provides information about the nature of the lesion and the adjacent normal structure and quantitatively assesses the lesion size, distance from the skin or mucosal surface, and relative proximity to the skin or mucosal surfaces [11].

Clinical applications of USG as diagnostic aids or for evaluation of the treatment for OSF have been carried out exclusively in India [12–23]. Studies measured the submucosal thickness of the buccal and labial mucosal sites and reported that as the severity of the disease increased, the submucosal tissue thickness increased and the vascularity of OSF lesions decreased compared to controls. ◘ Figure 13.1 shows the submucosal thickness of buccal mucosa on USG. A systematic review of 12 studies [12–23] investigated the role of USG in evaluating OSF [24]. Although the results did not provide clear evidence of the clinical value of USG for the early diagnosis of OSF, USG is a safe and conventional modality to assess muscular and submucosal tissue thickness, especially in terms of availability and cost factors. The authors indicated that to precisely evaluate OSF using USG, a highly accurate intraoral probe should be used.

These findings were also useful for examining masseteric hypertrophy in OSF during the initial diagnosis or evaluation of treatment. Kamala et al. conducted a preliminary study to measure the masseter muscle thickness both at rest and at maximum clenching state by USG in patients with OSF and showed that the masseter muscle thickness increased as the duration and frequency of areca nut use increased and as the disease progressed clinically and histologically [12].

Peak systolic velocity (PSV) is measured by colored Doppler USG to assess vascular distribution of subcutaneous or submucosal tissues (◘ Fig. 13.2). Manjunath et al. conducted a study to elucidate the usefulness of USG (two-dimensional [2D] and duplex Doppler including color flow imaging) in the buccal mucosa for patients with OSF. This was assessed by measuring the PSV ratio before and after the medical treatment [13]. The study indicated that OSF tissues showed increased hyperechoic areas representing fibrous bands or diffuse fibrosis and reduced vascularity and PSV.

Dupare and Dhole [20] conducted a study to evaluate the role of USG in OSF patients (grades I–IV). They examined submucosal thickness and vascularity by PSV, bilaterally on buccal and labial mucosae. The results showed a decrease in PSV with the progression of OSF severity, and in ultrasonographic diagnosis of OSF, the reported submucosal thickness had a sensitivity, specificity, PPV, NPV, and accuracy of 80%, 100%, 100%, 71.4%, and 87%, respectively, but PSV was unable to classify lesions.

A biopsy of an OSF patient is not 100% representative of OSF disease severity because OSF is a diffuse disease and may vary in severity across oral subsites in the same patient [14]. Multiple or serial biopsies to detect dysplastic or malignant changes are difficult for patients. USG may facilitate both diagnosis and monitoring of OSF patients chairside and may also be used to evaluate treatment outcomes without patient discomfort. For clear evidence of USG efficacy in patients with OSF, the correlation of USG assessment to clinical grading and histopathological findings should be examined [21]. More well-designed clinical trials are needed to elucidate the effectiveness of USG on OSF.

Overall, the utility of ultrasonography as a noninvasive diagnostic adjunctive technique is limited in patients with OSF. Diagnostic performance varies depending on the objectives and needs standardized image interpretation skills.

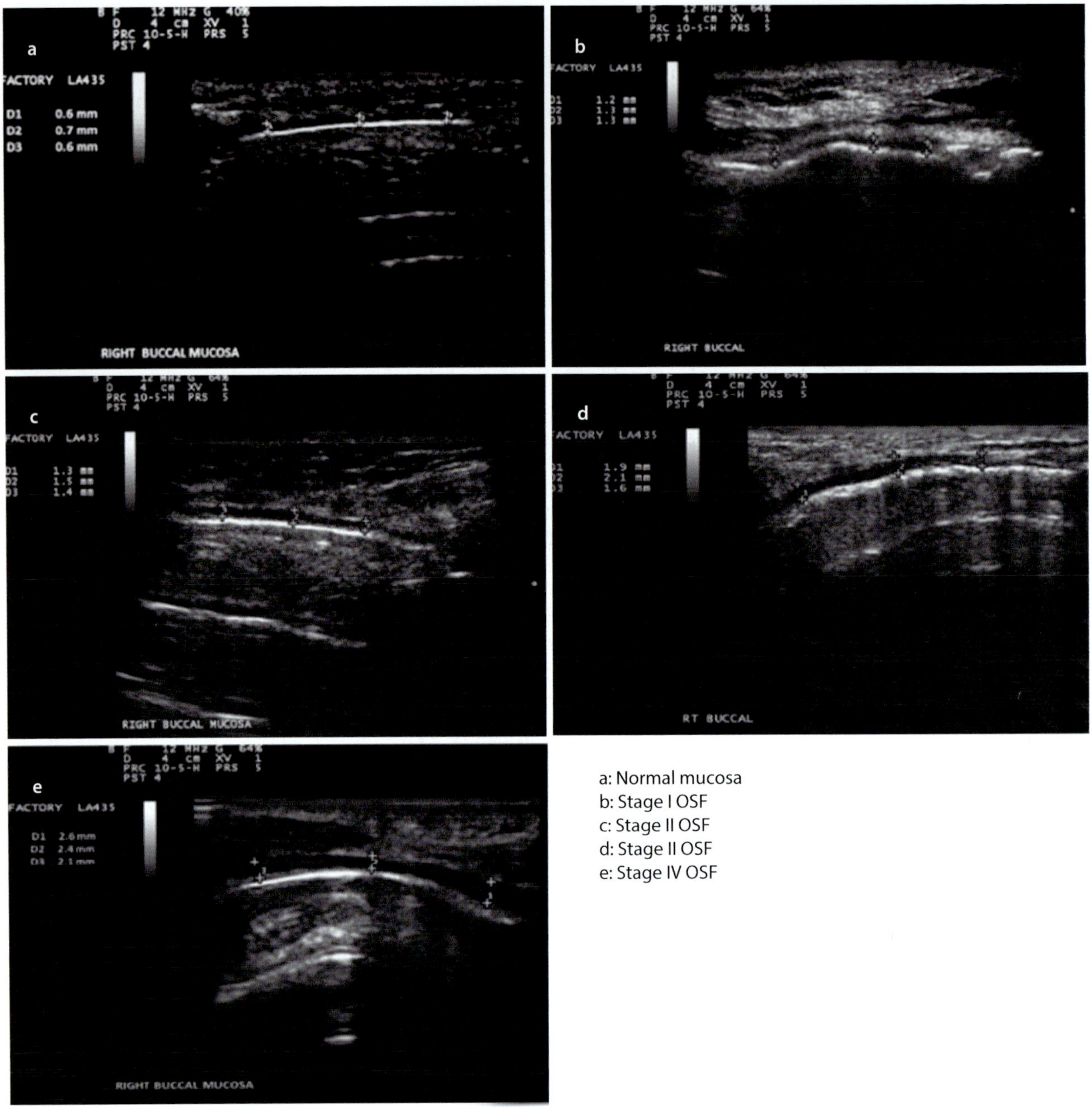


**Fig. 13.1** Submucosal thickness of buccal mucosa on ultrasonography (By courtesy of Dr. Aditya Dupare)
Submucosal thickness measurements in millimeters (mm) are taken at three points: the anterior (D1), middle (D2), and posterior (D3) for buccal mucosa

As the severity of the disease increased from grade I b**B** to IV e the thickness of the submucosal tissue increased compared to the normal control **a** point D1 (**a**–**e** 0.6 mm, followed by 1.2, 1.3, 1.9, and 2.6 mm, respectively), point D2 (**a**–**e** 0.7 mm, followed by 1.3, 1.5, 2.1, and 2.4 mm, respectively), and point D3 (**a**–**e** 0.6 mm, followed by 1.3, 1.4, 1.6, and 2.1 mm, respectively)

### 13.3.3 ATR-FTIR Spectroscopy

Fourier transform infrared (FTIR) spectroscopic imaging is used for the analysis of biochemical components (e.g., proteins, carbohydrates, and nucleic acids) and has been proposed as an adjunct to current histopathological techniques [25]. FTIR imaging provides a nondestructive image of the sample and does not require staining. Attenuated total reflection-Fourier transform infrared spectroscopy (ATR-FTIR) has been used to diagnose cancer in biofluids, such as the serum, plasma, urine, and saliva; however, its clinical translation is still under development [26, 27]. Shaikh et al. used ATR-FTIR spectroscopy to measure total protein estimation in saliva to discriminate patients with OSF from healthy controls [28] (Table 13.1).

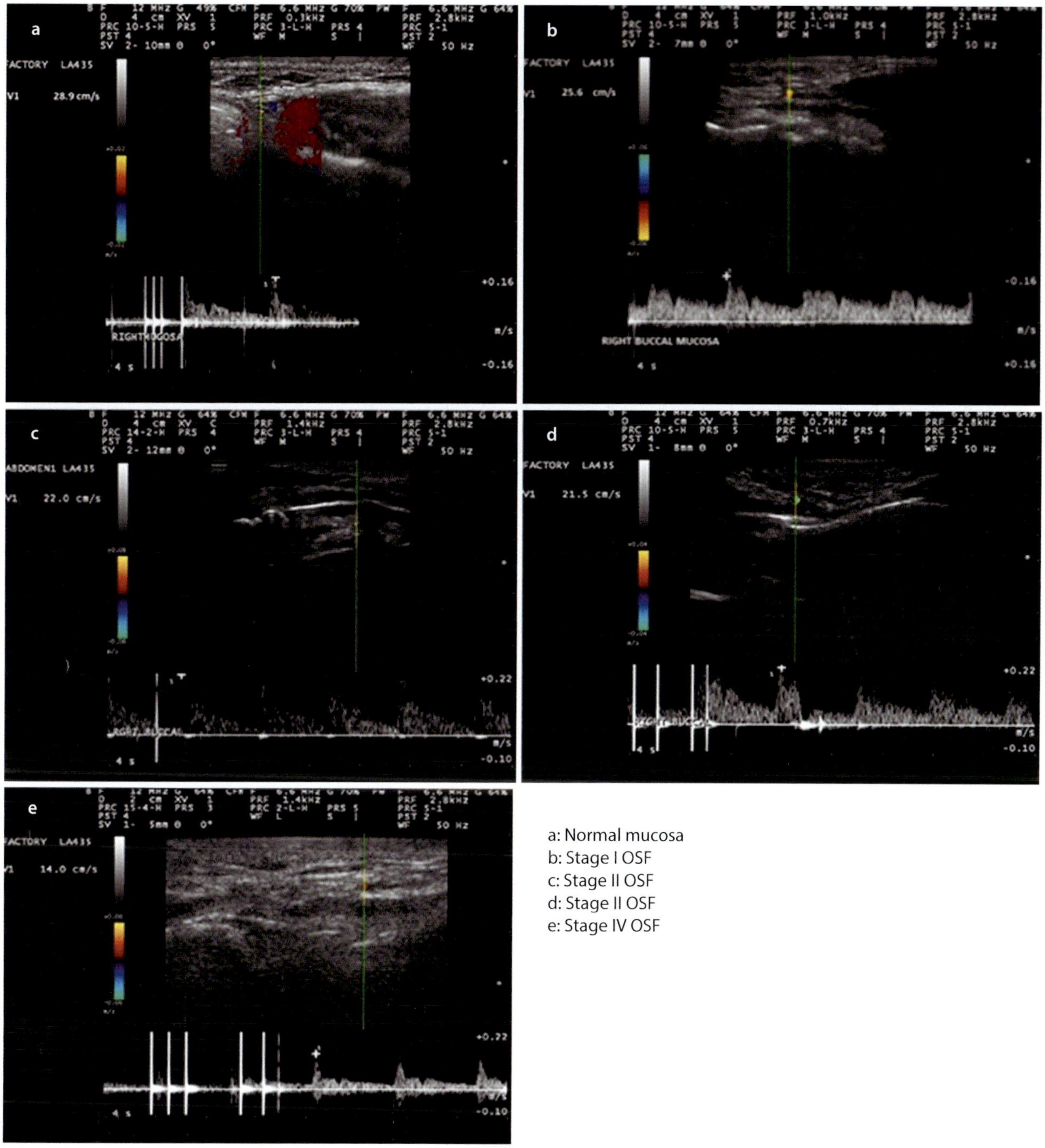


a: Normal mucosa
b: Stage I OSF
c: Stage II OSF
d: Stage II OSF
e: Stage IV OSF

**Fig. 13.2** Peak systolic velocity (PSV) on colored Doppler ultrasonography (By courtesy of Dr. Aditya Dupare)
Vascular distribution by peak systolic velocity (PSV) measured on colored Doppler USG of right buccal mucosa shows a decrease as the severity of OSF progresses from grade I b to IV **E** e-compared to normal control **a** (**a**–**e** 28.9 cm/s, followed by 28.9, 22.0, 21.5, and 14.0 cm/s, respectively)

The study showed that the specific infrared spectrum of patients with OSF could be distinguished from the healthy controls based on the spectral shift of proteins/amide II, carbohydrates, and nucleic acids using a principal component analysis and hierarchical cluster analysis. However, there were study limitations due to the small sample size. Therefore, further studies should be conducted to assess the ATR-FTIR using saliva for the assessment as a screening tool to support early diagnostic aid of OSF.

**Table 13.1** Noninvasive diagnostic techniques in oral submucous fibrosis

| Instrument/method | | Test objectives | Outcomes | Time value of test | Ease of introduction to the chairside of clinics[a] | Maintaining test accuracy | Diagnostic performance |
|---|---|---|---|---|---|---|---|
| Measurement of mouth opening | | OSF diagnosis degree of severity<br>Monitoring therapeutic effect | Functional staging by mouth-opening grade: severity of OSF | Real time | High | Easy measurement but needs standardization | High but indirect procedure |
| Optical instrument | Autofluorescence spectroscopy<br>optical coherence tomography<br>Contact endoscopy ultrasonography | Early diagnosis<br>Monitoring therapeutic effect<br>Degree of severity<br>Monitoring susceptibility to cancer | Optical inspection images (unclear threshold): detection of malignancies, blood flow pattern, presence of fibrotic bands | Real time | Low to high | Needs standardized image interpretation skill | Low to moderate (depending on the objectives) insufficient evidence |
| Biomarkers in saliva | Lactate dehydrogenase (LDH)<br>Trace elements oxidative stress markers<br>Micronutrients predictive tumor markers | OSF diagnosis degree of severity<br>Monitoring susceptibility to cancer<br>Therapeutic effect and prognosis | Biological or genetic evaluation (unclear threshold): detection of malignancies, grading of OSF | Real time but time consuming depending on instruments | Low | Standardized | Insufficient evidence<br>Not specific to OSF |
| X-ray (lateral cephalometric analysis) | | OSF diagnosis<br>Degree of severity | Morphological change images of lateral soft palate and uvula: severity of OSF, comorbidities in patients with OSF such as sleep apnea syndrome, dysphagia, and other disorders | Moderate time | High: conventional methods in dentistry | Standardized and needs X-ray interpretation skill | High for late stage but not for early stage |

[a]In low- and middle-income countries

### 13.3.4 Optical Coherence Tomography

Optical coherence tomography (OCT) is a high-resolution cross-sectional imaging modality analogous to ultrasound imaging except that it uses light instead of sound [29]. In OCT, distance and microstructure measurements are performed by backscattering and backscattering light waves from various microstructure features within a material or tissue [30]. Imaging depths are not as deep as ultrasound, up to 2–3 mm deep; however, the OCT resolution is >10–100 times finer than ultrasound [31]. A study was conducted to elucidate the possibility of using OCT to identify differences in oral and oropharyngeal mucosal and submucosal tissue in patients with benign and malignant processes in the oral cavity and oropharynx [32], and the results showed that disruption of tissue structure was observed as the pathological tissues invade healthy areas, clearly demonstrating the transition from normal epithelium with an intact basement membrane to invasive tumors. Tsai et al. [33] developed a handheld OCT system for in vivo oral cavity imaging, enabling the identification of the different structures, epithelium, lamina propria layers, fungiform papilla, and salivary gland, and the observation of the microcirculation patterns across various oral mucosal types, including non-keratinized, keratinized (masticatory), and specialized mucosae.

According to clinical scans of a swept source OCT (SS-OCT) system, the following parameters were identified to facilitate the clinical diagnosis of oral lesions [34]: epithelial (EP) thickness, standard deviation (SD) of A-mode scan intensity profile of the EP layer, and decay constants of the spatial domain spectrum of the A-mode scan profile. Lee et al. conducted a study in Taiwan to elucidate the effectiveness of the SS-OCT system for clinical diagnosis of OSF [4]. The results of the study showed that the EP layer was thinner and the SD of the A-mode scan intensity in the lamina propria (LP) layer was reduced in OSF compared to healthy controls (◘ Fig. 13.3, ◘ Table 13.1). The EP thickness cutoff values of 350 and 400 μm achieved 100% sensitivity and specificity, and the SD value of 0.21 in the LP layer achieved 90.9% sensitivity and 84.1% specificity for OSF. On the other hand, as the lesion begins to progress from epithelial hyperplasia to dysplasia, the EP layer thickens if the EP/LP boundary is still identified. When early OSCC coexists with OSF, the surface features are unclear, and variable EP thickness can make distinguishing between healthy tissues, other OPMDs, OSCC, and OSF difficult. The researchers categorized OSF patients into three groups based on the maximum mouth opening (MMO) and showed that EP thickness and average LP SD in the LP layer may be a more effective OSF diagnostic method than measuring MMO [4] (◘ Fig. 13.4).

Some limitations of OCT include the following: (1) pathologists should interpret and evaluate the acquired live histology images; (2) images do not provide quantitative information and require subjective visual assessment; and (3) due to the small size of the OCT probe, only a very small area can be inspected at a time [35]. Overall, although OCT is good at diagnosing OSF, clinical application of OCT remains challenging in patients with OSF in terms of early detection of malignant changes.

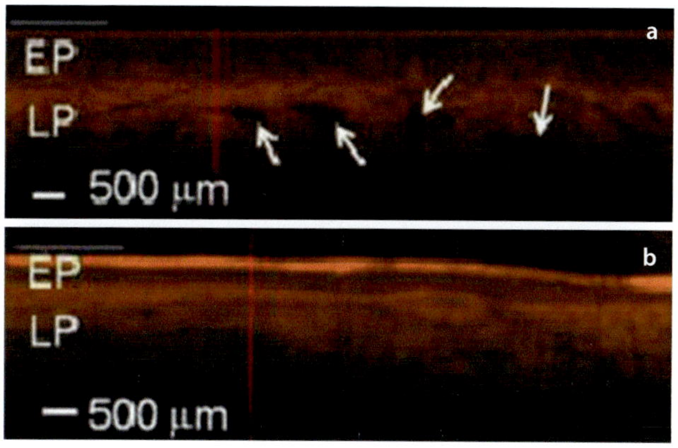


◘ **Fig. 13.3** Swept source OCT (SS-OCT) scanning images: **a** healthy mucosa, **b** OSF mucosa
In healthy mucosa, glands or blood vessels can be observed as black spots as indicated by arrows. *EP* epithelial, *LP* lamina propria (Reproduced from Lee et al. Diagnosis of oral submucous fibrosis with optical coherence tomography. J Biomed Opt. 2009; 14:054008 [4])

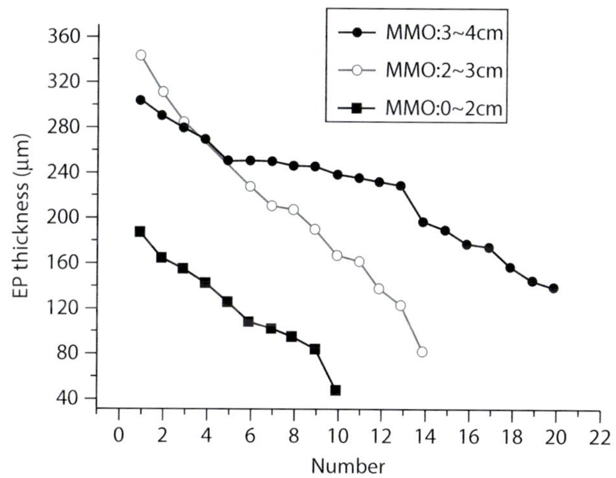


◘ **Fig. 13.4** EP thickness data points of OSF samples grouped according to different MMO ranges
EP thickness is related to MMO. (Reproduced from Lee et al. Diagnosis of oral submucous fibrosis with optical coherence tomography. J Biomed Opt. 2009; 14:054008 [4])

### 13.3.5 Contact Endoscopy

Contact endoscopy (CE) is a noninvasive optical detection technique first used in minimally invasive gynecologic surgery [36] and has subsequently been applied in urology, bronchoscopy, arthroscopy, and otolaryngology. This technique enables real-time evaluation of the superficial cell layers of the epithelium and magnifies the images. Mishra et al. examined the diagnostic accuracy of CE in the detection of oral mucosal lesions and OSCC, including OSF [37] (◘ Table 13.1). CE showed 84.2% sensitivity and 94.4% specificity for the diagnosis of malignancies of oral mucosal lesions compared to histopathological diagnosis; however, no malignancy was detected in OSF due to the small sample size ($n = 7$). The results did not include CE images indicating OSF.

One of the types of contact endoscopy, colposcopy, is designed as a gynecological diagnostic technique to evaluate changes in mucosal surface topography and vascular patterns of the cervix. Parameters include vascular pattern, intercapillary distance, surface pattern, color tone, opacity, and clarity of the mucosal lesion demarcation [38]. This technique has been applied to patients with OPMDs and OSCC to distinguish between benign, dysplastic, and malignant diagnoses and to assist in biopsy site selection [39–42]. Ujwara et al. used this technique to diagnose OSCC in 90 cases of OPMDs, including 30 patients with OSF, following the application of acetic acid and Lugol's iodine, and showed that colposcopy was useful in outlining the most suspicious lesion for histopathological diagnosis by biopsy [42] (◘ Table 13.1). However, colposcopy did not help reveal clinical patterns of dysplastic or malignant changes in OSF, and the iodine application did not show uniform uptake even in dysplastic lesions. Overall, colposcopy may not be useful in defining early-stage malignancy in patients with OSF.



## 13.4 Biomarkers in Saliva

Saliva contains a wide range of proteins/peptides, nucleic acids, electrolytes, and hormones from multiple local and systemic sources [43] and may be useful for multiplexed assays developed as point-of-care devices [44]. Saliva may be reflective of the serum or contain biomarkers that are shed from the surface of the oral mucosa. Several studies have been conducted using unstimulated saliva for OSF diagnosis, monitoring of treatment, and surveillance of patients for progression and malignant transformation [45–62] (◘ Table 13.2).

### 13.4.1 Lactate Dehydrogenase

Lactate dehydrogenase (LDH) is an enzyme found in the cytoplasm of a number of body tissues [58, 63], which converts lactate to pyruvate. It is also a nonspecific marker of tissue turnover, a normal metabolic process. It's increase can serve as a prognostic marker for the progression of different types of cancer [63]. In a meta-analysis [64], 2 out of 13 studies [58, 59] evaluated salivary LDH in patients with OSF and showed that standardized mean difference (SMD) of salivary LDH levels was higher in the OSF group than in healthy control, but this was not statistically significant (SMD 25.83; 95% CI: −1.74 to 53.40).

### 13.4.2 Trace Elements

Among trace elements, tissue copper levels were determined to be elevated in patients with OSF [65–67]. Copper acts as an initiating factor for OSF and plays a role in stimulating fibrosis by upregulating lysyl oxidase activity [65]. A meta-analysis showed a significant increase in the copper levels and a significant decrease in zinc and iron levels in patients with OSF [68]. A significant difference was observed in the mean salivary copper [45, 46, 48], zinc [46, 47], iron [45–47], and copper/zinc levels [46, 47] of OSF patients when compared to the normal controls (◘ Table 13.2). However, there is a limitation in that the influence of dietary intake was not investigated in most studies.

### 13.4.3 Oxidative Stress/Micronutrients

Saliva serves as the primary defense against free radicals generated in the oral cavity during various physiological processes, and several oxidative markers have been analyzed in unstimulated saliva from both OSF and control groups (◘ Table 13.2). Serum and saliva ascorbic acid (vitamin C) levels consistently decreased with the increased severity of OSF [49, 53, 69]. A case-control study was conducted in India to determine the correlation between oxidative stress marker levels and OSF severity as defined according to the mouth-opening grade, fibrotic bands, and histopathological grades [53]. The results showed that vitamins A, C, and E levels and salivary superoxide dismutase (SOD) and glutathione peroxidase (GPx) activities were significantly lower in OSF patients than in controls. These changes were significantly correlated with increased histopathological grades of OSF and clinical staging of mouth opening, reflecting increased oxidative stress as the disease progressed.

Salivary malondialdehyde, one of the final byproducts of lipid peroxidation, levels were significantly higher in OSF patients than in controls and increased as the clinical stage [54] as well as the histopathological grade of OSF worsened [56].

The level of salivary 8-hydroxy-2-deoxyguanosine (8-OHdG), one of the reactive oxygen species and a potential DNA damage biomarker, is significantly higher in patients with OSCC or OSF than that in the control group [55, 57]. Salivary lipid peroxide, conjugated diene, hydroxyl radicals, and superoxide dismutase levels were higher, and

Table 13.2 Biomarkers in saliva for diagnostic aids of oral submucous fibrosis

| Purpose | Biomarkers | | Age range or mean, SD | Outcome values (mean, SD) | | Unit | Number (OSF, control) | Significance ($p$-value) | Diagnostic confirmation of OSF | Note | Year | References |
|---|---|---|---|---|---|---|---|---|---|---|---|---|
| | | | | OSF | Healthy control | | | | | | | |
| OFS diagnosis | Salivary lactate dehydrogenase (LDH) | | 18- | 606.83, 60.01 | 80.73, 12.06 | U/L | 30, 30 | <0.001 | Clinicopathological | | 2015 | Sivarakrishnan [58] |
| | | | 20–70 | 608.28, 30.22 | 182.21, 34.85 | Unstated | 25, 10 | <0.001 | Clinical | | 2016 | Kallalli [79] |
| | | | 28.63, 10.39 | 1057.30, 640.12 | 668.25, 498.45 | μg/dl | 20, 20 | 0.04 | Clinical | | 2018 | Mishra [80] |
| | | | 18–70 | 350.43, 5.90 | 86.12, 7.05 | IU/L | 30, 30 | Not indicated | Clinicopathological | Grade I-IV OSF | 2019 | Mantri [81] |
| | | | – | 631.67, 7.67 | 140.62, 8.87 | Unstated | 40, 40 | <0.001 | Clinical | | 2020 | Panda [82] |
| Monitoring susceptibility to cancer | Salivary trace elements | Cu | 30–50 | 0.13, 0.015 | 0.15, 0.016 | ppm/L | 35, 35 | <0.05 | Clinicopathological | | 2012 | Chitra [45] |
| | | | – | 87.45, 2.67 | 46.07, 4.56 | μg/dl | 50, 50 | 0.001 | Clinicopathological | | 2015 | Shetty [46] |
| | | | 16–60 | 0.087, 0.162 | 0.051, 0.06 | ppm/L | 30, 30 | NS | Clinical | | 2015 | Okade [47] |
| | | | 20–63 | 27.023, 14.498 | 8.393, 2.256 | μg/dl | 30, 30 | 0.005 | Clinicopathological | Grade I-III OSF | 2015 | Mohammed [48] |
| | | Zn | 35–50 | 0.15, 0.017 | 0.13, 0.014 | ppm/L | 35, 35 | NS | Clinicopathological | | 2012 | Chitra [45] |
| | | | – | 24.67, 4.86 | 35.78, 3.97 | μg/dl | 50, 50 | 0.001 | Clinicopathological | | 2015 | Shetty [45] |
| | | | 16–60 | 0.100, 0.214 | 0.100, 0.295 | ppm/L | 30, 30 | <0.05 | Clinical | | 2015 | Okade [47] |

(continued)

**Table 13.2** (continued)

| Purpose | Biomarkers | | Age range or mean, SD | Outcome values (mean, SD) | | Unit | Number (OSF, control) | Significance ($p$-value) | Diagnostic confirmation of OSF | Note | Year | References |
|---|---|---|---|---|---|---|---|---|---|---|---|---|
| | | Cu/Zn ratio | 35–50 | 1 | 1 | | 35, 35 | NS | Clinicopathological | | 2012 | Chitra [45] |
| | | | – | 3.53 | 1.28 | μg/dl | 50, 50 | 0.001 | Clinicopathological | | 2015 | Shetty [46] |
| | | | 16–60 | 3.78, 4.13 | 10.91, 15.89 | ppm/L | 30, 30 | <0.05 | Clinical | | 2015 | Okade [47] |
| | | Fe | 35–50 | 0.4, 0.05 | 0.10, 0.02 | ppm/L | 35, 35 | <0.05 | Clinicopathological | | 2012 | Chitra [45] |
| | | | 20–40 | 107.448, 28.932 | 119.898, 31.519 | Unstated | 65, 21 | NS | Clinicopathological | | 2012a | Shetty [49] |
| | | | 16–60 | 0.149, 0.242 | 0.524, 0.143 | ppm/L | 30, 30 | <0.05 | Clinical | | 2015 | Okade [47] |
| | | | – | 35.67, 1.34 | 76.07, 3.65 | μg/dl | 50, 50 | 0.001 | Clinicopathological | | 2015 | Shetty [46] |
| | Salivary predictive tumor markers | S100A7 | 28.2 (mean) for OSF, 26.9 for control | 0.28, 0.9 | 0.19, 0.03 | ng/ml | 30, 30 | <0.001 | Clinical | | 2019 | Raffat [50] |
| | | MMP-12 | 33.27, 12.43 | 12.53, 3.2 | 0.82, 0.45 | ng/ml | 30, 30 | <0.001 | Clinical | | 2021 | Saleem [51] |
| | | microRNAs | 34.1, 13.4 | 14.31, 23.33 | 0.50, 0.30 | | 61, 63 | <0.001 | Clinical | miRNA expression fold | 2020 | Prasad [52] |
| Monitoring therapeutic effect and prognosis | Salivary oxidative stress markers | LPO | 20–70 | 197.22, 64.5 | 15.86, 4.63 | μM of MDA/ml | 63, 63 | <0.001 | Clinicopathological | Grade I-IV OSF | 2018 | Divyambika [53] |
| | | GSH | | 464.51, 84.15 | 474.6, 47.2 | μM/ml | | NS | | | | |
| | | SOD | | 0.72, 0.22 | 1.42, 0.28 | U/100 mg protein | | <0.001 | | | | |

| | | | | | | | | | | | | |
|---|---|---|---|---|---|---|---|---|---|---|---|---|
| | | GPX | | 0.85, 0.33 | 1.41, 0.38 | mM of GSH reduced/min/mg protein | | <0.001 | | | | |
| | | Malondialdehyde | 20–40 | 0.434 | 0.224 | nmol/mg | 65, 21 | <0.001 | Clinicopathological | | 2012b | Shetty [54] |
| | | | 41–60 | 0.43, 0.07 | 0.08, 0.07 | µM/ml | 40, 40 | <0.005 | Clinicopathological | | 2016 | Kaur [55] |
| | | | Unstated | 0.359, 0.06 | 0.179, 0.04 | nmol/mg | 40, 40 | <0.05 | Clinicopathological | Grade I-III OSF | 2021 | Ganta [56] |
| | | 8-OHdG | 41–60 | 0.49, 0.08 | 0.07, 0.07 | ng/dl | 40, 40 | <0.005 | Clinicopathological | | 2016 | Kaur [55] |
| | | | 31–60 | 13.89, 1.96 | 6.59, 1.47 | ng/dl | 30, 30 | <0.0001 | Clinicopathological | | 2020 | Nandakumar [57] |
| | Salivary micronutrients | Ascorbic acid (vitamin C) | 20–70 | 226.91, 77.34 | 302.65, 95.32 | µg/ml | 63, 63 | <0.01 | Clinicopathological | Grade I-IV OSF | 2018 | Divyambika [53] |
| | | | 20–40 | 0.665, 0.282 | 0.936, 0.274 | Unstated | 65, 21 | <0.05 | Clinicopathological | | 2012a | Shetty [49] |
| | | | 41–60 | 0.53, 0.12 | 1.2, 0.6 | µg/L | 40, 40 | <0.005 | Clinicopathological | | 2016 | Kaur [55] |

*LPO* oxidative markers of lipid peroxides, *GSH* reduced glutathione, *SOD* superoxide dismutase, *GPx* glutathione peroxidase, *8-OHdG* 8-hydroxy-2-deoxyguanosine, *NS* not significant hydrogen peroxide and sodium levels were lower in patients with OSF than those in normal healthy controls [45]. Measuring these markers may help predict the severity of oral diseases, but it is not specific to OSF patients.

### 13.4.4 Predictive Tumor Markers

S100A7 (Psoriasin) is a signaling molecule that regulates cell function and is highly expressed in hyperproliferative skin conditions [70]. High S100A7, which expresses in the oral mucosa, is found in dysplasia associated with a high risk of cancer development among OPMDs including OSF patients [71]. Salivary S100A7 in OSF was examined in Pakistan and showed a significant positive association between salivary S100A7 levels and duration of gutkha use and mouth opening [50]. However, no sensitivity and specificity were calculated because no histological examination was performed, and the threshold for diagnostic S100A7 levels in OSF remains unclear.

Matrix metalloproteinases-12 (MMP-12) has been shown to have important sensitivity and specificity to qualify as a diagnostic biomarker for OSCC [72]. Salleem et al. showed that salivary MMP-12 expression was higher in patients with OSF or OSCC than that in the healthy controls [51] (◘ Tables 13.1 and 13.2). They also showed that salivary MMP-12 in OSF was significantly lower than that of OSCC, explaining that MMP-12 increases as OSF progresses to OSCC.



Salivary microRNAs have been explored as possible predictive biomarkers for malignant transformation of OPMDs [73]. miRNA-21 overexpression in OSF has been suggested to be due to areca nut stimulation mediated by the TGF-β pathway [74]. A recent study analyzed the salivary miRNA-21 in areca nut users with OSF compared to areca nut users without OSF. They showed that miRNA-21 was overexpressed in the OSF patients; however, expression levels were not significantly associated with disease severity [52].

Although salivary biomarkers can be used as sensitive diagnostic and disease progression markers for OSF, it should be noted that they are not OSF specific. Furthermore, analyte concentration in saliva can be affected by stimulating or non-stimulating sampling procedures, fluid intake, and ingestion of some drugs [75]. Overall, evidence on the utility of biomarkers in saliva was insufficient for the diagnosis of OSF. In the future, saliva tests hold promise both as a screening tool and as a marker for predicting the progression of malignant transformation in OSF.

## 13.5 X-Ray (Lateral Cephalometric Analysis)

OSF can also cause changes in the morphology and function of the soft palate. The morphology of the soft palate in normal individuals according to digital cephalometric studies falls into six types [76]. Studies evaluating the morphology of soft palate in patients with OSF using a digital lateral cephalogram showed that the soft palate in areca nut users changes from an elongated to a short and thick morphology as the disease progresses [77–80] (◘ Fig. 13.5). These changes are due to fibro-

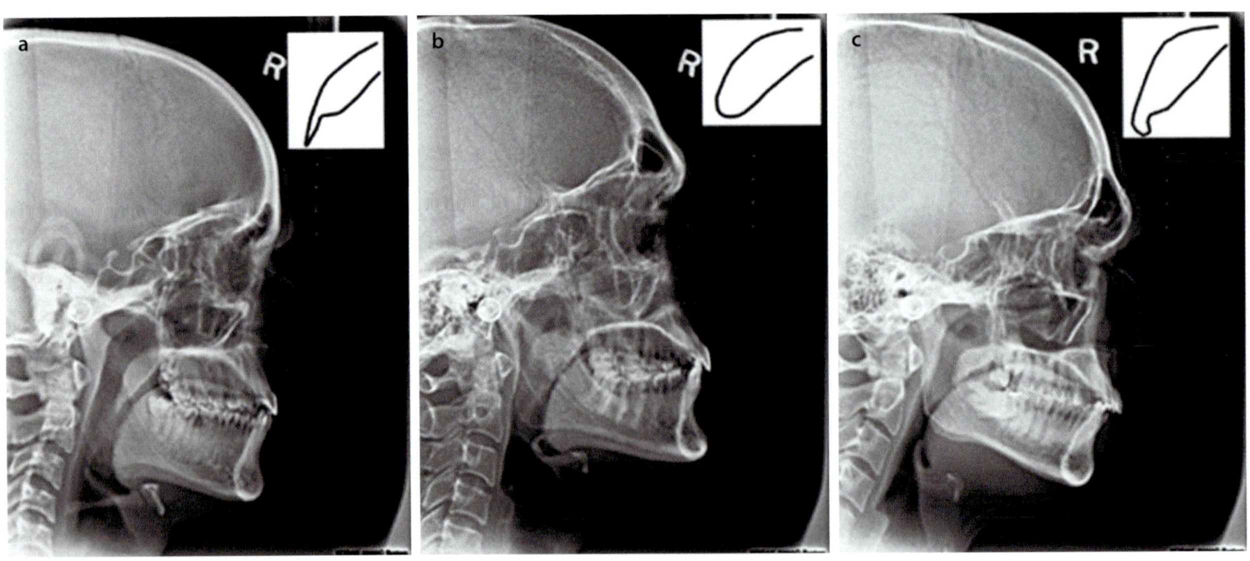


◘ **Fig. 13.5** Lateral ► cephalogram for morphology of the soft palate of OSF
**a**: type 1 (leaf-shaped), **b**: type 3 (butt shaped), and **c**: type 6 (crook shaped) soft palates (Reproduced from Shankar et al. Morphometric evaluation of soft palate in oral submucous fibrosis--a digital cephalometric study. J Craniomaxillofac Surg. 2014; 42:48–52 [77])

sis in the soft palate and uvula [81], which functionally impairs speech, respiratory, and auditory function. The uvula shrinks and hooks up, exhibiting a shape known as the "hockey-stick uvula" [82], which is confirmed not only by visual examination but also by lateral cephalogram (as type 6 by Shankar et al. [77]). Verification of soft palate cephalometric findings helps identify the likelihood of developing comorbidities in patients with OSF, including obstructive sleep apnea syndrome, dysphagia, and other disorders. The X-ray examinations by lateral cephalometric analysis of OSF patients may be morphologically and functionally useful in the late stages, but not in the early stages. X-ray interpretation skills and standardization of the tests are needed for this analysis. Radiation exposure is a limitation of repeated examinations.

## 13.6 Discussion

The key objectives of using noninvasive diagnostic techniques for patients with OSF include early detection of OSF, assessment and monitoring of OSF severity (and response to treatment), and risk stratification or monitoring of OSF patients for malignant transformation (i.e., OSCC). Point-of-care diagnostic techniques for OSF must demonstrate utility, accuracy, and ease to deploy in both primary and secondary settings (i.e., in rural areas).

Most studies have evaluated the effectiveness of adjunctive diagnostic aids in patients with OSF in cohort studies with heterogeneous populations including OSCC and other OPMDs rather than specifically addressing OSF patients alone. The diagnostic adjunctive techniques presented in this chapter are based on the results of non-randomized controlled trials (mostly case-control) with small sample size, suggesting that the evidence of their effectiveness is low (i.e., due to the high risk of biases, such as selection bias in normal control, and the case group (diagnosis of OSF) itself). Nevertheless, some promising adjunctive diagnostic methods have been reported for OSF.

Early diagnosis of OSF is challenging but critical given that some children use areca nut (Chap. 5). Change in clinical features of the oral mucosa is an important sign of early exposure to areca nut products. A simple history and clinical examination with standardized measuring MMO remain the most important way to detect OSF. There is insufficient evidence that other noninvasive adjunctive diagnostic techniques can play a role here.

Optical instruments and X-rays used chairside can help patients visually understand the nature of the disease without harm or adverse events, although these diagnostic techniques add little overall value to the current assessment, risk stratification, and monitoring of patients with OSF. Perturbations in various salivary markers have been identified from patients with OSF; however, cutoff values are not well defined, and the current body of evidence to support their use is low. In addition, the use of time-consuming and costly diagnostic techniques is also unsupported by the evidence, particularly in lower resource countries where betel quid and areca nut use are a social problem and the prevalence of OSF is high.

> **Summary**
> The potential utility of noninvasive diagnostic techniques in oral submucous fibrosis (OSF) includes early detection, assessment of OSF severity (and response to treatment), and monitoring of OSF patients for malignant transformation. Numerous adjunct techniques, including optical techniques, ultrasonography, and salivary biomarkers, have been evaluated but have demonstrated limited utility in primary and secondary settings. Many adjunctive techniques require expensive equipment or laboratory testing. The development of low-cost point-of-care testing for monitoring patients with OSF is needed in low- and middle-income countries where the use of areca nut is widespread.

## References

1. Cox SC, Walker DM. Establishing a normal range for mouth opening: its use in screening for oral submucous fibrosis. Br J Oral Maxillofac Surg. 1997;35:40–2.
2. Ranganathan K, Davi U, Joshua E, Bhardwaj A, Rooban T, Viswanathan R. Mouth opening, cheek flexibility and tongue protrusion. Parameters of 800 normal patients in Chennai. South India J Indian Dent Assoc. 2001;7:78–80.
3. Chiu CJ, Lee WC, Chiang CP, Hahn LJ, Kuo YS, Chen CJ. A scoring system for the early detection of oral submucous fibrosis based on a self-administered questionnaire. J Public Health Dent. 2002;62:28–31.
4. Lee CK, Tsai MT, Lee HC, Chen HM, Chiang CP, Wang YM, et al. Diagnosis of oral submucous fibrosis with optical coherence tomography. J Biomed Opt. 2009;14:054008.
5. Gillenwater A, Jacob R, Ganeshappa R, Kemp B, El-Naggar AK, Palmer JL, et al. Noninvasive diagnosis of oral neoplasia based on fluorescence spectroscopy and native tissue autofluorescence. Arch Otolaryngol Head Neck Surg. 1998;124(11):1251–8.
6. Chen HM, Wang CY, Chen CT, Yang H, Kuo YS, Lan WH, et al. Auto-fluorescence spectra of oral submucous fibrosis. J Oral Pathol Med. 2003;32(6):337–43.
7. Haris PS, Balan A, Jayasree RS, Gupta AK. Autofluorescence spectroscopy for the in vivo evaluation of oral submucous fibrosis. Photomed Laser Surg. 2009;27(5):757–61.
8. Chaturvedi P, Majumder SK, Krishna H, Muttagi S, Gupta PK. Fluorescence spectroscopy for noninvasive early diagnosis of oral mucosal malignant and potentially malignant lesions. J Cancer Res Ther. 2010;6:497–502.

9. Wang CY, Tsai T, Chiang CP, Chen HM, Chen CT. Improved diagnosis of oral premalignant lesions in submucous fibrosis patients with 5-aminolevulinic acid induced PpIX fluorescence. J Biomed Opt. 2009;14(4):044026.
10. Shah S, Waknis P, Saha A, Setiya S, Ratra T, Vaswani V. The use of Velscope to assess cellular changes occurring in oral premalignancy. J Oral Biol Craniofac Res. 2020;10(2):99–103.
11. Rangaiah P, Annigeri RG, Lingappa A. Transcutaneous ultrasonographic assessment of oral submucous fibrosis: a preliminary study. Int J Oral Med Sci. 2010;9:137–47.
12. Kamala KA, Annigeri RG, Ashok L. Ultrasonic diagnosis of masseteric hypertrophy in oral submucous fibrosis: a preliminary study. J Indian Acad Oral Med Radiol. 2010;22:197–200.
13. Manjunath K, Rajaram PC, Saraswathi TR, Sivapathasundharam B, Sabarinath B, Koteeswaran D, et al. Evaluation of oral submucous fibrosis using ultrasonographic technique: a new diagnostic tool. Indian J Dent Res. 2011;22:530–6.
14. Krithika C, Ramanathan S, Koteeswaran D, Sridhar C, Satheesh Krishna J, et al. Ultrasonographic evaluation of oral submucous fibrosis in habitual areca nut chewers. Dentomaxillofac Radiol. 2013;42:20120319.
15. Devathambi JR, Aswath N. Ultrasonographic evaluation of oral submucous fibrosis and masseteric hypertrophy. J Clin Imaging Sci. 2013;3(Suppl. 1):12.
16. Chakarvarty A, Panat SR, Sangamesh NC, Aggarwal A, Jha PC. Evaluation of masseter muscle hypertrophy in oral submucous fibrosis patients -an ultrasonographic study. J Clin Diagn Res. 2014;8:ZC45–ZC47.
17. Kant P, Bhowate RR, Sharda N. Assessment of cross-sectional thickness and activity of masseter, anterior temporalis and orbicularis oris muscles in oral submucous fibrosis patients and healthy controls: an ultrasonography and electromyography study. Dentomaxillofac Radiol. 2014;43:20130016.
18. Agarwal RK, Hebbale M, Mhapuskar A, Tepan M. Correlation of ultrasonographic measurements, histopathological grading, and clinical staging in oral submucous fibrosis. Indian J Dent Res. 2017;28:476–81.
19. Tiwari M, Deoghare A, Sharma A, Saha S, Poptani R. Evaluation of OSMF with ultrasonography. Int J Oral Health Dent. 2017;3:169–74.
20. Dupare A, Dhole A. Ultrasonographic evaluation of submucosal thickness in oral submucous fibrosis patients: a cross-sectional study. Pol J Radiol. 2018;83:e280–8.
21. Nadendla LK, Tatikonda VK, Bangi BB, Bhayya H, Devulapally RV, Pokala A. Sonographic imaging of fibrosis of oral mucosa and its correlation with clinical staging in oral submucous fibrosis. J Cancer Res Ther. 2018;14:394–7.
22. Mukul SK, Kumar S, Pandey S, Mokhtar EA, Kumar A. Ultrasound elastography as a potential diagnostic aid in oral submucous fibrosis. Natl J Maxillofac Surg. 2019;10:129–33.
23. Sadaksharam J, Mahalingam S. Evaluation of oral pentoxifylline in the management of oral submucous fibrosis—an ultrasonographic study. Contemp Clin Dent. 2017;8(2):200–4.
24. Patil SR, Maragathavalli G, Ramesh DNSV, Rao KA, Bandela V, Alam MK. Role of ultrasonography in evaluation of oral submucous fibrosis patients: a systematic review. Int Med J. 2021;28:254–7.
25. Walsh MJ, Kajdacsy-Balla A, Holton SE, Bhargava R. Attenuated total reflectance Fourier-transform infrared spectroscopic imaging for breast histopathology. Vib Spectrosc. 2012;60:23–8.
26. Elkins KM. Rapid presumptive "fingerprinting" of body fluids and materials by ATR FT-IR spectroscopy. J Forensic Sci. 2011;56:1580–7.
27. Sala A, Anderson DJ, Brennan PM, Butler HJ, Cameron JM, Jenkinson MD, et al. Biofluid diagnostics by FTIR spectroscopy: a platform technology for cancer detection. Cancer Lett. 2020;477:122–30.
28. Shaikh S, Yadav DK, Rawal R. Saliva based non invasive screening of Oral submucous fibrosis using ATR-FTIR spectroscopy. J Pharm Biomed Anal. 2021;203:114202.
29. Fujimoto JG, Pitris C, Boppart SA, Brezinski ME. Optical coherence tomography: an emerging technology for biomedical imaging and optical biopsy. Neoplasia. 2000;2:9–25.
30. Huang D, Swanson EA, Lin CP, Schuman JS, Stinson WG, Chang W, et al. Optical coherence tomography. Science. 1991;254(5035):1178–81.
31. Fujimoto JG. Optical coherence tomography for ultrahigh resolution in vivo imaging. Nat Biotechnol. 2003;21:1361–7.
32. Ridgway JM, Armstrong WB, Guo S, Mahmood U, Su J, Jackson RP, et al. In vivo optical coherence tomography of the human oral cavity and oropharynx. Arch Otolaryngol Head Neck Surg. 2006;132:1074–81.
33. Tsai MT, Chen Y, Lee CY, Huang BH, Trung NH, Lee YJ, et al. Noninvasive structural and microvascular anatomy of oral mucosae using handheld optical coherence tomography. Biomed Opt Express. 2017;8:5001–12.
34. Tsai MT, Lee HC, Lee CK, Yu CH, Chen HM, Chiang CP, et al. Effective indicators for diagnosis of oral cancer using optical coherence tomography. Opt Express. 2008;16:15847–62.
35. Olivo M, Bhuvaneswari R, Keogh I. Advances in bio-optical imaging for the diagnosis of early oral cancer. Pharmaceutics. 2011;3:354–78.
36. Hamou JE. Microhysteroscopy Acta Endosc. 1980;10:415–22.
37. Mishra AK, Nilakantan A, Sahai K, Datta R, Malik A. Contact endoscopy of mucosal lesions of oral cavity—preliminary experience. Med J Armed Forces India. 2014;70:257–63.
38. Kolstad P. Terminology and definitions. In: Kolstad P, editor. Atlas of colposcopy. 3rd ed. London: Churchill Livingstone; 1982. p. 21–31.
39. Gynther GW, Rozell B, Heimdahl A. Direct oral microscopy and its value in diagnosing mucosal lesions: a pilot study. Oral Surg Oral Med Oral Pathol Oral Radiol Endod. 2000;90:164–70.
40. Kumar A, Shankar YU, Prakash S, Radhika B, Fatima N. Colposcopy—a novel diagnostic technique for oral mucosal lesions. J Clin Diagn Res. 2014;8:ZE25-8.
41. Nayyar AS, Khan M, Bafna UD, Siddique A, Gayitri HC. Colposcopy: gynecological vision in viewing oral lesions. Indian J Pathol Microbiol. 2014;57:223–30.
42. Ujwala N, Singh NA, Milind N, Prafulla P, Vidhya P, Bhushan B, et al. Colposcopy in pre-malignant lesions and oral squamous cell carcinoma: linking threads of clinical, histopathological and colposcopic inferences. J Cancer Res Ther. 2016;12:295–301.
43. Chianeh YR, Prabhu K. Biochemical markers in saliva of patients with oral squamous cell carcinoma. Asian Pac J Trop Dis. 2014;4(Suppl. 1):S33–40.
44. Malamud D. Saliva as a diagnostic fluid. Dent Clin N Am. 2011;55:159–78.
45. Chitra S, Balasubramaniam M, Hazra J. Effect of α-tocopherol on salivary reactive oxygen species and trace elements in oral submucous fibrosis. Ann Clin Biochem. 2012;49:262–5.
46. Shetty SR, Babu S, Kumari S, Shetty P, Hegde S, Karikal A. Status of trace elements in saliva of oral precancer and oral cancer patients. J Cancer Res Ther. 2015;11:146–9.
47. Okade AR, Hallikeri KS, Trivedi DJ. Salivary estimation of copper, iron, zinc and manganese in oral submucous fibrosis patients: a case-control study. Clin Cancer Invest J. 2015;4:302–3016.
48. Mohammed F, Manohar V, Jose M, Thapasum AF, Mohamed S, Shamaz BH, et al. Estimation of copper in saliva and areca

13

nut products and its correlation with histological grades of oral submucous fibrosis. J Oral Pathol Med. 2015;44:208–13.
49. Shetty SR, Babu S, Kumari S, Shetty P, Vijay R, Karikal A. Evaluation of micronutrient status in serum and saliva of oral submucous fibrosis patients: a clinicopathological study. Indian J Med Paediatr Oncol. 2012a;33(4):224–6.
50. Raffat MA, Hadi NI, Hosein M, Zubairi AM, Ikram S, Akram Z. Differential expression of salivary S100A7 in oral submucous fibrosis. Saudi Dent J. 2019;31:39–44.
51. Saleem Z, Shaikh AH, Zaman U, Ahmed S, Majeed MM, Kazmi A, et al. Estimation of salivary matrix metalloproteinases- 12 (MMP- 12) levels among patients presenting with oral submucous fibrosis and oral squamous cell carcinoma. BMC Oral Health. 2021;21:205.
52. Prasad SR, Pai A, Shyamala K, Yaji A. Expression of salivary miRNA 21 in Oral submucous fibrosis (OSMF): an observational study. Microrna. 2020;9:295–302.
53. Divyambika CV, Sathasivasubramanian S, Vani G, Vanishree AJ, Malathi N. Correlation of clinical and histopathological grades in oral submucous fibrosis patients with oxidative stress markers in saliva. Indian J Clin Biochem. 2018;33:348–55.
54. Shetty SR, Babu SG, Kumari S, Rao V, Vijay R, Karikal A. Malondialdehyde levels in oral sub mucous fibrosis: a clinicopathological and biochemical study. N Am J Med Sci. 2012b;4:125–8.
55. Kaur J, Politis C, Jacobs R. Salivary 8-hydroxy-2-deoxyguanosine, malondialdehyde, vitamin C, and vitamin E in oral pre-cancer and cancer: diagnostic value and free radical mechanism of action. Clin Oral Investig. 2016;20:315–9.
56. Ganta SR, Chittemsetti S, Sravya T, Guttikonda VR. Salivary malondialdehyde in oral submucous fibrosis—a marker for oxidative damage. J Oral Maxillofac Pathol. 2021;25:82–7.
57. Nandakumar A, Nataraj P, James A, Krishnan R, Mahesh KM. Estimation of salivary 8-Hydroxydeoxyguanosine (8-OHdG) as a potential biomarker in assessing progression towards malignancy: a case-control study. Asian Pac J Cancer Prev. 2020;21:2325–9.
58. Sivaramakrishnan M, Sivapathasundharam B, Jananni M. Evaluation of lactate dehydrogenase enzyme activity in saliva and serum of oral submucous fibrosis patients. J Oral Pathol Med. 2015;44:449–52.
59. Kallalli BN, Rawson K, Muzammil SA, Awati MA, Shivhare P. Lactate dehydrogenase as a biomarker in oral cancer and oral submucous fibrosis. J Oral Pathol Med. 2016;45:687–90.
60. Mishra S, Kritika C, Bajoria AA, Choudhury P, Sahoo SK, Sangamesh NC. Estimation of salivary and serum lactate dehydrogenase in oral submucous fibrosis. J Int Soc Prev Commun Dent. 2018;8:289–95.
61. Mantri T, Thete SG, Male V, Yadav R, Grover I, Adsure GR, et al. Study of the role of salivary lactate dehydrogenase in habitual tobacco chewers, oral submucous fibrosis and oral cancer as a biomarker. J Contemp Dent Pract. 2019;20:970–3.
62. Panda A, Behura SS, Bhuyan L, Dash KC, Kumar V, Mukherjee S. Assessment of lactate dehydrogenase enzyme levels in saliva and serum of oral submucous fibrosis and leukoplakia patients. J Oral Maxillofac Pathol. 2020;24(1):183.
63. Farhana A, Lappin SL (2021). Biochemistry, lactate dehydrogenase. 2021 May 7. In: StatPearls. Treasure. Island, FL: StatPearls Publishing
64. Iglesias-Velázquez Ó, López-Pintor RM, González-Serrano J, Casañas E, Torres J, Hernández G. Salivary LDH in oral cancer and potentially malignant disorders: a systematic review and meta-analysis. Oral Dis. 2020; https://doi.org/10.1111/odi.13630.
65. Trivedy CR, Warnakulasuriya KA, Peters TJ, Senkus R, Hazarey VK, Johnson NW. Raised tissue copper levels in oral submucous fibrosis. J Oral Pathol Med. 2000;29:241–8.
66. Ayinampudi BK, Narsimhan M. Salivary copper and zinc levels in oral pre-malignant and malignant lesions. J Oral Maxillofac Pathol. 2012;16:178–82.
67. Kode MA, Karjodkar FR. Estimation of the serum and the salivary trace elements in OSMF patients. J Clin Diagn Res. 2013;7:1215–8.
68. Sachdev PK, Freeland-Graves J, Beretvas SN, Sanjeevi N. Zinc, copper, and iron in oral submucous fibrosis: a meta-analysis. Int J Dent. 2018;2018:3472087.
69. Bhat S, Babu SG, Bhat SK, Castelino RL, Rao K, Madi M. Status of serum and salivary ascorbic acid in oral potentially malignant disorders and oral cancer. Indian J Med Paediatr Oncol. 2017;38:306–10.
70. Son ED, Kim HJ, Kim KH, Bin BH, Bae IH, Lim KM, et al. S100A7 (psoriasin) inhibits human epidermal differentiation by enhanced IL-6 secretion through IκB/NF-κB signalling. Exp Dermatol. 2016;25:636–41.
71. Kaur J, Matta A, Kak I, Srivastava G, Assi J, Leong I, et al. S100A7 overexpression is a predictive marker for high risk of malignant transformation in oral dysplasia. Int J Cancer. 2014;134:1379–88.
72. Choudhry N, Sarmad S, Waheed NUA, Gondal AJ. Estimation of serum matrix metalloproteinases among patients of oral squamous cell carcinoma. Pak J Med Sci. 2019;35:252–6.
73. Maheswari TNU, Venugopal A, Sureshbabu NM, Ramani P. Salivary micro RNA as a potential biomarker in oral potentially malignant disorders: a systematic review. Ci Ji Yi Xue Za Zhi. 2018;30:55–60.
74. Yang HW, Yu CC, Hsieh PL, Liao YW, Chu PM, Yu CH, et al. Arecoline enhances miR-21 to promote buccal mucosal fibroblasts activation. J Formos Med Assoc. 2021;120:1108–13.
75. Khoubnasabjafari M, Ansarin K, Vaez-Gharamaleki J, Jouyban A. Comments on "salivary 8-hydroxy-2-deoxyguanosine, malondialdehyde, vitamin C, and vitamin E in oral pre-cancer and cancer: diagnostic value and free radical mechanism of action". Clin Oral Investig. 2016;20(2):395–6.
76. You M, Li X, Wang H, Zhang J, Wu H, Liu Y, et al. Morphological variety of the soft palate in normal individuals: a digital cephalometric study. Dentomaxillofac Radiol. 2008;37:344–9.
77. Shankar VN, Hegde K, Ashwini NS, Praveena V, Ravi Prakash SM. Morphometric evaluation of soft palate in oral submucous fibrosis—a digital cephalometric study. J Craniomaxillofac Surg. 2014;42:48–52.
78. Raja Lakshmi C, Ayesha Thabusum D, Bhavana SM. An innovative approach to evaluate the morphological patterns of soft palate in oral submucous fibrosis patients: a digital cephalometric study. Int J Chronic Dis. 2016;2016:5428581.
79. Kaur Domir S, Gargava A, Deoghare A, Agrawal R. Morphometric evaluation of soft palate in OSMF patients using cephalometrics. Indian J Otolaryngol Head Neck Surg. 2019;71(Suppl. 1):1018–22.
80. Tripathy M, Anekar J, Ac R, Sandeepa NC, Napplli D, Lokanath P, Alharbi AN, Alsobil FM, et al. A digital cephalometric study on the morphometric evaluation of soft palate in oral submucous fibrosis. Asian Pac J Cancer Prev. 2020;21:2169–76.
81. Chaturvedi P. Uvular abnormalities in patients with submucous fibrosis. Oral Dis. 2009;15:516.
82. O'Riordan BC. Oral submucous fibrosis. Proc Royal Soc Medicine. 1974;67:876–8.

# Pathology of Oral Submucous Fibrosis

*Kannan Ranganathan and Kavitha Loganathan*

## Contents



© The Author(s), under exclusive license to Springer Nature Switzerland AG 2023
S. Warnakulasuriya, K. Ranganathan (eds.), *Oral Submucous Fibrosis*, Textbooks in Contemporary Dentistry,
https://doi.org/10.1007/978-3-031-12855-4_14

## 14.1 Introduction

Biopsy and histopathological examination, along with clinical features, not only confirm the clinical diagnosis in the early stages of the disease but are also important to assess the stage of oral submucous fibrosis (OSF), degree of epithelial dysplasia, and risk of malignant transformation. Hematoxylin and eosin-stained sections are routinely used to assess OSF. Special stains such as Masson's trichrome, reticulin, van Gieson's, and picrosirius red can be used to study changes in the connective tissue.

**Learning Goals**

- To understand both the classic and less commonly seen histopathological changes in OSF

### 14.1.1 General Aspects

OSF is a collagen metabolic disorder characterised by increased deposition of collagen in the oral mucosa, that results from exposure to areca nut alkaloids. Histopathological changes in OSF include inflammation, progressive fibrosis of the lamina propria and deeper connective tissue, loss of fibroelasticity with epithelial hyperplasia or atrophy, and varying degrees of keratinization and dysplasia [1]. This chapter discusses the spectrum of mucosal histopathological changes seen in OSF.



**Histopathological features of oral submucous fibrosis (OSF)**

| | Classic OSF | Variations in OSF |
|---|---|---|
| Epithelium | Hyperkeratosis | Subepithelial vesicles |
| | Atrophy | Hyperplasia |
| | Flattened epithelium-connective tissue interface | Epithelial dysplasia |
| | | Intracellular edema<br>Signet ring appearance |
| Connective tissue | "Juxta-epithelial" hyalinization | Lichenoid reaction |
| | Fibrosis (Dense collagen fibre bundles) | Mast Cells |
| | Reduced blood vessels | Oral squamous cell carcinoma |
| | Minimal inflammatory cell infiltrate<br>Muscle degeneration (Advanced stages) | |

## 14.2 Epithelial Changes

Epithelial changes include variations in epithelial thickness and keratinization patterns, surface erosions and ulcerations, dysplasia, and alterations of epithelium-connective tissue interface [1–3].

### 14.2.1 Epithelial Thickness

Epithelial atrophy is a common feature of OSF [4–7] as illustrated in Fig. 14.1. There is a gradual decrease in epithelial thickness with increasing clinical severity [8, 9]. In the early stages, there is epithelial hyperplasia with shortening of rete ridges (Fig. 14.2). This is followed

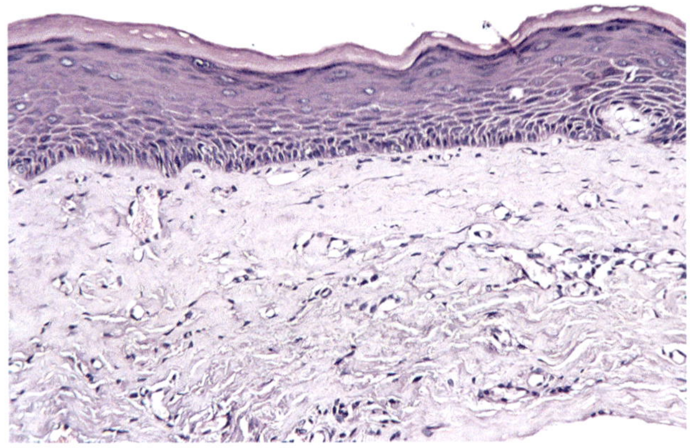

Fig. 14.1 OSF exhibiting epithelial atrophy (H and E; 20× magnification)

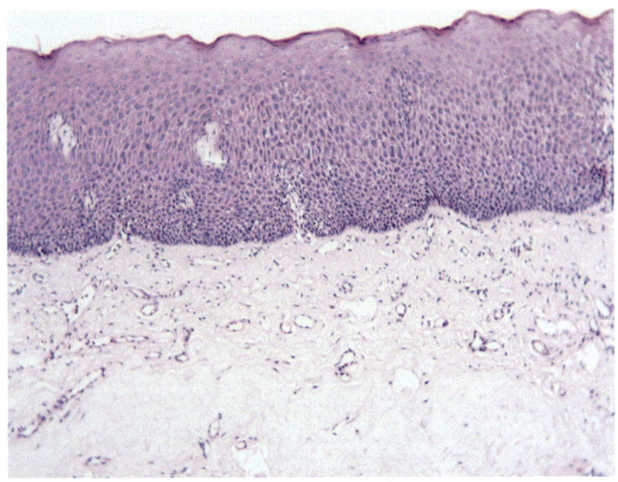

Fig. 14.2 OSF with epithelial hyperplasia (H and E; 10× magnification)

by loss of rete ridges progressing to marked atrophy in the advanced stages [2, 3, 10].

The thickness of the epithelium in OSF may vary from 3 to 12 cell layers compared with 26 ± 4.39 cell layers for normal epithelium [10]. Various reasons have been postulated to explain the epithelial atrophy in OSF. The most common hypothesis is that of ischemic atrophy, which is due to the decreased vascularity resulting from the fibrosis.

Other reasons for epithelial atrophy include

- Direct effect of the areca nut alkaloids, such as arecoline, on the epithelium [1, 2]
- Reduced proliferation of the oral epithelium due to cytotoxic and genotoxic effect of inducible nitric oxide synthase (iNOS), which is released by areca nut constituents [11]
- Reduction in salivary mucous secretion by minor salivary glands, leading to decreased lubrication of the surface epithelial cells resulting in rapid exfoliation, which contributes to atrophy of oral epithelium [12]
- Atrophy secondary to subepithelial inflammation, fibrosis, tissue ischemia, and hypoxia in the connective tissue [1, 2, 12]
- Atrophy secondary to nutritional deficiency, malnutrition, and anemia, which occurs because of the restricted mouth opening and difficulty in chewing and swallowing food [13, 14]

The epithelium may also show hyperplasia, with or without dysplasia [1, 2, 15–20]. Epithelial hyperplasia may occur as an adaptive response to local irritants from abrasive effects of areca products [21]. In a study of 104 OSF cases, it was shown that 82% of those who also used tobacco exhibited hyperplastic epithelium [17]. Hyperplastic changes include hyperkeratosis, acanthosis, basal cell hyperplasia, papillomatosis, and less commonly pseudoepitheliomatous hyperplasia [22].

### 14.2.2 Vesicles and Erosions

Blisters (subepithelial vesicles) may precede the onset or occasionally occur in the early stages of OSF (◘ Fig. 14.3). The vesicles occur on the buccal mucosa or palate, vesicles rupture resulting in surface erosion and ulcerations which heal by formation of granulation tissue and fibrosis [2, 15, 23–26], and rarely there may be necrosis and suppuration [22]. Vesicles could indicate an allergic response to the contents of the areca nut products [2]. Microbiologic culture studies of the vesicular fluid have shown no microorganisms [15, 24].

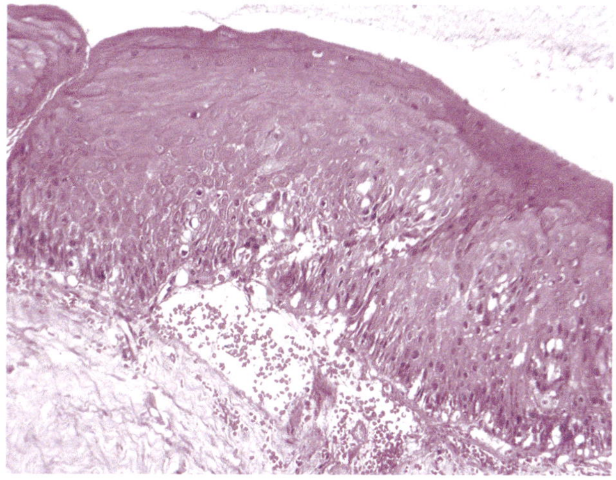

◘ **Fig. 14.3** OSF with subepithelial vesiculation (H and E; 20× magnification)

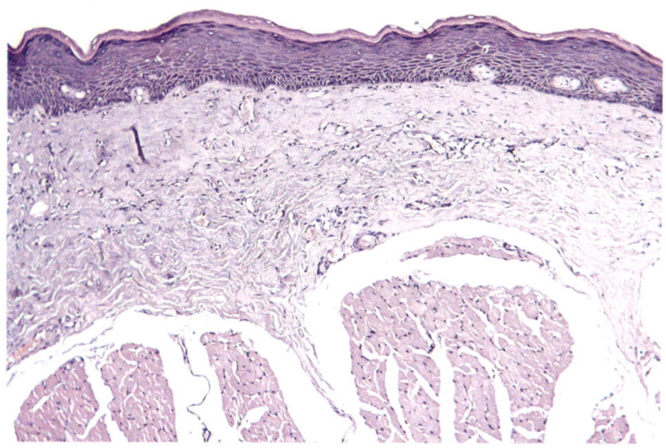

◘ **Fig. 14.4** Epithelial atrophy with hyperkeratosis in OSF (H and E; 10× magnification)

### 14.2.3 Keratinization

The affected buccal mucosa may exhibit hyperkeratosis, orthokeratosis, or parakeratosis [5, 6, 22] (◘ Fig. 14.4). The epithelial cells respond to the local irritation due to the areca nut product with faster turnover rate and keratinization [12]. The keratinization pattern is influenced by the site of the lesion and the type of the areca nut used. Changes involving the palate predominantly show orthokeratosis (42%) and those of the buccal mucosa, parakeratosis (45%) [17]. It has been reported that epithelial atrophy in OSF is associated with hyperorthokeratosis (69%), whereas cases with hyperplastic epithelium are associated with hyperparakeratosis (89%) [12, 27].

Parakeratosis manifesting with clinical leukoplakia has been suggested to predispose to carcinoma [2, 28].

### 14.2.4 Epithelial Dysplasia

Identification of oral epithelial dysplasia (OED) by light microscopy is the current gold standard for the prediction of malignant transformation [29–31]. Epithelial dysplasia has been reported to occur in 7–43% of OSF in different studies (◘ Figs. 14.5 and 14.6). Tissue hypoxia, as evidenced by significant expression of hypoxia inducible factor-alpha (HIF-alpha), is an important factor for initiating epithelial dysplasia in OSF [32].

The high mitotic count in the parakeratotic epithelium in OSF suggests a predisposition to carcinoma [2, 28]. In a study from the Tata Institute of Fundamental Research, Mumbai, in 1970, epithelial atypia was diagnosed in 22.6% (12 out of 53 biopsies) of clinically diagnosed OSF patients and one case had oral squamous cell carcinoma. Epithelial dysplastic features included irregular epithelial stratification, increased number of mitotic figures, nuclear pleomorphism and hyperchromatism, loss of polarity of cells, and presence of signet ring cells in the basal layers (◘ Fig. 14.7). Spongiosis was seen in 75% of the cases with atypia in the basal cell layers and in 52.5% of cases without atypia [28]. Other reported dysplastic changes in OSF are variation in cell size and shape, large nuclei, prominent nucleoli, and increased mitotic activity [22].

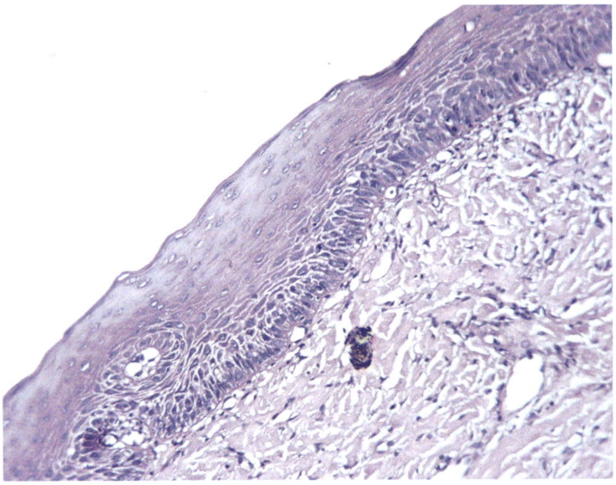

◘ **Fig. 14.5** Mild epithelial dysplasia in OSF (H and E; 20× magnification)

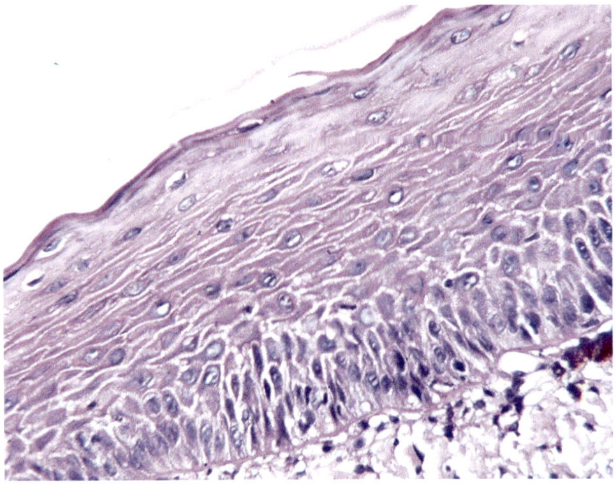

◘ **Fig. 14.6** Mild epithelial dysplasia in OSF (H and E; 40× magnification)

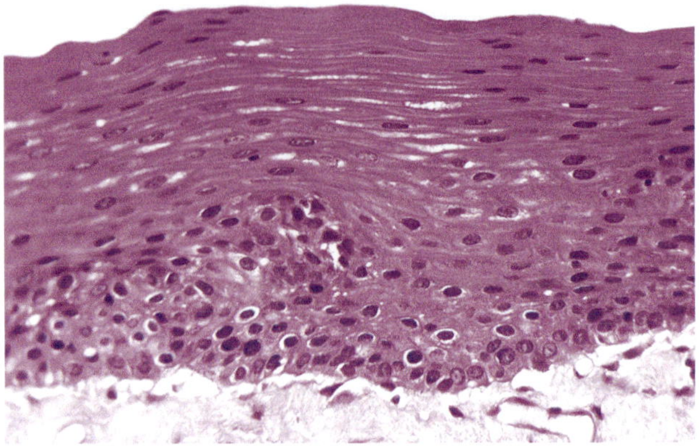

◘ **Fig. 14.7** Loss of epithelial stratification in OSF (H and E; 20× magnification)

It has been suggested that OSF lesions that have greater fibrosis are also more likely to present with epithelial dysplasia. In one study from Sri Lanka, OSF cases with moderate dysplasia exhibited thicker fibrosis compared to the cases which showed mild dysplasia. The mean thicknesses of fibrosis of the non-dysplastic lesions and dysplastic lesions were 0.91 ± 0.41 mm and 1.17 ± 0.52 mm (mean ± standard deviation [SD]), respectively. Focal budding rete morphology is conspicuous in OSF with epithelial dysplasia as opposed to cases without dysplasia which present with epithelial atrophy. Increasing degree of collagen cross-linking and connective tissue hyalinization increases the risk of epithelial dysplasia in OSF [12, 33].

Applying the WHO criteria for grading OED in OSF tissue specimens is difficult because of the epithelial atrophy. Reduced epithelial thickness and absence of clear demarcation between different strata of epithelium in OSF, especially in the advanced stages (III and IV), make grading of OED challenging [8, 34]. This further raises the dilemma of interpreting whether malignancy in OSF arises subsequent to OED or without any dysplastic changes [34].

14

### 14.2.5 Cellular Changes in Keratinocytes and Non-keratinocyte Cells

#### 14.2.5.1 Keratinocytes and Keratinization

The direct contact of the oral mucosa with areca nut contents including alkaloids disrupts the proteolytic equilibrium in collagen synthesis and degradation leading to fibrosis [12]. Cytomorphometric analysis of keratinocytes shows a decrease in cytoplasmic area and increase in nuclear area, ratio of nuclear area to cytoplasmic area, and nuclear dimension to cytoplasmic dimension in OSF compared to normal mucosa. These morphometric changes in advanced OSF are similar to those seen in OSCC (Oral Squamous Cell Carcinoma) [35].

Normal oral keratinocytes express matched pairs of type I and type II keratin (K) polypeptides that are site specific [36–38]. Immunohistochemical studies have shown an increase in K1, K10, and K17 and complete loss of K19 in the epithelium of OSF patients [39], and aberrant expression of K8 with decrease in K5, K14, and high-molecular-weight cytokeratin, a marker of keratinized surface epithelium [40].

**Signet ring cells:** "Signet ring" cells are cells that present with a large cytoplasmic vacuole, which compresses the nucleus in the form of a crescent, with variable contents within the vacuole (e.g., mucin, lipid, or glycogen) (◘ Fig. 14.8). The vacuoles could represent cytoplasmic lumen, cytoplasmic pseudoinclusion, intracellular edema, or hydropic swelling of mitochondria [41, 42].

Early studies on OSF done in 1963 and 1964 by Pindborg and Sirsat have shown atrophic epithelium exhibiting signet cells in 13% of cases [43]. A study done on 53 biopsies of suspected OSF cases in 51 Indian villagers revealed signet cells, mostly in the basal layer in 19.2% biopsies of OSF [28]. In another study from India, signet cell degeneration has been reported in the spinous cell layer associated with liquefaction in the basal cell layer [27].

#### 14.2.5.2 Non-keratinocytes

**Oral Melanocytes**

Melanocytes are the melanin-producing dendritic cells found in the basal layers of the epithelium. These cells decrease in number with advancing stages of OSF [3]. There is marked loss of melanin from the basal epithelial cell layers and increase in melanin accumulation in the subepithelial lamina propria, a process described as melanin fallout [44], as illustrated in ◘ Fig. 14.9. Depigmentation of oral mucosa has been reported as an early manifestation of oral submucous fibrosis in Sri Lankan preschool children with areca nut-chewing habit [45] (see also ▶ Chap. 10).

**Langerhans Cells**

Langerhans cells (LCs) are dendritic cells present in the suprabasal layers of the oral epithelium. LCs are antigen-presenting cells that induce specific T cell reaction by the interaction of the MHC class II with the CD4+ cells. It has been suggested that tissue changes in OSF are either due to direct stimulation from exogenous antigens like areca alkaloids or by changes in tissue antigenicity leading to an autoimmune response [46].

Persistent antigenic challenge in this process leads to significant increases in LCs. Alterations in the number of LCs have been reported to play a role in OSF progression and malignant transformation [47–49].

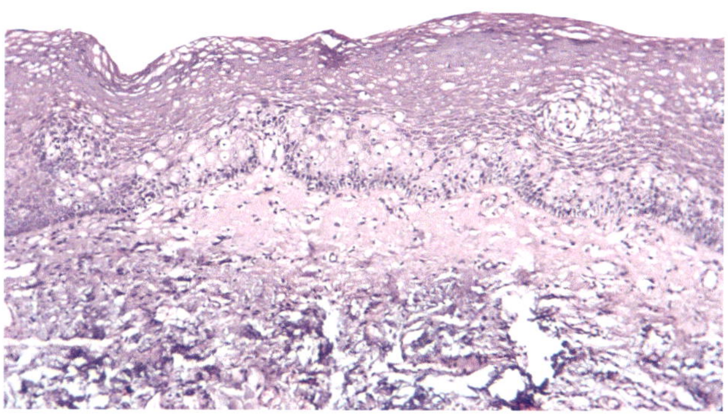

◘ **Fig. 14.8** Intracellular edema with signet ring appearance of cells in OSF (H and E; 10× magnification)

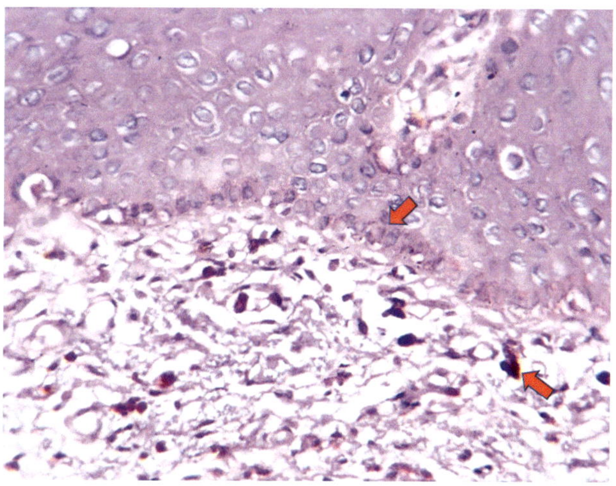

◘ **Fig. 14.9** Melanin pigmentation and incontinence in OSF (H and E; 40× magnification)

## 14.3 Connective Tissue Changes

Connective tissue changes in OSF include fibrosis, extracellular matrix remodeling, changes in fibroblasts, myofibroblasts, connective tissue thickness, and juxtaepithelial inflammation.

### 14.3.1 Fibrosis and Hyalinization

OSF is a collagen metabolic disorder where areca alkaloids cause a disequilibrium in the collagen metabolism leading to fibrosis and extracellular matrix remodeling (see ► Chap. 12). Fibrosis causes vascular rarefaction (vessel compression or obliteration), nutrient depletion, and tissue hypoxia leading to mucosal atrophy [50].

There is deposition of type I collagen in all stages of OSF [2, 6]. Fibrosis increases with increasing severity of OSF. Fibrosis starts in the submucosa and subsequently involves the lamina propria as the disease advances [51–53]. In early OSF, there is fibrosis immediately beneath the subepithelial zone (◘ Fig. 14.10). In the intermediate stage, fibrosis extends up to the muscle layer, compressing blood vessels, and hyalinization is seen as a subepithelial band. In the advanced stage, there is marked fibrosis and hyalinization that extends between muscle fibers causing muscle atrophy [6, 43] (◘ Fig. 14.11).

Subepithelial hyalinization is a characteristic feature of OSF. Hyalinization starts initially in the juxtaepithelial zone and spreads downwards with increasing intensity [6] (◘ Fig. 14.12). As the disease progresses, the connective tissue loses its fibrillar staining pattern and becomes amorphous. Hyalinization occurs due to increase in cross-linking of collagen, which leads to changes in the birefringence of the fibers [54–56].

14

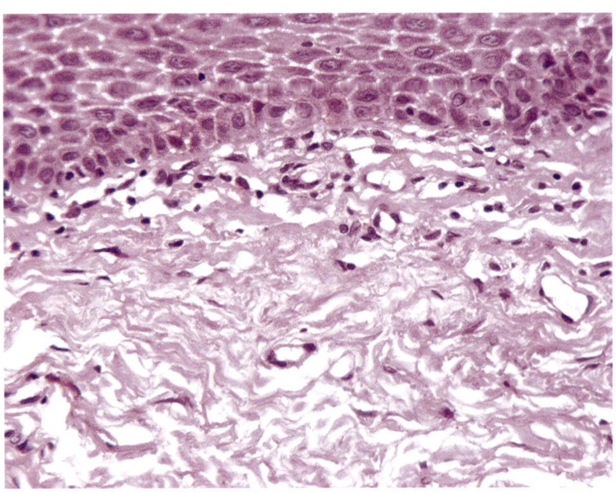

◘ **Fig. 14.10** Collagen fiber bundles—early stages of OSF (H and E; 40× magnification)

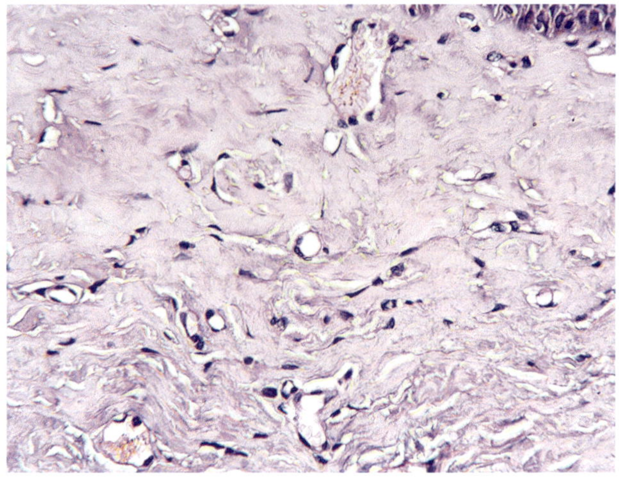

◘ **Fig. 14.11** Collagen fiber bundles—advanced stages of OSF (H and E; 40× magnification)

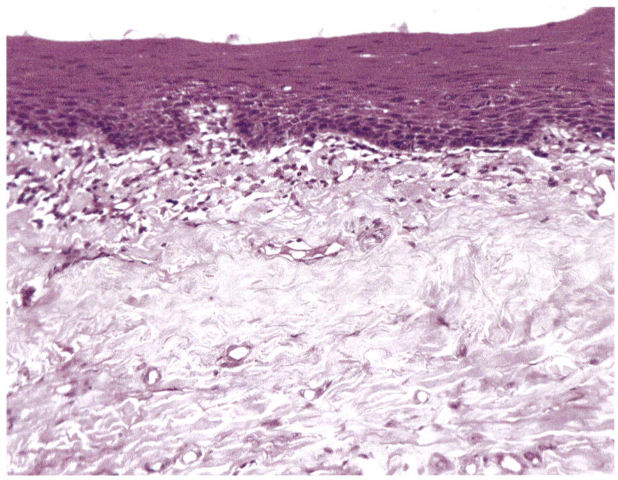

◘ **Fig. 14.12** Subepithelial hyalinization in OSF (H and E; 20× magnification)

The persistence of fibrin matrix due to reduced fibrinolytic activity, increased myofibroblastic activity, and reduced fibronectin phagocytosis contributes to fibrosis. The fibrosis in OSF has been compared to exuberant wound healing due to the chronic physical, chemical, or mechanical injury to the oral mucosa, as evidenced by the immunolocalization of matricellular proteins, perlecan, and fibronectin [56–59].

Remodeling of ECM shows enhancement of perlecan, tenascin, fibronectin, and collagen type III in the early stages of OSF. With the progression of OSF to advanced stages, all ECM molecules show degradation and complete replacement with type I collagen [1, 60]. There is a reduction in the levels of matrix metalloproteinases (MMPs) secreted by buccal mucosal fibroblasts, particularly MMP-2 and MMP-9, and an increase in the levels of tissue inhibitor of MMP-1 [50].

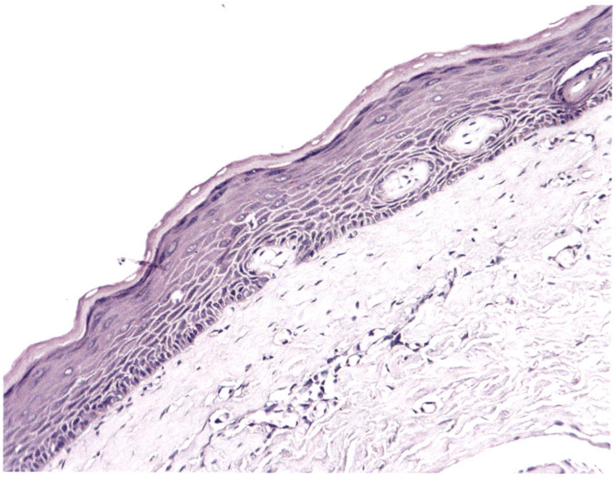

**Fig. 14.13** Reduced vascularity in OSF (H and E; 20× magnification)

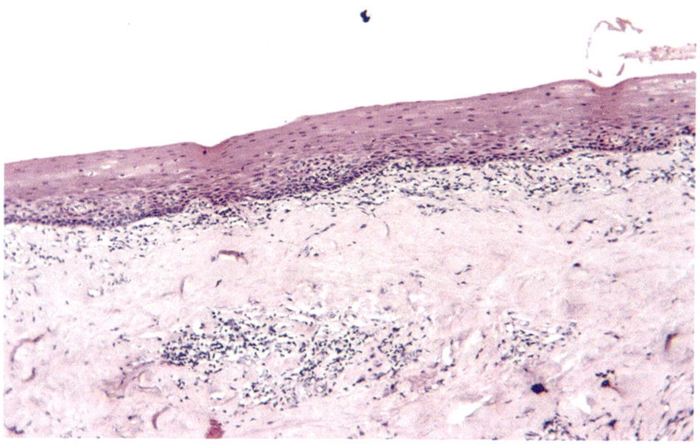

**Fig. 14.14** Subepithelial inflammatory infiltrate associated with OSF (H and E; 10× magnification)

### 14.3.2 Vascularity

Vascularity increases in the early stage of OSF and decreases in the advanced stages [16, 61–65] as illustrated in Fig. 14.13. As fibrosis progresses, there is a decrease in microvessel density [16, 61]. Mast cells which are actively involved in angiogenesis rise in number during the early stages of OSF and eventually decrease in number in the advanced stages.

Interestingly, it has been shown that as connective tissue gets denser, due to fibrosis, the resultant physical and biochemical restriction to blood vessel growth can paradoxically induce angiogenic activity. This phenomenon explains the neo-angiogenesis seen during the malignant transformation of OSF [1, 2].

### 14.3.3 Inflammation

The coarse granules of areca nut and associated substances injure the oral mucosa causing microtrauma. This facilitates ingression of chemical irritants leading to inflammation and activation of macrophages and influx of cytokines. There is enhanced expression of pro-inflammatory cytokines, interleukin-1 and -6, and tumor necrosis factor-alpha, along with a decrease in antifibrotic interferons in OSF. Transforming growth factor-β (TGF-β) is a major cytokine involved in OSF progression (vide ► Chap. 12). It regulates the expression of α-SMA and deposition of type 1 collagen [12, 66]. The inflammatory cells seen are predominantly lymphocytes and plasma cells [2] (Fig. 14.14).

The continuous contact of the oral mucosa with areca alkaloids results in a state of chronic inflammation leading to activation of macrophages and T cells and an increase in the level of cytokines such as interleukin-6, tumor necrosis factor-alpha, interferon-alpha, and TGF-β [67]. Macrophages are cells of the mononuclear phagocyte system that function to remove cellular debris, protect the body against foreign antigens, and provide innate immunity [68].

There is an increase in the number of macrophages in the intermediate and advanced stages of OSF compared to normal tissues [69]. Fibrogenic cytokines secreted by activated macrophages and T lymphocytes are important in the development of fibrosis [70] (see ► Chap. 12).

### 14.3.4 Myofibroblast

Myofibroblasts are a unique group of cells phenotypically intermediate between smooth muscle cells and fibroblasts. They display prominent cytoplasmic actin microfilaments (stress fibers) and are connected to each other by adherens and gap junction. Myofibroblasts originate from three sources: local recruitment from the surrounding connective tissue during wound healing, from pericytes or vascular smooth muscle cells around blood vessels, and in epithelial-mesenchymal transition (EMT) [71]. Myofibroblasts in wounds of normal mucosa originate from local recruitment of fibroblasts from the surrounding tissue [50], and as healing occurs, the myofibroblasts undergo apoptosis. In OSF, however, there is persistence of myofibroblasts.

In OSF, myofibroblasts are recruited in response to the tissue injury caused by areca alkaloids. Loss of rete ridges due to atrophy decreases the surface area of epithelial connective tissue interface, changing and concentrating force vectors on fibroblasts and stimulating their differentiation into myofibroblasts [58].

Persistence of myofibroblast in OSF and production of TGF-β stimulate proto-myofibroblasts in the connective tissue to express α-SMA, which in turn creates larger surface adhesion with ECM and formation of the myofibroblasts that can withstand higher contractile forces [71, 72]. Myofibroblasts increase the production of collagen (COL 1A1, 1A2) and modulate ECM turnover favoring the progression of OSF [72].

### 14.3.5 Mast Cells

Mast cells have a significant role in mitogenesis, extracellular matrix degradation, angiogenesis, and augmentation of microvascular hyperpermeability and recruitment of inflammatory cells including macrophages [68, 73] (◘ Fig. 14.15).

Areca alkaloids cause mast cell accumulation, activation, and degranulation [74]. They release proteases (tryptase, chymase, and cathepsin G), histamine, serotonin, acid hydrolases, and cytokines like TNF-α and IL-16, which cause the initial inflammatory signs of burning sensation, stomatitis, and glossitis in OSF, with occasional vesicle formation [73]. Mast cell mediators like prostaglandins and leukotrienes are potent secretagogues for serous and mucous cells, which contribute to the increased salivation that may occur in OSF.

The densities of mast cells are higher in OSF than in normal buccal mucosa and increase with disease severity suggesting a role in the initiation and progression of OSF [73]. Mild, moderate, and severe inflammation in OSF shows increased number of typical (TMCs), atypical (AMCs), and granular mast cells (GMCs), respectively [75–77].

The angiogenic factors secreted by mast cells, including histamine, heparin, VEGF, β-FGF, and tryptase, promote the migration and/or proliferation of endothelial cells. These may have a role in the angiogenesis seen during the neoplastic transformation of OSF.

14

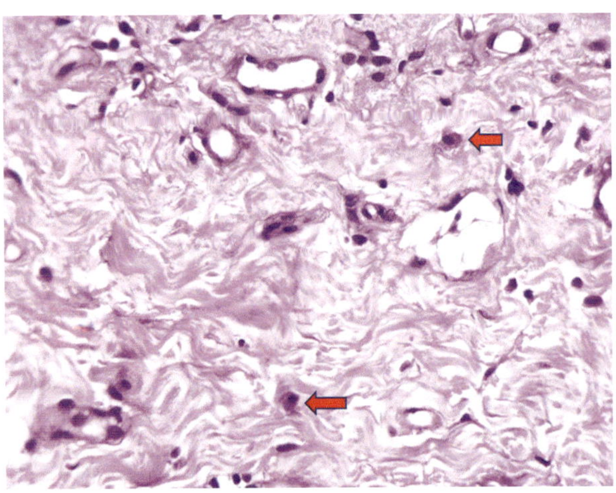

◘ Fig. 14.15 Mast cells in OSF (H and E; 20× magnification)

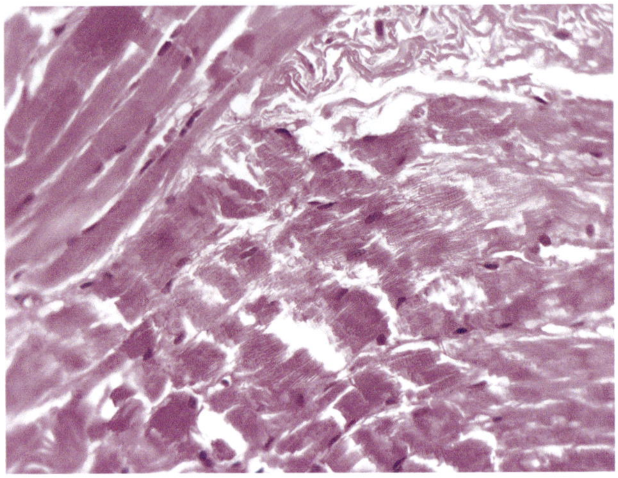

◘ Fig. 14.16 Muscle degeneration in advanced OSF (H and E; 40× magnification)

### 14.3.6 Muscles

There is histological evidence of fibrosis and degeneration of muscle fibers in OSF [78, 79] (◘ Fig. 14.16). Palatal and paratubal muscles show evidence of muscle damage in the form of edema, loss of striations, and atrophy, causing Eustachian tube dysfunction and hearing impairment in some.

Histological changes indicative of muscle damage include loss of striations, muscle fiber fragmentation, nucleus internalization, and multiple nuclei. The damage is more severe in advanced OSF. Reduction in the muscle-epithelial distance is a significant predictor of OSF progression [80, 81].

## 14.4 Electron Microscopic (EM) Features in OSF

EM studies of oral mucosa in areca nut chewers show cytoplasmic projections of the basal cells into the subepithelial stroma with frequent gaps in the basal membrane. Other findings are encroachment of the blood vessels by collagen fibers, compression of blood vessels by excessive fibrosis, and thinner collagen fiber bundles in the superficial part of lamina propria compared to those deeper [82].

Ultrastructural study of muscle fibers found evidence of damage to the muscle fibers, such as muscle atrophy, necrosis, sarcolemmal folding, reduplicated basement membrane, hypercontraction of muscle fibers, and autophagic vacuoles [81]. Findings suggest that restricted mouth opening in OSF is also due to muscle degeneration, in addition to submucosal fibrosis [83, 84].

Scanning electron microscopic (SEM) studies show that the interepithelial spaces are widened and unusual microvilli are present on epithelial cell surfaces. Intercellularly, crystalloid material of unknown origin has been reported [85]. A 3D assessment of OSF by SEM revealed progressive patchy degenerative connective tissue cores with advancing grades of the condition [86]. The normal pattern of uniformly sized collagen fibrils, gathered in bundles, is replaced by many fine (immature) fibrils in an interfibrillar matrix [87, 88]. Destruction and necrosis of muscle were seen in OSF cases with limited mouth opening [83, 84]. Studies have also shown collagen fibers with frayed ends and degenerated cores [53].

## 14.5 Special Stains

Collagen assessment using Mallory and Weigert resorcin-fuchsin stains demonstrates thickened collagen bundles and uneven staining pattern [88]. With van Gieson's stain, the juxta-epithelial connective tissue band in OSF is amorphous and hyalinized and stains faint grayish pink, rather than the normal deep red [24]. Though traditional stains such as van Gieson and trichrome are used to study collagen fibers, polarizing microscopy using picrosirius red demonstrates both thin and thick collagen fibers. Picrosirius red stains the thin fibers intensely and increases their birefringence. Mixed birefringence indicates an increase in both type I and type III collagen, while yellowish orange to reddish orange indicates type I collagen that is arranged in thick bundles. Collagen fibers showed mixed birefringence with a shift in polarization from yellow to red-orange in lamina propria, around muscle and blood vessels [55, 89–91]. Parallel arrangement of fibers is observed with van Gieson, but picrosirius red-stained sections reveal predominantly parallel type I fibers along with some perpendicular type III fibers [92]. Unidirectional collagen fibers have been demonstrated in OSF by polarizing microscopy [54, 93, 94].

The thickness and degree of keratinization and subepithelial changes are best demonstrated with Mallory's stain. The changes in blood vessels can be seen with van Gieson's and Mallory's staining. Areas of muscle degeneration, especially in deeper connective tissue, are better seen with Mallory's and Masson's stain as compared to van Gieson's stain [78, 95]. Verhoeff-van Gieson stain is used to demonstrate very fine elastic fibers [96].

Tissue copper content can be assessed by the rhodamine staining technique. Tissue copper is higher in OSF than leukoplakia and OSCC and can be used as a prognostic indicator for the assessment of disease progression [97].

**Box 14.1 Histological Staging Systems: Described in** **▶ Chap. 6**

**Commonly used histological staging systems in oral submucous fibrosis**

| | |
|---|---|
| Pindborg and Sirsat (1966 [43]; based on the connective tissue changes) | Very early stage<br>Early stage<br>Moderately advanced stage<br>Advanced stage |
| Khanna and Andrade (1995 [3]; based on both clinical and histopathological features) | Group I very early cases<br>Group II early cases<br>Group III moderately advanced cases<br>Group IV advanced cases<br>– IVA: advanced cases<br>– IVB: advanced cases with premalignant/malignant changes |
| Utsunomiya, Tilakaratne, Oshiro et al. (2005 [60]; based on the gain or loss of extracellular matrix molecules using immunohistochemistry) | Early stage<br>Intermediate stage<br>Advanced stage |

## 14.6 Lesions Associated with OSF

### 14.6.1 Leukoplakia and OSF

Leukoplakia occurs in around 25% of cases with OSF in the advanced stages [98]. There has been one report of oral proliferative verrucous leukoplakia with oral submucous fibrosis. Studies have shown a higher risk of malignant transformation of OSF with oral leukoplakia [99].

### 14.6.2 Verrucous Hyperplasia and OSF

Exophytic growth in the background of OSF ranges from simple benign hyperplastic lesions to oral verrucous hyperplasia (OVH) to verrucous carcinoma and exophytic OSCC [100, 101]. The fibrosis of connective tissue stroma offers resistance to the process of downward proliferation of dysplastic/transformed epithelium leading to exophytic proliferation. Jayasinghe and colleagues [100] reported, for the first time, five cases of exophytic verrucous hyperplasia in OSF with features of mild-to-moderate dysplasia. Shah et al. [101] reported a case series of six patients who presented with verrucopapillary exophytic lesions mimicking frank malig-

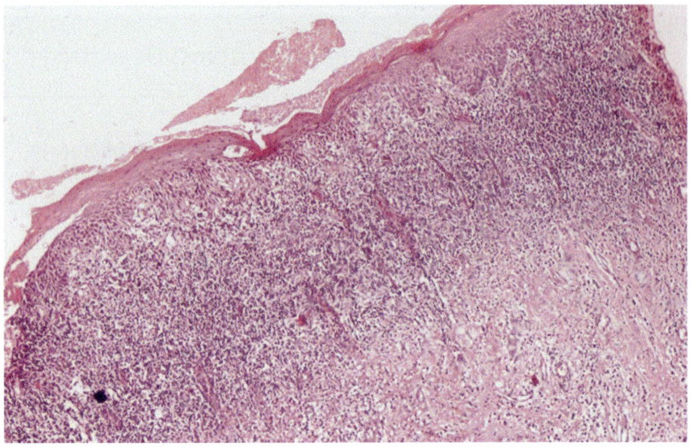

Fig. 14.17 Lichenoid reaction coexistent with OSF (H and E; 10× magnification)

nancy in the background of OSF without any dysplasia. In a Taiwanese study, out of 60 OVH lesions, 51 were reported to be areca chewers (91%) [102].

► Chapter 4 provides a detailed description of these associated conditions.

### 14.6.3 Coexistence of Lichenoid Features and Fibrosis

Prolonged contact of areca nut/tobacco quid with the mucosa of patients leads to the development of contact oral lichenoid lesion, referred to as quid-associated oral lichenoid lesion (Fig. 14.17). Clinically, these lesions appear as white, linear, wavy parallel non-elevated streaks, which may radiate from a central erythematous area [103, 104]. Histologically, in addition to fibrosis, there is a subepithelial diffuse dense inflammatory cell infiltrate along with degeneration of the basal cells. Quid-associated oral lichenoid lesions are known to regress after the stoppage of habit, though it may not be the case for OSF patients [105].

## 14.7 Oral Cancer and OSF

In addition to the morbidity associated with fibrosis, OSF is a potentially malignant condition (Fig. 14.18). Numerous reports have highlighted the progression of OSF to oral cancer (squamous cell carcinoma). The malignant transformation rate of OSF ranges from 7% to 13% [106]. In 1956, Paymaster first described the development of a slow-growing OSCC in one-third of the cases of OSF seen among patients in Bombay [107]. Murti et al. (1985) in a follow-up study of OSF for a period of 17 years recorded a malignant transformation rate of 7.6% [108]. Betel leaf with areca nut (pan) chewing accounts for 31% of oral cancers in a study from Madras (Chennai), South India [109].

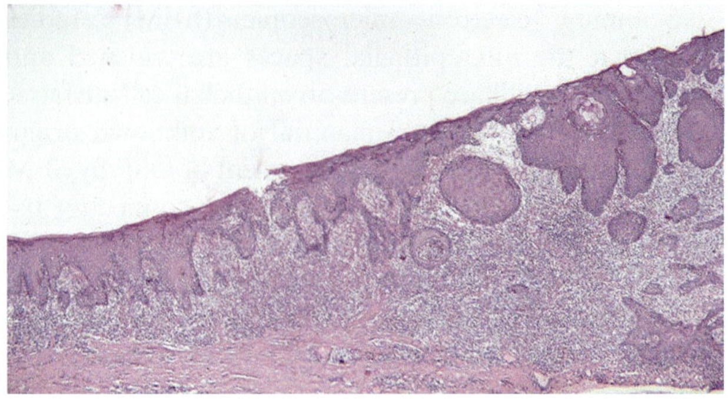

Fig. 14.18 Malignant transformation of OSF to OSCC (H and E; 10× magnification)

Some of the proposed mechanisms of malignant transformation in OSF are the following:

(a) The atrophic epithelium first becomes hyperkeratotic (clinically leukoplakic); basal cell hyperplasia then develops, followed by epithelial atypia and OSCC [6].
(b) Alkaloids in betel quid cause fibrosis and tissue ischemia. Reduced blood flow leads to hypoxia and lack of nutrition, which augments the permeability of the epithelium to carcinogens in areca products [1, 32].
(c) Arecoline is a desiccating agent that causes shrinkage of cells and enlargement of intercellular spaces, which permits the percolation of chemical mutagens through the epithelium to basal layer inducing epithelial dysplasia and neoplastic cellular transformation [1, 32].
(d) Epithelial changes (epithelial atrophy, hyperplasia or hyperkeratosis, and dysplasia) and connective tissue changes (excessive collagenization, which further leads to hyalinization, angiogenesis, and inflammatory infiltration) favor the progression of OSF to OSCC [1, 12].
(e) The epithelial and connective tissue changes mutually contribute to events in epithelial-mesenchymal transition [1, 12] and malignant transformation.

OSCC arising in a background of OSF has a better grade of differentiation than OSCC occurring without OSF [110] and hence has a better prognosis with low postoperative recurrence and better survival rate. It has been suggested that this is because the molecular mechanisms involving cell cycle regulation, hypoxia, DNA double-strand breaks, and cell senescence in areca nut-induced malignant transformation are different from those due to tobacco and other causes of oral cancer [106].

### 14.7.1 Histological Markers for Genetic Damage and Malignant Transformation in OSF

#### 14.7.1.1 Micronucleus

Micronuclei (MNs) are extranuclear cytoplasmic DNA bodies formed by genotoxic agents that damage chromosomes. They are formed by the exclusion of chromosome fragments or whole chromosomes lagging at mitosis. MN assay in exfoliated buccal cells in OSF has been used as a biomarker for genotoxicity. Studies have shown that OSF has more MN compared to leukoplakia [111–119]. A study where comet assay was used to assess tissue micronucleus content showed that the mean micronucleus tail length was the highest in OSCC (25 ± 4.5) followed by OSF (14 ± 1.8) and normal mucosa (7.0 ± 2.2) [120].

#### 14.7.1.2 Silver Staining Nucleolar Organizing Region (AgNOR)

Nucleolar organizer regions (NORs) are loops of DNA that encode ribosomal RNA and are vital for the synthesis of proteins. The NORs are morphological sites around which the nucleolus develops at the end of mitosis and AgNOR staining reflects the rapidity of cell replication. NORs are located on the short arms of acrocentric chromosomes, 13, 14, 15, 21, and 22. The mean number and size of AgNORs gradually increase from normal to oral leukoplakia to oral submucous fibrosis to oral squamous cell carcinoma [121].

As the grade of dysplasia increases, the mean AgNOR count also increases [121]. High AgNOR counts in OSF are indicative of an increased risk of malignant transformation [123–130].

**Summary**

Epithelial atrophy and collagen deposition in the submucosa are the key histopathologic features in OSF. A thorough understanding of the histopathological changes, both epithelial and connective tissue, is essential for the classification and assessment of the disease progression that will aid in the diagnosis and help in appropriate clinical management and follow-up of the patient.

## References

1. Ray JG, Ranganathan K, Chattopadhyay A. Malignant transformation of Oral submucous fibrosis: overview of histopathological aspects. Oral Surg Oral Med Oral Pathol Oral Radiol. 2016;122(2):200–9.
2. Rajendran R. Oral submucous fibrosis: etiology, pathogenesis, and future research. Bull World Health Organ. 1994;72(6): 985–96.
3. Khanna JN, Andrade NN. Oral submucous fibrosis: a new concept in surgical management report of 100 cases. Int J Oral Maxillofac Surg. 1995;24:433–9.
4. Rao ABN. Idiopathic palatal fibrosis. Brit J Surg. 1962;30:23–5.
5. Pindborg JJ, Chawla TN, Srivastava AN, Gupta D. Epithelial changes in oral submucous fibrosis. Acta Odontol Scand. 1965;23:277–86.
6. Pindborg JJ, Odont D, Poulsen HE, Zachariah J. Oral epithelial changes in thirty Indians with oral cancer and submucous fibrosis. Cancer. 1967;20:1141–6.
7. Canniff JP, Harvey W, Harris M. Oral submucous fibrosis: its pathogenesis and management. Br Dent J. 1986;160:429–34.
8. Sarode SC, Sarode GS. Better grade of tumor differentiation of oral squamous cell carcinoma arising in background of oral submucous fibrosis. Med Hypotheses. 2013;81:540–3.
9. Rathore AS, Gupta A, Shetty DC, Kumar K, Dhanapal R. Redefining epithelial characterization in oral submucous fibrosis using morphometric analysis. J Oral Maxillofac Pathol. 2017;21:36–40.
10. Desai RS, Mamatha GS, Khatri MJ, Shetty SJ. Immunohistochemical expression of CD34 for characterization and quantification of mucosal vasculature and its probable role in malignant transformation of atrophic epithelium in oral submucous fibrosis. Oral Oncol. 2010;46:553–8.
11. Rajendran R, Varkey S. Inducible nitric oxide synthase expression is upregulated in oral submucous fibrosis. Indian J Dent Res. 2007;18:94–100.
12. Hande AH, Chaudhary MS, Gawande MN, Gadbail AR, Zade PR, Bajaj S, et al. Oral submucous fibrosis: an enigmatic morpho-insight. J Can Res Ther. 2019;15:463–9.
13. Rajendran R, Vijayakumar T. An alternative pathogenetic pathway for oral submucous fibrosis. Med Hypotheses. 1989;30: 35–7.
14. Ganapathy KS, Gurudath S, Balikai B, Sushmini Hegde S, Sujatha D. Role of iron deficiency in oral submucous fibrosis: an initiating or accelerating factor. J Indian Acad Oral Med Radiol. 2011;23(1):25–8.
15. DeSa JV. Submucous fibrosis of the palate and cheek. Ann Otol Rhinol Laryngol. 1957;66:1143–51.
16. Debnath S, Mitrab B, Paul B, Saha TN, Maity A. Morphometric analysis of oral submucous fibrosis and its correlation with histological staging and clinical severity of trismus. Egypt J Ear Nose Throat Allied Sci. 2013;14:85–90.
17. Wahi PN, et al. Submucous fibrosis of the oral cavity: histomorphological studies. Br J Cancer. 1966;20:676–87.
18. Sharan J. Histopathological observations on cases of submucous fibrosis of the oral cavity. Indian J Pathol Bacterial. 1959;2: 150–2.
19. Garg N, Mehrotra RR. Morphometric analysis of epithelial thickness and blood vessels in different grades of oral submucous fibrosis. Malays J Pathol. 2014;36(3):189–93.
20. Prestin S, Rothschild SI, Betz CS, Kraft M. Measurement of epithelial thickness within the oral cavity using optical coherence tomography. Head Neck. 2012;34:1777–81.
21. Tilakaratne WM, Ekanayaka RP, Herath M, Jayasinghe RD, Sitheeque M, Amarasinghe H, et al. Intralesional corticosteroids as a treatment for restricted mouth opening in oral submucous fibrosis. Oral Surg Oral Med Oral Pathol Oral Radiol. 2016;122:224–31.
22. Isaac U, Isaac JS, Khoso NA. Histopathologic features of oral submucous fibrosis: a study of 35 biopsy specimens. Oral Surg Oral Med Oral Pathol Oral Radiol Endod. 2008;106:556–60.

23. Hayes PA, et al. Oral submucous fibrosis in a 4-year-old girl. Oral Surg Oral Med Oral Pathol. 1985;59(5):475–8.
24. Hamner JE, et al. Altered staining reaction of connective tissues in 53 submucous fibrosis patients. J Dent Res. 1971;50:388–92.
25. Jani YV, Dudhia BB. The clinicohistopathologic study of oral submucous fibrosis: a new staging system with treatment strategies. J Indian Acad Oral Med Radiol. 2016;28:111–8.
26. Gupta D, Sharma SC. Oral submucous fibrosis-a new treatment regimen. J Oral Maxillofac Surg. 1988;46(10):830–3. https://doi.org/10.1016/0278-2391(88)90043-2.
27. Mani NJ, Singh B. Studies on oral submucous fibrosis III. Epithelial changes. Oral Surg. 1976;41:203–14.
28. Pindborg JJ, Mehta FS, Daftary DK. Occurrence of epithelial atypia in 51 Indian villagers with oral submucous fibrosis. Br J Cancer. 1970;24(2):253–7.
29. van der Waal I. Potentially malignant disorders of the oral and oropharyngeal mucosa; terminology, classification and present concepts of management. Oral Oncol. 2009;45:317–23.
30. Reibel J. Prognosis of oral pre-malignant lesions: significance of clinical, histopathological, and molecular biological characteristics. Crit Rev Oral Biol Med. 2003;14:47–62.
31. Warnakulasuriya S, Kovacevic T, Madden P, et al. Factors predicting malignant transformation in oral potentially malignant disorders among patients accrued over a 10-year period in south East England. J Oral Pathol Med. 2011;40:677–83.
32. Tilakaratne WM, Iqbal Z, Ariyawardana A, et al. Upregulation of HIF1a in malignant transformation of oral submucous fibrosis. J Oral Pathol Med. 2008;37:372–7.
33. Jayasooriya PR, Jayasinghe KAN, Tilakaratne WM. Relationship between thickness of fibrosis and epithelial dysplasia in oral submucous fibrosis. J Investig Clin Dent. 2011;2:171–5.
34. Shirsat PM, et al. Letter to the editor: oral epithelial dysplasia in oral submucous fibrosis: a challenge. Oral Oncol. 2016; 54:e19.
35. Kemtur P, Acharya S, Hallikeri K. Keratinocytes in oral submucous fibrosis: a cytomorphometric analysis using computer aided image analyser. Saudi J Oral Sci. 2015;2:86–93.
36. Moll R, Franke WW, Schiller DL, Geiger B, Krepler R. The catalog of human cytokeratins: patterns of expression in normal epithelia, tumors and cultured cells. Cell. 1982;31:11–24.
37. Vaidya MM, Sawant SS, Borges AM, Ogale SB, Bhisey AN. Cytokeratin expression in precancerous lesions of the human oral cavity. Oral Oncol. 1998;34:261–4.
38. Schweizer J, Bowden PE, Coulombe PA, et al. New consensus nomenclature for mammalian keratins. J Cell Biol. 2006;174: 169–74.
39. Lalli A, Tilakaratne WM, Ariyawardana A, et al. An altered keratinocyte phenotype in oral submucous fibrosis: correlation of keratin K17 expression with disease severity. J Oral Pathol Med. 2008;37:211–20.
40. Ranganathan K, Kavitha R, Sawant SS, Vaidya MM. Cytokeratin expression in oral submucous fibrosis--an immunohistochemical study. J Oral Pathol Med 35 (2006) 25–32.
41. Altemani A, Costa AF, Montalli VA, Mosqueda-Taylor A, Paes de Almeida O, León JE, et al. Signet-ring cell change in adenoid cystic carcinoma: a clinicopathological and immunohistochemical study of four cases. Histopathology. 2013;62:531–42.
42. Sharma G, Kamboj M. The enigma of signet ring cells. J Oral Maxillofac Pathol. 2020;24:18–9.
43. Pindborg J, Sirsat S. Oral submucous fibrosis. Oral Surg Oral Med Oral Pathol. 1966;22:764–79.
44. Cox SC, Walker DM. Oral submucous fibrosis: a review. Aust Dent J. 1996;41:5.
45. Sitheeque M, Ariyawardana A, Jayasinghe R, Tilakaratne WM. Depigmentation of oral mucosa as the earliest possible manifestation of oral submucous fibrosis in Sri Lankan preschool children. J Investig Clin Dent. 2010;1:156–9.
46. Silva LC, Fonseca FP, Almeida OP, Almeida Mariz BALA, Lopes MA, Radhakrishnan R, et al. CD1a+ and CD207+ cells are reduced in oral submucous fibrosis and oral squamous cell carcinoma. Med Oral Patol Oral Cir Bucal. 2020;25(1):e49–55.
47. Narayanan B, Narasimhan M. Langerhans cell expression in Oral submucous fibrosis: an Immunohistochemical analysis. J Clin Diagn Res. 2015;9(7):ZC39–41.
48. Nyachhyon R, Nagaraj SK, Ongole R. Expression of CD1a by Langerhans cells in oral mucosa of submucous fibrosis patients and arecanut/gutkha chewers. J Nepal Dental Assoc. 2014;14:2.
49. Haque MF, Harris M, Meghji S, Speight PM. An immunohistochemical study of oral submucous fibrosis. J Oral Pathol Med. 1997;26:75–82.
50. Angadi PV, Rao SS. Areca nut in pathogenesis of oral submucous fibrosis: revisited. Oral Maxillofac Surg. 2011;15:1–9.
51. Wynn TA. Common and unique mechanisms regulate fibrosis in various fibroproliferative diseases. J Clin Invest. 2007;117:524–9.
52. Joseph AP, Rajendran R. Submucosa precedes lamina propria in initiating fibrosis in oral submucous fibrosis—evidence based on collagen histochemistry. OMPJ. 2010;1(1)
53. Kamath VV. The nature of collagen in oral submucous fibrosis: a systematic review of the literature. S J Oral Sci. 2014;1(2):57–64.
54. Parveen S, Ahmed SA, Tanveer S. A study on orientation of collagen fibres in oral submucous fibrosis. Int J Sci Res Publ. 2013;3:1–4.
55. Velidandla S, Gaikwad P, Ealla KK, Bhorgonde KD, Hunsingi P, Kumar A. Histochemical analysis of polarizing colors of collagen using Picrosirius red staining in oral submucous fibrosis. J Int Oral Health. 2014;6(1):33–8.
56. Yanjia H, Xinchun J. The role of epithelial-mesenchymal transition in oral squamous cell carcinoma and oral submucous fibrosis. Clin Chim Acta. 2007;383(1–2):51–6.
57. Sharma M, Radhakrishnan R. CTGF is obligatory for TGF-$\beta_1$ mediated fibrosis in OSMF. Oral Oncol. 2016;56:e10–1.
58. Sharma M, Shetty SS, Radhakrishnan R. Oral submucous fibrosis as an over healing wound: implications in malignant transformation. Recent Pat Anticancer Drug Discov. 2018;13:272–91.
59. Sarode G, Sarode SC, Deshmukh R, Raktade P, Patil S. Myofibroblasts could be recruited in a chemokine (C-C motif) ligand 2-dependent manner in pathogenesis of oral submucous fibrosis. J Oral Pathol Med. 2017;46(6):443–7.
60. Utsunomiya H, Tilakaratne WM, Oshiro K, Maruyama S, Suzuki M, Ida-Yonemochi H, et al. Extracellular matrix remodeling in oral submucous fibrosis: its stage-specific modes revealed by immunohistochemistry and in situ hybridization. J Oral Pathol Med. 2005;34:498–507.
61. Murgod VV, Kale AD, Angadi PV, Hallikerimath S. Morphometric analysis of the mucosal vasculature in oral submucous fibrosis and its comparison with oral squamous cell carcinoma. J Oral Sci. 2014;56:173–8.
62. Singh M, Chaudhary AK, Pandya S, Debnath S, Singh M, Singh PA, et al. Morphometric analysis in potentially malignant head and neck lesions: oral submucous fibrosis. Asian Pac J Cancer Prev. 2010;11:257–60.
63. Fang CY, Han WN, Fong DY. A morphometric study on the microvessel in oral submucous fibrosis. Hunan Yi Ke Da Xue Xue Bao. 2000;25:55–7.
64. Pandiar D, Shameena P. Immunohistochemical expression of CD34 and basic fibroblast growth factor(bFGF) in oral submucous fibrosis. J Oral Maxillofac Pathol. 2014;18:155–61.
65. Rajendran R, Paul S, Mathews PP, Raghul J, Mohanty M. Characterisation and quantification of mucosal vasculature in oral submucous fibrosis. Indian J Dent Res. 2005;16:83–91.


14

66. Shih YH, Wang TH, Shieh TM, Tseng YH. Oral submucous fibrosis: a review on Etiopathogenesis, diagnosis, and therapy. Int J Mol Sci. 2019;20:2940.
67. Sudarshan R, Annigeri RG, Sree VG. Pathogenesis of oral submucous fibrosis: the past and current concepts. Int J Oral Maxillofac Pathol. 2012;3:27–36.
68. Gartner LP, Hiatt JL. Chapter 6: Connective tissue. Color textbook of histology. 3rd ed. Saunders Elsevier Publication. Pennsylvania. p. 111–129.
69. Pereira T, Naik S, Tamgadge A. Quantitative evaluation of macrophage expression using CD68 in oral submucous fibrosis: an immunohistochemical study. Ann Med Health Sci Res. 2015;5:435–41.
70. Chiang CP, Wu HY, Liu BY, Wang JT, Kuo MY. Quantitative analysis of immunocompetent cells in oral submucous fibrosis in Taiwan. Oral Oncol. 2002;38:56–63.
71. Hinz B. Formation and function of the myofibroblast during tissue repair. J Invest Dermatol. 2007;127:526–37.
72. Wadhwan V, Venkatesh A, Reddy V, Malik S. The role of myofibroblasts in the progression of oral submucous fibrosis: a systematic review. J Oral Maxillofac Pathol. 2019;23:257–66.
73. Pujari R, Vidya N. Mast cell density in oral submucous fibrosis: a possible role in pathogenesis. Int J Health Sci (Qassim). 2013;7:23–9.
74. Huang S, Ling T, Wu H. Experimental study on aqueous areca nut extracts inducing oral submucous fibrosis in rats. II. Effection of mast cells on collagen metabolism. Hua Xi Kou Qiang Yi Xue Za Zhi. 1997;15:94–6.
75. Cheema VS, Ramesh V, Balamurali PD. Relevance of mast cells in oral squamous cell carcinoma. J Clin Diagn Res. 2012;6:1803–7.
76. DeBruin EJ, Gold M, Lo BC, Snyder K, Cait A, Lasic N, Lopez M, McNagny KM, Hughes MR. Mast cells in human health and disease. Methods Mol Biol. 2015;1220:93–119.
77. Hiromatsu Y, Toda S. Mast cells and angiogenesis. Microsc Res Tech. 2003;60:64–9.
78. Rooban T, Saraswathi TR, AL Zainab FH, Devi U, Elizabeth J, Ranganathan K. A light microscopic study of fibrosis involving muscle in oral submucous fibrosis. Indian J Dent Res. 2005;16:131.
79. Siriwardena BSMS, Jayawardena K, Senarath N, Tilakaratne WM. An evaluation of clinical and histopathological aspects of patients with oral submucous fibrosis in the background of oral squamous cell carcinoma. Biomed Res Int. 2018;2018:1–7. https://doi.org/10.1155/2018/4154165.
80. Gupta S, Khanna S, Singh M, Singh PA. Histological changes to palatal and paratubal muscles in oral submucous fibrosis. J Laryngol Otol. 2001;114:947–50. https://doi.org/10.1258/0022215001904428.
81. Chawla H, Urs A, Augustine J, Kumar P. Characterization of muscle alteration in oral submucous fibrosis-seeking new evidence. Med Oral Patol Oral Cirugia Bucal. 2015;20:e670. https://doi.org/10.4317/medoral.20656.
82. Tom A, Baghirath V, Krishna B, Ganepalli A, Kumar JV, Mohan SP. Ultrastructural changes of collagen in different histopathological grades of oral submucous fibrosis. J Pharm Bioallied Sci. 2019 May;11(Suppl. 2):S309–13. https://doi.org/10.4103/JPBS.JPBS_20_19.
83. El-Labban NG, Canniff JP. Ultrastructural findings of muscle degeneration in oral submucous fibrosis. J Oral Pathol. 1985;14:709–17.
84. Sumathi MK, Narayanan B, Malathi N. A prospective transmission electron microscopic study of muscle status in oral submucous fibrosis along with retrospective analysis of 80 cases of oral submucous fibrosis. J Oral Maxillofac Pathol. 2012;16:318–24.
85. Reichart P, Böning W, Srisuwan S, Theetranont C, Mohr U. Ultrastructural findings in the oral mucosa of betel chewers. J Oral Pathol. 1984;13(2):166–77. https://doi.org/10.1111/j.1600-0714.1984.tb01413.x.
86. Yoshimura K, Dissanayake UB, Nanayakkara D, Kageyama I, Kobayashi K. Morphological changes in oral mucosae and their connective tissue cores regarding oral submucous fibrosis. Arch Histol Cytol. 2005;68:185–92.
87. Binnie WH, Cawson RA. A new ultrastructural finding in oral submucous fibrosis. Br J Dermatol. 1972;86:286–90.
88. Sirsat SM, Pindborg JJ. Subepithelial changes in oral submucous fibrosis. Acta Pathol Microbiol Scand. 1967;70:161–73.
89. Ikram P, Jeddy N. Evaluation of fibrotic changes in OSMF: a retrospective study using special stains and polarizing microscopy. Int J Med Dent Sci. 2017;6(2):1518–24.
90. Ceena DE, Bastian TS, Ashok L, Annigeri RG. Comparative study of clinicofunctional staging of oral submucous fibrosis with qualitative analysis of collagen fibers under polarizing microscopy. Indian J Dent Res. 2009;20:271–6.
91. Arora KS, Nayyar A, Kaur P, Arora KS, Goel A, Singh S. Evaluation of collagen in leukoplakia, oral submucous fibrosis and Oral squamous cell carcinomas using polarizing microscopy and immunohistochemistry. Asian Pac J Cancer Prev. 2018;19(4):1075–80. https://doi.org/10.22034/APJCP.2018.19.4.1075.
92. Nishat R, Kumar H. Collagen fibres in oral submucous fibrosis—a polarizing microscopy study using two special stains. Indian J Pathol Microbiol. 2019;62(4):537–43. https://doi.org/10.4103/IJPM.IJPM_324_19.
93. Smitha BR, Donoghue M. Clinical and histopathological evaluation of collagen fibre orientation in patients with oral submucous fibrosis. J Oral Maxillofac Pathol. 2011;15:154–60.
94. Kamath VV, Satelur KP, Komali Y, Krishnamurthy SS. Image analyses of collagen types and thickness in oral submucous fibrosis stained with picrosirius red under polarizing microscope. J Orofac Sci 2013; 5:123–127.
95. Reshma V, Varsha BK, Rakesh P, Radhika MB, Soumya M, D'Mello S. Aggrandizing oral submucous fibrosis grading using an adjunct special stain: a pilot study. J Oral Maxillofac Pathol. 2016;20:36–46.
96. Mishra NSS, Wanjari SP, Parwani RN, Wanjari PV, Kaothalker SP. Assessment of collagen and elastic fibres in various stages of oral submucous fibrosis using Masson's trichrome, Verhoeff van Gieson and picrosirius staining under light and polarizing microscopy. J Dent Specialities. 2015;3(2):170–2.
97. Joshi PS, Hongal BP, Agnihotri NS, Kempwade RS. A retrospective study on qualitative assessment of copper content in oral leukoplakia, submucous fibrosis, and squamous cell carcinoma with rhodamine stain. J Interdiscipl Histopathol. 2015;3(3):105–9.
98. Pindborg JJ. Oral submucous fibrosis: a review. Ann Acad Med Singap. 1989 Sep;18(5):603–7.
99. Lian I-B, Tseng YT, Su CC, Tsai KY. Progression of precancerous lesions to oral cancer: results based on the Taiwan National Health Insurance Database. Oral Oncol. 2013;49(5):427–30.
100. Jayasinghe LA, Peiris PM, Tilakaratne WM, Attygalla AM, Jayasinghe RD, Sitheeque MA, et al. Clinically malignant exophytic lesions in the background of oral submucous fibrosis: report of five cases. Oral Surg Oral Med Oral Pathol Oral Radiol. 2016;122:210–5.
101. Shah AM, Bansal S, Shirsat PM, Prasad P, Desai RS. Exophytic verrucous hyperplasia in oral submucous fibrosis: a single-center study. J Oral Maxillofac Pathol. 2020;23:393–9.
102. Wang YP, Chen HM, Kuo RC, Yu CH, Sun A, Liu BY, Kuo YS, Chiang CP. Oral verrucous hyperplasia: histologic classifi-

cation, prognosis, and clinical implications. J Oral Pathol Med. 2009;38:651–6.

103. Zain RB, Ikeda N, Gupta PC, Warnakulasuriya S, van Wyk CW, Shrestha P, Axéll T. Oral mucosal lesions associated with betel quid, areca nut and tobacco chewing habits: consensus from a workshop held in Kuala Lumpur, Malaysia, November 25–27, 1996. J Oral Pathol Med. 1999;28(1):1–4.

104. Reichart PA, Warnakulasuriya S. Oral lichenoid contact lesions induced by areca nut and betel quid chewing: a mini review. J Investig Clin Dent 2012;3(3):163–166.132.

105. Yanduri S, Kumar VB, Suma S, Madhura MG. Lichenoid features and fibrosis: coexistence in Quid-induced Oral lesions. J Contemp Dent Pract. 2015;16(5):389–93.

106. Ekanayaka RP, Tilakaratne WM. Oral submucous fibrosis: review on mechanisms of malignant transformation. Oral Surg Oral Med Oral Pathol Oral Radiol. 2016;

107. Paymaster JC. Cancer of the buccal mucosa. A clinical study of 650 cases in Indian patients. Cancer. 1956;9(431–5):37.

108. Murti PR, Bhonsle RB, Pindborg JJ, Daftary DK, Gupta PC, Mehta FS. Malignant transformation rate in oral submucous fibrosis over a 17-year period. Community Dent Oral Epidemiol. 1985;13:340–1.

109. Jayanthi V, Probert CSJ, Sher KS, Mayberry JF. Oral submucosal fibrosis a preventable disease. Gut. 1992;33:4–6.

110. Gadbail AR, et al. Oral squamous cell carcinoma in the background of oral submucous fibrosis is a distinct clinicopathological entity with better prognosis. J Oral Pathol Med. 2017;46(6):448–53.

111. Gupta N, Rakshit A, Srivastava S, Suryawanshi H, Kumar P, Naik R. Comparative evaluation of micronuclei in exfoliated oral epithelial cells in potentially malignant disorders and malignant lesions using special stains. J Oral Maxillofac Pathol. 2019;23:157.

112. Gupta J, Gupta K, Agarwal R. Comparison of different stains in exfoliated oral mucosal cell micronucleus of potentially malignant disorders of oral cavity. J Can Res Ther. 2019;15:615–9.

113. Kohli M, Ahuja P, Mehendiratta M, Sharma M, Dutta J. Micronucleus assay: an early diagnostic tool to assess genotoxic changes in patients with tobacco use, Oral leukoplakia and Oral submucous fibrosis journal of clinical and diagnostic. Research. 2017;11(9):ZC28–32.

114. Palaskar S, Jindal C. Evaluation of micronuclei using Papanicolaou and may Grunwald Giemsa stain in individuals with different tobacco habits—a comparative study. J Clin Diagn Res. 2010;4:3607–13.

115. Kayalf JJ, Trivedi AH, Dave BJ, Nair J, Nair UJ, Bhlde SV, Goswami UC, Adhvaryu SC. Incidence of micronuclei in oral mucosa of users of tobacco products singly or in various combinations. Mutagenesis. 1993;8(1):31–3.

116. Fenech M, Kirsch-Volders M, Natarajan AT, Surralles J, Crott JW, Parry J, Norppa H, Eastmond DA, Tucker JD, Thomas P. Molecular mechanisms of micronucleus, nucleoplasmic bridge and nuclear bud formation in mammalian and human cells. Mutagenesis. 2011;26:125–32.

117. Adhvaryu SG, Dave BJ, Trivedi AH. Cytogenetic surveillance of tobacco-areca nut (mava) chewers, including patients with oral cancers and premalignant conditions. Mutat Res. 1991;261:41–9.

118. Joshi MS, Verma Y, Gautam AK, Shivgotra VK, Parmar G, Kumar S. Assessment of genetic damage among chewers of mixture containing mainly areca nut and tobacco. Asia Pac J Public Health. 2011;23:852–60.

119. Grover S, Ahmed MB, Telagi N, Shivappa AB, Nithin KP. Evaluation of diagnostic reliability of micronuclei in potentially malignant disorders of oral cavity. CHRISMED J Health Res. 2014;1:15–20.

120. Katarkar A, Mukherjee S, Khan MH, Ray JG, Chaudhuri K. Comparative evaluation of genotoxicity by micronucleus assay in the buccal mucosa over comet assay in peripheral blood in oral precancer and cancer patients. Mutagenesis. 2014;29(5):325–34. https://doi.org/10.1093/mutage/geu023.

121. Warnakulasuriya KA, Johnson NW. Nucleolar organiser region (NOR) distribution as a diagnostic marker in oral keratosis, dysplasia and squamous cell carcinoma. J Oral Pathol Med. 1993 Feb;22(2):77–81. https://doi.org/10.1111/j.1600-0714.1993.tb00048.x.

122. Khushbu BP, Chalisshazar M, Kale H, Baranwal M, Modi T. Quantitative and qualitative assessment of argyrophilic nucleolar organizer regions in normal, premalignant and malignant oral lesions. J Oral Maxillofac Pathol. 2017;21(3):360–6.

123. Sowmya GV, Nahar P, Astekar M, Agarwal H, Singh MP. Analysis of silver binding nucleolar organizer regions in exfoliative cytology smears of potentially malignant and malignant oral lesions. Biotech Histochem. 2017;92(2):115–21.

124. Ankathil R, Vijayakumar T, Nesy EA, Chandini R, Beena VT, Abraham E, Nair MK. Interphase nucleolar organizer region distribution in the tissues of oral leukoplakia, oral submucous fibrosis and oral cancer: evaluation of diagnostic and prognostic implications. Oncol Rep. 1997;4:187–90.

125. Chattopadhyay A. AgNORs in tumoral pathology. Review of literature and observations on the technic and reaction in normal oral epithelium. Indian J Dent Res. 1993;4:47–53.

126. Chattopadhyay A, Chawda JG, Doshi JJ. Silver-binding nucleolar organizing regions: a study of oral leukoplakia and squamous cell carcinoma. Int J Oral Maxillofac Surg. 1994;23:374–7.

127. Chattopadhyay A, Ray JG, Caplan DJ. AgNOR count as objective marker for dysplastic features in oral leukoplakia. J Oral Pathol Med. 2002;31:512–7.

128. Chattopadhyay A, Ray JG. AgNOR cut-point to distinguish mild and moderate epithelial dysplasia. J Oral Pathol Med. 2008;37:78–82.

129. Ray JG, Chattopadhyay A, Caplan DJ. Usefulness of AgNOR counts in diagnosing epithelial dysplasia. J Oral Pathol Med. 2003;32:71–6.

130. Chauhan GR, Shah V, Shah S, Pradip C, Chauhan B. Epithelial dysplasia and silver binding nucleolar organizer region proteins (AgNORs) in oral submucous fibrosis. Int J Biol Med Res. 2012;3:2261–8.

# Biomarkers in Oral Submucous Fibrosis

*Kannan Ranganathan and Kavitha Loganathan*

## Contents



© The Author(s), under exclusive license to Springer Nature Switzerland AG 2023
S. Warnakulasuriya, K. Ranganathan (eds.), *Oral Submucous Fibrosis*, Textbooks in Contemporary Dentistry,
https://doi.org/10.1007/978-3-031-12855-4_15

## 15.1 Introduction

A biomarker is "a biological molecule found in blood, other body fluids, or tissues that is a sign of a normal or abnormal process, or of a condition or disease". Biomarkers differentiate an affected patient from a person without the disease [1]. Biomarkers can potentially predict response to specific therapeutic interventions (predictive), inform clinicians regarding the risk of clinical outcomes such as cancer recurrence or disease progression in the future (prognostic), and identify the disease as early as possible (diagnostic) [2].

**Table 15.1** Biomarkers in oral submucous fibrosis

| Epithelial markers | Connective tissue markers | Proliferative markers | Stemness markers | Markers of cell signaling | Other markers (transcription factors, enzymes, glycoproteins, and metabolic markers) |
|---|---|---|---|---|---|
| Annexin A4 (ANXN A4)<br>Beta-catenin<br>CD1a, CD207, CD303<br>Cytokeratins (CK-5/6, CK-10, CK8, CK18, CK14)<br>E-cadherin (E-cad)<br>Epidermal growth factor receptor (EGFR)<br>Filamin A (FLMN A)<br>Loricrin | Alpha-smooth muscle actin ($\alpha$-SMA)<br>Bone morphogenetic protein-7 (BMP-7)<br>CD34, CD68, CD105, CD147<br>Collagen (Col 1, Col 3, collagen IV)<br>Connective tissue growth factor (CTGF)<br>Decorin<br>Fibroblast growth factor (bFGR, FGF2, and its receptors FGFR2 and FGFR3)<br>Fibronectin<br>Hypoxia-inducing factors (HIF-1$\alpha$, HIF-2$\alpha$)<br>Mast cell chymase, mast cell tryptase<br>Matrix metalloproteinases (MMP-1, MMP-2)<br>N-cadherin (N-cad)<br>Osteopontin<br>Podoplanin<br>S100A4<br>STRO1<br>Syndecan-1<br>Tenascin-C<br>Transforming growth factor-$\beta$ (TGF-$\beta$, TGF-$\beta$1, TGF-$\beta$2)<br>Tissue inhibitors of matrix metalloproteinases (TIMPs; TIMP-1, TIMP-2)<br>Transglutaminase-2<br>TWIST<br>Vascular endothelial growth factor (VEGF)<br>Vimentin | Bax<br>Bmi1<br>Budding uninhibited by benzimidazole-related 1 (BUBR1)<br>Caspase 3<br>c-Jun<br>c-met<br>c-Myc<br>Cyclin D1<br>Fragile histidine triad protein (FHIT)<br>Human telomerase reverse transcriptase (hTERT)<br>Insulin-like growth factor II mRNA-binding protein 3 (IMP3)<br>Ki67<br>Microtubule-associated protein light chain 3 (LC3)<br>Mouse double-minute 2 homolog (MDM2)<br>p16, p53, p62, p63<br>Proliferating cell nuclear antigen (PCNA)<br>Polo-like kinase (PLK)<br>Phosphatase and tensin homolog deleted on chromosome 10 (PTEN)<br>Survivin | Aldehyde dehydrogenase 1 (ALDH1)<br>CD133<br>Stage-specific embryonic antigen (SSEA-4)<br>SRY (sex-determining region on Y chromosome) type homeobox genes (SOX2) | Dickkopf WNT signaling pathway inhibitor 3 (DKK3)<br>Phosphorylated extracellular signal-regulated kinases (pERK)<br>Glioma-associated oncogene homolog 1 (GLI1)<br>Sonic hedgehog (Shh)<br>WNT inhibitory factor 1 (WIF1) | Alpha enolase (ENO1)<br>Beta-integrin<br>Calreticulin<br>C–C motif chemokine ligand 2 (CCL2)<br>Cyclooxygenase-2 (COX-2)<br>Cyclophilin A<br>Fatty acid synthase (FASN)<br>Fibrinogen alpha-chain precursor (FGA)<br>Glucose transporter 1 (GLUT1)<br>Heat-shock protein (Hsp70)<br>Hexokinase-2<br>4-Hydroxynonenal (4-HNE)<br>Mucin 1 (MUC1)<br>Organic cation transporter-3 (OCT3)<br>Secreted frizzled-related proteins (SFRPs) |

Immunohistochemistry (IHC) is a versatile tool used to identify cell or tissue antigens, ranging from amino acids and proteins to infectious agents and specific cellular populations [3]. IHC helps in classifying the cellular origin of tumors, identifying tumor subtypes, determining treatment efficacy, predicting prognosis, and ascertaining the malignant transformation potential of oral potentially malignant disorders (OPMDs), such as OSF [4]. OSF has a malignant transformation rate of 1.2–23% [5]. Here, we discuss our current understanding of the use of immunohistochemical biomarkers in understanding the pathogenesis, progression, and malignant transformation of OSF.

**Learning Goals**

- To have an understanding of the biomarkers and their role in OSF
- An overview of the different types of biomarkers are categorized as (◘ Table 15.1)

The biomarkers discussed are listed in ◘ Table 15.1.

## 15.2 Epithelial Markers

### 15.2.1 Annexin A4 (ANXN A4)

Annexins are calcium-dependent phospholipid-binding proteins located in the nucleus, cytoplasm, or cell membrane. It helps in vesicle aggregation, regulation of ion channels, cell cycle, and cell differentiation [6]. ANXN A4 is associated with loss of cell adhesion and plays an important role in the apoptosis, cell migration, carcinogenesis, chemoresistance, and invasion of cancer cells. It also facilitates the repair of cell membrane damage and influences cell shape in wound healing.

ANXN A4 expression is upregulated in epithelial tumors such as cancer of kidneys, breast, larynx, pancreas, and OSCC. Its overexpression is associated with advanced tumor stage and poor prognosis. ANXN A4 with protein kinase C plays an important role in buccal squamous cell carcinoma (BSCC) pathogenesis [6]. Liu et al. show an increased expression of ANXN A4 in OSF (72.34%; 68/94), with localization of expression in the spinous and corneal layer of the epithelium. Annexin A4 expression levels are greater in OSCC compared to OSF [6].

### 15.2.2 Beta-Catenin (β-Catenin)

β-Catenin is a pivotal component of the cadherin complex and is a key mediator of canonical Wnt signaling. Its activation is important in tumor development and progression. β-Catenin binds to the T cell factor/lymphoid enhancer factor (TCF/LEF-1) family of transcription factors and activates target genes involved in the Wnt signaling pathway [7, 8]. β-Catenin is involved in the stabilization of the adherens junction along with E-cadherin and also functions as a nuclear oncogenic transcription factor. In OSCC, aberrant expression of β-catenin is associated with epithelial-mesenchymal transition (EMT), poor survival, and nodal metastases [8]. Bag et al. observed downregulation of β-catenin in OSF with dysplasia (52.8%; 19/36), but no significant difference in expression was observed in OSF without dysplasia (47.2%; 17/36). A similar downregulation of β-catenin was observed in OSCC cases; this downregulation was associated with decreases in epithelial maturation [7].

### 15.2.3 CD1a, CD303, and CD207

These markers are expressed by dendritic cells. Dendritic cells (DCs) are of three types: Langerhans (CD1a, CD207), myeloid (CD1c, CD141), and plasmacytoid (CD303, CD304) type. They have an important role in the stimulation or suppression of immune response.

Langerhans cells (LCs) are clear cells present in the suprabasal layer of the oral mucosa. They are antigen-presenting cells (APCs) that trigger T cell activation. These cells are essential for immune surveillance function against antigens involved in allergic reactions and the antigens expressed during malignant transformation [9, 10]. LCs are derived from myeloid stem cells of bone marrow. They are APCs that interact with the major histocompatibility complex (MHC) class II and CD4+ cells to provoke a specific T cell reaction [11, 12]. CD1a is a specific marker for immature DCs and LCs.

CD207, also called Langerin, is the hallmark of active epidermal Langerhans cells (LCs). The expression of the CD207 receptor in DCs is suggestive of effective coupling of antigen with MHC-I and MHC-II, a process that activates the CD8+ and CD4+ T cells. Downregulation of CD207 might indicate a suppression of the T cell response [12, 13].

CD303 or blood dendritic cell antigen (BDCA) is a type II lectin used in the identification of plasmacytoid DC. Plasmacytoid DC resides in lymphoid and nonlymphoid organs and is involved in the production of large amounts of type I interferon (IFN) [12, 14].

In OSF, the genotoxic components of betel quid alter the structure of DNA, proteins, and lipids resulting in the production of antigens. This stimulus triggers LCs which are responsible for antigen processing and induction of T cell-mediated immune response [12, 15].

Increased activation of LCs in the dysplastic epithelium has also been reported in leukoplakia [16]. This may indicate the presence of acquired antigens from dysplastic cells. An increase in the number of CD303+ cells is associated with OSCC and poor prognosis of melanoma [14]. CD1a, CD303, and CD207 expressions are altered in OSF and OSCC. da Silva et al. reported a decrease in CD1a+ (57 ± 42.9) and CD207+ (35.7 ± 25.7) cells in OSF compared to normal epithelium (CD1a+: 101.3 ± 58.2; C207+: 71.1 ± 47.9). In contrast, a gradual increase in CD303+ cells was observed for OSF (0.2 ± 0.6), OSF-OSCC (2.2 ± 2.5), and OSCC (2.7 ± 4.8), respectively, when compared to the control (0.1 ± 0.4). The Langerhans-type DCs are decreased in OSCC and OSCC-OSF, while the plasmacytoid-type DCs are increased in OSCC compared to OSF. This difference reflects a shift in the type of immune response in the progression to OSCC.

### 15.2.4 Cytokeratins (CKs)

Cytokeratins (CKs) are the major intermediate filaments in squamous epithelium, which have a role in cell stabilization, cell shape, intracellular signaling, and cell transport. CKs are present in all epithelial cells and neoplasms derived from them [17, 18]. They are broadly divided into types I and II, with more than 20 subtypes [19].

Type I: (CKs 9 through 23) acidic and low molecular weight (40–64 kDa) [17–19]

Type II: (CKs 1 through 8) basic or neutral with high molecular weight (52–68 kDa) [17–19]

CKs are sensitive markers for carcinoma. The low-molecular-weight (LMW) CKs are seen in simple non-stratified epithelia, and the high-molecular-weight (HMW) CKs are seen in complex stratified squamous epithelia and in the tumors arising from the corresponding epithelium. Alteration in CK patterns has been reported in dysplastic lesions, OSF, and OSCC [17, 18].

CK10 expression in the keratinized epithelium is a marker for terminal differentiation and maturation of epithelial cells [20]. The combined overexpression of CK5 and CK14 is seen in the basal cells of stratified squamous epithelium and squamous cell carcinomas of the head and neck. The expression of CK5 and CK14 persists even in lower grades of malignancy [21].

CK8 and CK18 are the most common members of the large intermediate filament expressed in "simple" epithelial tissues. They are associated with dysplasia and are indicative of an unfavorable prognosis for patients with OSCC. Loss of CK8 phosphorylation increases cell migration and tumor spread in OSCC, and loss of CK8 and 18 leads to alterations in α6β4-integrin-mediated signaling and alteration in tumor progression [21]. CK8 and CK18 are increased in OSCC compared to OSF indicating a shift to low-molecular-weight CK expression, with malignant transformation [22]. This shift is associated with a poor prognosis in cancer.

Increased intensity of staining for PanCK and HMWCK, aberrant expression of CK8, and decreased expression of CKs 5 and 14 occur in OSF [18]. A significant association has been reported between the expression of low-molecular-weight CK8/18 and 19 and a high tumor grade. HMWCKs, CK1, 5/6, 10, and 14 are significantly associated with the expression of p21 and Hsp70 in OSF [21].

Vaidya et al. reported that out of 7 OSF cases, positive expression of CK5, CK14, and CK8 was seen in 2 (28.57%), 5 (71.43%), and 3 (42.86%) cases, respectively [23]. Ranganathan et al. reported on panCK, CK8, CK18, CK4, and CK1 in 50 cases of OSF. Their findings were as follows: 35 (70%) exhibited mild, 11 (22%) moderate, and 4 (8%) intense staining of PanCK-cytokeratin. In OSF, 26 (52%) cases showed mild, while 19 (38%) and 3 (6%) showed moderate and intense staining of HMWCK. In OSF, all the six (12%) cases that stained positive exhibited only mild staining of CK18. One case of OSF showed mild staining of CK14. Five (10%) of OSF exhibited CK8 staining. Intense, moderate, and mild staining of CK5 was exhibited in 8 (16%), 25 (50%), and 15 (30%) of OSF cases. In OSF, 37 (74%) and 2 (4%) cases exhibited mild and moderate staining of CK4, respectively. In OSF, 13 (26%) showed mild staining of CK1 [18].

Lalli et al. reported cytokeratin profile in 28 OSF patients. CK16 staining was entirely suprabasal with similar expression in all OSF. In OSF, CK6 was detectable in both the basal and the suprabasal layers. This increase in expression in the basal layer of OSF epithelium was highly significant ($p < 0.001$), while the suprabasal CK6 expression was unaffected. There was no expression of CK19 in any OSF samples whether from keratinized or non-keratinized sites, suggesting a highly significant reduction in site-matched non-keratinized epithelia ($p < 0.001$) compared with the normal controls. CK14 staining was present homogenously throughout the basal and suprabasal layers, while CK15 was detected in the entire basal layer of both normal and OSF samples implying that the disease did not influence these two keratins. No staining for CK7, CK8, CK18, or CK8/CK18 complex was observed in normal or OSF samples [24].

### 15.2.5 E-Cadherin (E-Cad)

E-cad is a calcium-dependent cell surface adhesion molecule involved in the transduction of signals controlling various cellular events, including polarity, differentiation, growth, and cell migration. It can inhibit cell proliferation by upregulating p27 through epidermal growth factor receptors. Loss of E-cad expression has been correlated with cancer progression, and its reduced expression in cancer correlates with aggressive behavior, high proliferation, invasion, metastasis, and poor prognosis. The epithelial-mesenchymal transition (EMT) signature of low E-cad and high vimentin is associated with greater metastasis in primary head and neck squamous cell carcinomas [25, 26]. E-cad expression levels are decreased in OSF and OSCC, and a significant loss of E-cad is seen with increasing grades of dysplasia in OSF [25, 26].

Das et al. and Sridevi et al. show a gradual decrease in E-cadherin from normal to OSF to OSCC. E-cadherin exhibited membranous staining in basilar cells, parabasal cells, superficial cells (intermediate cells), and corneal cells [18, 27, 28].

### 15.2.6 Epidermal Growth Factor Receptor (EGFR)

Epidermal growth factor receptor (EGFR) belongs to the ErbB family of receptor tyrosine kinases. EGFR is a 170 kDa transmembrane glycoprotein on chromosome 7p11.2. Overexpression of EGFR indicates high intrinsic proliferative activity [29]. Meka et al. studied EGFR expression in 10 cases of OSF and reported that 4/10 (40%) cases showed strong expression, while 3/10 (30%) cases showed mild and moderate expression of EGFR. An overexpression of EGFR has been reported in the membrane and cytoplasm of basal and suprabasal cells and keratin layer of epithelium in OSF. EGFR expression levels help to predict the malignant transformation potential of dysplastic tissues [29]. Aberrant EGFR expression is linked to oncogenic transformation, autonomous cell growth, invasion, angiogenesis, and metastases in several cancers. EGFR overexpression is also predictive of disease-free survival independent of cervical lymph node status in cancer [29].

### 15.2.7 Filamin A (FLNA)

FLNA is an actin filament cross-linking protein involved in cytoskeletal rearrangement. FLNA interacts with more than 90 functionally diverse binding partners to regulate cellular functions and processes by its scaffolding action [6].

Persistent mechanical shear stress caused by areca nut chewing in OSF leads to upregulation of FLNA as a defensive mechanism to prevent cellular damage. Dysregulation of FLNA results in mutagenic DNA double-strand breaks [6]. It is also known to suppress ribosomal gene transcription. FLNA has a role in cell mobility, cell-extracellular matrix (ECM) interactions, cell signaling, and DNA damage response. Its cytoplasmic overexpression promotes tumor invasion and metastasis. Liu et al. report an overexpression of FLNA in 62/94 (65.96%) cases of OSF, with localization in the lower spinous and basal layer of the epithelium. FLNA is increased in OSF and OSCC, with higher expression in OSCC [6].

### 15.2.8 Loricrin

Loricrin is a major component of the cornified cell envelope (CE) keratins, which belongs to a multigene family coded by more than 30 intermediate filament genes. Interaction of loricrin with keratin intermediate filaments provides flexibility to the CE. Loricrin also protects against mechanical stress by its association with nectin and calcium [30].

Chewing areca causes both mechanical and chemical stress that leads to increased expression of loricrin. Areca nut is usually taken along with lime (calcium hydroxide), and the increased calcium concentration influences loricrin expression. Variation in loricrin expression in the different stages of OSF is attributed to the adapting capacity of the epithelium towards a new stimulus. Nithya et al. report positive expression of loricrin in 20/30 (66.7%) cases of OSF, with localization in the granular and corneal layer of epithelium. Increase in loricrin levels in OSF has been suggested to be useful in the early identification of malignant transformation [30, 31].

## 15.3 Connective Tissue Markers

### 15.3.1 Alpha-Smooth Muscle Actin (α-SMA)

α-SMA is an actin isoform of smooth muscle actin protein that plays an important role in fibrogenesis, wound healing, and tissue repair. It is expressed in smooth muscle cells and myofibroblasts. Its expression indicates the transformation of fibroblast to myofibroblast [32].

Myofibroblasts (MFs) are a unique group of phenotypically intermediate cells: between smooth muscle cells and fibroblasts. They are identified by the expression of α-SMA and are essential for the production of extracellular matrix (ECM) after injury, tissue homeostasis, and repair. Altered myofibroblasts have been implicated in disease with increased extracellular matrix (ECM) deposition and fibrosis [32]. MFs are major effector cells in many fibrotic disorders like scleroderma, hepatic and pancreatic fibrosis, and pulmonary fibrosis

[32]. They are prominent in scarring and fibrosis [33]. Transdifferentiation of fibroblasts to MFs is a crucial event in tumorigenesis. MFs stimulate tumor progression by stimulating the growth of cancer cells, sustaining angiogenesis, and attenuating cancer cell death. MFs also promote invasion and metastasis by proteolysis and mechanical propulsive force [34]. MFs are present in the stroma of cancers of the breast, kidney, liver, bladder, colon, and prostate, and OSCC [35].

Fibroblasts in close proximity to cancer cells are called cancer-associated fibroblasts (CAFs). α-SMA-expressing myofibroblasts are activated CAFs. Activated CAFs can express several molecular markers, including α-smooth muscle actin (α-SMA), fibroblast activation protein-α (FAPα), and fibroblast-specific protein-1 (FSP-1). CAFs not only produce type I collagen fibers but also release lysyl oxidase (LOX) for the cross-linking of fibers that cause matrix stiffness that influences cancer invasion [36].

In OSF, chronic mechanical and chemical irritation caused by the areca nut and the alkaloids, respectively, induces the production of inflammatory mediators and transdifferentiation of mucosal fibroblast to myofibroblast [37]. OSF is considered by some to be an exuberant healing process [38]. Transforming growth factor (TGF)-β1 stimulates proto-myofibroblasts to express α-SMA [39].

There is a significant increase in the intensity of α-SMA expression in OSCC compared to normal and OSF [34, 35, 40, 41]. Angadi et al., Sarode et al., Gupta et al., and Anura et al. report significantly high α-SMA in OSF and OSCC compared to normal oral mucosal tissues [32–35]. In subjects with OSCC arising in OSF, α-SMA is significantly higher in the advanced clinical TNM stage and correlates inversely with 3-year patient survival. α-SMA expression increases with increasing severity of dysplasia and advancing grades of OSF and OSCC [41, 42].



### 15.3.2 Bone Morphogenetic Protein-7 (BMP7)

Bone morphogenetic protein (BMP) is a member of the family of transforming growth factor-β (TGF-β). BMP plays an important role in regulating cell proliferation, apoptosis, cell differentiation, migration, and invasion [43]. BMP7 is a negative modulator of ECM, collagen production, and fibrosis induced by TGF-β. BMP7 prevents or reverses fibrosis by reducing pSMAD2 accumulation in the nucleus. Upregulation of profibrotic TGF-β and downregulation of antifibrotic BMP7 are important events in the pathogenesis of OSF. Khan et al. reported this inverse relation in 70% (11/16) of OSF cases and found that BMP7 is predominantly localized in the cytoplasm and extracellular matrix [43].

### 15.3.3 CD34

CD34 (human hematopoietic progenitor cell antigen) is a 110 kDa transmembrane surface glycoprotein. It is expressed on hematopoietic stem cells, endothelium, interstitial cells of Cajal, and dendritic cells present in the dermis, around blood vessels, and in nerve sheath. CD34 is an important marker of tissue vascularization and microvascular density in the tissue [44, 45]. CD34 expression is increased in angiogenesis seen in OSCC and during malignant transformation of OSF [45, 46].

Sharma et al. report that the mean microvascular density was more in OSF (12.5 ± 4.5) compared to normal subjects (3.8 ± 0.5). Mean vascular density (MVD) represented by CD34 expression increases in the early stage and decreases in the advanced stages of OSF [44, 47]. This indicates that there is an increase in the number of vessels in the early stage of OSF, which decreases in later stages as the severity of fibrosis escalates [48]. CD105 expression increases gradually from mild, moderate, and severe dysplasia to OSCC [35].

### 15.3.4 CD68

CD68 is a pan-macrophage marker. Macrophages are derived from circulating monocytes and play an important role in innate and adaptive immunity [49]. Fibrogenic cytokines secreted by activated macrophages are important in fibrotic disorders. In OSF, the continuous contact of areca and its components with the oral mucosa causes chronic inflammation and induces macrophages and T cells to produce cytokines such as interleukin-6 (IL-6), tumor necrosis factor (TNF), interferon-α (IFN α), and transforming growth factor-beta (TGF-β). Pereira et al. observed that the mean macrophage cell density in the epithelium (13.4 ± 2.9) and subepithelial connective tissue (60.9 ± 2.1) of OSF cases was significantly higher than that of normal control group (epithelium: 0.1 ± 0.2; connective tissue: 17.3 ± 19.1) [50]. An increase in CD68-positive macrophages in OSF may be involved in local and systemic upregulation of fibrogenic cytokines and downregulation of antifibrotic cytokine in the pathogenesis of OSF [49, 50].

The presence of CD68-positive tumor-associated macrophages (TAMs) is associated with decreased 5-year survival rates in several malignancies including those of thyroid, lung, liver, and esophagus [51, 52].

### 15.3.5 CD105

CD105 (endoglin) is encoded by the gene located on chromosome 9q34. It is a hypoxia-induced protein and a potential marker for activated endothelial cells. It promotes angiogenesis via TGF-β1 signaling by binding to its specific receptor and initiating the Smad pathways. CD105 is strongly expressed in the blood vessels of OSF and OSCC, with a higher expression in OSCC [35, 41, 46, 52]. Pammar et al. reported that 12 out of 30 OSF cases (40%) showed CD105 positivity, whereas in normal oral mucosa, only 1 out of 15 cases (6.67%) showed positivity for CD105 [46].

### 15.3.6 CD147

CD147, also termed as extracellular matrix metalloproteinase inducer (EMMPRIN), is a highly glycosylated transmembrane protein and a member of the immunoglobulin (Ig) superfamily. It is expressed on the surface of epithelial, endothelial, and immune cells. CD147 plays a significant role in organ fibrosis of the liver, kidney, and lungs. CD147 stimulates matrix metalloproteinase production in stromal cells. CD147 expression positively correlates with TGF-β1 expression involved in the pathogenesis of OSF. Wang et al. showed that CD147 staining is cytoplasmic and membranous. It is predominantly restricted to the lower spinous layer in OSF compared to the normal tissue, where it is confined to the basal layer. CD147 is upregulated in OSF and is a potential predictor of OSCC progression [53, 54]. The mean levels of CD147 and TGF-β1 are significantly lower in early OSF than in intermediate/advanced OSF [54].

### 15.3.7 Collagen

Collagen is a major component of the extracellular matrix that provides tensile strength to the tissue [35, 55]. In OSF, tissue changes include an increase in insoluble collagen deposition and a decrease in collagen degradation. Anura et al. studied the ultrastructural features of collagen in OSF using atomic force microscopy (AFM) and showed that the papillary layer of OSF had concentrated extracellular matrix with dense collagen deposition. The collagen fibrils were closely packed in the form of bundles with collagen hyalinization which was absent in normal tissues. A similar change was also observed in the reticular layer of OSF where the thin and thick bundles of collagen fibrils were more tightly packed and arranged in a single planar direction. The number of fibroblasts in OSF was diminished, and the blood vessels were constricted and pushed towards the juxta-epithelial area of the connective tissue [35].

Collagen degradation and its decreased synthesis allow invasion of tumor cells through the stroma [56]. ECM proteomics reveal that dormant cancer cells assemble a type III collagen-enriched ECM niche. Tumor-derived type III collagen is required to sustain tumor dormancy, as its disruption restores tumor cell proliferation through DDR1-mediated STAT1 signaling. Type III collagen levels are increased in tumors from patients with lymph node-negative head and neck squamous cell carcinoma compared to those with positive lymph nodes [57].

### 15.3.8 Connective Tissue Growth Factor (CTGF)

Connective tissue growth factor (CTGF) is an extracellular matrix protein of the CCN (Cyr61: cysteine-rich protein 61) family of extracellular matrix-associated heparin-binding proteins. CTGF is a key regulatory molecule involved in cell proliferation, angiogenesis, wound healing, and tissue fibrosis [58]. CTGF can sustain fibrotic response even in the absence of the profibrogenic TGF-β. CTGF expression in fibrosis has been reported in the skin, lung, cardiac, liver, kidney, peritoneum, muscle, conjunctiva, and gingiva. It is highly upregulated during tissue remodeling such as in wound healing, fibrotic disorders, angiogenesis, and EMT [59]. Shah et al. report that in their study all the cases of OSF (100%; 40/40) overexpressed CTGF with no expression in normal mucosa. A gradual increase in expression was observed in the epithelium from stage 1 OSF to stage 4 OSF. CTGF expression showed an increase in CTGF expression from normal to OSF to OSCC in OSF. There was a statistically significant difference in CTGF connective tissue expression when normal and OSF were compared with all well differentiated squamous cell carcinoma with or without OSF ($p < 0.05$) [59].

### 15.3.9 Decorin

Decorin plays a pivotal role in the extracellular matrix assembly and cell cycle regulation [60]. Decorin prevents cell proliferation and metastasis of tumor cells by downregulating the epidermal growth factor receptor tyrosine kinase. Decorin is expressed predominantly in the tumor stroma but may be expressed in the cancer cells. Cytoplasmic localization of decorin is indicative of negative regulation of cell proliferation and angiogenesis. Its expression is downregulated from OPMDs (OSF and leukoplakia) to OSCC [60]. Cytoplasmic decorin functions as a natural inhibitor of angiogenesis, which may have clinical application in the development of antiangiogenic therapy. Nayak et al. report that in their study, expression of decorin in the epithelium was greater in OSF (69%; 20/29) compared to OSCC (5.6%; 6/108) and normal controls (38.5%; 20/52). The connective tissue associated with the dysplastic epithelium showed lower expression in OSF (65.5%; 19/29) cases compared to OSCC (56.5%; 61/108) and normal subjects (98.1%; 51/52) [60].

### 15.3.10 Fibroblast Growth Factor (FGF) and Its Receptors (bFGF, FGF2, FGFR2, and FGFR3)

Fibroblast growth factors (FGFs) are heparin-binding proteins that interact with cell surface-associated heparan sulfate proteoglycans. They promote epithelium-connective tissue signaling and regulate the growth and differentiation of a wide variety of tissues including epithelium [61]. The FGF receptor family constitutes four members, which include FGFR-1, FGFR-2, FGFR-3, and FGFR-4. FGF-2 induces angiogenesis, and its receptors influence collagen formation, and it is involved in the invasion of cancer cells and the proliferation of fibroblasts around cancer cells. Nayak et al. observed that FGF-2, FGFR-2, and FGFR-3 were upregulated in OSF (FGF-2: 3%, 9/29; FGFR-2: 24%, 7/29; FGFR-3: 38%; 11/29), leukoplakia (FGF-2: 32.6%, 14/43; FGFR-2: 39.5%, 17/43; FGFR-3: 41.9%; 18/43), and OSCC (FGF-2: 5.1%, 53/108; FGFR-2: 57.4%, 62/108; FGFR-3: 8%; 81/108) [61]. Pandiar et al. studied mean vascular density (MVD) using bFGF and observed that MVD in controls, stage 2 OSF, stage 3 OSF, stage 4 OSF, OSF with dysplasia, and OSF turning malignant was 32.5, 15.6, 14, 14.5, 11, and 34, respectively. The difference in MVD between cases and controls was statistically significant (*P*-value 0.000) [45].

15

### 15.3.11 Fibronectin

Fibronectin is a multifunctional glycoprotein expressed by fibroblasts during development and wound healing. It is an extracellular matrix (ECM) component that is organized in a fibrillary network. It exists in a soluble form produced by the hepatocytes, which is a major component of blood plasma and a less soluble cellular form synthesized by the fibroblasts, as a component of ECM [62, 63]. Fibronectin regulates cell adhesion, migration, growth, and differentiation [59]. It binds to integrin receptors of the cell surface and is a key player in the communication between the intra- and the extracellular environment [63].

Remodeling of ECM is associated with increased production of perlecan, tenascin, fibronectin, and collagen type III in early stages of OSF [64]. Fibronectin in tumor stroma correlates with poor prognosis or aggressive phenotypes of colorectal cancer, urothelial carcinoma, breast cancer, and OSCC. Anura et al. have reported that in normal mucosa, fibronectin was present throughout the subepithelium with high intensity near blood vessels and below the basement membrane. However, their expression was diminished in OSF [35].

### 15.3.12 Hypoxia-Inducible Factor (HIF)

HIFs are transcription factors that mediate the adaptive responses to hypoxia. HIFs are involved in carcinogenesis through regulation of genes involved in angiogenesis and glycolytic metabolism. HIFs are involved in the malignant transformation of epithelia in the breast and prostate and show marked upregulation in OSF [65, 66].

HIF-1α is a transcription factor that binds specifically to a 5-RCGTG-3 hypoxia response element on the promoter region of various hypoxia-inducible genes. It is involved in angiogenesis, oxygen transport, iron metabolism, glycolysis, glucose uptake, growth factor signaling, apoptosis, invasion, and metastasis. Increased fibrosis and reduction of vascularity result in hypoxia and overexpression of HIF-1α in OSF [66, 67]. HIF-1α is associated with the upregulation of various growth factors that promote tumor progression such as vascular endothelial growth factor (VEGF), TGF-β, fibroblast growth factor (FGF), platelet-derived growth factor (PDGF), and epidermal growth factor receptor (EGFR). [66] HIF-1α expression is significantly increased in OSF and OSCC with OSCC showing a greater expression than OSF [68].

Tilakaratne report that in their study, 17 of 48 cases (35.4%) of OSF cases with dysplasia showed positive expression of HIF-1α. Twenty-two (45.8%) cases of OSF without dysplasia did not express HIF-1α in the epithelium, while nine cases (18.8%) without dysplasia showed mild positivity [66].

HIF-2α (also called EPAS1/HRF/HLF/MOP2) is a mammalian basic helix-loop-helix per-aryl hydrocarbon receptor nuclear translocator (ARNT)-Sim (bHLH-PAS) protein similar to HIF-1α. Both HIF-1α and HIF-2α are related structurally, sharing 48% of overall amino acid identity. HIF-2α is expressed prominently in vascular endothelial cells during embryonic development, liver hepatocytes, kidney fibroblasts, epithelial cells of intestinal lumen, pancreatic interstitial cells, interstitial cells of heart myocytes, and lung type II pneumocytes. Further, it has been shown to be expressed in vascular cells, parenchymal cells, and infiltrating macrophages in the tumor microenvironment. HIF-2α binds to ARNT, and its function is to transactivate the hypoxia-responsive genes, that target erythropoietin and VEGF and may have an important role in tumorigenesis [65]. Joseph et al. reported varying intensities in the expression of HIF-2α in OSF. Mild and moderate intensities of HIF-2α were observed in 45% (5 of 11) and 55% (6 of 11) of cases. The mean labeling index in OSF (11 ± 19.2) was lesser than normal mucosa (12.2 ± 24.1), but not statistically significant [65].

### 15.3.13 Mast Cell Tryptase and Mast Cell Chymase

Mast cells (MCs) are immune cells of myeloid lineage found in the connective tissue throughout the body. In response to immunological/non-immunological stimuli, they release inflammatory mediators, which degrade the connective tissue matrix and facilitate neovascular sprouts and tumor angiogenesis [27, 69].

MCs when activated secrete profibrotic cytokines such as TGF-β, FGF, PDGF, interleukin-1 and -6, and TNF-α, which are known to cause fibrosis of lungs, liver, skin, and kidney. Yadav et al. showed that early OSF shows a significant increase in the number of tryptase-positive MCs subepithelially and deeper distribution of tryptase-positive MCs in OSCC and advanced stages of OSF. Sabarinath et al. have shown an increase in mean mast cell density from normal mucosa to different grades of OSF [69]. However, the total mast cell count was found to be lesser in OSF (8.10) compared to normal oral mucosa (11.68). The mean mast cell tryptase- and chymase-positive cells in OSF were 4.9 and 3.7 in subepithelial and deeper OSF tissues, respectively, which was less than that in normal mucosa (subepithelial 9.8 and deep 6.2) [27].

### 15.3.14 Matrix Metalloproteinase (MMP; MMP-1, MMP-13)

Matrix metalloproteinases (MMPs) are zinc- and calcium-dependent endopeptidases that degrade extracellular matrix [55] and along with tissue inhibitors of MMPs (TIMPs) play an essential role in the remodeling of the extracellular matrix [70]. MMPs are involved in wound healing, tissue inflammation and degeneration, tumor growth, and metastasis.

MMPs are produced by fibroblasts, macrophages, and neutrophils. MMPs include interstitial collagenases, gelatinases, stromelysin, and membrane-bound MMPs. An imbalance between MMPs and TIMPs results in conditions with abnormal matrix turnover, such as keloid, OSF, gingival overgrowth, and plantar fibromatosis. Elevated MMP-13 levels have been reported in several malignancies and correlate with the clinical course of cancer and its prognosis [55]. Mishra et al. reported an increase in staining intensity of MMP-1 in the epithelium (40%; 12 of 30) and connective tissue (43.3%; 13 of 30) of OSF patients compared to the normal subjects (epithelium: 20%, 2 of 10; connective tissue: 10%, 1 of 10) [71]. Illeperuma et al. found that only 21.1% (9 of 42) OSF cases showed over 70% MMP-1 expression compared to the 77.8% (6 of 8) normal cases [72].

### 15.3.15 Tissue Inhibitors of Matrix Metalloproteinases (TIMPs; TIMP-1, TIMP-2)

Tissue inhibitors of metalloproteinases (TIMPs), a multigene family, regulate MMPs that degrade the extracellular matrix. The balance between MMPs and TIMPs is important for the maintenance of extracellular matrix organization [72]. MMP-2 and TIMP-2 levels increase with progressing stages of OSF [70]. Shrestha et al. observed a heterogeneous pattern of staining of MMP-2 and TIMP-2 in OSF. Out of 14 early-stage cases of OSF, MMP-2-positive expression was seen in 64.2% (9 of 14) and TIMP-2 in 78.5% (11 of 14), both in the epithelium and connective tissue. All 16 moderately advanced-stage OSF expressed positive immunostaining to MMP-2 and TIMP-2, both in the epithelium and connective tissue [70].

### 15.3.16 N-Cadherin (N-Cad)

N-Cad is a member of the calcium-dependent adhesion molecule family of classical cadherins. They are expressed in neural cells, endothelial cells, stromal cells, and osteoblasts. They mediate homotypic and heterotypic cell-cell adhesion and play a significant role in cell motility. The hallmark of EMT is the upregulation of N-Cad followed by the downregulation of E-cadherin. Das et al. studied EMT markers in 55 OSF cases (25 OSF without dysplasia and 30 OSF with dysplasia) and in normal oral mucosa and reported that in OSF, N-Cad along with TWIST was overexpressed in the basal layer of epithelium and has a role in facilitating EMT [73].

### 15.3.17 Osteopontin

Osteopontin, a major sialoprotein of the extracellular matrix, binds to calcium and functions in the early-stage mineralization of bone and dentin. It is an important component of type 1 immunity, and it mediates angiogenesis and inhibits apoptosis in soft tissues. It contains Arg-Gly-Asp (RGD) sequence, which binds certain integrins (αvβ1, αvβ3, αvβ5) and influences cell migration. Expression of osteopontin has been reported in lung, esophagus, breast, and salivary gland tumors and their metastasis. Routray et al. report that, osteopontin expression was decreased in OSF with positive expression in 35% (14 of 40) cases and increased in OSCC compared to normal oral mucosa with positive expression in 60% (12 of 20) cases [74].

### 15.3.18 Podoplanin

Human podoplanin is a 38 kDa type 1 transmembrane sialomucin-like glycoprotein consisting of 162 amino acids. It is an IHC biomarker for lymphatic endothelial cells [75]. Podoplanin is expressed in a wide variety of normal as well as tumor cells. It remodels actin in the cytoskeleton of tumor cells, causing increased motility of tumor cells, facilitating invasion. Podoplanin is also expressed in the epithelial cells of oral dysplastic and hyperplastic lesions, which have an increased risk of malignant transformation [76]. Its expression gradually increases with increasing grades of dysplasia in OSF [75]. Deepa et al. reported that 90% (18 of 20) cases of OSF had positive expression of podoplanin [76].

### 15.3.19 S100A4

15

S100A4 is a member of the S100 calcium-binding protein family, also termed metastasin (Mts1), pEL-98, 18A2, 42A, p9Ka, CAPL, calvasculin, and fibroblast-specific protein. It is involved in the regulation of cell proliferation and differentiation, apoptosis, calcium homeostasis, and energy metabolism. S100A4 is involved in liver fibrosis, kidney fibrosis, pulmonary fibrosis, and cardiac fibrosis. S100A4 is found to be increased in OSF. Yu et al. reported that 83% (25 of 30) of OSF cases showed a strong positive expression of S100A4 compared to normal buccal mucosa, which exhibited weak positivity in 80% (8 of 10) cases [77]. Tumor cells acquire invasive phenotype following downregulation of E-cadherin by S100A4. S100A4 protein also contributes to tumor angiogenesis by stimulating the motility of endothelial cells [78].

### 15.3.20 Syndecan-1

Syndecan-1 is a transmembrane proteoglycan with three extracellular attachment sites. The primary core protein consists of four different syndecans: syndecan-1, -2, -3, and -4. It participates in cell-to-cell and cell-to-matrix interaction. Aberrant expression or function of syndecan-1 has been implicated in tumor development, tumor cell differentiation, invasion, and metastasis. Syndecan-1 expression is mild in basal layer, strong in spinous and granular layer, and almost absent in the uppermost layer. Kamat et al. showed that 70% (7 of 10) of OSF tissue showed strong immunostaining and 30% (3 of 10) showed intermediate immunostaining for syndecan-1 [79].

### 15.3.21 Tenascin-C

The principal extracellular matrix glycoproteins are fibronectin, tenascin, and undulin. Tenascin is synthesized by fibroblasts, muscle cells, and epithelial cells. Several isomers of tenascin are differentially expressed during embryogenesis and tumorigenesis [80]. Tenascin is upregulated in inflammation, tissue repair, and OSF. Immunohistochemical staining intensity of tenascin-C decreases from early to advanced stages of OSF [80]. Tak et al. report that among early OSF cases, 90% exhibited both bright and continuous deposition of tenascin as a band at the epithelial-connective tissue junction (ECJ). In moderate OSF cases, the tenascin band at ECJ was bright in 80% and continuous in 70% of the sections. In OSF sections of advanced grade, 90% sections showed weak, discontinuous tenascin deposition at ECJ [80].

Secretion of tenascin is induced by TGF-β. Tenascin is present in the blood vessel walls in moderate and advanced stages of OSF and around the plump endothelial cells (new vascular channels) in the early phase of OSF [80–82]. Increased deposition of tenascin has been reported in the tumor stroma of epithelial malignancies including those arising from the breast, uterus (both the cervix and body), ovary, prostate, pancreas, colon, stomach, oral cavity, larynx, lung, urinary tract, and skin [83].

### 15.3.22 Transforming Growth Factor-Beta (TGF-β; TGF-β1, TGF-β2)

TGF-β is a profibrotic growth factor that increases the synthesis of collagen and decreases the degradation of collagen. It has a pivotal role in extracellular matrix organization [69, 81]. TGF-β stimulates fibroblast proliferation, fibrosis, and scar formation. TGF-β is an important factor in chronic fibrosis of many organs, including lung, kidney, liver, or skin. A significant increase in TGF-β expression is seen in OSF [50, 69, 84, 85]. Ileperuma reported increased TGF-β1 expression in 71% of OSF cases (30 of 42)

[72]. TGF-β1 expression increases as OSF progresses showing more than 70% connective tissue expression in intermediate and advanced stages [72]. TGF-β controls several functions of the cells involved in the fibrotic tissue and tumor microenvironment. It promotes myofibroblast differentiation, favors recruitment of immune cells, inhibits the anti-tumor immune responses, and regulates epithelial and endothelial cell differentiation [72].

### 15.3.23 Transglutaminase-2 (TGM-2)

Tissue transglutaminases include a family of calcium-dependent enzymes that catalyze the formation of γ-glutamyl cross-links. These proteins serve as tissue scaffolds, maintain membrane integrity, regulate cell adhesion, and modulate signal transduction [86, 87]. TGM-2 cross-links extracellular collagen and fibronectin, making them more resistant to degradation, and promotes fibrosis in kidney, liver, lung, and cyclosporine A-induced gingival overgrowth [84]. In a Taiwanese study of 40 OSF and 10 normal mucosal tissues, transglutaminase expression was significantly higher in OSF specimens compared to normal specimens ($p < 0.005$). TGM-2 is observed mainly in the cytoplasm of fibroblasts in OSF specimens. Fibroblasts derived from OSF exhibit higher TGM-2 expression than Buccal mucosal fibroblasts in protein levels ($p < 0.05$) [88].

### 15.3.24 TWIST

The TWIST1 gene encodes for a transcription factor containing a basic helix-loop-helix (bHLH) domain that binds the Nde1 E-box element that activates or represses multiple genes. It is important in early embryogenesis for mesoderm specification and differentiation [73, 89]. TWIST1 promotes EMT by repressing E-cadherin expression. It is associated with aggressive breast cancer, hepatocellular carcinoma, and cancer of prostate, stomach, esophagus, bladder, and pancreas. TWIST1 can override oncogene-induced cell senescence and apoptosis, augment cancer cell resistance to chemotherapy, enhance cancer stem cell (CSC) population, and promote cancer cell invasion and metastasis. Das et al. reported that TWIST gene expression was upregulated in OSF with dysplasia ($n = 30$) compared to OSF without dysplasia ($n = 25$) and normal subjects ($n = 16$) ($p < 0.0001$) [73, 89].

### 15.3.25 Vascular Endothelial Growth Factor (VEGF)

Vascular endothelial growth factor (VEGF), also known as vascular permeability factor (VPF), plays a vital role in the regulation of blood and lymphatic vessel development and homeostasis. They promote vascular development by endothelial cell proliferation. VEGFs and their receptors, VEGFR 1 and VEGFR 2, are essential molecules in the development of vasculature [46].

VEGF expression is significantly increased in OSF and OSCC [28, 46]. VEGF significantly increases with increasing grades of dysplasia in OSF. It has been suggested that serum VEGF levels may be a surrogate marker for tissue expression of VEGF [28]. There is a positive correlation between deregulated expression of E-cadherin and increased VEGF expression in OSF, and this increases with increasing grades of dysplasia [90]. Tumor angiogenesis and expression of VEGF are important prognostic factors in OPMDs and OSCC [91]. Nirmal et al. observed a statistically significant increase in MVD from OSF without any epithelial dysplasia (23.2 ± 9.4) to OSF with evidence of epithelial dysplasia (24.0 ± 8.3) and OSF cases with either micro-invasion or invasion (38.9 ± 5.1) [91].

### 15.3.26 Vimentin

Vimentin is a type III intermediate filament protein of mesenchymal cells with a molecular weight of 54 kDa. It is involved in the regulation of cell attachment, migration, cell signaling, and tumor metastases [92]. Nayak et al. and Sharma et al. reported an upregulation of vimentin expression in OSF and an increase in OSCC compared to OSF [43, 89]. A significant increase in vimentin expression is seen in mild and severe dysplasia in OSF [93]. The tissue localization of vimentin especially in the invasive fronts of the tumor stroma has better prognostic value rather than their cellular expression levels [93].

## 15.4 Proliferative, Apoptosis, and Senescence Markers

### 15.4.1 Bax

The pro-apoptotic protein, Bax, plays an important role in defense against oncogenic events as it mediates apoptosis in response to genotoxic stress. Bax is expressed in normal epithelium. It has been shown that Bax can bind to Bcl-2, resulting in the inactivation of the anti-apoptotic action of Bcl-2. Bax expression is reported to increase in OSF and OSCC compared to normal subjects. OSCC has a greater expression of Bax compared to OSF. Ranganathan et al. reported that the staining intensity for Bax in the suprabasal layer showed significant difference between normal, OSF, and cancer. 56% (28 of 50) of OSF cases showed no suprabasal Bax immunoreactivity compared to no expression in 20% (2 of 10) of normal cases. The absence of Bax in the suprabasal region in OSF may be an indicator of abnormal proliferation, predisposing to malignant transformation [94, 95].

### 15.4.2 Budding Uninhibited by Benzimidazole-Related 1 (BUBR1)

BUBR1 protein is a key component of the spindle assembly checkpoint (SAC) machinery, which restrains cells from entering anaphase until all chromosomes are attached to bipolar spindles. BUBR1 gene expression is usually undetectable in normal tissue [96]. Hseigh et al. reported an overexpression of BUBR1 in OPMDs compared to normal oral mucosa. BUBR1 staining was not detected in any samples of normal oral mucosa (9 of 9); in contrast, cytoplasmic BUBR1 staining with occasional nuclear staining was detected at suprabasal layer of 63% (12 of 19) of OSF cases. Upregulation of BUBR1 expression has been reported in OSF and OSCC. OSCC cases show a greater expression of BUBR1 compared to OSF [93]. Overexpression of BUBR1 in OSCC cells results in chromosome mis-segregation during mitosis, contributing to genomic instability. Overexpression of BUBR1 is also associated with loss of heterozygosity (LOH) and aneuploidy due to weakened SAC activity, which is implicated in tumor initiation in the colorectum, urinary bladder, breast, lung, and head and neck [97].



### 15.4.3 Caspases

Cell apoptosis is initiated by the stimulation of one of the two distinct pathways: the intrinsic death receptor-independent pathway and the extrinsic death receptor-dependent pathway. Both the pathways require the sequential functioning of cysteine proteases known as caspases [98].

Caspases cleave many vital cellular proteins and degrade the nuclear scaffold and cytoskeleton. Activated caspase-3 is the main executor of apoptosis. A difference in the localization pattern of caspase-3 was reported by Zhu et al. In normal oral mucosal tissues, caspase-3-positive cells were mainly present in the spinous and granular layers and were minimally expressed in the basal layer. However, caspase-3 expression levels were expressed in the basal layer in OSF epithelial tissues [99]. Caspase-3 expression in OSF epithelial tissues is significantly higher than that of normal oral mucosal tissues, and its expression increases with advancing stages of OSF [99, 100].

### 15.4.4 C-Jun

Human c-Jun is a 3.1 kb intron-less proto-oncogene localized on chromosome region 1p31–32. c-Jun is essential for the progression of cells through the G1 phase of the cell cycle. It exerts direct transcriptional control on the cyclin D1 gene, which provides a molecular link between growth factor signaling and cell cycle proteins regulating G1 progression [101, 102].

In OSF, there is persistent induction of the c-Jun proto-oncogene by areca nut alkaloids leading to an increase in its expression [103]. Dysregulated activation and aberrant expression of c-Jun have been observed in several human neoplasms including the malignant transformation of OPMDs. In a study by Shraddha et al., the average nuclear labeling index (LI) of c-Jun expression in normal, OSF, epithelial dysplasia, and OSCC was 35.0%, 35.6%, 89.1%, and 83.3%, respectively. The nuclear positivity for c-Jun was expressed in all the cases of OSF (15 of 15). Nuclear staining was predominantly in basal and parabasal layers [102].

### 15.4.5 Mesenchymal-Epithelial Transition Factor (c-Met)

c-Met plays a crucial role in morphogenic organization during embryogenesis. It controls cell migration and proliferation necessary for tissue repair [104, 105]. c-Met is the only known high-affinity receptor for hepatocyte growth factor (HGF) [103]. Bazarsad et al. demonstrated a significant increase in the expression of c-Met in OSF and OSCC arising from OSF and in the transformation of normal mucosa to epithelial dysplasia and OSCC ($p = 0.03$). c-Met expression was undetectable in the normal mucosa. Sixteen (51.6%) of 31 OSF samples without transformation exhibited the same expression pattern as that of the normal mucosa. In contrast, all cases of OSF with transformation showed a definite cytoplasmic staining in the basal and suprabasal layers [105]. The HGF/c-Met signaling pathway promotes proliferation, migration, survival, angiogenesis, and invasion in a broad range of human solid tumors, including ovarian, stomach, lung, breast, liver, and brain tumors [103].

### 15.4.6 C-Myc

c-Myc is a helix-loop-helix motif-containing transcription factor that regulates cellular proliferation, differentiation, cellular metabolism, and apoptosis [106, 107]. c-Myc and p53 function together to maintain tissue homeostasis by balancing cell proliferation, apoptosis, and differentiation [107]. c-Myc expression has been reported in the epithelium of OSF with dysplasia. Anura et al. observed that deregulated c-Myc expression in the dysplastic epithelium in OSF indicates impaired epithelial differentiation, improved proliferative potential, and potential for oncogenic transformation. They also showed that in normal oral mucosa, c-Myc was faintly expressed in the nucleus of basal and parabasal layers of epithelium, whereas the proliferative layer of OSF showed c-Myc positivity in nuclei with high intensity. c-Myc-positive nuclei were detected diffusely in OSF with hyperplastic epithelium and OSF with dysplasia [107]. c-Myc also mediates activation of TGF-β1, MMP-9, insulin receptor, and insulin-like growth factor 1 receptor, which is essential for cell proliferation, anti-apoptosis, and invasion of oral cancer cells [108].

### 15.4.7 Cyclin D1

Cyclins are a group of proteins responsible for the activation of cell division transitional points. Protein kinases called cyclin-dependent kinases (CDKs) exert their enzymatic activity in the presence of cyclins. The activation of specific cyclin-CDK complex results in a cascade of protein phosphorylation that is required for cell cycle progression [109]. Cyclin D1, expressed in the G1-S phase of the cell cycle, plays an important role in apoptosis. Cyclin D1 along with its CDK partners, CDK 4 and 6, acts on the E2F transcription factor enabling the cells to enter the S phase [93]. Bazarsad et al. reported that proliferating index of cyclin D1 was 4–9% in normal mucosa and most cases of OSF showed no positive expression of cyclin D1 [105]. There is increasing evidence that aberrant activity of cell cycle proteins, cyclins, plays a critical role in head and neck neoplasms [105].

### 15.4.8 Fragile Histidine Triad Protein (FHIT)

The human fragile histidine triad (FHIT) gene is a putative tumor suppressor gene located at chromosome 3p14.2. FHIT is a member of histidine triad (HIT) proteins, which includes a small family of nucleotide-binding and hydrolyzing proteins [110]. It acts as a genome caretaker by regulating cellular DNA repair. FHIT loss leads to replicative stress and accumulation of double-strand breaks in DNA [111]. The deletion or loss of its transcription has been observed in head and neck, gastrointestinal, cervical, lung, breast, kidney, and hematopoietic tumors [110]. Xiaomin et al. found that the FHIT expression significantly decreases in OSF and OSCC arising in a background of OSF ($p < 0.05$), suggesting that downregulation of FHIT in OSF may have a role in malignant transformation [112].

### 15.4.9 Human Telomerase Reverse Transcriptase (hTERT)

Telomeres are nucleoprotein complexes present at the ends of the chromosome, consisting of multiple TTAGGG repeats. Normal cells have limited replicative potential due to the shortening of the telomeres during successive replication. Telomerase is a specific enzyme that prevents the shortening of telomeres. Telomerases have a catalytic subunit hTERT (human telomerase reverse transcriptase) and an RNA unit (hTR). hTR expression is found to be positive in most of the cells, rendering it nonspecific for assessing telomerase activity. Higher expression of hTERT has been observed in germ cells, embryonic cells, as well as cancer cells. Upregulation of telomerase activity is reported in OSCC as well as OPMDs [113].

Raju et al. observed that the mean labeling score of hTERT in OSF was 6.2 ± 1.9, which increased with advancing histologic grade. Thirty percent (6 of 20) cases of OSF displayed a mild staining intensity, and 70% (14 of 20) cases showed moderate staining intensity. Combined nuclear and cytoplasmic hTERT staining was observed in 85% (17/20) cases, and the remaining 3 cases showed cytoplasm staining. Eighty-five percent of the cases showed expression throughout the thickness of the epithelium, and the rest displayed expression restricted to basal and suprabasal layers. Early OSF shows a weak-to-moderate positive hTERT expression restricted to the basal and suprabasal layers. Moderately advanced OSF and advanced OSF show moderate nuclear and cytoplasmic expression throughout the epithelium [113]. OSCC shows a significant increase in hTERT expression compared to OSF and normal oral mucosa [113, 114]. Increased hTERT expression is associated with E-cadherin reduction and upregulation of vimentin and EMT transcription factors such as Slug and TWIST1 [115, 116].

### 15.4.10 Insulin-Like Growth Factor II mRNA-Binding Protein 3 (IMP3)

IMP3 is an oncofetal protein that promotes tumor cell proliferation, invasion, and metastasis [117]. In a Sri Lankan study including 36 OSF tissue specimens, IMP3 is found to be significantly increased in OSF compared to normal mucosa ($p < 0.05$) [105]. IMP3 is specific for malignant and potentially malignant conditions and is not found in benign pathologies [118].

### 15.4.11 Ki67

Ki67 is a specific and sensitive biomarker of cell proliferation, active in all phases of the cell cycle (G1, S, G2, M phase only) [94]. Ki67 expression is increased in OSF with and without dysplasia [41, 94, 119]. Ranganathan et al. observed a progressive increase in the mean labeling index of Ki67 from normal (5.3 ± 3.6) to OSF (19.1 ± 7.6) to OSCC (29.1 ± 8.8) tissues [94]. Gadbail et al. reported an increase in the expression of Ki67 from healthy mucosa to oral epithelial dysplasia and OSCC. In OSCC arising in OSF, Ki67, CD105, and α-SMA are significantly higher in the advanced clinical TNM stage and are associated with poor prognosis [41].

### 15.4.12 Microtubule-Associated Protein Light Chain 3 (LC3)

LC3, a human homolog of yeast Atg8, is an essential component of autophagy. LC3 plays an important role in degradation pathways in which components of autophagy are coupled with phagocytosis by LC3-associated phagocytosis (LAP) [120]. There is increase in LC3 expression with increasing severity of OSF. Zhu et al. found a difference in the localization pattern of LC3 in OSF and normal subjects. In normal oral mucosal tissues, LC3 was mainly present in the spinous and granular layers and was minimally expressed in the basal layer. However, in OSF, its expression was elevated in the basal layer [99, 121]. High expression of LC3 has also been reported in esophageal, gastric, and pancreatic cancers [122].

15

### 15.4.13 Mouse Double-Minute 2 Homolog (MDM2)

MDM2 protein is the primary negative regulator of p53 protein. MDM2 maintains the stability of the p53 signaling pathway by ligating the p53 protein through its E3 ubiquitin ligase. Ubiquitinated p53 is transferred to the cytoplasm and degraded by proteasomes [123]. Xiaomin et al. reported an overexpression of MDM2 expression in OSF and OSCC-OSF compared to healthy mucosa ($p < 0.05$) [112]. MDM2 amplification is observed in many human malignancies, including lung cancer and colon cancer [124].

### 15.4.14 p16

p16 is a tumor suppressor gene that inhibits cyclin-dependent kinase 4A. In normal conditions, it serves to regulate the cells passing through G1 to S phase of the cell cycle [125]. An increase in p16 protein expression has been reported in OSF and OSF with dysplasia. Bazarsad et al. studied p16 expression in OSF undergoing malignant transformation. High expression was detected in 40% (2 of 5) OSF samples with transformation compared to normal mucosa [105]. A similar finding was reported by Sudhakaran et al. where an overexpression of p16 was seen in OSCC arising in OSF compared to normal mucosa and OSF without malignant transformation [125].

### 15.4.15 p53

p53 is a tumor suppressor encoded by the gene TP53 located on the short arm (p) of chromosome 17. p53 protein prevents the accumulation of genetic damage in cells, either by allowing for repair of the damage before cell division or by causing the death of the cell [126].

Mutations in p53 impair the ability of the cells to repair and undergo apoptosis in response to DNA damage, which leads to uncontrolled cell growth in OPMD and malignancies [105]. Ranganathan et al., Varun et al. and Humanyun et al. report a significant increase in mutated p53 expression in OSF, OSF with dysplasia, and OSCC, suggesting that p53 in the malignant transformation of OSF to OSCC [94, 105, 126, 127].

### 15.4.16 p62

p62, an autophagy marker protein, is associated with different ubiquitin-tagged cargos which are degraded by autophagosome/lysosome fusions [128]. As p62 is constantly degraded in autolysosomes, it is a reliable marker to monitor autophagic flux. A decrease in p62 is observed as OSF progresses in severity. A difference in the localization of p62 was observed between the OSF tissue and normal mucosa. p62-positive cells were found in the entire epithelial layer of the normal oral mucosa, but were restricted to the basal layer in advanced stage of OSF [99]. Cytoplasmic p62 is higher in OSCC cells than normal oral mucosa [128].

### 15.4.17 p63

p63 gene, a member of the p53 family, is located on chromosome 3q27–29. It has a transactivation domain at N-terminal, a core DNA-binding domain, and an oligomerization domain at the carboxy-terminal. p63 protein is essential for maintaining the turnover and regulation of epithelial cell maturation [129]. p63 along with its promoter variants/isoforms (TA and ΔN p63) and splice variants (i.e., α, β, and γ) plays a vital role in the development and maintenance of the stratified epithelia [51, 73, 90, 127]. The p63 gene is frequently altered in epithelial dysplasia and OSCC [94]. Upregulation of p63 has been reported in OSF and OSCC with OSCC showing a greater expression compared to OSF [48, 51, 73, 127, 128]. p63 expression is seen in basal and suprabasal layers of all cases of OSF. Sinha et al. and Varun et al. found a significant increase in mean labeling index of p63 in OSF compared to normal subjects [124, 126]. Das et al. also demonstrated that p63 expression progressively increases in OSF with advancing grades of dysplasia (% of p63-positive nuclei: normal: 80.8 ± 64.2, OSF with mild: 80.8 ± 64.2, moderate: 93.5 ± 69.9, and severe dysplasia: 99.2 ± 62) [7, 27, 48].

### 15.4.18 Proliferating Cell Nuclear Antigen (PCNA)

PCNA, a 36 kDa acidic nuclear protein, and cofactor of DNA polymerase, plays an important role in DNA synthesis, DNA repair, cell cycle progression, and cell proliferation. An increase in PCNA expression occurs during the S phase and declines during the G2/M phase of the cell cycle. It is found in the nucleus of both normal and proliferating cells undergoing transformation, but not in resting cells [130].

PCNA is involved in DNA excision repair, and its expression increases following DNA damage induced by areca quid components [130]. PCNA expression is elevated in OSF and OSCC. Kaur et al. and Illeperuma et al. observed an increase in PCNA expression in OSF compared to normal oral mucosa [72, 131]. PCNA expression correlates with prognosis and survival in several malignancies including colorectal cancer, breast cancer, and OSCC [131].

### 15.4.19 Polo-Like Kinase (PLK)

PLK1, a member of the serine/threonine protein kinase family, is a pivotal regulator of the cell cycle and is involved in centrosome maturation, regulation of anaphase-promoting complex, and bipolar spindle formation. PLK1 is expressed in highly proliferative tissues such as developing embryos, testis, thymus, and spleen [132, 133].

Aberrant PLK1 function in human cells leads to prometaphase/metaphase-like arrest. PLK inhibitors induce mitotic chaos and severely disrupt cell cycle progression, resulting in cancer cell death [114]. The overexpression of PLKs is observed in human tumors but is seldom seen in healthy, non-dividing cells. Vittal et al. reported that 10% (3 of 30) cases of OSF showed positive expression of PLK1 and about 90% (27 of 30) OSCC cases showed positive PLK1 expression [133]. Dysregulation of PLK1 is reported in various types of human cancers such as glioma, thyroid carcinoma, head and neck squamous cell carcinoma (HNSCC), melanoma, colorectal cancers, esophageal carcinoma, ovarian carcinoma, breast cancer, and prostate cancer [134].

### 15.4.20 Phosphatase and Tensin Homolog Deleted on Chromosome 10 (PTEN)

PTEN is a tumor suppressor gene and a negative regulator of the PI3K/AKT (phosphatidyl inositol-3-kinase/AKT) pathway. PTEN controls cell proliferation, apoptosis (cell death), cell cycle regulation, and cell adhesion and migration [135]. Angadi et al. report a decrease in PTEN immunohistochemical expression in OSF and OSCC. A progressive loss of PTEN was observed from normal to OSF to OSCC. Loss of PTEN expression was observed in 20% (6 of 30) cases of OSF. PTEN exhibits a strong nuclear expression in the epithelium [135]. Inactivation of PTEN results in the proliferation and reduction in apoptosis, predisposing to malignant transformation.

Germline mutations of PTEN are reported in patients with multiple hamartoma syndrome. Somatic mutations or deletion resulting in loss of PTEN is seen in several potentially malignant conditions and malignancies, including glioblastomas, melanoma, breast, prostate, endometrial carcinomas and HNSCC. PTEN has also been implicated in the pathogenesis of several fibrotic disorders, including scleroderma, hepatic fibrosis, and kidney, pulmonary, and cardiac fibrosis [132]. Total suppression of the PTEN gene expression is lethal to embryonic cells, and partial suppression leads to carcinogenesis [136].

### 15.4.21 Survivin

Survivin is the smallest member of the inhibitor of apoptosis protein (IAP) family that suppresses caspase activity. Survivin is a multifunctional protein involved in the regulation of cytokinesis and cell cycle progression. It participates in p53, Wnt, hypoxia, TGF-beta, and Notch signaling pathways. In embryonic tissues, survivin is highly expressed during the G2-M phase of the cell cycle [137]. Survivin expression is significantly increased in OSF and OSCC with greater expression in OSCC compared to OSF. Zhou et al. observed that survivin expression was localized in the basal/parabasal and prickle cell layers in OSF. Twenty-four out of 50 OSF cases (48%) showed cytoplasmic survivin positivity [138]. Survivin is one of the few proteins that are overexpressed in virtually every human cancer. It is a potential early predictor of malignant transformation in oral epithelial dysplasia and oral leukoplakia [137–139].

## 15.5 Stemness Markers

### 15.5.1 Aldehyde Dehydrogenase (ALDH1)

ALDH1 is an isoform of aldehyde dehydrogenase (ALDH). It is a cytosolic, detoxifying isoenzyme that oxidizes intracellular aldehydes and contributes to the oxidation of retinol to retinoic acid in early stem cell differentiation [140]. Chatterjee et al. studied the correlative network of hypoxia-associated oxidative stress and EMT in OSF ($n = 12$) and OSCC ($n = 14$) and normal subjects ($n = 10$). A negative expression of ALDH1 was seen in OSF and normal tissues and a positive expression in metastatic OSCC ($p < 0.05$) [68]. An increase in ALDH expression has been reported in various tumors of stomach, lung, breast, pancreas, and HNSCC. Tumors with high ALDH1 expression have high invasive potential and carry the risk of lymph node metastasis [141].

### 15.5.2 B-Cell-Specific Moloney Murine Leukemia Virus Insertion Site 1 (Bmi1)

15

Bmi1 is a member of the polycomb group of chromatin-modifier proteins. Bmi1 is involved in the transcriptional repression of Hox genes. Bmi1 mediates gene silencing by regulating chromatin structure and plays a central role in cell cycle regulation, cell immortalization, cell senescence, and EMT [142]. Bmi1 is a stem cell marker that plays a key role in the functioning of endogenous stem cells and cancer stem cells (CSCs) [143]. Bmi1 expression correlates with several cancer stem cell markers, including ALDH1, CD44, Oct4, SOX2, Nanog, and ABCG2 [79].

In human cancers, Bmi1 overexpression drives stem-like properties associated with the induction of the epithelial-mesenchymal transition that promotes invasion, metastasis, and poor prognosis. Overexpression of Bmi1 is related to tumor cell proliferation and survival in HNSCC [141]. Increased expression of Bmi-1 is observed in oral leukoplakia and OSF. Xie et al. reported that Bmi1 was highly expressed during every stage of OSF, and as the pathological changes in fibrosis progress, the expression level of Bmi1 in the epithelium is dramatically upregulated, especially in the middle ($p < 0.0001$) and late stages ($p < 0.0001$) [119, 142].

### 15.5.3 CD133

CD133, a 5-transmembrane domain glycoprotein, is a hematopoietic stem cell and endothelial progenitor marker involved in angiogenesis [142, 143]. CD133 expression serves as a prognostic signature for various tumor stages in leukemia, brain tumors, retinoblastoma, renal tumors, pancreatic tumors, colon carcinoma, prostate carcinoma, hepatocellular carcinoma, thyroid carcinoma, melanoma, and OSCC. Its expression positively correlates with tumor progression and recurrence and negatively correlates with the prognosis of patients with OSCC [144].

CD133-positive cells in dysplastic cells of OPMD are three times more likely to undergo malignant transformation than CD133-negative cells [145]. Chatterjee et al. observed a negative expression of CD133 in OSF and normal tissues, whereas a positive expression was observed in OSCC metastatic knots ($p < 0.05$) [68]. The expression of CD133 in oral epithelium increases from normal epithelium, through dysplasia, to carcinoma [68, 146].

### 15.5.4 Stage-Specific Embryonic Antigen (SSEA4)

Stage-specific embryonic antigen 4 (SSEA4), a sialyl-glycolipid, is a well-known cell surface marker for embryonic stem cells and pluripotent stem cells. Yu et al. found that SSEA4 was overexpressed in 88.8% (31 of 35) of OSF cases. Increased SSEA4 expressions are also observed in keloid and cancer stem cells [147].

### 15.5.5 STRO1 (in Fibroblasts and Myofibroblasts)

STRO1, a mesenchymal stem cell (MSC) marker, was the first antibody used to prospectively select a population of immune cells from human bone marrow that included the entire clonogenic colony-forming fibroblastic population. In the oral cavity, STRO1 has been utilized for the selection of stem cells from periodontium, dental pulp, and periapical regions. STRO1 is significantly higher in OSF compared with buccal mucosal fibroblasts. Yu et al. observed that STRO1 staining in OSF was stronger than normal buccal mucosa, which exhibited only a faint expression. In normal tissues, there was almost no expression in the epithelial cells, endothelial cells, and lamina propria. In OSF, increased staining for STRO1 expression was observed in the epithelial cells (60%; 18 of 30), endothelial cells (30%; 3 of 30), inflammatory cells (60%; 18 of 30), and fibroblasts (70%; 21 of 30). STRO1 plays an important role in the pathogenesis of fibrotic changes [148].

### 15.5.6 SRY (Sex-Determining Region on Y Chromosome) Type Homeobox Genes (SOX2)

The SOX2 protein is a high-mobility SRY-related HMG box transcription factor. SOX2 is involved in multiple signal transduction pathways that regulate cell proliferation, migration, invasion, stemness, tumorigenesis, anti-apoptosis, and chemoresistance. SOX2 confers self-renewal capability to cancer stem cells. It facilitates tumor growth and treatment resistance. Upregulation of SOX-2 expression is observed in OSF, with a higher expression in OSF tissue with dysplasia. Xie et al. report that the expression of SOX2 was slightly upregulated in the early-stage ($n = 27$, $p = 0.0553$) and mid-stage ($n = 28$, $p = 0.0356$) OSF epithelium, and the expression level of SOX2 protein was significantly upregulated in the late-stage OSF epithelium ($n = 26$, $p = 0\ 0.0019$). A positive correlation among SOX2, Bmi1, and Ki67 expression in the OSF epithelium has been reported [119].

## 15.6 Markers of Signaling Pathway Alterations

### 15.6.1 Dickkopf WNT Signaling Pathway Inhibitor 3 (DKK3)

The dickkopf (DKK) family includes Wnt antagonists, comprising five members, DKK1, DKK2, DKK3, DKK4, and DKKL1, which act as inhibitors of the canonical Wnt pathway [149]. DKK3 is a putative Wnt signaling inhibitor. DKK3 is localized on 11p15, a locus often deleted in cancerous cells [150]. Hypermethylation of its promoter correlates with the occurrence of cancers. Zhou et al. report that 33% (6 of 15) of normal oral mucousa cases showed DKK3 positivity in the cytoplasm compared to 77.8% (35 of 45) of OSF, and 96.4% (53 of 55) of OSCC. The average values of DKK3 expression varied in the different tissue samples, with a mean score of 1.73 in normal oral mucosal tissues, 3.73 in OSF tissues, and 4.45 in OSCC tissues. DKK3 expression level gradually increased from normal oral mucosa to OSF to OSCC [ 150].

### 15.6.2 Phosphorylated Extracellular Signal-Regulated Kinases (pERK)

Extracellular signal-regulated kinases (ERK) are members of the mitogen-activated protein kinase (MAPK) family [151]. Phosphorylation of ERK occurs during oxidative stress that drives EMT. ERK signaling pathway plays a critical role in regulating cell proliferation, differentiation, survival, and apoptosis in malignant tumors. Chatterjee et al. observed an increase of p-ERK in the epithelial cells of buccal mucosa in OSF ($n = 12$; $p < 0.01$) and OSCC ($n = 14$; $p < 0.001$) as compared to that of normal oral mucosal tissues ($n = 10$) [68].

### 15.6.3 Glioma-Associated Oncogene Homolog 1 (GLI1)

GLI1, a protein-coding gene, is a transcriptional effector at the terminal end of the hedgehog signaling (Hh) pathway. It regulates embryogenesis and tissue patterning/differentiation. GLI1 induced by Hh signaling is necessary for cellular proliferation, stemness, and cellular survival in various organs [152]. GLI1 regulates cell cycle, DNA replication, and DNA damage repair processes. The consequences of GLI1 oncogenic activity surrounding DNA damage repair proteins, such as NBS1, and cell cycle proteins, such as CDK1, correlate with tumorigenesis and chemoresistance [152]. Chatterjee et al. studied 10 normal, 12 OSF, and 14 OSCC tissue specimen and reported a sequential increase of nuclear expression of GLI1 from normal to OSF to OSCC [68].

### 15.6.4 Sonic Hedgehog (Shh)

The hedgehog (Hh) pathway is one of the principal signal transduction pathways in embryonal development. The Hh ligands that initiate signal transduction of the hedgehog pathway include Sonic, Indian, and Desert Hh in vertebrates [153]. Interaction of Shh with specific receptors, namely, Smo and Patched, leads to the activation and nuclear translocation of GLI1 for transcriptional regulation. Shh-GLI1 signaling axis plays a vital role in promoting the process of EMT during carcinogenesis. Shh-GLI1 signaling facilitates the acquisition of stemness as well as the maintenance of CSC population. Chatterjee et al. report an increase in Shh in OSF ($p < 0.001$) and OSCC ($p < 0.01$), with higher expression in OSCC [68].

### 15.6.5 WNT Inhibitory Factor 1 (WIF1)

Wnt inhibitory factor 1 (WIF1), a secreted Wnt antagonist, inhibits Wnt/β-catenin signaling by directly binding to Wnt proteins. The Wnt signaling pathway plays an important role in embryonic development, tissue regeneration, cell proliferation, and cell differentiation. The Wnt/β-catenin signaling pathway plays a vital role in human malignancies including OSCC. Abnormal activation of Wnt results in many types of cancers, such as colon cancer, liver cancer, lung cancer, breast cancer, and childhood T cell acute lymphoblastic leukemia [154].

WIF1 silencing may be an early event in tumorigenesis. WIF1, either at the protein or mRNA level, is seen in normal oral mucosal tissues and gradually decreases in the progressive stages of OSF and OSCC tissues. Also, WIF1 is frequently methylated in OSCC tissues. In the study by Zhou et al., normal oral mucosa exhibited strongly positive WIF1 protein expression in the nucleus. OSF tissues from early-stage and moderately advanced-stage showed WIF1-positive expression in the cytoplasm and nucleus. OSF in advanced-stage showed a weak WIF1 expression in cytoplasm. Primary OSCC showed very weak cytoplasmic immunoreaction for WIF1. Ninety-three percent (14 of 15) normal oral mucosa showed nuclear WIF1 positivity, compared to 73.3% (33 of 45) in OSF and 36.4% (20 of 55) in OSCC. The average values of WIF1 expression gradually reduced from normal oral mucosa to OSF to OSCC tissues with mean scores of 5.37, 3.29, and 1.27, respectively [157].

## 15.7 Inflammatory Markers, Glycoproteins, and Enzymes

15

### 15.7.1 Alpha-Enolase (ENO1)

Alpha-enolase or enolase-1 (ENO1) is a multifunctional protein and a glycolytic enzyme, which acts as a plasminogen receptor on the cell surface [154, 157]. The differential expression of ENO1 is related to several pathologies including cancer, Alzheimer's disease, and rheumatoid arthritis. ENO1 promotes many oncogenic events involving protein-protein interactions, glycolysis, and signaling pathways leading to chemoresistance [154]. ENO1 is highly expressed in OSF and OSCC compared to normal tissues [159]. Bag et al. reported that ENO1 has a higher expression in OSF with dysplasia (86.2 ± 2.9) and OSCC (94.7 ± 3.3) compared to OSF without dysplasia (24.3 ± 1.9) and normal subjects (33.6 ± 3.4). Among the total OSF with dysplasia ($n = 23$) patients, 11 patients (47.82%) showed high level (positive cell count >85%) of α-enolase expression, indicating its potential as a biomarker in predicting malignant transformation of OSF [137].

### 15.7.2 Beta-Integrin (β-Integrin)

Integrins are transmembrane proteins that link the cell cytoskeleton to the extracellular matrix. They play an important role in cell signaling. β1-Integrin acts along with growth factors in the regulation of the cell cycle through transmembrane proteins called tetraspanins [68]. Beta-integrin controls the S-phase progression in the epithelium, which parallels Jak/Stat and EGFR signaling pathways. It mediates signal transduction and adhesion following the phosphorylation of focal adhesion kinase [160]. β1-Integrin is downregulated in OSF and OSCC arising in OSF. Veeravarmal et al. observed that the percentage of β1-integrin-positive cells in normal epithelium ranged from 14% to 30%. The staining intensity was mild in all normal mucosal tissues (15 of 15; 100%) and was observed in the rete pegs and rete ridge areas. In OSF, the β1-integrin-positive cells were present in the basal and suprabasal layers. The percentage of β1-integrin-positive cells ranged from 8% to 70% in early OSF, 2% to 71% in moderate OSF, and 2% to 66% in advanced OSF [160].

### 15.7.3 Calreticulin

Calreticulin is a calcium-binding chaperone protein, which participates in many cellular processes [161]. Upregulation of calreticulin is observed in various malignancies such as OSCC, ductal carcinoma, colorectal cancer, and prostate and vaginal carcinoma. High calreticulin expression is associated with a poor survival rate in pancreatic cancer and esophageal squamous cell carcinoma [161]. A proteomic analysis study by Das et al. demonstrated that 15 proteins were upregulated in the OSF tissues. Among the 15 overexpressed proteins, calreticulin was significantly upregulated in OSF compared to normal tissues ($p < 0.001$). Higher expression level of calreticulin was localized in the epithelial layer of the OSF tissue [161].

### 15.7.4 C–C Motif Chemokine Ligand 2 (CCL2)

Chemokines are leukocyte chemo-attractants that act with profibrotic cytokines in the development of fibrosis by recruiting myofibroblasts, macrophages, and other cells. Epithelial cells and fibroblasts are a major source of proinflammatory and profibrotic factors including CCL2 [33]. CCL2 expression has been identified in inflammatory and fibrotic diseases such as atherosclerosis, hepatic cirrhosis, pulmonary fibrosis, and glomerulosclerosis. Its neutralization reduces TGF-beta and procollagen synthesis that leads to fibrosis. CCL2 plays a key role in the recruitment of myofibroblasts, and it shows a higher expression in OSF. Sarode et al. studied 30 OSF and 10 normal mucosal tissues and reported that CCL2 expression in basal cells (CCL2-B) and connective tissue (CCL2-CT) was significantly greater in advanced OSF ($p = 0.0075$) [33].

### 15.7.5 Cyclooxygenase 2 (COX-2)

Prostaglandin-endoperoxide synthase or cyclooxygenase (COX) is a key regulatory enzyme in tissue inflammation and is present in two isoforms COX-1 and COX-2 [162]. COX-1 is found in blood vessels, interstitial cells, smooth muscle cells, platelets, and mesothelial cells. In contrast, COX-2 is predominantly seen in the parenchymal cells of many tissues [163]. COX-2 overexpression is associated with tumor promotion, activation of carcinogens, neoangiogenesis, tumor progression, and inhibition of apoptosis. OPMDs are preceded by alteration in COX gene expression. Upregulation of COX-2 is associated with increased angiogenesis and cancer stem cell proliferation. Rangaswamy et al. observed overexpression of COX-2 in OSF (66.67%) compared to normal tissues (17.5%), underlining the role of inflammation in tissue fibrosis [162].

### 15.7.6 Cyclophilin A

Cyclophilin A, a member of the peptidylprolyl cis-trans-isomerase (PPIse) family, is an 18 kDa protein with a broad range of functions in cell proliferation and apoptosis. CypA is a key regulator of fibroblast viability and contributes to OSF development probably through promoting fibroblast cell proliferation. Oxidative stress induces the upregulation of cyclophilin A. Upregulation of cyclophilin A is seen in lung cancer, cholangiocarcinoma, pancreatic cancer, myeloma, gastric carcinoma, and human oral cancer cell lines. An increase in the expression of cyclophilin A is seen in OSF. Hou et al. reported that 12% (3 of 25) of normal mucosa tissues were negative and 88% (22 of 25) weakly positive. In OSF, 16% (4 of 25) were weakly positive, 44% (11 of 25) were positive, and 40% (10 of 25) were strongly positive. The mRNA level of cyclophilin A was significantly greater in OSF tissues compared to normal mucosa [155, 163]. The CypA expression was higher in later OSF stages than early stages. OSCC tissues showed an even higher average CypA expression level than that in OSF tissues. A relatively weak CypA signal was detected in both epithelial and submucosa areas from normal and early-stage OSF tissues, while an intense CypA immunoreactivity was observed in both epithelial and submucosa areas from those OSF tissues from mid- and late stages [173].

### 15.7.7 Fatty Acid Synthase (FASN)

Fatty acid synthase (FASN) is an enzyme that initiates the synthesis of long-chain fatty acids from acetyl-CoA and malonyl-CoA. Lipid metabolism is an important cellular process of membrane biosynthesis [155]. There is increased expression of FASN in OSF. FASN provides lipids for membrane formation in fast-developing cancer cells and acts as a key enzyme in the progression to malignancy. Upregulation of FASN is reported in many cancers, including breast, prostate, ovarian, tongue, esophageal, and OSCC. Rai et al. observed an increase in FASN expression in OSF with dysplasia compared to normal mucosa. Higher expression of FASN was cytoplasmic in the basal layer and membranous in the upper layers of epithelium in OSF with dysplasia, compared to the normal mucosa [164].

### 15.7.8 Fibrinogen Alpha-Chain Precursor (FGA)

FGA is a protein encoded by the FGA gene in humans. FGA is a component of fibrinogen (FG), an important blood protein, regulated by calcium ions. FGA is consistently downregulated from normal buccal mucosal to OSF to OSCC [6].

### 15.7.9 Glucose Transporter 1

Glucose transporter 1 (GLUT1) is a protein that mediates glucose transport through the plasma membrane and is a key component in cellular metabolism. It facilitates diffusion of soluble ions, nutrients, and other metabolites across the hydrophobic cell membrane [165]. Cancer cells reprogram their metabolic activity to meet nutritional demands. This metabolic reprogramming initiates the production of metabolic intermediates, which results in the rapid proliferation of cancer cells. The important metabolic alterations in cancer cells include the Warburg effect, which is an increase in glucose uptake by aerobic glycolysis and lipid biosynthesis. GLUT1 transports the glucose required for aerobic glycolysis promoting Warburg effect in carcinogenesis.

As OSF progresses towards carcinogenesis, a complex metabolic ecosystem develops which consists of altered glycolytic pathways and lipid biosynthesis. A significant increase of GLUT1 in OSF with dysplasia compared to normal tissues was reported by Rai et al. The expression of GLUT1 was cytoplasmic in the basal layer and membranous in the upper layers, with membranous expression being continuous in OSF with dysplasia [164]. GLUT1 is commonly expressed in OSCC, and its expression positively correlates to tumor stage, treatment resistance, and poor prognosis [164, 165].

### 15.7.10 Heat-Shock Protein 70 (Hsp70)

Heat-shock proteins (Hsp) are a large and heterogeneous group of chaperon molecules, whose synthesis is induced by both physiological and pathological conditions, such as heat shock, oxidative stress, inflammation, infection, and neoplastic transformation. They play an important role in cellular homeostasis. The absence of Hsp70 leads to cell apoptosis [161, 166]. Hsp70 is overexpressed in a wide range of human cancers and is implicated in tumor cell proliferation, differentiation, and metastasis. A significant increase in the expression of Hsp70 is observed in tissues progressing from OSF to OSCC, suggesting a role for Hsp70 in malignant transformation of OSF. The high copper content of areca nut generates reactive oxygen species, which upregulates Hsp70 in OSF [161]. There is a positive correlation between Hsp70 and severity of oral epithelial dysplasia [166].

### 15.7.11 Hexokinase 2 (HK2)

15

Hexokinases catalyze the intake of glucose into glucose-6-phosphate in the first step of glycolysis. HK1, HK2, HK3, and HK4 are the isoforms of hexokinase. Among them, HK1 is ubiquitously expressed in most mammalian tissues, and HK2 is detected in adipose, skeletal, and cardiac muscles, whereas HK3 and HK4 show relatively low expression in mammalian tissues. HK2 is rarely expressed in normal tissues. A high level of HK2 expression has been reported in OSF and many solid tumors and is associated with tumor progression, poor overall survival, and treatment resistance. HK2 expression has been reported in various types of cancers, including esophageal, lung, uterine, breast, pancreatic, glioblastoma, and OSCC [164, 167]. Rai et al. report a significant overexpression of HK2 in OSF with dysplasia compared to normal subjects, suggesting the role of glycolysis in malignant transformation of OSF. Hexokinase showed both cytoplasmic and membranous expression in the upper layers of the epithelium [164].

### 15.7.12 Hydroxynonenal (4-HNE)

4-Hydroxy-2-nonenal (4-HNE) is a lipid peroxidation product that represents one of the most bioactive lipid alkenals. 4-HNE modulates several signaling processes through the formation of covalent adducts with nucleophilic functional groups in proteins, nucleic acids, and membrane lipids [166]. 4-HNE alterations in carcinogenesis reduce membrane integrity, affect cytosol protein function, cause nuclear and mitochondrial DNA damage, inhibit electron transport chain activity, activate mitochondrial uncoupling, reduce tricarboxylic acid cycle activity, and inhibit ALDH2. Chatterjee et al. studied the expression of oxidative stress markers in 12 OSF tissues. They found an increase in the expression of 4-HNE in OSF ($p < 0.01$) and OSCC ($p < 0.001$), with a significant escalation of 4-HNE expression in OSCC compared to OSF and normal subjects [68, 168]. Strong correlation ($r = 0.9837$) between 4-HNE and HIF-1α expressions depicted the association of oxidative stress and hypoxia during OSF and OSCC [68].

### 15.7.13 Mucin-1 (MUC1)

Mucins are highly glycosylated proteins that act as molecular surface barriers. They are involved in morphogenetic signal transduction pathways at the epithelial surface. Mucin glycosylation determines the biochemical and biophysical properties of viscoelastic secretions and plays an important role in diverse biological functions, such as cell differentiation, cell adhesion, immune response, and cell signaling [169, 170]. Alterations in mucin expression and its glycosylation are associated with the development and progression of malignancies. Kumar et al. reported a steady increase in mucin expression from normal to OPMDs including OSF and leukoplakia to OSCC. Of 10 cases of OSF, 9 (90%) cases showed immunoreactivity in the basal, parabasal, and spinous layer cells [169].

### 15.7.14 Organic Cation Transporter 3 (OCT3)

Organic cation transporter 3 (OCT3) is a membrane transporter, which regulates cellular metabolic homeostasis by transporting endogenous and exogenous cation compounds across the membrane. They belong to the SLC22 family, which includes OCT1 (SLC22 A1), OCT2 (SLC22 A2), and OCT3 (SLC22 A3). OCT1 and OCT2 are highly expressed in the liver and kidneys, and OCT3 is widely expressed in a variety of tissues. An increase in OCT3 is seen in OSF and OSCC with greater expression in OSCC compared to OSF. OCT3 is upregulated in oral, liver, rectal, and cervical cancers but downregulated in prostate cancer. In a study from Central South University of Changsha, Hunan, China, the staining index scores of OCT3 were studied in 13 normal mucosal specimen, 13 OSF, and 30 OSCC tissues. They observed a gradual increase in expression from the normal to OSF to OSCC-OSF groups ($p < 0.0001$) [171]. OCT3 expression is positively associated with the grade of malignancy and its prognosis [171].

### 15.7.15 Secreted Frizzled-Related Proteins (SFRPs)

SFRPs contain around 300 amino acids, including an N-terminal cysteine-rich domain (CRD) and a hydrophilic heparin-binding region in the C-terminal domain. SFRPs include SFRP1, 2, 3, 4, and 5 that inhibit the Wnt signaling pathway through binding to the Wnt ligand and competing with frizzled (Fz) receptors [170]. The mRNA levels of SFRPs are in a reduced state in many malignancies including OSCC. Deregulation of SFRPs by promoter CpG methylation has been reported in oral, nasopharyngeal, esophageal, lung, gastric, colorectal, hepatocellular, breast, ovarian, endometrial, cervical, renal, and bladder carcinomas. Methylated SFRPs mediate tumor cell proliferation, differentiation, apoptosis, and progression. Deregulation of SFRPs that act as Wnt antagonists is considered a primary step in the multiple-step tumorigenesis of OSCC. Zhou et al. reported that 80% (12 of 15) of normal oral mucosa showed SFRP1 positivity, which was nuclear. In OSF, 66.7% (30 of 45) showed SFRP1 expression, which was cytoplasmic. SFRP5 nuclear expression was seen in 86.7% (13 of 15) of normal oral mucous tissues, whereas cytoplasmic SFRP5 was detected in 73.3% (33 of 45) of OSF tissues. SFRP expression decreases from normal to OSF to OSCC [172].

**Summary**

The markers discussed above are summarized in ◘ Table 15.2. Our understanding of these changes and their clinical implication is evolving, and this chapter gives an overview of the current state of our understanding of IHC markers in OSF and OSCC.

◘ **Table 15.2** Summary of biomarkers in oral submucous fibrosis (OSF)

| S. No. | Biomarkers in OSF | Reference | Expression levels (IHC) | Localization in tissue<br>Epithelium/connective tissue |
|---|---|---|---|---|
| Epithelial markers | | | | |
| 1 | Annexin A4 (ANXN A4) | Liu et al. [6] | Upregulated | Epithelium (spinous layer of epithelial cells) |
| 2 | Beta-catenin (β-catenin) | Bag et al. [7] | Downregulated | Epithelium (a component of cadherin complex) |
| | | Chatterjee et al. [68] | Upregulated | |
| 3 | CD1a | da Silva et al. [12] | Downregulated | Epithelium (Langerhans cells) |
| 4 | CD207 | da Silva et al. [12] | Downregulated | Epithelium (Langerhans cells) |
| 5 | CD303 | Narayanan et al. [11]<br>da Silva et al. [12] | Upregulated | Plasmacytoid dendritic cells |
| 6 | Cytokeratins (CK) | | | Epithelium |
| | CK-5/6 | Bag et al. [7] | Upregulated | |
| | CK10 | Bag et al. [7] | Upregulated | |
| | CK8 | Nanda et al. [22] | Upregulated | |
| | CK18 | Nanda et al. [22] | Upregulated | |
| 7 | E-cadherin (E-cad) | Sharada et al. [25]<br>Sridevi et al. [26]<br>Das et al. [52]<br>Chatterjee et al. [68]<br>Das et al. [73]<br>Anura et al. [90] | Downregulated | Epithelium |

(continued)

**Table 15.2** (continued)

| S. No. | Biomarkers in OSF | Reference | Expression levels (IHC) | Localization in tissue Epithelium/connective tissue |
|---|---|---|---|---|
| 8 | Epidermal growth factor receptor (EGFR) | Meka et al. [29] | Upregulated | Epithelium |
| 9 | Filamin A (FLNA) | Liu et al. [6] | Upregulated | Epithelium (lower spinous layer and basal cell layer) |
| 10 | Loricrin | Nithya et al. [30] | Upregulated | Stratum corneum and stratum granulosum of the keratinized epithelium; absent in non-keratinized epithelium |
| Connective tissue markers | | | | |
| 1 | Alpha-smooth muscle actin (α-SMA) | Angadi et al. [32]<br>Sarode et al. [33]<br>Gupta et al. [34]<br>Anura et al. [35]<br>Jayaraj et al. [36]<br>Gadbail et al. [41]<br>Gandhi et al. [42] | Upregulated | Connective tissue (myofibroblasts and blood vessels) |
| 2 | Bone morphogenetic protein 7 (BMP7) | Khan et al. [43] | Downregulated | Connective tissue (extracellular matrix) |
| 3 | CD34 | Desai et al. [44]<br>Sharma et al. [47]<br>Tekade et al. [48] | Upregulated | Connective tissue (endothelial cells/blood vessels) |
| | | Pandiar et al. [45]<br>Pammar et al. [46]<br>Madhavan Nirmal et al. [91] | Downregulated | |
| 4 | CD105 | Anura et al. [35]<br>Gadbail et al. [41]<br>Pammar et al. [46]<br>Das et al. [52] | Upregulated | Connective tissue (endothelial cells/blood vessels) |
| 5 | CD68 | Pereira et al. [50] | Upregulated | Connective tissue (macrophages) |
| 6 | CD147 | Wang et al. [54] | Upregulated | Epithelium (basal layer and lower parts of stratum spinosum) |
| 7 | Collagen | | | Connective tissue (collagen is present throughout the lamina propria) |
| | • Col 1 | Anura et al. [35] | Upregulated | |
| | • Col 3 | Anura et al. [35] | Upregulated | |
| 8 | Connective tissue growth factor (CTGF) | Shah et al. [59] | Upregulated | Epithelium and connective tissue (stromal fibroblasts; around blood vessels and in skeletal muscles) |
| 9 | Decorin | Nayak et al. [60] | Upregulated | Predominantly in connective tissue (endothelial cells and stroma); also found in epithelial nests of tumor |

■ **Table 15.2** (continued)

| S. No. | Biomarkers in OSF | Reference | Expression levels (IHC) | Localization in tissue<br>Epithelium/connective tissue |
|---|---|---|---|---|
| 10 | Fibroblast growth factor (FGF) and its receptors | | | |
| | • FGF2, FGFR2, and FGFR3 | Nayak et al. [61] | Downregulated | FGF-2: Basal, parabasal layers in tissues with lining epithelium, tumor cells and also in the stroma<br>FGF2R: Full thickness of the epithelium, tumor cells, and stromal cells;<br>FGFR-3: upper and midstratum layer of lining epithelium, stromal fibroblast cells, tumor cells, and seldom in endothelium of tumor stroma |
| | • bFGF | Pandiar et al. [45] | Downregulated | Connective tissue |
| 11 | Fibronectin | Anura et al. [35] | Upregulated | Connective tissue (fibroblasts, extracellular matrix) |
| 12 | Hypoxia-inducible factor-2α (HIF-2α) | Joseph et al. [65] | Downregulated | Epithelium (basal and suprabasal layers) and connective tissue |
| | Hypoxia inducible factor-1α (HIF-1α) | Tilakaratne et al. [66]<br>Ekanayaka et al. [67]<br>Chatterjee et al. [68] | Upregulated | Epithelium |
| 13 | Mast cell chymase | Sabarinath et al. [69] | Upregulated | |
| | | Yadav et al. [27] | Downregulated | Connective tissue |
| 14 | Matrix metalloproteinase (MMP) | | | Predominantly in connective tissue (stromal fibroblasts, macrophages, endothelial cells); some epithelial cells |
| | • MMP-1 | Mishra et al. [71] | Upregulated | |
| | • MMP-1 | Illeperuma et al. [72] | Downregulated | |
| | • MMP-2 | Shrestha et al. [70] | Upregulated | |
| 15 | N-cadherin | Das et al. [73] | Upregulated | Epithelium (basal layer) |
| 16 | Osteopontin | Routray et al. [74] | Downregulated | Connective tissue (extracellular matrix) |
| 17 | Podoplanin | Karunagaran et al. [75] | Upregulated | Connective tissue (lymphatics and endothelial cells) and epithelium |
| | | Deepa et al. [76] | Upregulated | |
| 18 | S100A4 | Yu et al. [77] | Upregulated | Connective tissue |
| 19 | Syndecan-1 | Kamat et al. [79] | Downregulated | Epithelium (modest in basal layer, strong in spinous and granular layer) |
| 20 | Tenascin-C | Tak et al. [80] | Downregulated | Weak expression at the epithelial connective tissue junction; diffusely in deeper connective tissue |
| 21 | Transforming growth factor-beta (TGF-β) | | | Connective tissue (fibroblasts, inflammatory cells) and epithelium |
| | • TGF-β | Khan et al. [43] | Upregulated | |
| | • TGF-β1 | Wang et al. [54]<br>Illeperuma et al. [72]<br>Kamath et al. [84] | Upregulated | |
| | • TGF-β2 | Kamath et al. [84] | Upregulated | |

(continued)

**Table 15.2** (continued)

| S. No. | Biomarkers in OSF | Reference | Expression levels (IHC) | Localization in tissue Epithelium/connective tissue |
|---|---|---|---|---|
| 22 | Tissue inhibitors of matrix metalloproteinases (TIMPs) | | | Connective tissue (fibroblasts, endothelial cells) and epithelium |
| | • TIMP-1 | Illeperuma et al. [72] | Downregulated | |
| | • TIMP-2 | Shrestha et al. [70] | Upregulated | |
| 23 | Transglutaminase-2 | Lim et al. [88] | Upregulated | Connective tissue (fibroblasts) |
| 24 | TWIST | Das et al. [73] | Upregulated | Epithelium (basal layer) |
| 25 | Vascular endothelial growth factor (VEGF) | Sharada et al. [25]<br>Nayak et al. [28]<br>Sharma et al. [47]<br>Anura et al. [90]<br>Madhavan Nirmal et al. [91] | Upregulated | Connective tissue (stromal components such as fibroblasts, inflammatory cells, and muscles) and epithelium |
| 26 | Vimentin | Chatterjee et al. [68]<br>Nayak et al. [92]<br>Sawant et al. [93] | Upregulated | Epithelium (suprabasal layers) |
| Proliferative markers | | | | |
| 1 | Bax | Ranganathan et al. [94] | Upregulated | Epithelium |
| 2 | BUBR1 | Hsieh et al. [96] | Upregulated | Epithelium |
| 3 | Caspase 3 | Zhu et al. [99] | Upregulated | Epithelium |
| | | Veeravarmal et al. [100] | Downregulated | |
| 4 | c-Jun | Shraddha et al. [102] | Upregulated | Epithelium |
| 5 | c-met | Bazarsad et al. [105] | Upregulated | Epithelium |
| 6 | Cyclin D1 | Bazarsad et al. [105] | Downregulated | Epithelium |
| 7 | c-Myc | Anura et al. [107] | Upregulated | Epithelium |
| 8 | Fragile histidine triad protein (FHIT) | Yin et al. [112] | Downregulated | Epithelium |
| 9 | Human telomerase reverse transcriptase (hTERT) | Raju et al. [113] | Upregulated | |
| | | Mishra et al. [114] | Downregulated | |
| 10 | Insulin-like growth factor II mRNA-binding protein 3 (IMP3) | Bazarsad et al. [105] | Upregulated | Epithelium |
| 11 | Ki67 | Gadbail et al. [41]<br>Ranganathan et al. [94]<br>Xie et al. [119] | Upregulated | Epithelium (basal and suprabasal layers) |
| | | Bazarsad et al. [105]<br>Humayun et al. [126] | Downregulated | |
| 12 | Microtubule-associated protein light chain 3 (LC3) | Zhu et al. [99] | Upregulated | Epithelium (spinous and granular layers were minimally expressed in the basal layer) |
| 13 | Mouse double-minute 2 homolog (MDM2) | Yin et al. [112] | Upregulated | Epithelium |
| 14 | p16 | Bazarsad et al. [105]<br>Sudhakaran et al. [125] | Upregulated | Epithelium |

15

**Table 15.2** (continued)

| S. No. | Biomarkers in OSF | Reference | Expression levels (IHC) | Localization in tissue Epithelium/connective tissue |
|---|---|---|---|---|
| 15 | p53 | Ranganathan et al. [94]<br>Bazarsad et al. [105]<br>Humayun et al. [126]<br>Varun et al. [127] | Upregulated | Epithelium (in this study only basal and suprabasal layers were evaluated—Ranganathan et al.) |
| 16 | p62 | Zhu et al. [99] | Downregulated | Epithelium |
| 17 | P63 | Das et al. [52]<br>Das et al. [73]<br>Anura et al. [90]<br>Varun et al. [127]<br>Sinha et al. [129] | Upregulated | Epithelium |
| 18 | Proliferating cell nuclear antigen (PCNA) | Kaur et al. [130]<br>Sheelam et al. [131] | Upregulated | Epithelium |
| 19 | Polo-like kinase (PLK) | Vittal et al. [133] | Upregulated | Epithelium |
| 20 | Phosphatase and tensin homolog deleted on chromosome 10 (PTEN) | Angadi et al. [135] | Downregulated | Epithelium |
| 21 | Survivin | Chatterjee et al. [68]<br>Zhou et al. [138] | Upregulated | Epithelium |
| Stemness markers | | | | |
| 1 | Aldehyde dehydrogenase 1 (ALDH1) | Chatterjee et al. [68] | Not expressed | Metastatic islands of OSCC |
| 2 | Bmi1 | Xie et al. [119] | Upregulated | Epithelium |
| 3 | CD133 | Chatterjee et al. [68] | Not expressed | Metastatic islands of OSCC |
| 4 | Stage-specific embryonic antigen (SSEA4) | Yu et al. [147] | Upregulated | Connective tissue (fibroblasts) |
| 5 | SRY (sex-determining region on Y chromosome) type homeobox genes (SOX2) | Xie et al. [119] | Upregulated | Epithelium |
| 6 | STRO1 (in fibroblasts and myofibroblasts) | Yu et al. [148] | Upregulated | Connective tissue (mesenchymal stem cells) |
| Markers involved in cell signaling | | | | |
| 1 | Dickkopf WNT signaling pathway inhibitor 3 (DKK3) | Zhou et al. [150] | Upregulated | Epithelium |
| 2 | Glioma associated oncogene homolog 1 (GLI1) | Chatterjee et al. [68] | Upregulated | Epithelium |
| 3 | Phosphorylated extracellular signal-regulated kinase (pERK) | Chatterjee et al. [68] | Upregulated | Epithelium |
| 4 | Sonic hedgehog (Shh) | Chatterjee et al. [68] | Upregulated | Epithelium |
| 5 | WNT inhibitory factor 1 (WIF1) | Zhou et al. [157] | Downregulated | Epithelium |
| Other markers (transcription factors, enzymes, glycoproteins, and metabolic markers) | | | | |
| 1 | Alpha enolase ($\alpha$-enolase) | Bag et al. [159] | Upregulated | Data not available |

(continued)

Table 15.2 (continued)

| S. No. | Biomarkers in OSF | Reference | Expression levels (IHC) | Localization in tissue Epithelium/connective tissue |
|---|---|---|---|---|
| 2 | Beta-integrin (β-integrin) | Veeravarmal et al. [160] | Downregulated | Epithelium (basal and suprabasal layers) |
| 3 | Calreticulin | Das et al. [161] | Upregulated | Epithelium |
| 4 | C–C motif chemokine ligand 2 (CCL2) | Sarode et al. [33] | Upregulated | Connective tissue (subepithelial layer) |
| 5 | Cyclooxygenase 2 | Rangaswamy et al. [162] | Upregulated | Epithelium and connective tissue |
| 6 | Cyclophilin A | Hou et al. [155]<br>Yuan et al. [173] | Upregulated | Epithelium and connective tissue |
| 7 | Fatty acid synthase (FASN) | Rai et al. [164] | Upregulated | Epithelium |
| 9 | Glucose transporter 1 (GLUT1) | Rai et al. [164] | Upregulated | Epithelium |
| 10 | Heat shock protein 70 (Hsp70) | Das et al. [161] | Upregulated | Epithelium |
| 11 | Hexokinase-2 | Rai et al. [164] | Upregulated | Epithelium |
| 12 | 4-Hydroxynonenal (4-HNE) | Chatterjee et al. [68] | Upregulated | Epithelium |
| 13 | Mucin-1 (MUC1) | Kumar et al. [169] | Upregulated | Epithelium |
| 14 | Organic cation transporter 3 (OCT3) | Hu et al. [171] | Upregulated | Epithelium and tumor nest within the connective tissue |
| 15 | Secreted frizzled-related proteins (SFRPs) | Zhou et al. [172] | Downregulated | Epithelium |

## References


1. Henry NL, Hayes DF. Cancer biomarkers. Mol Oncol. 2012;6(2):140–6. https://doi.org/10.1016/j.molonc.2012.01.010.
2. Goossens N, Nakagawa S, Sun X, Hoshida Y. Cancer biomarker discovery and validation. Transl Cancer Res. 2015;4(3):256–69.
3. Matos LL, Trufelli DC, de Matos MG, da Silva Pinhal MA. Immunohistochemistry as an important tool in biomarkers detection and clinical practice. Biomark Insights. 2010;5:9–20. https://doi.org/10.4137/bmi.s2185.
4. Chong Y, Thakur N, Lee JY, et al. Diagnosis prediction of tumours of unknown origin using ImmunoGenius, a machine learning-based expert system for immunohistochemistry profile interpretation. Diagn Pathol. 2021;16:19. https://doi.org/10.1186/s13000-021-01081-8.
5. Shen YW, Shih YH, Fuh LJ, Shieh TM. Oral submucous fibrosis: a review on biomarkers, pathogenic mechanisms, and treatments. Int J Mol Sci. 2020;21(19):7231. https://doi.org/10.3390/ijms21197231.
6. Liu W, Zeng L, Li N, Wang F, Jiang C, Guo F, Chen X, Su T, Xu C, Zhang S, Fang C. Quantitative proteomic analysis for novel biomarkers of buccal squamous cell carcinoma arising in background of oral submucous fibrosis. BMC Cancer. 2016;16:584.
7. Bag S, Pal M, Chaudhary A, Das RK, Paul RR, Sengupta S, Chatterjee J. Connecting cyto-nanoarchitectural attributes and epithelial molecular expression in oral submucous fibrosis progression to cancer. J Clin Pathol. 2015;68(8):605–13.
8. Valenta T, Hausmann G, Basler K. The many faces and functions of β-catenin. EMBO J. 2012;31(12):2714–36. https://doi.org/10.1038/emboj.2012.150.
9. Chandavarkar V, Mishra MN, Sangeetha R, Premalatha BR. The current understanding on Langerhans' cells and its role in oral lesions. Contemp Clin Dent. 2020;11:211–6.
10. Lombardi T, Hauser C, Budtz-Jörgensen E. Langerhans cells: structure, function and role in oral pathological conditions. J Oral Pathol Med. 1993;22:193–202.
11. Narayanan B, Narasimhan M. Langerhans cell expression in oral submucous fibrosis: an immunohistochemical analysis. J Clin Diagn Res. 2015;9(7):ZC39–41.
12. da Silva LC, Fonseca FP, de Almeida OP, de Almeida Mariz BAL, Lopes MA, Radhakrishnan R, Sharma M, Kowalski LP, Vargas PA. CD1A+ and CD207+ cells are reduced in oral submucous fibrosis and oral squamous cell carcinoma. Med Oral Patol Oral Cir Bucal. 2020;25(1):e49–55.
13. De Monte A, Olivieri CV, Vitale S, Bailleux S, Castillo L, Giordanengo V, Maryanski JL, Segura E, Doglio A. CD1c-related DCs that express CD207/Langerin, but are distinguishable from Langerhans cells, are consistently present in human tonsils. Front Immunol. 2016;7:197. https://doi.org/10.3389/fimmu.2016.00197.

14. Pellicioli ACA, Bingle L, Farthing P, Lopes MA, Martins MD, Vargas PA. Immunosurveillance profile of oral squamous cell carcinoma and oral epithelial dysplasia through dendritic and T-cell analysis. J Oral Pathol Med. 2017;46(10):928–33. https://doi.org/10.1111/jop.12597.
15. Nyachhyon R, Nagraj SK, Ongole R. Expression of CD1a by Langerhans cells in oral mucosa of submucous fibrosis patients and arecanut/gutkha chewers. J Nepal Dental Assoc. 2014;14(2):1.
16. Öhman J, Magnusson B, Telemo E, Jontell M, Hasséus B. Langerhans cells and T cells sense cell dysplasia in oral leukoplakias and oral squamous cell carcinomas--evidence for immunosurveillance. Scand J Immunol. 2012;76(1):39–48. https://doi.org/10.1111/j.1365-3083.2012.02701.x.
17. Belaldavar C, Mane DR, Hallikerimath S, Kale AD. Cytokeratins: its role and expression profile in oral health and disease. J Oral Maxillofacial Surg Med Pathol. 2016;28:77–84.
18. Ranganathan K, Kavitha R, Sawant SS, Vaidya MM. Cytokeratin expression in oral submucous fibrosis--an immunohistochemical study. J Oral Pathol Med. 2006;35(1):25–32. https://doi.org/10.1111/j.1600-0714.2005.00366.x.
19. Bragulla HH, Homberger DG. Structure and functions of keratin proteins in simple, stratified, keratinized and cornified epithelia. J Anat. 2009;214(4):516–59. https://doi.org/10.1111/j.1469-7580.2009.01066.x.
20. Jacques CM, Pereira AL, Maia V, Cuzzi T, Ramos-e-Silva M. Expression of cytokeratins 10, 13, 14 and 19 in oral lichen planus. J Oral Sci. 2009;51(3):355–65. https://doi.org/10.2334/josnusd.51.355.
21. Frohwitter G, Buerger H, VAN Diest PJ, Korsching E, Kleinheinz J, Fillies T. Cytokeratin and protein expression patterns in squamous cell carcinoma of the oral cavity provide evidence for two distinct pathogenetic pathways. Oncol Lett. 2016;12(1):107–13. https://doi.org/10.3892/ol.2016.4588.
22. Nanda KD, Ranganathan K, Devi U, Joshua E. Increased expression of CK8 and CK18 in leukoplakia, oral submucous fibrosis, and oral squamous cell carcinoma: an immunohistochemistry study. Head Neck Pathol. 2012;6(3):314–21.
23. Vaidya MM, Sawant SS, Borges AM, Ogale SB, Bhisey AN. Cytokeratin expression in precancerous lesions of the human oral cavity. Oral Oncol. 1998;34(4):261–4.
24. Lalli A, Tilakaratne WM, Ariyawardana A, Fitchett C, Leigh IM, Hagi-Pavli E, Cruchley AT, Parkinson EK, Teh MT, Fortune F, Waseem A. An altered keratinocyte phenotype in oral submucous fibrosis: correlation of keratin K17 expression with disease severity. J Oral Pathol Med. 2008;37(4):211–20. https://doi.org/10.1111/j.1600-0714.2007.00609.x.
25. Sharada P, Swaminathan U, Nagamalini BR, Kumar KV, Ashwini BK, Lavanya V. Coalition of E-cadherin and vascular endothelial growth factor expression in predicting malignant transformation in common oral potentially malignant disorders. Asian Pac J Cancer Prev. 2018;19(4):1075–80.
26. Sridevi U, Jain A, Nagalaxmi V, Kumar UV, Goyal S. Expression of E-cadherin in normal oral mucosa, in oral precancerous lesions and in oral carcinomas. Eur J Dent. 2015;9(3):364–72.
27. Yadav A, Desai RS, Bhuta BA, Singh JS, Mehta R, Nehete AP. Altered immunohistochemical expression of mast cell tryptase and chymase in the pathogenesis of oral submucous fibrosis and malignant transformation of the overlying epithelium. J Investig Clin Dent. 2014;5(3):214–9.
28. Nayak S, Goel MM, Chandra S, Bhatia V, Mehrotra D, Kumar S, Makker A, Rath SK, Agarwal SP. VEGF-A immunohistochemical and mRNA expression in tissues and its serum levels in potentially malignant oral lesions and oral squamous cell carcinomas. Oral Oncol. 2012;48:233–9.
29. Meka JN, Ugrappa S, Velpula N, Kumar S, Maloth KN, Kodangal S, Lalitha CH, Goyal S. Quantitative Immunoexpression of EGFR in Oral potentially malignant disorders: oral leukoplakia and oral submucous fibrosis. J Dent Res Dent Clin Dent Prospect. 2015;9(3):166–74.
30. Nithya S, Joshua E, K R, Thavarajah R, Rao UK. Loricrin expression and its implication in oral submucous fibrosis, hyperkeratosis and normal mucosa with association to habits—an immunohistochemical study. J Oral Biol Craniofac Res. 2019;9(3):226–231.
31. Nithya S, Radhika T, Jeddy N. Loricrin: an overview. J Oral Maxillofac Pathol. 2015;19(1):64–8. https://doi.org/10.4103/0973-029X.157204.
32. Angadi PV, Kale AD, Hallikerimath S. Evaluation of myofibroblasts in oral submucous fibrosis: correlation with disease severity. Natl J Maxillofac Surg. 2011;2(1):38–46.
33. Sarode G, Sarode SC, Deshmukh R, Raktade P, Patil S. Myofibroblasts could be recruited in a chemokine (C-C motif) ligand 2-dependent manner in the pathogenesis of oral submucous fibrosis. J Oral Maxillofac Pathol. 2016;20(3):445–52.
34. Gupta K, Metgud R, Gupta J. Evaluation of stromal myofibroblasts in oral leukoplakia, oral submucous fibrosis, and oral squamous cell carcinoma--an immunohistochemical study. Indian J Cancer. 2015;52(1):87–92.
35. Anura A, Das D, Pal M, Paul RR, Das S, Chatterjee J. Nanomechanical signatures of oral submucous fibrosis in sub-epithelial connective tissue. J Oral Pathol Med. 2017;46(6):431–8.
36. Jayaraj G, Sherlin HJ, Ramani P, Premkumar P, Natesan A. Stromal myofibroblasts in oral squamous cell carcinoma and potentially malignant disorders. J Oral Biol Craniofac Res. 2015;5(3):165–72.
37. Son GM, Kwon MS, Shin DH, Shin N, Ryu D, Kang CD. Comparisons of cancer-associated fibroblasts in the intratumoral stroma and invasive front in colorectal cancer. Medicine (Baltimore). 2019;98(18):e15164. https://doi.org/10.1097/MD.0000000000015164.
38. Chang YC, Tsai CH, Lai YL, Yu CC, Chi WY, Li JJ, et al. Arecoline-induced myofibroblast transdifferentiation from human buccal mucosal fibroblasts is mediated by ZEB1. J Cell Mol Med. 2014;18:698–708.
39. Sharma M, Shetty SS, Radhakrishnan R. Oral submucous fibrosis as an overhealing wound: implications in malignant transformation. Recent Pat Anticancer Drug Discov. 2018;13(3):272–91. https://doi.org/10.2174/1574892813666180227103147.
40. Wadhwan V, Venkatesh A, Reddy V, Malik S. The role of myofibroblasts in the progression of oral submucous fibrosis: a systematic review. J Oral Maxillofac Pathol. 2019;23:257–66.
41. Gadbail AR, Chaudhary MS, Sarode SC, Gondivkar SM, Belekar L, Mankar-Gadbail MP, Dande R, Tekade SA, Yuwanati MB, Patil S. Ki67, CD105 and α-smooth muscle actin expression in disease progression model of oral submucous fibrosis. J Investig Clin Dent. 2019;10(4):e12443.
42. Gandhi P, Prasad UC. Evaluation of myofibroblasts in oral submucous fibrosis and oral squamous cell carcinoma: the pathogenesis and correlation. Dent Res J (Isfahan). 2017;14(5):314–20.
43. Khan I, Agarwal P, Thangjam GS, Radhesh R, Rao SG, Kondaiah P. Role of TGF-b and BMP7 in the pathogenesis of oral submucous fibrosis. Growth Factors. 2011;29(4):119–27.
44. Desai RS, Mamatha GS, Khatri MJ, Shetty SJ. Immunohistochemical expression of CD34 for characterization and quantification of mucosal vasculature and its probable role in malignant transformation of atrophic epithelium in oral submucous fibrosis. Oral Surg Oral Med Oral Pathol Oral Radiol Endod. 2010;109(2):257–67.

45. Pandiar D, Shameena PM. Immunohistochemical expression of CD34 and basic fibroblast growth factor (bFGF) in oral submucous fibrosis. J Oral Maxillofac Pathol. 2014;18:155–61.
46. Pammar C, Nayak RS, Kotrashetti VS, Hosmani J. Comparison of microvessel density using CD34 and CD105 in oral submucous fibrosis and its correlation with clinicopathological features: an immunohistochemical study. J Oral Maxillofac Pathol. 2018;22(2):281.
47. Sharma E, Tyagi N, Gupta V, Narwal A, Vij H, Lakhnotra D. Role of angiogenesis in oral submucous fibrosis using vascular endothelial growth factor and CD34: an immunohistochemical study. J Cancer Res Ther. 2018;14(6):1180–3.
48. Tekade SA, Chaudhary MS, Tekade SS, Sarode SC, Wanjari SP, Gadbail AR, Wanjari PV, Gawande MN, Korde-Choudhari S, Zade P. Early stage oral submucous fibrosis is characterized by increased vascularity as opposed to advanced stages. J Clin Diagn Res. 2017;11(5):ZC92–6.
49. Kalogirou EM, Tosios KI, Christopoulos PF. The role of macrophages in oral squamous cell carcinoma. Front Oncol. 2021;11:611115. https://doi.org/10.3389/fonc.2021.611115.
50. Pereira T, Naik S, Tamgadge A. Quantitative evaluation of macrophage expression using CD68 in oral submucous fibrosis: an Immunohistochemical study. Ann Med Health Sci Res. 2015;5(6):435–41.
51. Bdewi AT, Alkadir Mohamed Labib AA, Drobie BF, Abdullah BH, Omar M. Evaluation of CD68 in oral squamous cell carcinoma and their relation with clinicopathological parameters—an immunohistochemical study. Int J Curr Microbiol Appl Sci. 2020;9(07):3832–9. https://doi.org/10.20546/ijcmas.2020.907.448.
52. Das RK, Pal M, Barui A, Paul RR, Chakraborty C, Ray AK, Sengupta S, Chatterjee J. Assessment of malignant potential of oral submucous fibrosis through evaluation of p63, E-cadherin and CD105 expression. Oral Oncol. 2010;46(7):553–8.
53. Sahaf R, Naseem N, Rehman A-U, Anjum R, Nagi AH. EMMPRIN (CD147) as a potential predictor of oral squamous cell carcinoma progression: a study from Pakistan. J Histol Histopathol. 2017;4:8. https://doi.org/10.7243/2055-091X-4-8.
54. Wang W, Xiong H, Hu Z, Zhao R, Hu Y, Chen W, Han Y, Yang L, Hu X, Wang C, Mao T, Xia K, Su T. Experimental study on TGF-β1-mediated CD147 expression in oral submucous fibrosis. Oral Dis. 2018;24(6):993–1000.
55. Akhtar R, Sherratt MJ, Cruickshank JK, Derby B. Characterizing the elastic properties of tissues. Mater Today (Kidlington). 2011;14(3):96–105. https://doi.org/10.1016/S1369-7021(11)70059-1.
56. Arora KS, Nayyar A, Kaur P, Arora KS, Goel A, Singh S. Evaluation of collagen in leukoplakia, oral submucous fibrosis and oral squamous cell carcinomas using polarizing microscopy and immunohistochemistry. Asian Pac J Cancer Prev. 2018;19(4):1075–80. https://doi.org/10.22034/APJCP.2018.19.4.1075.
57. Di Martino JS, Nobre AR, Mondal C, et al. A tumor-derived type III collagen-rich ECM niche regulates tumor cell dormancy. Nat Cancer. 2021;3:90. https://doi.org/10.1038/s43018-021-00291-9.
58. Chen Z, Zhang N, Chu HY, Yu Y, Zhang ZK, Zhang G, Zhang BT. Connective tissue growth factor: from molecular understandings to drug discovery. Front Cell Dev Biol. 2020;8:593269. https://doi.org/10.3389/fcell.2020.593269.
59. Shah AM, Jain K, Desai RS, Bansal S, Shirsat P, Prasad P, Bodhankar K. The role of increased connective tissue growth factor in the pathogenesis of Oral submucous fibrosis and its malignant transformation-an Immunohistochemical study. Head Neck Pathol. 2021;15(3):817–30. https://doi.org/10.1007/s12105-020-01270-9.
60. Nayak S, Goel MM, Bhatia V, Chandra S, Makker A, Kumar S, Agrawal SP, Mehrotra D, Rath SK. Molecular and phenotypic expression of decorin as modulator of angiogenesis in human potentially malignant oral lesions and oral squamous cell carcinomas. Dent Res J (Isfahan). 2013;10(3):321–7.
61. Nayak S, Goel MM, Makker A, Bhatia V, Chandra S, Kumar S, Agarwal SP. Fibroblast growth factor (FGF-2) and its receptors FGFR-2 and FGFR-3 may be putative biomarkers of malignant transformation of potentially malignant Oral lesions into Oral squamous cell carcinoma. PLoS One. 2015;10(10):e0138801.
62. Sundquist E, Kauppila J, Veijola J, et al. Tenascin-C and fibronectin expression divide early stage tongue cancer into low- and high-risk groups. Br J Cancer. 2017;116:640–8. https://doi.org/10.1038/bjc.2016.455.
63. Parisi L, Toffoli A, Ghezzi B, Mozzoni B, Lumetti S, Macaluso GM. A glance on the role of fibronectin in controlling cell response at biomaterial interface. Jpn Dent Sci Rev. 2020;56(1):50–5. https://doi.org/10.1016/j.jdsr.2019.11.002.
64. Hande AH, Chaudhary MS, Gawande MN, Gadbail AR, Zade PR, Bajaj S, Patil SK, Tekade S. Oral submucous fibrosis: an enigmatic morpho-insight. J Can Res Ther. 2019;15:463–9.
65. Joseph I, Elizabeth J, Rao UK, Ranganathan K. Study of hypoxia-inducible factor-2 alpha expression in the malignant transformation of Oral submucous fibrosis. J Oral Maxillofac Pathol. 2020;24(1):33–9.
66. Tilakaratne WM, Iqbal Z, Teh MT, Ariyawardana A, Pitiyage G, Cruchley A, Stewart JE, Hagi-Pavli E, Lalli A, Waseem A, Parkinson EK, Fortune F. Upregulation of HIF-1alpha in malignant transformation of oral submucous fibrosis. J Oral Pathol Med. 2008;37(6):372–7. https://doi.org/10.1111/j.1600--0714.2007.00625.x.
67. Ekanayaka RP, Tilakaratne WM. Oral submucous fibrosis: review on mechanisms of malignant transformation. Oral Surg Oral Med Oral Pathol Oral Radiol. 2016;122(2):192–9. https://doi.org/10.1016/j.oooo.2015.12.018.
68. Chatterjee R, Ghosh B, Mandal M, Nawn D, Banerjee S, Pal M, Paul RR, Banerjee S, Chatterjee J. Pathophysiological relationship between hypoxia associated oxidative stress, epithelial-mesenchymal transition, stemness acquisition and alteration of Shh/ Gli-1 axis during oral sub-mucous fibrosis and oral squamous cell carcinoma. Eur J Cell Biol. 2021;100(1):151146. https://doi.org/10.1016/j.ejcb.2020.151146.
69. Sabarinath B, Sriram G, Saraswathi TR, Sivapathasundharam B. Immunohistochemical evaluation of mast cells and vascular endothelial proliferation in oral submucous fibrosis. Indian J Dent Res. 2011;22(1):116–21. https://doi.org/10.4103/0970-9290.80009.
70. Shrestha A, Carnelio S. Evaluation of matrix metalloproteinases-2 (MMP-2) and tissue inhibitors of metalloproteinases-2 (TIMP-2) in oral submucous fibrosis and their correlation with disease severity. Indian J Pathol Microbiol. 2013;56(3):204–10.
71. Mishra G, Ranganathan K. Matrix metalloproteinase-1 expression in oral submucous fibrosis: an immunohistochemical study. Indian J Dent Res. 2010;21(3):320–5.
72. Illeperuma RP, Ryu MH, Kim KY, Tilakaratne WM, Kim J. Relationship of fibrosis and the expression of TGF-beta1, MMP-1, and TIMP-1 with epithelial dysplasia in oral submucous fibrosis. Oral Med Pathology. 2010;15:21–8.
73. Das RK, Anura A, Pal M, Bag S, Majumdar S, Barui A, Chakraborty C, Ray AK, Sengupta S, Paul RR, Chatterjee J. Epithelio-mesenchymal transitional attributes in oral sub-

mucous fibrosis. Oral Surg Oral Med Oral Pathol Oral Radiol. 2012;113(2):245–53.
74. Routray S, Kheur SM, Kheur M. Osteopontin: a marker for invasive oral squamous cell carcinoma but not for potentially malignant epithelial dysplasias. Ann Diagn Pathol. 2013;17(5):421–4. https://doi.org/10.1016/j.anndiagpath.2013.03.005.
75. Karunagaran M, Murali P, Palaniappan V, Sivapathasundharam B. Expression and distribution pattern of podoplanin in oral submucous fibrosis with varying degrees of dysplasia – An immunohistochemical study. J Histotechnol. 42(2):80–6.
76. Deepa AG, Janardanan-Nair B, Varun BR. Podoplanin expression in oral potentially malignant disorders and oral squamous cell carcinoma. J Mech Behav Biomed Mater. 2017;65:705–15.
77. Yu C-C, Tsai C-H, Hsu H-I, Chang Y-C. Elevation of S100A4 expression in buccal mucosal fibroblasts by Arecoline: involvement in the pathogenesis of Oral submucous fibrosis. PLoS One. 2013;8(1):e55122.
78. Natarajan J, Hunter K, Mutalik VS, Radhakrishnan R. Overexpression of S100A4 as a biomarker of metastasis and recurrence in oral squamous cell carcinoma. J Appl Oral Sci. 2014;22(5):426–33. https://doi.org/10.1590/1678-775720140133.
79. Kamat SS, Kumar GS, Koshy AV. Immunohistochemical analysis of syndecan-1 in leukoplakia and oral submucous fibrosis. Ann Diagn Pathol. 2013;17(5):421–4.
80. Tak J, Rao NN, Chandra A, Gupta N. Immunohistochemical analysis of tenascin expression in different grades of oral submucous fibrosis. J Oral Maxillofac Pathol. 2015;19(3):291–6.
81. Luomanen M, Virtanen I. Distribution of tenascin in healing incision, excision and laser wounds. J Oral Pathol Med. 1993;22:41–5.
82. Shrestha P, Sakamoto F, Takagi H, Yamada T, Mori M. Enhanced tenascin immunoreactivity in leukoplakia and squamous cell carcinoma of the oral cavity: an immunohistochemical study. Eur J Cancer B Oral Oncol. 1994;30B:132–7.
83. Yoshida T, Akatsuka T, Imanaka-Yoshida K. Tenascin-C and integrins in cancer. Cell Adhes Migr. 2015;9(1–2):96–104. https://doi.org/10.1080/19336918.2015.1008332.
84. Kamath VV, Krishnamurthy S, Satelur KP, Rajkumar K. Transforming growth factor-β1 and TGFβ2 act synergistically in the fibrotic pathway in oral submucous fibrosis: an immunohistochemical observation. Indian J Med Paediatr Oncol. 2015;36(2):111–6.
85. Caja L, Dituri F, Mancarella S, et al. TGF-β and the tissue microenvironment: relevance in fibrosis and cancer. Int J Mol Sci. 2018;19(5):1294. https://doi.org/10.3390/ijms19051294.
86. Eckert RL, Kaartinen MT, Nurminskaya M, et al. Transglutaminase regulation of cell function. Physiol Rev. 2014;94(2):383–417. https://doi.org/10.1152/physrev.00019.2013.
87. Lee SS, Chen YJ, Tsai CH, Huang FM, Chang YC. Elevated transglutaminase-2 expression mediates fibrosis in areca quid chewing-associated oral submucocal fibrosis via reactive oxygen species generation. Clin Oral Investig. 2016;20(5):1029–34.
88. Lim E, Wu CH, Moi SH, Lui MT, Yang CH, Yang CC. The expression of transglutaminase 2 (TG-2) in oral squamous cell carcinoma and its clinical significance. J Chin Med Assoc. 2017;80(8):515–20. https://doi.org/10.1016/j.jcma.2017.05.004.
89. Qin Q, Xu Y, He T, et al. Normal and disease-related biological functions of Twist1 and underlying molecular mechanisms. Cell Res. 2012;22:90–106. https://doi.org/10.1038/cr.2011.144.
90. Anura A, Das RK, Pal M, Paul RR, Ray AK, Chatterjee J. Correlated analysis of semi-quantitative immunohistochemical features of E-cadherin, VEGF and CD105 in assessing malignant potentiality of oral submucous fibrosis. PLoS One. 2014;9(5):e98719.
91. Madhavannirmal R, Veeravarmal V, Bhavani S, Srinivasan P, Austin RD. Evaluation of MicroVessel density (MVD) and vascular endothelial growth factor (VEGF) as possible indicator of malignant transformation in Oral submucous fibrosis. IOSR J Dental Med Sci (IOSR-JDMS). 2016;15(11):72–7.
92. Nayak MT, Singh A, Desai RS, Vanaki SS. Immunohistochemical analysis of vimentin in oral submucous fibrosis. J Cancer Epidemiol. 2013;2013:549041.
93. Sawant SS, Vaidya MM, Chaukar DA, Alam H, Dmello C, Gangadaran P, Kannan S, Kane S, Dange PP, Dey N, Ranganathan K, D'Cruz AK. Clinical significance of aberrant vimentin expression in oral premalignant lesions and carcinomas. Oral Dis. 2014;20(5):453–65.
94. Ranganathan K, Kavitha R. Proliferation and apoptosis markers in oral submucous fibrosis. Indian J Dent Res. 2011;22(2):362.
95. Thongsuksai P, Pruegsanusak K, Boonyaphiphat P. Prognostic significance of p16, p53, Bcl-2, and Bax in oral and oropharyngeal squamous cell carcinoma. Asian Biomed. 2014;8(2):255–62.
96. Hsieh PC, Chen YK, Tsai KB, Shieh TY, Chang YY, Chang JG, Wu HL, Lin SF. Expression of BUBR1 in human oral potentially malignant disorders and squamous cell carcinoma. Oral Surg Oral Med Oral Pathol Oral Radiol Endod. 2010;109(2):257–67.
97. Teixeira JH, Silva P, Faria J, Ferreira I, Duarte P, Delgado ML, Queirós O, Moreira R, Barbosa J, Lopes CA, Do Amaral JB, Monteiro LS, Bousbaa H. Clinicopathologic significance of BubR1 and Mad2 overexpression in oral cancer. Oral Dis. 2015;21(6):713–20. https://doi.org/10.1111/odi.12335.
98. Wong RS. Apoptosis in cancer: from pathogenesis to treatment. J Exp Clin Cancer Res. 2011;30:87. https://doi.org/10.1186/1756-9966-30-87.
99. Zhu B, Jiang Q, Que G, Dai Z, Wu Y. Role of autophagy and apoptosis in atrophic epithelium in oral submucous fibrosis. J Oral Sci. 2020;62(2):184–8.
100. Veeravarmal V, Austin RD, Siddavaram N, Thiruneelakandan S, Nassar MH. Caspase-3 expression in normal oral epithelium, oral submucous fibrosis and oral squamous cell carcinoma. J Oral Maxillofac Pathol. 2016;20(2):214–8.
101. Wisdom R, Johnson RS, Moore C. C Jun regulates cell cycle progression and apoptosis by distinct mechanisms. EMBO J. 1999;18:188–97.
102. Shraddha KS, Niranjan KC, Hallikeri K. Immunolocalization of c-Jun in normal mucosa, oral submucous fibrosis, epithelial dysplasia, and oral squamous cell carcinoma: a comparative study. J Can Res Ther. 2018;14:1180–3.
103. Sun Z, Liu Q, Ye D, Ye K, Yang Z, Li D. Role of c-met in the progression of human oral squamous cell carcinoma and its potential as a therapeutic target. Oncol Rep. 2018;39(1):209–16. https://doi.org/10.3892/or.2017.6073.
104. Brusevold IJ, Soland TM, Khuu C, Christoffersen T, Bryne M. Nuclear and cytoplasmic expression of met in oral squamous cell carcinoma and in an organotypic oral cancer model. Eur J Oral Sci. 2010;118:342–9.
105. Bazarsad S, Zhang X, Kim KY, Illeperuma R, Jayasinghe RD, Tilakaratne WM, Kim J. Identification of a combined biomarker for malignant transformation in oral submucous fibrosis. J Oral Pathol Med. 2017;46(6):431–8.
106. Eilers M, Eisenman RN. Myc's broad reach. Genes Dev. 2008;22(20):2755–66.
107. Anura A, Kazi A, Pal M, Paul RR, Sengupta S, Chatterjee J. Endorsing cellular competitiveness in aberrant epithelium of oral submucous fibrosis progression: neighborhood analy-

sis of immunohistochemical attributes. Indian J Dent Res. 2018;29(2):171–5.
108. Wang T, Cai B, Ding M, Su Z, Liu Y, Shen L. C-Myc overexpression promotes Oral cancer cell proliferation and migration by enhancing Glutaminase and glutamine Synthetase activity. Am J Med Sci. 2019;358(3):235–42. https://doi.org/10.1016/j.amjms.2019.05.014.
109. Moharil RB, Khandekar S, Dive A, Bodhade A. Cyclin D1 in oral premalignant lesions and oral squamous cell carcinoma: an immunohistochemical study. J Oral Maxillofac Pathol. 2020;24:397.
110. Hassan MI, Naiyer A, Ahmad F. Fragile histidine triad protein: structure, function, and its association with tumorogenesis. J Cancer Res Clin Oncol. 2010;136(3):333–50. https://doi.org/10.1007/s00432-009-0751-9.
111. Bellon M, Bialuk I, Galli V, Bai XT, Farre L, Bittencourt A, Marçais A, Petrus MN, Ratner L, Waldmann TA, Asnafi V, Gessain A, Matsuoka M, Franchini G, Hermine O, Watanabe T, Nicot C. Germinal epimutation of fragile histidine triad (FHIT) gene is associated with progression to acute and chronic adult T-cell leukemia diseases. Mol Cancer. 2021;20(1):86. https://doi.org/10.1186/s12943-021-01370-2.
112. Yin X, Wen C, Han Y, Gao Y, Tang Z. Expression of FHIT and MDM2 in oral submucous fibrosis and canceration tissues. Zhong nan Da Xue Xue Bao Yi Xue Ban Chinese. 2010;35(6):572–5. https://doi.org/10.3969/j.issn.1672-7347.2010.06.006.
113. Raju KL, Haragannavar VC, Patil S, Rao RS, Nagaraj T, Augustine D, Venkatesiah SS, Nambiar S. Expression of hTERT in oral submucous fibrosis and oral squamous cell carcinoma—an Immunohistochemical analysis. Pathol Oncol Res. 2020;26(3):1573–82.
114. Mishra N, Tandon N, Fatima N, Srivastava AN, Lal N, Kumar V. Immunohistochemical expression of human telomerase reverse transcriptase in oral cancer and precancer: a case–control study. J Oral Maxillofac Pathol. 2019;23:412–7.
115. Zhao T, Hu F, Qiao B, et al. Telomerase reverse transcriptase potentially promotes the progression of oral squamous cell carcinoma through induction of epithelial-mesenchymal transition. Int J Oncol. 2015;46:2205–15. https://doi.org/10.3892/ijo.2015.2927.
116. Boscolo-Rizzo P, Da Mosto MC, Rampazzo E, et al. Telomeres and telomerase in head and neck squamous cell carcinoma: from pathogenesis to clinical implications. Cancer Metastasis Rev. 2016;35:457–74. https://doi.org/10.1007/s10555-016-9633-1.
117. Cornejo K, Shi M, Jiang Z. Oncofetal protein IMP3: a useful diagnostic biomarker for leiomyosarcoma. Hum Pathol. 2012;43(10):1567–72. https://doi.org/10.1016/j.humpath.2011.12.020.
118. Li HG, Han JJ, Huang ZQ, Wang L, Chen WL, Shen XM. IMP3 is a novel biomarker to predict metastasis and prognosis of tongue squamous cell carcinoma. J Craniofac Surg. 2011;22(6):2022–5. https://doi.org/10.1097/SCS.0b013e3182319750.
119. Xie C, Feng H, Zhong L, Shi Y, Wei Z, Hua Y, Ji N, Li J, Tang Z, Chen Q. Proliferative ability and accumulation of cancer stem cells in oral submucous fibrosis epithelium. Oral Dis. 2020:1–10.
120. Dhingra A, Alexander D, Reyes-Reveles J, Sharp R, Boesze-Battaglia K. Microtubule-associated protein 1 light chain 3 (LC3) isoforms in RPE and retina. Adv Exp Med Biol. 2018;1074:609–16. https://doi.org/10.1007/978-3-319-75402-4_74.
121. Li J, Zhao TT, Zhang P, Xu CJ, Rong ZX, Yan ZY, Fang CY. Autophagy mediates oral submucous fibrosis. Exp Ther Med. 2016;11(5):1859–64.
122. Tang JY, Hsi E, Huang YC, Hsu NC, Chu PY, Chai CY. High LC3 expression correlates with poor survival in patients with oral squamous cell carcinoma. Hum Pathol. 2013;44(11):2558–62. https://doi.org/10.1016/j.humpath.2013.06.017.
123. Oliner JD, Saiki AY, Caenepeel S. The role of MDM2 amplification and overexpression in tumorigenesis. Cold Spring Harb Perspect Med. 2016;6(6):a026336. https://doi.org/10.1101/cshperspect.a026336.
124. Ye C, Tang H, Zhao Z, Lei CT, You CQ, Zhang J, Gao P, He FF, Chen S, Wang YM, Zhang C, Su H. MDM2 mediates fibroblast activation and renal tubulointerstitial fibrosis via a p53-independent pathway. Am J Physiol Renal Physiol. 2017;312(4):F760–8. https://doi.org/10.1152/ajprenal.00528.2016.
125. Sudhakaran A, Hallikeri K, Babu B. p16 as an independent marker for detection of high-risk HPV in oral submucous fibrosis and oral squamous cell carcinoma. Indian J Pathol Microbiol. 2019;62(4):523–8.
126. Humayun S, Prasad VR. Expression of p53 protein and ki-67 antigen in oral premalignant lesions and oral squamous cell carcinomas: an immunohistochemical study. Natl J Maxillofac Surg. 2011;2(1):38–46.
127. Varun BR, Ranganathan K, Rao UK, Joshua E. Immunohistochemical detection of p53 and p63 in oral squamous cell carcinoma, oral leukoplakia, and oral submucous fibrosis. J Investig Clin Dent. 2014;5(3):214–9. https://doi.org/10.1111/jicd.12038.
128. Liang L, Luo H, He Q, You Y, Fan Y, Liang J. Investigation of cancer-associated fibroblasts and p62 expression in oral cancer before and after chemotherapy. J Craniomaxillofac Surg. 2018;46(4):605–10. https://doi.org/10.1016/j.jcms.2017.12.016.
129. Sinha A, Chandra S, Raj V, Zaidi I, Saxena S, Dwivedi R. Expression of p63 in potentially malignant and malignant oral lesions. Indian J Med Paediatr Oncol. 2015;36(2):111–6.
130. Kaur M, Saxena S, Bansal P. Expression of proliferating cell nuclear antigen in normal oral mucosa, oral submucous fibrosis and leukoplakia with or without dysplasia. Int J Oral-Med Sci. 2011;10(3):149–55.
131. Sheelam S, Reddy SP, Kulkarni PG, Nandan S, Keerthi M, Raj GS. Role of cell proliferation and vascularity in malignant transformation of potentially malignant disorders. J Oral Maxillofac Pathol. 2018;22(1):40–7.
132. de Cárcer G. The mitotic cancer target polo-like kinase 1: oncogene or tumor suppressor? Genes (Basel). 2019;10(3):208. https://doi.org/10.3390/genes10030208.
133. Vittal K, Pandian SS, Joseph LD, Raj SG. Immunohistochemical expression of polo-like kinase 1 in oral squamous cell carcinoma and oral submucous fibrosis. Oral Surg Oral Med Oral Pathol Oral Radiol. 2018; pii: S2212–4403(18)30045–2
134. Liu Z, Sun Q, Wang X. PLK1, a potential target for cancer therapy. Transl Oncol. 2017;10(1):22–32. https://doi.org/10.1016/j.tranon.2016.10.003.
135. Angadi PV, Krishnapillai R. Evaluation of PTEN immunoexpression in oral submucous fibrosis: role in pathogenesis and malignant transformation. J Oral Maxillofac Pathol. 2011;15(2):148–53.
136. Starzyńska A, Sejda A, Adamska P, et al. Prognostic value of the PIK3CA, AKT, and PTEN mutations in oral squamous cell carcinoma: literature review. Arch Med Sci. 2021;17(1):207–17. https://doi.org/10.5114/aoms.2020.100780.
137. Sekar B, Indrapriyadharshini K, Ambika M, Saranya R, Nirmal M, Manzoor S. Survivin expression in metastatic and nonmetastatic oral squamous cell carcinoma: a comparative study. J Adv Oral Res. 2021;12(1):75–80.
138. Zhou S, Qu X, Yu Z, Zhong L, Ruan M, Ma C, Wang M, Zhang C, Jian X. Survivin as a potential early marker in the

carcinogenesis of oral submucous fibrosis. Oral Surg Oral Med Oral Pathol Oral Radiol Endod. 2010;109(4):575–81.
139. Sakthivel R, Ramamoorthy A, Jeddy N, Singaram M. Evaluation and expression of Survivin in potentially malignant lesions and squamous cell carcinoma: a comparative study. Cureus. 2020;12(4):e7551. https://doi.org/10.7759/cureus.7551.
140. Feng JQ, Xu ZY, Shi LJ, Wu L, Liu W, Zhou ZT. Expression of cancer stem cell markers ALDH1 and Bmi1 in oral erythroplakia and the risk of oral cancer. J Oral Pathol Med. 2013;42(2):148–53. https://doi.org/10.1111/j.1600-0714.2012.01191.x.
141. Rao RS, Raju KL, Augustine D, Patil S. Prognostic significance of ALDH1, Bmi1, and OCT4 expression in Oral epithelial dysplasia and Oral squamous cell carcinoma. Cancer Control. 2020;27(1):1073274820904959. https://doi.org/10.1177/1073274820904959.
142. Klein IP, Meurer L, Danilevicz CK, Squarize CH, Martins MD, Carrard VC. BMI-1 expression increases in oral leukoplakias and correlates with cell proliferation. J Appl Oral Sci. 2020;28:e20190532. https://doi.org/10.1590/1678-7757-2019-0532.
143. He Q, Liu Z, Zhao T, Zhao L, Zhou X, Wang A. Bmi1 drives stem-like properties and is associated with migration, invasion, and poor prognosis in tongue squamous cell carcinoma. Int J Biol Sci 2015;11(1):1–10. doi:https://doi.org/10.7150/ijbs.10405.
144. Yu CC, Hu FW, Yu CH, Chou MY. Targeting CD133 in the enhancement of chemosensitivity in oral squamous cell carcinoma-derived side population cancer stem cells. Head Neck. 2016;38(Suppl. 1):E231–8. https://doi.org/10.1002/hed.23975.
145. Liu W, Wu L, Shen XM, Shi LJ, Zhang CP, Xu LQ, et al. Expression patterns of cancer stem cell markers ALDH1 and CD133 correlate with a high risk of malignant transformation of oral leukoplakia. Int J Cancer. 2013;132(4):868–74. https://doi.org/10.1002/ijc.27720.
146. Ravindran G, Devaraj H. Aberrant expression of CD133 and musashi-1 in preneoplastic and neoplastic human oral squamous epithelium and their correlation with clinicopathological factors. Head Neck. 2012;34(8):1129–35. https://doi.org/10.1002/hed.21896.
147. Yu CC, Yu CH, Chang YC. Aberrant SSEA-4 upregulation mediates myofibroblast activity to promote pre-cancerous oral submucous fibrosis. Sci Rep. 2016;6:37004. https://doi.org/10.1038/srep37004.
148. Yu CC, Liao YW, Yu CH, Chang YC. STRO-1 confers myofibroblast transdifferentiation in fibroblasts derived from oral submucous fibrosis. J Oral Pathol Med. 2018;47(3):299–305.
149. Katase N, Nagano K, Fujita S. DKK3 expression and function in head and neck squamous cell carcinoma and other cancers. J Oral Biosci. 2020;62(1):9–15. https://doi.org/10.1016/j.job.2020.01.008.
150. Zhou S, Zhu Y, Mashrah M, Zhang X, He Z, Yao Z, Zhang C, Guo F, Hu Y, Zhang C. Expression pattern of DKK3, dickkopf WNT signaling pathway inhibitorÂ 3, in the malignant progression of oral submucous fibrosis. Oncol Rep. 2017;37(2):979–85.
151. Theocharis S, Kotta-Loizou I, Klijanienko J, Giaginis C, Alexandrou P, Dana E, Rodriguez J, Patsouris E, Sastre-Garau X. Extracellular signal-regulated kinase (ERK) expression and activation in mobile tongue squamous cell carcinoma: associations with clinicopathological parameters and patients survival. Tumour Biol. 2014;35(7):6455–65. https://doi.org/10.1007/s13277-014-1853-9.
152. Avery JT, Zhang R, Boohaker RJ. GLI1: a therapeutic target for cancer. Front Oncol. 2021;11:673154. https://doi.org/10.3389/fonc.2021.673154.
153. Srinath S, Iyengar AR, Mysorekar V. Sonic hedgehog in oral squamous cell carcinoma: an immunohistochemical study. J Oral Maxillofac Pathol. 2016;20(3):377–83. https://doi.org/10.4103/0973-029X.190906.
154. Xie J, Huang L, Lu YG, Zheng DL. Roles of the Wnt signaling pathway in head and neck squamous cell carcinoma. Front Mol Biosci. 2021;7:590912. https://doi.org/10.3389/fmolb.2020.590912.
155. Hou X, Liu R, Huang C, Jiang L, Zhou Y, Chen Q. Cyclophilin a was revealed as a candidate marker for human oral submucous fibrosis by proteomic analysis. Cancer Biomark. 2017;20(3):345–56.
156. Baillie R, Tan ST, Itinteang T. Cancer stem cells in Oral cavity squamous cell carcinoma: a review. Front Oncol. 2017;7:112. https://doi.org/10.3389/fonc.2017.00112.
157. Zhou S, Chen L, Mashrah M, Zhu Y, He Z, Hu Y, Xiang T, Yao Z, Guo and Zhang C. Expression and promoter methylation of Wnt inhibitory factor-1 in the development of oral submucous fibrosis. Oncol Rep 2015; 34: 2636–2642.
158. Almaguel FA, Sanchez TW, Ortiz-Hernandez GL, Casiano CA. Alpha-enolase: emerging tumor-associated antigen, cancer biomarker, and oncotherapeutic target. Front Genet. 2021;11:614726. https://doi.org/10.3389/fgene.2020.614726.
159. Bag S, Dutta D, Chaudhary A, Sing BC, Pal M, Ray AK, Banerjee R, Paul RR, Basak A, Das AK, Chatterjee J. Identification of alpha-enolase as a prognostic and diagnostic precancer biomarker in oral submucous fibrosis. J Clin Pathol. 2018;71(3):228–38.
160. Veeravarmal V, Austin RD, Nagini S, Nassar MHM. Expression of Beta-1 integrin in normal epithelium, oral submucous fibrosis and oral squamous cell carcinoma. Pathol Res Pract. 2018;214(2):273–80.
161. Das T, Prodhan C, Patsa S, Ray JG, Chaudhuri K. Identification of over expressed proteins in oral submucous fibrosis by proteomic analysis. J Cell Biochem. 2018;119(6):4361–71.
162. Rangaswamy S, Chikkalingaiah RG, Sharada P, Kumar VK. Expression of cyclooxygenase 2 in oral submucous fibrosis: an immunohistochemical pilot study. J Oral Maxillofac Pathol. 2019;23(2):301.
163. Zidar N, Odar K, Glavac D, Jerse M, Zupanc T, Stajer D. Cyclooxygenase in normal human tissues--is COX-1 really a constitutive isoform, and COX-2 an inducible isoform? J Cell Mol Med. 2009;13(9B):3753–63. https://doi.org/10.1111/j.1582-4934.2008.00430.x.
164. Rai V, Bose S, Mukherjee R, Sarbajna A, Chakraborty C. Evaluation of aberrant metabolism related proteins in oral submucous fibrosis: a pilot study. J Oral Biosci. 2018;60(4):87–91.
165. Botha H, Farah CS, Koo K, Cirillo N, McCullough M, Paolini R, Celentano A. The role of glucose transporters in Oral squamous cell carcinoma. Biomol Ther. 2021;11(8):1070. https://doi.org/10.3390/biom11081070.
166. Priyanka KP, Majumdar S, Kotina S, Uppala D, Balla H. Expression of heat shock protein 70 in Oral epithelial dysplasia and Oral squamous cell carcinoma: an Immunohistochemical study. Contemp Clin Dent. 2019;10(2):185–90. https://doi.org/10.4103/ccd.ccd_101_18.
167. Li WC, Huang CH, Hsieh YT, Chen TY, Cheng LH, Chen CY, Liu CJ, Chen HM, Huang CL, Lo JF, Chang KW. Regulatory role of hexokinase 2 in modulating head and neck tumorigenesis. Front Oncol. 2020;10:176. https://doi.org/10.3389/fonc.2020.00176. Erratum in: Front Oncol. 2020;10:410
168. Zhong H, Yin H. Role of lipid peroxidation derived 4-hydroxynonenal (4-HNE) in cancer: focusing on mitochon-

dria. Redox Biol. 2015;4:193–9. https://doi.org/10.1016/j.redox.2014.12.011.

169. Kumar MH, Sanjai K, Kumarswamy J, Keshavaiah R, Papaiah L, Divya S. Expression of MUC1 mucin in potentially malignant disorders, oral squamous cell carcinoma and normal oral mucosa: an immunohistochemical study. J Oral Maxillofac Pathol. 2016;20(2):214–8.

170. Narashiman S, Narasimhan M, Venkatraman G. Expression of mucin 4 in leukoplakia and oral squamous cell carcinoma: an immunohistochemical study. J Oral Maxillofac Pathol. 2014;18(1):25–31. https://doi.org/10.4103/0973-029X.131887.

171. Hu Y, Qian Y, Lin L, Chen W, Yang L, Hu X, Tian K, Xia K, Su T. Differential expression of organic cation transporter 3 in oral submucous fibrosis-associated buccal squamous cell carcinoma. Pathol Res Pract. 2018;214(2):273–80.

172. Zhou S, Chen L, Mashrah M, Zhu Y, Liu J, Yang X, He Z, Wang L, Xiang T, Yao Z, Guo F, Yang W, Zhang C. Deregulation of secreted frizzled-related proteins is associated with aberrant β-catenin activation in the carcinogenesis of oral submucous fibrosis. Onco Targets Ther. 2015;8:2923–31.

173. Yuan Y, Hou X, Feng H, Liu R, Xu H, Gong W, Deng J, Sun C, Gao Y, Peng J, Wu Y, Li J, Fang C, Chen Q. Proteomic identification of cyclophilin A as a potential biomarker and therapeutic target in oral submucous fibrosis. Oncotarget. 2016;7(37):60348–65. https://doi.org/10.18632/oncotarget.11254.

# Management of Oral Submucous Fibrosis

Contents

# Medical Management of Oral Submucous Fibrosis

*Kavitha Loganathan and Kannan Ranganathan*

## Contents



© The Author(s), under exclusive license to Springer Nature Switzerland AG 2023
S. Warnakulasuriya, K. Ranganathan (eds.), *Oral Submucous Fibrosis*, Textbooks in Contemporary Dentistry,
https://doi.org/10.1007/978-3-031-12855-4_16

**Learning Goals**

- Medical treatment has been shown to be of some benefit in the early stages of oral submucous fibrosis, while surgical treatment is reserved for advanced cases. The various medical therapeutic agents, their route of administration, and the current understanding of their effectiveness are discussed in this chapter.

## 16.1 Introduction

Oral submucous fibrosis (OSF) is an insidious, chronic, progressive, and debilitating disease characterized by fibrotic changes in the oral mucosa. The pathogenesis of oral submucous fibrosis (OSF) involves areca nut alkaloids causing disequilibrium in the regulation of matrix metalloproteinase and tissue inhibitors of matrix metalloproteinase resulting in the deposition of abnormal extracellular matrix (ECM) [1]. The cessation of areca nut habit is the most significant step in the management of OSF in areca nut users. In addition to habit cessation activities, various medical treatment modalities have been researched. These include dietary supplements (micronutrients, vitamins, and antioxidants), immunomodulatory/anti-inflammatory agents (corticosteroids), proteolytic agents (such as hyaluronidase and placental extracts), vasodilators, immunomodulators, and anticytokines. They have been administered orally, topically, or through submucosal injection. Herbal preparations containing substances like aloe vera, tulsi/basil, turmeric, and spirulina have also been used in the medical management of OSF [2–4]. Research related to oral submucous fibrosis that have been undertaken using these various agents are presented in ◘ Table 16.1.

The objectives of medical treatment are to eliminate the symptoms of burning sensation, to stabilize and improve mouth opening, and in the long term to prevent malignant transformation.

Surgery is reserved for patients in the advanced stages of the disease. Physical therapy acts synergistically with other treatment modalities. The complex nature of diseases and the lack of a universal treatment protocol makes the management of OSF a challenging process. We discuss here the results of different agents reported in the literature for the treatment of OSF and their limitations.

This chapter aims

1. To comprehensively present and discuss the medical interventions reported in the literature in the management of OSF.
2. To understand the mechanism of action of medicinal agents used.
3. To emphasize the applications and side effects of each of the medicinal regimens used to alleviate the signs and symptoms in OSF.

### 16.1.1 Medical Management of OSF

#### 16.1.1.1 Pharmaceutical Agents

**1. Systemic agents**

- Levamisole (capsules; Immunomodulator).
- Antioxidant (capsules; Immunomodulator).
- Betamethasone (intralesional injections; corticosteroids).
- Hydrocortisone (intralesional injections; corticosteroids).
- Triamcinolone (intralesional injections; corticosteroids).
- Methylprednisolone (intralesional injections; corticosteroids).
- Hyaluronidase (intralesional injections; fibrinolytic enzyme).
- Placental extract (intralesional injections; biogenic stimulation).
- Vitamin E (capsules; Vitamins).
- Micronutrient supplements (capsules; vitamins, minerals, and omega-3 fatty acids).
- Pentoxifylline (tablets; vasodilator).
- Isoxsuprine (tablets; vasodilator).
- Lycopene (capsules; antioxidant).

**2. Topical agents**

- Triamcinolone acetonide (oromucosal pastes; corticosteroids).
- Clobetasol propionate (oromucosal pastes; corticosteroids).

#### 16.1.1.2 Herbal Remedies

**1. Systemic agents**

- Curcumin (tablets/lozenges; anti-inflammatory and antioxidant).
- Oxitard (capsules; immunomodulation, anti-inflammatory, anti-anxiety, anti-convulsive, and anti-arthritic properties).
- Spirulina (tablets; antioxidant).
- Colchicine (tablets; anti-inflammatory).

**2. Topical agents**

- Aloe vera (gel; antioxidant, antibacterial, and provides hydration).
- Curcumin (gel; anti-inflammatory and antioxidant).

Table 16.1 Research studies on oral submucous fibrosis using various medical therapies

| Authors | Type of study[a] | Sample | Intervention | Duration of treatment/ Follow-up | Mouth opening assessment (Measured with vernier caliper)<br>B: baseline;<br>A: after intervention;<br>F: after follow-up | Burning sensation assessment (Measured with visual analog scale, VAS)<br>B: baseline;<br>A: after the intervention;<br>F: after follow-up | Observations reported by authors |
|---|---|---|---|---|---|---|---|
| Immunomodulators: Levamisole | | | | | | | |
| Jirge et al. [12] | Randomized, single-blind study<br>Levamisole<br>Antioxidant<br>Levamisole + Antioxidant | 45 OSF patients<br>Counseled to quit areca nut practice | **Group I:** ($n = 15$)<br>Levamisole 50 mg tablets (Vermisol)—one tablet three times daily, for three consecutive days in a week for three alternate weeks<br>**Group II:** ($n = 15$)<br>Antioxidant capsules (ANTOXID) one capsule two times daily for 6 weeks<br>**Group III:** ($n = 15$)<br>Combination of group I and II treatments | 6 weeks of treatment<br>Post-treatment follow-up for 2 months | **Group I:** Levamisole<br>B: 2.8 ± 0.6 cm<br>A: 3.0 ± 0.7 cm<br>**Group II:** Antioxidant<br>B: 3.0 ± 1.1 cm<br>A: 3.2 ± 1.0 cm<br>**Group III:** Combination<br>B: 2.5 ± 1.0 cm<br>A: 2.7 ± 1.0 cm | **Group I:** Levamisole<br>B: 51.7 ± 19.9<br>A: 1.0 ± 2.8<br>**Group II:** Antioxidant<br>B: 58.0 ± 29.7<br>A: 10.1 ± 13.8<br>**Group III:** Combination<br>B: 39.3 ± 16.9<br>A: 2.7 ± 6.8 | Authors inferred that treatment of OSF with levamisole, antoxid, and the combination produced statistically significant improvement in mouth opening and reduction in burning sensation. Overall, a better response was seen to levamisole alone, than to antoxid and combination therapy. |
| Shinge et al. [13] | Randomized control trial<br>Levamisole<br>Antioxidant<br>Levamisole + Antioxidant | 60 OSF subjects<br>Divided into four groups according to OSF stages, then randomly subdivided into three groups based on treatments. | **Group A:** ($n = 30$)<br>Levamisole 150 mg (Tab. Vermisol) once a day for 3 consecutive days in a week for the following 3 alternate weeks<br>**Group B:** ($n = 20$)<br>Antioxidant capsules (Antoxid)<br>2 times daily for 6 weeks<br>**Group C:** ($n = 20$)<br>Combination of levamisole 150 mg + antioxidant capsules | 60 days | Improvement in mouth opening (%)<br>**Group A:** Levamisole<br>Stage 1: 10%<br>Stage 2: 22%<br>Stage 3: 18%<br>Stage 4: 7%<br>**Group B:** Antoxid<br>Stage 1: 10%<br>Stage 2: 16%<br>Stage 3: 18%<br>Stage 4: 12.5%<br>**Group C:** Combination<br>Stage 1: 20%<br>Stage 2: 22%<br>Stage 3: 20%<br>Stage 4: 5% | Evaluation of reduction (%)<br>**Group A:** Levamisole<br>Stage 1: 54%<br>Stage 2: 64%<br>Stage 3: 54%<br>Stage 4: 20%<br>**Group B:** Antoxid<br>Stage 1: 32%<br>Stage 2: 34%<br>Stage 3: 32%<br>Stage 4: 15%<br>**Group C:** Combination<br>Stage 1: 66%<br>Stage 2: 66%<br>Stage 3:54%<br>Stage 4: 17% | Combination drugs fared better than individual treatment groups. Further, being economical, non-invasive, safe and efficacious, levamisole and antioxidants can be considered an effective treatment protocol. |

| | | | | | | | |
|---|---|---|---|---|---|---|---|
| Anti-inflammatory: Corticosteroids | | | | | | | |
| Goel et al. [10] | Clinical longitudinal study<br>Lycopene<br>Betamethasone<br>Control | 270 OSF patients<br>Two treatment groups and a control group (90 in each group)<br>Counseled to quit areca nut practice.<br>Patients of each treatment group were further subdivided into three clinical stages of OSF (Stages I, II, III:). | **Lycopene group:** ($n = 90$)<br>2 mg of capsule lycopene per day (Lycored™) twice daily<br>**Betamethasone group:** ($n = 90$)<br>Intralesional injection of betamethasone 4 mg/ml diluted in 1.0 ml of 2% xylocaine (Injection Betnesol) biweekly with half dose on each side<br>**Control group:** ($n = 90$) | 6 months of treatment<br>6 months of follow-up | Post-treatment average improvement<br>**Lycopene group:**<br>Stage I: 3.00 ± 1.11 mm<br>Stage II: 6.07 ± 2.00 mm<br>Stage III: 6.53 ± 1.45 mm<br>**Betamethasone group:**<br>Stage I: 3.30 ± 1.51 mm<br>Stage II: 9.47 ± 2.47 mm<br>Stage III: 3.27 ± 1.36 mm<br>**Control group:**<br>Stage I: 0.00 ± 0.00 mm<br>Stage II- 0.00 ± 0.00 mm<br>Stage III- 0.00 ± 0.00 mm | ----------- | A positive clinical response was seen in all three clinical stages in both the test groups when compared with the control group.<br>Lycopene and betamethasone injection were seen to be efficacious, safe, and reliable drugs in the management of OSF. |
| Kisave et al. [95] | Prospective clinical study<br>Placentrex<br>Hydrocortisone | 60 OSF patients<br>Grade II and Grade III<br>Counseled to quit the areca nut practice.<br>Physiotherapy and multivitamins were advised. | **Group A:** ($n = 30$)<br>2 ml of placentrex, 2 injections per week<br>**Group B:** ($n = 30$)<br>2 ml of hydrocortisone, 2 injections per week | 3 months | **Group A:** Placentrex<br>B: 24.81 ± 1.11 mm<br>A: 30.00 ± 0.86 mm<br>**Group B:** Hydrocrotisone<br>B:23.14 ± 1.25 mm<br>A: 34.83 ± 0.85 mm | **Group A:** Placentrex<br>B: Mild-32.3%; moderate-35.5%; severe- 32.3%<br>A: absent-32.3% mild- 29.0%<br>**Group B:** Hydrocortisone<br>B: mild-27.6%; moderate-34.5%, severe-37.9%<br>A: absent-17.2% mild-48.3% | Overall, hydrocortisone seems to be a better regimen to improve mucosal health and increase mouth opening as compared to placentrex regimen.<br>However, placentrex is better than hydrocortisone in reducing the burning sensation. |
| Antioxidant: Lycopene | | | | | | | |
| Chole et al. [17] | Randomized controlled trial<br>Lycopene<br>Lycopene + Triamcinolone<br>Placebo | 90 OSF patients<br>Areca nut practice cessation was ascertained.<br>Groups 1,2,3 (Khanna and Andrade's classification) were included;<br>Group 4a and 4b were advised surgery. | **Group A:** ($n = 25$)<br>16 mg of lycopene (Cap Lycored)<br>**Group B:** ($n = 25$)<br>16 mg of lycopene + topical triamcinolone acetonide 0.1% (Cap Lycored + Ointment Kenacort)<br>**Group C:** ($n = 25$)<br>Placebo | 3 months | **Group A** showed 87% increase in mouth opening while **Group B** showed 93% and **Group C** showed 16% increase in mouth opening. | **Group A** showed 75%, **Group B** showed 94% and **Group C** showed 12% decrease in burning sensation in mouth | Lycopene was effective in improving mouth opening and alleviating pain and burning sensation when used in combination with triamcinolone acetonide 0.1%.<br>No side effects or intolerance to lycopene were reported. |

(continued)

**Table 16.1** (continued)

| Author | Type of study[a] | Sample | Intervention | Duration of treatment/ Follow-up | Mouth opening assessment (Measured with vernier caliper)<br>B: baseline; A: after intervention; F: after follow-up | Burning sensation assessment (Measured with visual analog scale, VAS)<br>B: baseline;<br>A: after the intervention; F: after follow-up | Observations reported by authors |
|---|---|---|---|---|---|---|---|
| Karemore et al. [31] | Randomized controlled trial<br>Lycopene<br>Placebo | 92 OSF patients | **Lycopene group:** (*n* = 46)<br>8 mg soft gel Lycored™ orally per day in two divided doses of 4 mg each<br>**Placebo group:** (*n* = 46) soft gel placebo twice a day orally | 3 months | **Lycopene group:**<br>Improvement at exit: 32 (69.56%)<br>No improvement at exit: 14 (30.63%)<br>Mean diff. in MO: 4.46 ± 3.65 mm<br>**Placebo group:**<br>Improvement at exit: 6 (13.04%)<br>No improvement at exit: 40 (86.95%)<br>Mean diff. in MO: 1.13 ± 1.6 mm | **Lycopene group:** Baseline:<br>Present 46, Absent 0, Reduced 0<br>Exit:<br>Present 1, Absent 31, Reduced 14<br>**Placebo group:** Baseline:<br>Present 46, Absent 0, Reduced 0<br>Exit:<br>Present 1, Absent 7, Reduced 38 | Lycopene appears to be a very promising drug in the management of OSF. |
| Selvam et al. [35] | Randomized controlled trial<br>Lycopene + Dexamethasone + Hyaluronidase<br>Antioxidant + Dexamethasone + Hyaluronidase<br>Dexamethasone + Hyaluronidase | 45 OSF patients | **Group A** (*n* = 15):<br>Oral Lycopene capsules 16 mg (Lycostar®, Lycopene 5000 µg + micronutrients), one capsule/day along with biweekly intralesional injections of Dexamethasone 1.5 ml and Hyaluronidase 1500 IU mixed with lignocaine.<br>**Group B** (*n* = 15)<br>Oral antioxidant capsules (Multivitamin A–Z soft capsules), one capsule/day along with biweekly intralesional injections of Dexamethasone 1.5 ml and Hyaluronidase 1500 IU mixed with lignocaine.<br>**Group C** (*n* = 15):<br>Biweekly intralesional injections of Dexamethasone 1.5 ml and Hyaluronidase 1500 IU with lignocaine | 6 weeks | Improvement in mouth opening between baseline and end of 6 weeks<br>**Group A:** 4.9 ± 2.5 mm<br>**Group B:** 4.3 ± 0.8 mm<br>**Group C:** 3.4 ± 0.5 mm | **Group A:**<br>B: 7.5<br>A: 0<br>**Group B:**<br>B: 7.0<br>A: 0<br>**Group C:**<br>B: 7.5<br>A: 0 | Lycopene with intralesional steroids showed greater improvement in mouth opening than antioxidants with intralesional steroids. However, the results of both groups did not differ enough to be statistically significant (‘p’ > 0.05). Lycopene in combination with intralesional steroids and hyaluronidase is highly efficacious in improving mouth opening and reducing other symptoms. |

| | | | | | | | |
|---|---|---|---|---|---|---|---|
| Singh et al. [28] | Prospective, randomized, and blinded controlled study<br>Lyocpene<br>Betamethasone | 44 OSF patients<br>Oral prophylaxis advised.<br>Counseled to quit the areca nut practice. | **Group I:** ($n = 22$)<br>10,000 mcg of lycopene (*Lyconex soft gels*) daily in two equally divided doses<br>**Group II:** ($n = 22$)<br>Intralesional injections of betamethasone (1 mL ampule of 4 mg each) twice weekly | Duration of treatment:<br>2 months<br>Follow-up<br>2 months after completion of treatment; total duration 4 months | **Group I:** Lycopene<br>B: 3.19 ± 0.55 mm<br>A: 4.39 + 0.29 mm<br>**Group II:** Betamethasone<br>B: 3.00 ± 0.82 mm<br>A: 3.39 ± 0.63 mm | **Group I:** Lycopene<br>B: 51.82 ± 24.08.<br>A: 94.5% reduction<br>**Group II:** Betamethasone<br>B: 49.55 ± 24.15.<br>A: 54.1% reduction | Lycopene capsules (Lyconex; lycopene with vitamins) are better than intralesional betamethasone injections in improving mouth opening and decreasing burning sensation. |
| Elizabeth et al. [36] | Randomized controlled trial<br>Lycopene +<br>Triamcinolone +<br>Hyaluronidase<br>Triamcinolone +<br>Hyaluronidase | 38 OSF patients<br>Complete oral prophylaxis and counseling on improving oral hygiene and motivated to stop areca nut use. | **Group 1:** ($n = 19$):<br>Oral Lycopene capsules 16 mg, one capsule/day along with intralesional injections of Triamcinolone (Kenacort) 40 mg/ml, 1 ml and Hyaluronidase 1500 IU mixed with 2% lignocaine once a week.<br>**Group 2:** ($n = 19$):<br>Intralesional Injections of Triamcinolone (Kenacort) 40 mg/ml, 1 ml, and Hyaluronidase 1500 IU mixed with 2% Lignocaine once a week. | Duration of treatment:<br>6 weeks<br>Follow-up post-treatment:<br>6 months | **Group 1:** Lycopene + corticosteroid injections<br>B: 1.5 cm<br>F: 4.5 ± 1.5 cm<br>**Group 2:** Corticosteroid injections<br>F: 3.5 ± 1.5 cm | -------- | Lycopene in combination with intralesional steroids and hyaluronidase is highly efficacious in improving the mouth opening compared to intralesional steroid and hyaluronidase injections alone. |
| Subramaniam et al. [37] | Randomized controlled trial<br>Lycopene<br>Ultrasound +<br>Muscle kneading exercises | 30 OSF patients | **Group A** ($n = 15$):<br>16 mg of lycopene (Lycored) daily in 2 equally divided doses (8 mg each)<br>**Group B** ($n = 15$):<br>15 consecutive sittings of therapeutic ultrasound of 5 min to left and right cheek each for 15 consecutive days, with permissible 1 day off each week. (Frequency of 3 MHz and Intensity 0.8 to 1.5 W/cm$^2$). Muscle kneading exercises: buccinator stretch, finger kneading and TMJ mobilization (anterior capsule stretch, TMJ joint mobility exercises) were given. | Duration of treatment:<br>6 weeks<br>Followed up until 3 months | Mean improvement in mouth opening (mm)<br>**Group A:** Lycopene<br>F: 5.10 mm<br>**Group B:** Ultrasound<br>F: 6.20 mm | Mean improvement in burning sensation<br>**Group A:** Lycopene<br>F: 2.73<br>**Group B:** Ultrasound<br>F: 1.4 | The mean improvement in tongue protrusion and burning sensation is significantly better with lycopene compared to therapeutic ultrasound.<br>The mean improvement in mouth opening is better in ultrasound group but the difference is not statistically significant.<br>The authors suggest that lycopene in isolation can be used as the initial treatment modality of OSF to relieve burning sensation, but if used in conjunction with therapeutic ultrasound will improve mouth opening. |

(continued)

**Table 16.1** (continued)

| Author | Type of study[a] | Sample | Intervention | Duration of treatment/ Follow-up | Mouth opening assessment (Measured with vernier caliper) B: baseline; A: after intervention; F: after follow-up | Burning sensation assessment (Measured with visual analog scale, VAS) B: baseline; A: after the intervention; F: after follow-up | Observations reported by authors |
|---|---|---|---|---|---|---|---|
| Arshad et al. [39] | Randomized controlled trial<br>Methylprednisolone<br>Lycopene<br>Methylprednisolone + Lycopene | 45 OSF patients | **Group A** ($n = 15$):<br>Methylprednisolone 20 mg/0.5 ml preparation was injected every month, at a single site on the buccal mucosa, bilaterally (40 mg in total)<br>**Group B** ($n = 15$):<br>Lycopene 10 mg soft gels<br>**Group C** ($n = 15$):<br>Intralesional methylprednisolone and lycopene capsules | Duration of treatment: 6 months<br>Follow-up post-treatment: 6 months | **Group A:**<br>B: 15.67 ± 6.46 mm<br>A: 19.13 ± 6.79 mm<br>**Group B:**<br>B: 17.07 + 4.2 mm<br>A: 19.53 ± 4.54 mm<br>**Group C:**<br>B: 17.87 ± 5.23 mm<br>A: 24.87 + 5.9 mm | ----------- | The most favorable response in terms of clinical efficacy was derived from the combination of intralesional steroid and oral antioxidant therapy in patients abstaining from areca nut habit and indulging in rigorous physiotherapy. |
| Kopuri et al. [44] | Randomized controlled trial<br>Lycopene<br>Curcumin | 30 OSF patients | **Group A** ($n = 15$):<br>Lycopene capsules Lycored 8 mg/day in 2 divided doses (Lycopene (2000 mcg), zinc (7.5 mg), and selenium (35 mcg)).<br>**Group B** ($n = 15$):<br>Curcumin Haridra 800 mg/day in 2 divided doses (Curcuma longa 400 mg) | 3 months | **Group A:** Lycopene<br>B: 24.26 ± 1.53 mm<br>A: 30.07 ± 1.1 mm<br>**Group B:** Curcumin<br>B: 26.07 ± 2.66 mm<br>A: 29 ± 2.27 mm | **Group A:** Lycopene<br>B: Mild 0, Moderate 11, Severe 4<br>A: Mild 8, Moderate 7, Severe 0<br>**Group B:** Curcumin<br>B: Mild 0, Moderate 13, Severe 2<br>A: Mild 13, Moderate 15, Severe 0 | Lycopene has produced better improvement in mouth opening and reduction in fibrous bands than curcumin. Curcumin has produced better improvement in burning sensation and blanching. Overall, a better response was seen to lycopene, than to curcumin. |
| Saran et al. [34] | Randomized clinical trial<br>Lycopene<br>Curcumin | 60 OSF patients Counseled to quit the areca nut practice. | **Group A:** ($n = 30$)<br>lycopene capsules (Cap Lycored; lycopene: 4 mg, zinc: 7.5 mg, selenium: 35 mg) orally given per day in two divided doses<br>**Group B:** ($n = 30$)<br>curcumin tablets (Turmix; curcuma longa extract: 300 mg and piper nigrum: 5 mg) one tablet thrice daily per day | 3 months | **Group A:** Lycopene<br>B: 3.17 ± 0.08 cm<br>A: 3.52 ± 0.07 cm<br>**Group B:** Curcumin<br>B: 3.32 ± 0.07 cm<br>A: 3.52 ± 0.08 cm | **Group A:** Lycopene<br>B: 65.83 ± 3.98<br>A: 0.00 ± 0.00<br>**Group B:** Curcumin<br>B: 62.33 ± 5.22<br>A: 0.00 ± 0.00 | Lycopene showed better results than curcumin in improving mouth opening; both drugs were equally effective in decreasing burning sensation in OSF patients. Lycopene and curcumin were safe, nontoxic, and effective alternatives to conventional drugs. |

| | | | | | | | |
|---|---|---|---|---|---|---|---|
| Johny et al. [33] | Nonrandomized controlled trial<br>Lycopene<br>Lycopene + hyaluronidase | 45 OSF patients (with Grade 2 OSF) | **Group A:** ($n$ = 15):<br>LycoRed™, containing 100% natural lycopene, with zinc, selenium, and phytonutrients) 16 mg daily<br>**Group B:** ($n$ = 15):<br>LycoRed™ along with hyaluronidase (Hynidase) intralesional injection 1500 IU twice weekly<br>**Group C:** ($n$ = 15):<br>Placebo capsules | 6 months | % in improvement<br>**Group A:** Lycopene<br>100% complete response<br>**Group B:** Lycopene with hyaluronidase<br>100% complete response<br>**Group C:** Placebo<br>46.2% | % in improvement<br>**Group A:** Lycopene<br>100% partial response<br>**Group B:** Lycopene with hyaluronidase<br>7.2% complete response and remaining partial response<br>**Group C:** Placebo<br>38.5%—partial response, 30.8% stable, 30.8% showed progression | Hyaluronidase with lycopene when compared with lycopene only showed better results but it was not statistically significant. The authors suggest that lycopene appears to be a very promising antioxidant in the management of oral submucous fibrosis, both in clinical and symptomatic improvement. |
| Bhowmick et al. [40] | Clinical prospective study<br>Lycopene<br>Lycopene + Hyaluronidase | 50 OSF patients<br>Counseled to quit the areca nut practice.<br>Mouth exercises advised. | **Group A:** ($n$ = 25)<br>Lycopene (Cap Lycored™) 8 mg daily in two equally divided dose<br>**Group B:** ($n$ = 25)<br>Lycopene (Cap Lycored™) 8 mg daily in two equally divided doses + intralesional injections of 1500 IU of Hyaluronidase (Hynidase) weekly | 3 months | **Group A:** Lycopene<br>B: 25.20 ± 3.01 mm<br>A: 29.36 ± 3.17 mm<br>**Group B:** Lycopene + Hyaluronidase<br>B: 24.58 ± 3.90 mm<br>A: 32.41 ± 3.22 mm | **Group A:** Lycopene<br>B: 7.16 ± 0.96<br>A: 0.88 ± 0.72<br>**Group B:** Lycopene + Hyaluronidase<br>B: 6.47 ± 1.10<br>A: 0.20 ± 0.12 | Combination therapy of lycopene with intralesional corticosteroids was comparatively more effective in relieving clinical symptoms. |
| Antioxidant: Curcumin | | | | | | | |
| Hazarey et al. [53] | Randomized clinical trial<br>Curcumin<br>Clobetasol propionate | 30 OSF patients with mouth opening 15–30 mm<br>Counseled to quit the areca nut practice<br>Physiotherapy for both groups using a mouth exercise device (MED). The patients were instructed to exercise for 20 min (10 min on each side) with the help of the MED three times a day for 3 months. | **Test group:** ($n$ = 15)<br>400 mg curcumin (Longvida lozenges) 2 g of daily dosage<br>**Control group:** ($n$ = 15)<br>Topical clobetasol propionate (Tenovate™) 3 times daily | 3 months | **Test group:** Curcumin<br>B: 21.13 ± 4.54 mm<br>A:27.06 ± 4.80 mm<br>**Control group:** clobetasol propionate<br>B: 23.93 ± 2.98 mm<br>A:26.6 ± 4.06 mm | **Test group:** Curcumin<br>B: 64 (42–73)<br>A: 7 (3–24)<br>**Control group:** clobetasol propionate<br>B: 34 (14.5–64.5)<br>A: 8 (3.5–37) | Curcumin was effective and the results achieved were sustained through a follow-up span of 9 months.<br>A combination strategy comprising curcumin treatment + physiotherapy + areca nut cessation provides favorable outcome. |

(continued)

**Table 16.1** (continued)

| Author | Type of study[a] | Sample | Intervention | Duration of treatment/ Follow-up | Mouth opening assessment (Measured with vernier caliper) B: baseline; A: after intervention; F: after follow-up | Burning sensation assessment (Measured with visual analog scale, VAS) B: baseline; A: after the intervention; F: after follow-up | Observations reported by authors |
|---|---|---|---|---|---|---|---|
| Piyush et al. [52] | Randomized placebo-controlled parallel clinical study<br>Curcumin<br>Lycopene<br>Placebo | 90 OSF patients | **Group A:** ($n$ = 30)<br>curcumin (300 mg) twice daily<br>**Group B:** ($n$ = 30)<br>Lycopene capsules (8 mg) twice daily<br>**Group C:** ($n$ = 30)<br>Placebo capsules once daily | Active treatment:6 months<br>Clinical evaluation:<br>9 months | **Group A:** Curcumin<br>B:25.40 ± 7.2 mm<br>A:29.35 ± 8.8 mm<br>**Group B:** Lycopene<br>B:24.43 ± 6.6 mm<br>A: 28.57 ± 7.2 mm<br>**Group C:** Placebo<br>B:28.97 ± 9.7 mm<br>A:30.37 ± 10.7 mm | **Group A:** Curcumin<br>B: 6.03 ± 3.1<br>A: 1.17 ± 1.2<br>**Group B:** Lycopene<br>B:6.80 ± 2.2<br>A: 1.77 ± 1.5<br>**Group C:** Placebo<br>B:5.80 ± 2.4<br>A:4.23 ± 2.2 | The therapeutic efficacy of curcumin and lycopene therapeutic were found to be almost equal. |
| Antioxidant: Aloe vera | | | | | | | |
| Patil et al. [63] | Prospective study<br>Lycopene<br>Aloe vera | 120 OSF patients<br>Counseled to quit the areca nut practice. | **Group A:** ($n$ = 60)<br>8 mg lycopene (Lycored™) in two divided doses of 4 mg<br>**Group B:** ($n$ = 60)<br>5 mg aloe vera gel topically thrice daily | 3 months | **Group A:** Lycopene<br>B: 18.2 ± 2.1 mm<br>A: 25.9 ± 2.3 mm<br>**Group B:** Aloe vera<br>B: 17.7 ± 2.2 mm<br>A: 22.1 ± 1.9 mm | **Group A:** Lycopene<br>B: present: 60<br>A: present:7, absent:32, reduced:21<br>**Group B:** Aloe vera<br>B: present: 60<br>A: present:9, absent:29, reduced:22 | Lycopene comparatively showed better improvements than aloe vera. Though few patients reported nausea with lycopene, it was well tolerated. |
| Nerkar Rajbhoj et al. [54] | Randomized clinical trial<br>Curcumin<br>Aloe vera | 60 OSF patients<br>Counseled to quit the areca nut practice. | **Group A:** ($n$ = 30)<br>5 mg curcumin gel (Curenext oral gel) 1 mg applied 3–4 times a day to achieve a total of 5 mg per day<br>**Group B:** ($n$ = 30)<br>5 mg Aloe Vera gel (1 mg of gel 3–4 times a day) | 6 months | **Group A:**<br>Curcumin gel<br>B: 30.5 ± 6.30 mm<br>A: 32.23 ± 6.25 mm<br>**Group B:** Aloe Vera gel<br>B: 31.500 ± 6.74 mm<br>A: 32.867 ± 6.66 mm | **Group A:** Curcumin<br>B: 7.50 ± 1.55<br>A: 4.43 ± 1.81<br>**Group B:** Aloe Vera<br>B: 7.33 ± 1.47<br>A: 2.83 ± 1.66 | Reduction in burning sensation was statistically significant in the aloe vera group when compared to the curcumin group. Both can be an effective alternative to conventional treatment. |
| Antioxidant: Spirulina | | | | | | | |
| Shetty et al. [66] | Intervention study<br>Spirulina + Betamethasone<br>Placebo + Betamethasone | 40 OSF patients<br>Counseled to quit the areca nut practice. | **Group A:** ($n$ = 20)<br>Spirulina 500 mg orally twice daily<br>**Group B:** ($n$ = 20)<br>placebo capsules orally twice daily<br>Inj. Betamethasone 4 mg/ml biweekly for both groups | 3 months | **Group A**: Spirulina<br>B: 31.05 mm<br>A: 36.8 mm<br>**Group B**: Placebo<br>B: 32.95 mm<br>A: 35.8 mm | **Group A:** Spirulina<br>B: 5.8<br>A:4.6<br>**Group B:** Placebo<br>B:5.3<br>A:2.65 | Comparatively better improvement in clinical symptoms was observed in Spirulina group. |

| | | | | | | | |
|---|---|---|---|---|---|---|---|
| Mulk et al. [65] | Randomized clinical trial<br>Pentoxifylline<br>Spirulina | 40 OSF patients<br>20 min of mouth exercise was advised. | **Group 1:** ($n$ = 20)<br>Oral pentoxifylline 400 mg twice daily<br>**Group 2:** ($n$ = 20)<br>Oral spirulina capsules 0.5 g twice daily | 4 months | **Group 1:**<br>Pentoxifylline<br>B:2.63 ± 0.78 mm<br>A:2.93 ± 0.77 mm<br>**Group 2:**<br>Spirulina<br>B:3.38 ± 1.29 mm<br>A:3.73 ± 1.26 mm | **Group 1:**<br>Pentoxifylline<br>B:6.05 ± 1.67<br>A:1.60 ± 0.94<br>**Group 2:**<br>Spirulina<br>B:6.95 ± 1.00<br>A:1.55 ± 1.32 | Spirulina fared better in reducing burning sensation while statistically nonsignificant results were recorded with mouth opening.<br>The authors state that spirulina is relatively safe over pentoxifylline as it is known to cause adverse effects. |
| Patil et al. [64] | Randomized clinical trial<br>Spirulina<br>Aloe vera | 42 OSF patients<br>Counseled to quit the areca nut practice. | **Group A:** ($n$ = 21)<br>500 mg spirulina in two divided doses<br>**Group B:** ($n$ = 21)<br>Aloe vera gel 5 mg topically thrice daily | 3 months | **Group A:** Spirulina<br>B: 19.9 ± 2.1 mm<br>A: 25.8 ± 2.5 mm<br>**Group B:** Aloe vera<br>B: 19.1 ± 2.7 mm<br>A: 23.9 ± 1.9 mm | **Group A:** Spirulina<br>B: present:21<br>A: present:3, absent:12, reduced:6<br>**Group B:** Aloe vera<br>B: present:21<br>A: present:5, absent:9, reduced: 7 | Though similar reduction in burning sensation was noted, spirulina fared better in improving mouth opening. |
| Vasodilators: Pentoxifylline (PTX) | | | | | | | |
| Mehrotra et al. [75] | Randomized controlled trial<br>Placebo (Multivitamin)<br>Pentoxifylline | 62 OSF patients<br>Counseled to quit the areca nut practice. | **Group A:** ($n$ = 30)<br>placebo (multivitamin) therapy<br>**Group B:** ($n$ = 32)<br>Tab. Pentoxifylline 400 mg for 7 months (inductive regime for the initial 30 days at a reduced dosage of 2 tablets daily followed by 3 tablets daily for 6 more months) | Treatment duration:<br>7 months<br>Clinical follow-up:<br>18 months | Mouth opening improved by 15.4% in placebo group and 35.7% in PTX | Burning sensation improved by 39.4% in placebo group and 86.6% in PTX. | Authors reported a statistically significant improvement in PTX group.<br>No local or systemic side effect were found in the placebo treatment group. However, side effects were observed with the use of PTX. The most frequent side effects were dyspepsia and nausea, which were observed in 24% of the patients.<br>Bloating and flatus were the complaints of 18% of patients and headache, vomiting, anxiety, and tremors were observed in 2% of patients. These symptoms were relatively mild in nature, lasted for 1–2 weeks, and settled on their own without cessation of drug or requiring medication. |

(continued)

**Table 16.1** (continued)

| Author | Type of study[a] | Sample | Intervention | Duration of treatment/ Follow-up | Mouth opening assessment (Measured with vernier caliper) B: baseline; A: after intervention; F: after follow-up | Burning sensation assessment (Measured with visual analog scale, VAS) B: baseline; A: after the intervention; F: after follow-up | Observations reported by authors |
|---|---|---|---|---|---|---|---|
| Patil et al. [85] | Prospective study<br>Pentoxifylline<br>Placebo<br>(Multivitamin) | 106 OSF patient | **Group A:** ($n$ = 53)<br>400 mg pentoxifylline twice daily<br>**Group B:** ($n$ = 53)<br>Placebo (Multivitamins) | 3 months | **Group A:** PTX<br>B: 20.2 ± 2.1 mm<br>A: 27.1 ± 2.3 mm<br>**Group B:** Placebo<br>B: 20.9 ± 2.1 mm<br>A: 24.9 ± 2.1 mm | **Group A:** PTX<br>B: present 53, absent 0, reduced 0<br>A: present 16, absent 23, reduced 14<br>**Group B:** Placebo<br>B: present 53, absent 0, reduced 0<br>A: present 27, absent 17, reduced 9 | The patients in PTX group showed significant improvement in all the parameters measured, mouth opening, tongue protrusion, pain associated with the condition, burning sensation, and difficulty in speech and swallowing.<br>However, few patients from PTX complained of bloating, nausea, anxiety, and dyspepsia. |
| Prabhu et al. [83] | Randomized clinical trial<br>Pentoxifylline + Conventional therapy<br>Conventional therapy | 30 OSF patients | **Interventional group:** ($n$ = 15)<br>PTX initial 15 days of 2 tablets daily followed by 3 tablets daily + Conventional therapy (intralesional corticosteroid, hyaluronidase, and placentrix injections + local heat therapy and mouth stretching exercises)<br>**Control group:** ($n$ = 15)<br>conventional therapy alone | 4 months | **Interventional group:** PTX<br>B: 19.93 ± 3.13 mm<br>A:21.00 ± 4.12 mm<br>**Control group:**<br>Conventional therapies<br>B:22.93 ± 3.56 mm<br>A:23.80 ± 2.91 mm | **Interventional group:** PTX<br>B: 0.93 ± 0.88<br>A:0.40 ± 0.51<br>**Control group:** Conventional therapies<br>B:1.00 ± 0.85<br>A:0.33 ± 0.49 | PTX presented vasodilatation at the histological level; however clinical improvement is at par with other drugs.<br>Its use is questionable given the long duration of treatment and its response. |

| | | | | | | | |
|---|---|---|---|---|---|---|---|
| Sadaksharam et al. [86] | Single-blinded randomized clinical trial<br>Pentoxifylline<br>Dexamethasone + Hyaluronidase | 30 OSF patients Counseled to quit the areca nut practice. | **Group A:** ($n$ = 15)<br>Oral pentoxifylline 400 mg thrice daily after meals for 3 months<br>**Group B:** ($n$ = 15)<br>0.5 ml of local anesthesia with 2 ml of dexamethasone + 1500 I.U of hyaluronidase biweekly for 6 weeks | Clinical follow-up: 6 months | **Group A:** PTX<br>B: 25.66 ± 5.33 mm<br>A: 30.20 ± 6.03 mm<br>**Group B:**<br>Dexamethasone + Hyaluronidase<br>B: 27.20 ± 5.70 mm<br>A: 29.93 ± 5.80 mm | **Group A:** PTX<br>B: 6.66 ± 2.58<br>A: 0.00 ± 0.00<br>**Group B:**<br>Dexamethasone + Hyaluronidase<br>B: 6.53 ± 2.26<br>A: 0.13 ± 0.35 | Both groups reported satisfactory improvement. A highly significant reduction in burning sensation, improvement in mouth opening, and changes in submucosal thickness were noticed in both groups, and significant improvement in echogenicity in both groups was noticed. However, the pentoxifylline group showed marginally better improvement than the dexamethasone group. PTX being well tolerated, noninvasive, and cost-effective could be considered as an alternative where intralesional steroids or hyaluronidase is contraindicated. |
| Bhambal et al. [87] | Prospective case-control clinical study<br>Pentoxifylline<br>Multivitamin | 80 OSF patients Counseled to quit the areca nut practice. | **Experimental drug group (EDX):** ($n$ = 40)<br>Pentoxifylline (Trental) 200 mg thrice daily for the first 30 days followed by 400 mg thrice daily for 2 more months<br>**Standard drug group (SDX):** ($n$ = 40)<br>Multivitamin capsules (B-complex one capsule before sleep daily) | 3 months | **EDX:** Pentoxifylline<br>B:26.79 ± 7.8 mm<br>A:29.13 ± 7.87 mm<br>**SDX:** Multivitamin<br>B:25.75 ± 7.93 mm<br>A:26.96 ± 7.33 mm | **EDX:**<br>Pentoxifylline<br>Mean ranks<br>B:33.97<br>A:26.94<br>**SDX:** Multivitamin<br>B:31.03<br>A:38.06 | Pentoxifylline was found to be a superior drug to the multivitamin drug. Hence it is suggested as an additional therapy in the routine management of OSF. |
| Bishnoi et al. [89] | Randomized clinical trial<br>Pentoxifylline<br>Multivitamin | 40 OSF patients Counseled to quit the areca nut practice. | **Study Group:** ($n$ = 20)<br>Pentoxifylline extended-release tablets, 400 mg twice daily<br>**Control group:** ($n$ = 20)<br>Multivitamin capsule twice daily after food | 3 months | **Study group:** Pentoxifylline<br>B: 26.32 ± 4.34 mm<br>A: 30.48 ± 4.28 mm<br>**Control group:** Multivitamin<br>B: 25.57 ± 3.97 mm<br>A: 26.17 ± 3.61 mm | **Study group:** Pentoxifylline<br>B: 4.1 ± 1.34<br>A: 2.3 ± 1.31<br>**Control group:** Multivitamin<br>B: 4.3 ± 1.53<br>A: 3.9 ± 1.95 | Pentoxifylline showed a significant increase in mouth opening, decrease in burning sensation, and pain as compared with multivitamin capsules. However, occasional gastrointestinal disturbances reported may lead to poor patient compliance. Pentoxifylline can be safer and better alternative treatment for oral submucous fibrosis. |

(continued)

16

**Table 16.1** (continued)

| Author | Type of study[a] | Sample | Intervention | Duration of treatment/ Follow-up | Mouth opening assessment (Measured with vernier caliper) B: baseline; A: after intervention; F: after follow-up | Burning sensation assessment (Measured with visual analog scale, VAS) B: baseline; A: after the intervention; F: after follow-up | Observations reported by authors |
|---|---|---|---|---|---|---|---|
| Vasodilators: Isoxsuprine | | | | | | | |
| Bhadage et al. [91] | Randomized controlled trial<br>Isoxsuprine<br>Dexamethasone + Hyaluronidase<br>Placebo (fine sugar) | 40 OSF patients<br>Counseled to quit the areca nut practice.<br>Physiotherapy was advised. | **Group A:** ($n = 15$)<br>Oral 10 mg isoxsuprine tablets (Tablet Duvadilan) 4 times a day<br>**Group B:** ($n = 15$)<br>intralesional injections of 2 ml dexamethasone (Injection Dexona) + 1500 IU hyaluronidase (Injection Hyalase) twice a week bilaterally<br>**Group C:** ($n = 10$)<br>orally placebo capsules containing fine sugar | Duration of treatment: 6 weeks<br>Follow-up: 4 months | **Group A:** Isoxsuprine<br>B: 26.5 ± 8.5 mm<br>A: 29.2 ± 8.9 mm<br>F: 29.5 ± 8.9 mm<br>Average improvement: 4 mm<br>**Group B:** Dexamethasone + Hyaluronidase<br>B: 22.9 ± 3.5 mm<br>A: 26.7 ± 3.1 mm<br>F: 26.9 ± 3.1 mm<br>Average improvement: 3 mm<br>**Group C:** Placebo<br>B: 28.3 ± 6.7 mm<br>A: 28.5 ± 6.8 mm<br>F: 29.0 ± 7.1 mm | **Group A:** Isoxsuprine<br>B: 5.53 ± 3.13<br>A: 0.53 ± 1.41<br>F: 0.67 ± 1.80<br>**Group B:** Dexamethasone + Hyaluronidase<br>B: 5.80 ± 2.93<br>A: 0.00 ± 0.00<br>F: 0.00 ± 0.00<br>**Group C:** Placebo<br>B: 5.80 ± 1.03<br>A: 5.20 ± 1.62<br>F: 0.00 ± 0.00 | Though dexamethasone and hyaluronidase injections alleviate pain at a faster pace, the benefit of isoxsuprine is that it does not require frequent visits to the clinic.<br>Oral isoxsuprine, as well as dexamethasone with hyaluronidase injections combined with physiotherapy, alleviate symptoms of oral submucous fibrosis. significantly more efficiently than physiotherapy alone.<br>They suggest that dexamethasone and hyaluronidase may hold a risk of tissue atrophy and injury while isoxsuprine may present with systemic effects with large doses of administration. |
| Biogenic stimulation: Placental extract | | | | | | | |
| Katharia et al. [94] | Prospective study<br>Placental extract | 22 OSF patients | 2 ml of Inj. Placental extract (Inj.Placentrex) was given locally in predetermined areas once a week | 1 month | Based on mouth opening scores<br>B: 5.13 ± 0.29 mm<br>A: 3.68 ± 0.25 mm | B: 2.81 ± 0 10<br>A: 1.68 ± 0.13 | Maximum improvement (40.21%) was observed in burning sensation followed by 38.55% in mucosal color; 30.59% in fibrous bands; 28.26% in mouth opening and 18.46% in protrusion of the tongue. Statistically significant changes were observed with improvement in mouth opening, change in color, and reduction in fibrous band. |

| | | | | | | | |
|---|---|---|---|---|---|---|---|
| Naik et al. [97] | Comparative case series analysis<br>Triamcinolone + Hyaluronidase<br>Placental extract | 60 OSF patients | **Group A:** ($n = 30$)<br>Triamcinolone acetonide (10 mg/ml) + hyaluronidase (1500 IU) at weekly intervals<br>**Group B:** ($n = 30$)<br>2 ml of placentrex injection intralesionally at weekly interval | 8 weeks | **Group A:** Corticosteroid<br>B: 16.27 mm<br>A: 35.9 mm<br>**Group B:**<br>Placentrex<br>B: 15.83 mm<br>A: 33.8 mm | **Group A:** Corticosteroid<br>B:2.36<br>A: 0.96<br>**Group B:**<br>Placentrex<br>B:2.56<br>A: 0.86 | A combination of triamcinolone acetonide and intralesional hyaluronidase was more effective than intral-esional placental extract in the treatment of OSF. However, placental extract injections are cost-effective. No side effects were seen in both study groups. |
| Raj et al. [98] | Longitudinal study<br>Placental extract | 24 OSF patients | **Group A:** ($n = 12$)<br>patients with inter-incisal mouth opening (MO) of less than 25 mm (moderately advanced OSF).<br>**Group B:** ($n = 12$)<br>patients with inter-incisal mouth opening between 26 and 30 mm (moderate OSF).<br>Patients of both groups received 2 ml of placental extract submucosal injection alternatively on right and left buccal mucosa once a week. | 10 weeks | **Group A:**<br>MO < 25 mm<br>B: 22.5 mm<br>A: 27.08 mm<br>Avg.increase:4.58 mm<br>**Group B:**<br>MO 26–30 mm<br>B: 27.5 mm<br>A: 33.67 mm<br>Avg.increase: 6.16 mm | All the patients had moderate to severe burning sensations during their first visit. After treatment, there was reduction in the severity of the burning sensation; with occurrence of mild burning sensation while having spicy food. | The authors conclude that the treatment of OSF with placental extract injection is more effective in moderate fibrosis compared to moderately advanced fibrosis. The placental extract is also helpful in reducing the burning sensation in OSF patients. |
| Dinesh et al. [99] | Prospective study<br>Placental extract | 30 OSF patients | 2 ml of Inj. Placentrex (0.1–0.8 gm, % nitrogen/ml) is given submucosally using a 2 ml syringe with a 24-gauge needle retromolar trigone once a week | 4 weeks | Mean inter-incisal distance (Mean ± SD)<br>B: 2.13 ± 0.74 cm<br>A: 2.74 ± 0.78 cm<br>Improvement (%): 28.63% | B: 2.2 ± 0.71<br>A: 0.9 ± 0.88<br>Improvement (%): 51% | Significant improvement in mouth opening, color of the mucosa, tongue protrusion, and reduction in burning sensation is observed with the use of the placental extract. The authors conclude that placental extract produces long-standing effects and can be used in the early stages of oral submucous fibrosis with good results. |
| Shah et al. [101] | Retrospective study<br>Placental extract + Dexamethasone<br>Hyaluronidase + Dexamethasone | 25 OSF patients (Stage III OSF) | **Group A:** ($n = 15$)<br>placental extract (2 ml) + dexamethasone (4 mg/ml)<br>**Group B:** ($n = 10$)<br>hyaluronidase (1500 IU) + dexamethasone (4 mg/ml) | 8 weeks | **Group A:**<br>B: 26.5 ± 6.52 mm<br>A: 30.03 ± 6.42 mm<br>**Group B:**<br>B: 21.7 ± 6.29 mm<br>A: 25.35 ± 7.11 mm | **Group A:**<br>B: 6.67 ± 0.97<br>A: 1.53 ± 0.99<br>**Group B:**<br>B: 6.40 ± 1.17<br>A: 1.50 ± 1.71 | The pre- and post-treatment differences were found to be statistically significant for both groups ($p < 0.05$). Both the treatment regimens studied were equally effective in the treatment of OSF. |

(continued)

**Table 16.1** (continued)

| Author | Type of study[a] | Sample | Intervention | Duration of treatment/ Follow-up | Mouth opening assessment (Measured with vernier caliper) B: baseline; A: after intervention; F: after follow-up | Burning sensation assessment (Measured with visual analog scale, VAS) B: baseline; A: after the intervention; F: after follow-up | Observations reported by authors |
|---|---|---|---|---|---|---|---|
| Priyankar et al. [100] | Randomized single-blinded comparative study<br>Placental extract<br>Dexamethasone<br>Hyaluronidase | 30 OSF patients (stage II) | **Group A:** ($n = 10$)<br>2 ml intralesional placental extract (Placentrex) mixed with 2 ml of 2% lignocaine HCL weekly<br>**Group B:** ($n = 10$)<br>Intralesional injection of dexamethasone 1.5 ml, mixed with 2 ml of 2% lignocaine HCL weekly.<br>**Group C:** ($n = 10$)<br>Intralesional hyaluronidase 1500 IU mixed with 2 ml of 2% lignocaine HCL weekly.<br>Patients were advised to do mouth opening exercises for 30 min daily without any dropout | 2 months | **Group A:** Placentrex<br>B: 18.49 ± 2.75 mm<br>A: 26.51 ± 4.10 mm<br>Avg. improvement: 8.02 mm<br>**Group B:** Dexamethasone<br>B: 17.11 ± 3.15 mm<br>A: 24.39 ± 4.43 mm<br>Avg. improvement: 7.28 mm<br>**Group C:** Hyaluronidase<br>B: 16.94 ± 2.45 mm<br>A: 26.14 ± 3.05 mm<br>Avg. improvement: 9.20 mm | **Group A:** Placentrex<br>B: 8.00 ± 0.65<br>A: 3.10 ± 1.05<br>**Group B:** Dexamethasone<br>B: 8.70 ± 1.05<br>A: 2.00 ± 0.35<br>**Group C:** Hyaluronidase<br>B: 8.70 ± 0.65<br>A: 5.50 ± 1.01 | Improvement in mouth opening was observed maximum with intralesional injection of hyaluronidase followed by placental extract and then dexamethasone.<br>Improvement in burning sensation was observed maximum with intralesional injection of dexamethasone followed by placental extract and comparatively less improvement was seen with hyaluronidase. |
| Shinde et al. [102] | Prospective randomized single-blinded study<br>Placental extract<br>Triamcinolone acetonide | 40 OSF patients<br>Counseled to quit the areca nut practice. | **Group P:** ($n = 20$)<br>intralesional injections of 2 ml aqueous placental extract bilaterally at weekly intervals<br>**Group T:** ($n = 20$)<br>triamcinolone acetonide (40 mg/ml; 1 ml) bilaterally at weekly intervals | 10 weeks | **Group P:** Placental extract<br>B:21.25 mm<br>A:25.15 mm<br>**Group T:** Triamcinolone<br>B:21.50 mm<br>A:25.20 mm | **Group P:** Placental extract<br>B: 67.50<br>A: 35.50<br>**Group T:** Triamcinolone<br>B:66.50<br>A:25.50 | Intralesional triamcinolone acetonide was found to be a superior intralesional drug when compared to placental extract. |
| Kale et al. [103] | Randomized clinical trial<br>Triamcinolone + Hyaluronidase<br>Placental extract | 60 cases diagnosed with OSF with mild to moderately restricted mouth opening | **Group A:** ($n = 30$)<br>Intralesional regimen of injection triamcinolone 40 mg and hyaluronidase 1500 IU<br>**Group B:** ($n = 30$)<br>2 ml injection of placental extract alone<br>Both the groups were treated with oral antioxidants and physiotherapy simultaneously along with intralesional injections. | 6 weeks<br>Follow-up: 3 months | Improvement in mouth opening (mm)<br>**Group A:** Corticosteroid—10 mm<br>**Group B:** Placental extract—7 mm | **Group A:** Corticosteroid<br>21 patients showed 75% improvement and 7 patients between 50 and 75%<br>**Group B:** Placental extract—14 patients showed 75% improvement and 11 patients between 50 and 75% | Improvement in mouth opening and reduction in burning sensation was better with the use of corticosteroid than placental extract.<br>However, no significant difference was observed between the two drug regimens.<br>The authors suggest that intralesional injection can give symptomatic relief and in addition, cessation of habits, antioxidants oral hygiene helps in the improvement of OSF. |

| | | | | | | | |
|---|---|---|---|---|---|---|---|
| Vitamins and micronutrients | | | | | | | |
| Thakur et al. [109] | Prospective clinical study<br>Micronutrient supplements + Physiotherapy exercises<br>Physiotherapy exercises<br>Micronutrient supplements | 64 OSF patients<br>Counseled to quit the areca nut practice. | **Group I:** ($n = 24$) micronutrient supplement (vitamins, minerals, and omega-three fatty acid) in the form of capsule MMO3 + physiotherapy exercises four times per day at an interval of 2–3 h<br>**Group II:** ($n = 24$): physiotherapy exercises four times per day at an interval of 2–3 h<br>**Group III:** ($n = 24$): micronutrients supplements alone | 6 weeks | Maximum improvement in group I followed by III and then group II. | Groups I and III showed improvement within the first week of intervention | Micronutrients along with physiotherapy substantially improved the mouth opening. |
| Nallapu et al. [106] | Comparative study<br>Dexamethasone + Hyaluronidase + Lignocaine<br>Dexamethasone + Hyaluronidase + Lignocaine + Vitamin E | 20 OSF patients | **Group A:** ($n = 10$)<br>Intralesional bilateral injections of dexamethasone 2 ml (2 mg/ml), hyaluronidase (1500 IU), and 0.2 cc lignocaine (2%) weekly once<br>**Group B:** ($n = 10$)<br>Intralesional injections of dexamethasone + hyaluronidase + lignocaine + oral vitamin E capsules of 400 IU once daily | 8 weeks | **Group A:** Dexamethasone + Hyaluronidase + Lignocaine<br>Post-treatment:<br>5-moderate, 4-mild,1-no improvement<br>**Group B:** Dexamethasone + Hyaluronidase + Lignocaine + Vitamin E<br>Post-treatment:<br>2-excellent, 5-moderate, 3-mild | **Group A:** Dexamethasone + Hyaluronidase + Lignocaine<br>B: Absent-0;<br>Present-10<br>A: Absent-9;<br>Present-1<br>**Group B:** Dexamethasone + Hyaluronidase + Lignocaine + Vitamin E<br>B: Absent-0; present-10<br>A: Absent-10; present-0 | Vitamin E with conventional therapy presented better results. |
| Nayak et al. [108] | Clinical prospective study<br>Lycopene<br>Lycopene + Vitamin E<br>Placebo | 72 OSF patients<br>Counseled to quit the areca nut practice. | **Group A:** ($n = 24$)<br>8 mg of lycopene soft gels (Lycored TM) in two equally divided doses<br>**Group B:** ($n = 24$)<br>8 mg of lycopene + vitamin E (400 I.U.) + selenium (200 mcg) in two equally divided doses (LYC-O-MATO soft gels)<br>**Group C:** Placebo capsules once daily | Treatment period:<br>3 months<br>Clinical follow-up:<br>2 months | **Group A:** Lycopene<br>B: 24.80 mm<br>A: 32.60 mm<br>**Group B:** Lycopene + Vitamin E<br>B: 24.60 mm<br>A: 33.60 mm<br>**Group C:** Placebo<br>B: 25.10 mm<br>A: 27.10 mm | **Group A:** Lycopene<br>A: present-4;<br>Absent-20<br>**Group B:** Lycopene + Vitamin E<br>A: present-2;<br>absent-22<br>**Group C:** Placebo<br>A: present- 8;<br>absent −16 | Lycopene when combined with vitamin E presented with better efficacy suggesting noninvasive management yielding significant improvement. |

(continued)

**Table 16.1** (continued)

| Author | Type of study[a] | Sample | Intervention | Duration of treatment/ Follow-up | Mouth opening assessment (Measured with vernier caliper) B: baseline; A: after intervention; F: after follow-up | Burning sensation assessment (Measured with visual analog scale, VAS) B: baseline; A: after the intervention; F: after follow up | Observations reported by authors |
|---|---|---|---|---|---|---|---|
| Raizada et al. [110] | An open-labeled randomized controlled trial<br>Placebo<br>Omega 3 | 48 clinically confirmed OSF patients | **Group A:** ($n$ = 24) placebo (lactose capsule) for 3 months<br>**Group B:** ($n$ = 24) 1gm of omega 3 (flaxseed oil) three times daily<br>Both the groups received biweekly intralesional injections of dexamethasone 1.5 ml and hyaluronidase 1500 IU mixed with lignocaine for 6 weeks | 3 months | Mean interincisal distance (Mean ± SD)<br>**Group A:** Placebo: 24.46 ± 5.43 mm<br>**Group B:** Omega 3: 25.46 ± 4.3 mm | Scoring with VAS<br>**Group A:** Placebo: 8.54 ± 1.53<br>**Group B:** Omega 3: 8.58 ± 1.5 | Statistically significant improvement in inter-incisal distance, burning sensation, tongue protrusion, and cheek flexibility was observed in patients receiving omega 3 when compared to those receiving placebo. Omega 3 in conjunction with intralesional injections is an effective therapy when compared to intralesional injections alone in treatment of patients with OSF (grade II and III) with no side effects. |
| Novel therapies:<br>Oxitard, a herbal antioxidant that contains the extracts of *Mangifera indica, Withania somnifera, Daucus carota, Glycyrrhiza glabra, Vitis vinifera,* powders of *Emblica officinalis* and *Yashada bhasma*, and oils of *Triticum sativum.* | | | | | | | |
| Patil et al. [117] | Prospective, randomized, and single-blind study<br>Oxitard<br>Aloe vera | 120 OSF patients Counseled to quit the areca nut practice. | **Group A:** ($n$ = 60) 2 oxitard capsules twice daily<br>**Group B:** ($n$ = 60) 5 mg aloe vera gel topically thrice daily | Medical management: 3 months<br>Clinical follow-up: 2 months | **Group A:** Oxitard<br>B: 19.1 ± 2.4 mm<br>A: 31.5 ± 2.9 mm<br>**Group B:** Aloe vera<br>B: 17.7 ± 2.2 mm<br>A: 22.1 ± 1.9 mm | Reported no significant improvement in burning sensation [$p$ = 0.002] among both the groups. | Significant improvement in mouth opening, burning sensation, tongue protrusion, difficulty in swallowing and speech, and pain associated with the lesion was reported in oxitard group compared to the aloe vera group. However, the authors reported that 8 patients in oxitard group experienced mild abdominal discomfort. No other side effects were reported. |

| | | | | | | | |
|---|---|---|---|---|---|---|---|
| Patil et al. [116] | Prospective study<br>Oxitard<br>Placebo | 120 OSF patients<br>Counseled to quit the areca nut practice. | **Group A:** ($n$ = 60)<br>2 oxitard capsules twice daily<br>**Group B:** ($n$ = 60)<br>placebo tablets twice daily | 3 months | **Group A:** Oxitard<br>B: 19.1 ± 2.4 mm<br>A: 31.5 ± 2.9 mm<br>**Group B:** Placebo<br>B: 20.1 ± 2.1 mm<br>A: 23.1 ± 1.9 mm | **Group A:** Oxitard<br>B: present:60, absent-0, reduced −0<br>A: present:3, absent-43, reduced −14<br>**Group B:** Placebo<br>B: present:60, absent-0, reduced −0<br>A: present:24, absent-20, reduced −16 | Oxitard capsules can bring about significant clinical improvements in the symptoms like mouth-opening, tongue protrusion, burning sensation, difficulty in swallowing and speech, and pain associated with the lesion thereby improving the quality of life of the affected individuals.<br>Changes in the severity of burning sensation, difficulty in swallowing and speech, and pain were noted but were poorly defined in the absence of a recognized and validated pain scale. |
| Novel therapies: Colchicine | | | | | | | |
| Krishnamoorthy et al. [19] | Randomized controlled trial<br>Colchicine + Hyaluronidase<br>Hyaluronidase + Hydrocortisone acetate | 50 OSF patients | **Group 1:**<br>Tablet colchicine orally, 0.5 mg twice daily and 0.5 ml intralesional injection Hyaluronidase 1500 IU into each buccal mucosa once a week.<br>**Group 2:**<br>0.5 ml intralesional injection Hyaluronidase 1500 IU and 0.5 ml intralesional injection Hydrocortisone acetate 25 mg/ml in each buccal mucosa once a week alternatively. | 12 weeks | ----------- | Thirty-three percent in group 1 got relief from burning sensation in the second week | Intergroup comparisons of increase in mouth opening and reduction in histological parameters indicated that patients who received colchicine with steroids responded better than patients who received corticosteroid injections alone. |
| Daga et al. [125] | Comparative study<br>Colchicine + Hyaluronidase<br>Colchicine + Triamcinolone acetonide | 30 OSF (Grade II) patients<br>Counseled to quit the areca nut practice. | **Group A:** ($n$ = 15)<br>Tablet colchicine 0.5 mg twice daily + intralesional injection of hyaluronidase 1500 IU weekly interval for 12 weeks<br>**Group B:** ($n$ = 15)<br>Tablet colchicine 0.5 mg twice daily + intralesional injection of triamcinolone acetonide 10 mg/ml at weekly intervals for 12 weeks. | Duration of treatment: 12 weeks<br>Outcome assessment was done at intervals of 3 weeks, 6 weeks, 3 months, and 6 months. | **Group A:**<br>increase of about 8 mm after 6 months of follow-up<br>**Group B:**<br>increase of about 5 mm after 6 months of follow-up | **Group A:**<br>Significant reduction except in 2 patients<br>**Group B:**<br>Persisted in 6 patients | The use of injection hyaluronidase with oral colchicine yielded better results in terms of increase in mouth opening and improvement in burning sensation without notable side effects. |

[a] Type of study: as described by the author

## 16.2 Anti-inflammatory Agents

### 16.2.1 Corticosteroids

OSF is characterized by an initial phase of inflammation that progresses to fibrosis in the advanced stages. A systematic review of the medical interventions of OSF conducted by More et al. [4] shows that among all the interventions, corticosteroids have been widely used to reduce the burning sensation and pain symptoms. Kerr et al. [2] reviewed a total of 21 studies that used immunomodulatory agents to reduce the inflammatory component: 16 of these used injectable corticosteroids and 19 studies included the use of proteolytic enzymes to reduce fibrosis of which seven studies used hyaluronidases [2]. In Indian studies, steroids are the most commonly adopted medical treatment for OSF. Steroids have immunosuppressive and anti-inflammatory properties. They inhibit the action of soluble factors released by sensitized lymphocytes following activation by specific antigens and facilitate apoptosis of inflammatory cells. They reduce profibrotic inflammation and enhance profibrolytic immune-mediated pathways.

Several corticosteroids such as short-acting (hydrocortisone), intermediate-acting (triamcinolone), and long-acting (betamethasone and dexamethasone) have been utilized for the treatment of oral submucous fibrosis [5]. Most authors report their use in the early stages when a patient presents with a burning sensation. The topical corticosteroids commonly used are triamcinolone acetonide (0.1%), or Betamethasone (0.5%) applied locally for 3 months. In the advanced stage of the disease when palpable fibrous bands appear, submucosal injection of dexamethasone—4 mg/ml or triamcinolone diacetate—10 mg/ml, is given at multiple sites of the fibrosis, twice a week for 3 months. Hydrocortisone and methylprednisolone (20 mg/0.5 ml) have also been used as submucosal injections [3, 6].

16

Hyaluronidase degrades hyaluronic acid and lowers the thickness of intercellular cemental substances. Combination of corticosteroid and hyaluronidase shows better results in OSF due to deeper penetration of the steroid [3, 7]. Veedu et al. compared the effects of two conventional therapies, namely, submucosal injections of hyaluronidase (1500 I.U), dexamethasone (8 mg), or a combination of both (750 I.U and 4 mg), for a duration of 5 weeks. The authors concluded that hyaluronidase provided relief of the symptoms more rapidly [8]. Panigrahi et al. in their prospective study found that submucosal injection of a combination of triamcinolone acetonide and hyaluronidase is superior to triamcinolone alone, with respect to improvement in symptoms and patient convenience [9]. Goel et al. performed a hospital-based longitudinal study, on 270 OSF patients for a duration of 2 years. They proposed that both submucosal betamethasone and oral lycopene resulted in a significant enhancement in mouth opening. In stage II OSF patients, they found that the betamethasone group showed greater improvement in mouth opening of 9.47 ± 2.47 mm than the lycopene group where the average improvement of mouth opening was 6.07 ± 2.00 mm ($p < 0.0001$). In stage III, the lycopene group had a significant average improvement of mouth opening of 6.53 ± 1.45 mm compared to injection betamethasone group patients who showed an average improvement in mouth opening of 3.27 ± 1.36 mm ($p < 0.0001$). In both test groups capsule lycopene showed better results compared to injection betamethasone [10]. Intralesional injections of dexamethasone, hyaluronidase, and chymotrypsin independently or in combinations show better outcomes than using a single drug regimen [5].

The limitation of injecting corticosteroids include pain, scar formation due to needle prick, and greater chances of relapse once the treatment is withdrawn. Topical formulations are not effective in the long-term. One study reported hypertrichosis from repeated triamcinolone injection [11].

## 16.3 Immunomodulators

### 16.3.1 Levamisole

Levamisole is an anthelmintic drug with a wide range of immunomodulatory actions which influence both humoral and cellular immunity. It has been reported to be beneficial in the early stages of OSF.

A randomized, single-blind clinical trial conducted by Jirge et al. compared 50 mg of oral levamisole, three times daily, for 3 consecutive days a week for 3 alternate weeks with an oral antioxidant [ANTOXID—containing beta carotene, selenium oxide, zinc sulfate, manganese, and copper]. The 45 participants included in this study were divided equally between three study groups: oral levamisole (group I), ANTOXID (group II), or a combination of oral levamisole with ANTOXID (group III). At the end of the intervention period of 15 weeks, there was an improvement in mouth opening by 7.1%, 6.7%, and 8.0% in groups I, II, and III, respectively. These gains were maintained on further evaluation 2 months later. There was also a significant reduction in burning sensations in all study groups. The levamisole group showed a significant reduction in burning sensation and improvement in mouth opening and also an improvement in serum IgA, IgM, and IgG levels [12]. Shinge et al. evaluated the efficacy of levamisole and antioxidants in 60 OSF patients as single and combined regimens. They found that the combined use of levamisole and antioxidant was more effective than use of levamisole or antioxidant alone [13].

### 16.3.2 Probiotic Agents

The use of probiotic agents, such as immunized cow's milk prepared by immunization of cows with human intestinal bacteria, has been proposed as a method of immunomodulation. Immunized milk contains vitamins such as vitamins A, C, B1, B2, B6, B12, nicotinic acid, pantothenic acid, folic acid, and elements iron, copper, and zinc. It suppresses inflammation and modulates cytokine production. 45 g of immunized milk powder twice a day for 3 months resulted in a significant improvement in the symptoms of OSF patients. The authors reported an increase of greater than 3 mm in mouth opening in 69% of their treated patients [6, 14–16].

## 16.4 Proteolytic/Fibrolytic Enzymes

Proteolytic enzymes are known to break down the cross-linking of collagen, which contributes to connective tissue fibrosis.

### 16.4.1 Hyaluronidase

Hyaluronidase degrades ECM hyaluronic acid, promotes the lysis of fibrin-formed coagulum, decreases the viscosity of intercellular cement substances, and decreases collagen synthesis. It is effective in reducing OSF symptoms and is often used in combination with steroids. It has been used as the first-line medical treatment in moderate grade of OSF [17, 18].

Krishnamoorthy et al. enrolled 50 patients and randomized them into two groups. Group 1 received intralesional injections of 1500 IU hyaluronidase mixed in 1 ml lignocaine (0.5 ml) injected submucosally into the buccal mucosa along with colchicine 0.5 mg twice daily and group 2 was given intralesional 0.5 ml of hydrocortisone acetate 25 mg/ml in addition to the hyaluronidase once a week for 12 weeks. Both groups received habit intervention. Thirty-three percent of patients in Group 1 had relief from the burning sensation in the second week. Group 1 patients responded better than Group 2 with an increase in mouth opening and improvement of histological parameters [19].

Cox and Zoellner compared the efficacy of physiotherapy and submucosal injections of a combination of hyaluronidase and corticosteroids in 54 Nepalese subjects. After 4 months, subjective and objective measures were compared with baseline. The physiotherapy group showed a significant increase in mouth opening but had no superior effect on subjective measures [20].

James et al. administered intralesional injection of dexamethasone 1.5 ml and hyaluronidase 1500 IU with 0.5 ml lignocaine biweekly for 4 weeks, to 27 OSF patients, with an average follow-up of 9 months. Improvement in mouth opening was observed with a net gain of 6 ± 2 mm (92%). There was a reduction in the burning sensation, pain, ulceration, and blanching of the oral mucosa. The authors concluded that submucosal injection of hyaluronidase with dexamethasone was an effective method of treating Grade III OSF [21].

### 16.4.2 Chymotrypsin

Chymotrypsin is a proteolytic enzyme (serine protease) found in the digestive systems of many organisms. It facilitates the cleavage of peptide bonds. Chymotrypsin is an end peptidase that hydrolyzes ester and peptide bonds. It has proteolytic and anti-inflammatory properties and has shown to provide some improvement in OSF symptoms [16, 22].

Ayub et al. compared the effectiveness of combined chymotrypsin and dexamethasone versus dexamethasone alone in patients with OSF. Their study included 146 OSF patients who were equally divided into two groups by a lottery method. Group A had 73 patients, treated with submucosal injection of a combination of chymotrypsin and dexamethasone, and group B, 73 patients treated with only dexamethasone, once a week for 1 month. Mouth opening was recorded on monthly follow-up without any other therapy for 3 months. Inter-incisal opening significantly increased by 3–5 mm in group A compared to group B suggesting that the combined regimen of chymotrypsin and dexamethasone was more effective than dexamethasone alone (74% vs. 57.5%) ($p = 0.036$) [23].

### 16.4.3 Collagenase

Collagenase is an enzyme capable of degrading various esters that are involved in the cross-linking of collagen. Clostridium histolyticum collagenase (Xiapex™) has been licensed for the treatment of fibrotic conditions, such as Dupuytren's contracture. It is highly potent in digesting collagen. Efficacy of collagenase in the treatment of Dupuytren's contracture was proven by Hurst et al. in their double-blind randomised control trial [24].

However, it is expensive, and the cost may preclude its availability in low-income countries.

Lin et al. studied the effect of collagenase treatment given as submucosal injections in 27 patients with well-developed OSF. They divided the patients into three groups (A, B, and C) with nine patients in each group: patients in group A, received phosphate-buffered saline (PBS) injection as a control; patients in group B were injected with 1 ml of triamcinolone diacetate (Ledercort) plus 1 ml of xylocaine and group C patients received 1 ml of collagenase (1% solution) mixed with 1 ml of xylocaine. All patients received their injections once a week for 6 weeks. The collagenase treatment not only resulted in a significant improvement of mouth opening, but also a striking reduction in hypersensitivity to spices, sour, cold and heat that helped restore normal eating in the study subjects. The mouth opening of patients who received PBS decreased approximately by 13–15% 6 weeks after the initial measurement. The OSF patients treated with triamcinolone diacetate or collagenase showed 9–13% and 64–82% increase in mouth opening, respectively. These results indicated that collagenase treatment was approximately fivefold more effective than triamcinolone diacetate alone [25].

## 16.5 Antioxidants in OSF

Constituents of betel quid generate substantial amounts of reactive oxygen species (ROS), which may create a biological imbalance between oxidants and antioxidants. OSF pathogenesis involves the accumulation of free radicals and production of lipid peroxides (LPO) [25]. On the basis of this hypothesis, several authors have used naturally occurring or synthetic antioxidants to treat OSF. Some of the agents that have been used include beta carotene, lycopene, tea pigments, aloe vera, curcumin, and spirulina.

16

### 16.5.1 Lycopene

Lycopene is a red carotenoid predominantly present in tomatoes and other pigment-containing vegetables and fruits [2–4]. It is a potent antioxidant and its antioxidant property is attributed to its high singlet oxygen quenching capacity with an increased propensity for quenching other free radicals *in vitro*. Experimental studies have established the role of lycopene in inhibiting cancer cell growth both *in vivo* and *in vitro* [27]. Lycopene has also been reported to be beneficial in the management of other potentially malignant oral disorders (e.g., oral leukoplakia and lichen planus) [16, 28, 29].

Kumar et al. recruited 83 participants who received either oral lycopene ($n = 21$; group A), oral lycopene with submucosal corticosteroids ($n = 19$; group B), or oral placebo tablets ($n = 18$; group C). The 2-month intervention period was completed by 58 people. Objective measurement of mouth opening improved with an average increase of 3.4 mm, 4.6 mm, and 0 mm for groups A, B, and C, respectively. The increases were maintained at 3- and 6-months follow-up. All patients who took lycopene reported relief of burning sensation within 2 weeks, whereas only one patient from the placebo group reported a similar improvement [30].

A randomized single-blind trial testing the effectiveness of lycopene was conducted in Maharashtra, India. Of the 92 participants enrolled, 46 were given 8 mg oral lycopene daily, and the rest were given a placebo tablet for 3 months and followed up for further 2 months. Significant improvement was reported with increase in mouth opening of 4.48 (±3.65) mm in the lycopene group compared with 1.13 (±1.6) mm in the control group, and 31% taking lycopene experienced a complete improvement in burning sensation compared with 7% in the control group [31].

A study by Beena et al. reported the effectiveness of dexamethasone and hyaluronidase to be superior to lycopene among 60 OSF patients [32]. However, as the lycopene group also showed improvement in mouth opening and reduction of burning sensation it may be used when dexamethasone is contraindicated due to medical comorbidities. Johny et al. evaluated the efficacy of lycopene and lycopene-hyaluronidase combination with placebo in the treatment of 45 OSF patients. There was a statistically significant improvement in mouth opening and burning sensation for lycopene and lycopene and hyaluronidase combination than in the placebo group in the treatment of OSF. The lycopene–hyaluronidase combination did not yield any statistically significant improvement when compared with lycopene alone [33]. Saran et al. compared the efficacy of oral lycopene with curcumin in 60 OSF patients. Lycopene showed better results than curcumin in improving mouth opening and both were equally effective in decreasing burning sensation in OSF patients [34]. Selvam et al. divided their cohort of 45 OSF patients into three groups: group A received oral lycopene with corticosteroid injections (dexamethasone + hyaluronidase), group B received oral antioxidant with corticosteroids, and group C received intralesional injections of dexamethasone and hyaluronidase. Lycopene used along with intralesional steroids was more effective in improving mouth opening compared to antioxidants with steroids [35]. Similarly, Elizabeth et al., in their study comparing the efficacy of lycopene with intralesional corticosteroids, found that lycopene in combination with intralesional steroids was more effective in improving mouth opening compared to intralesional steroid and hyaluronidase injections alone [36]. In a RCT of 30 OSF patients, Subramaniyam et al. found that the mean improvement in tongue protrusion (3.53 mm) and burning sensation (2.73 using VAS) was significantly better in patients who received lycopene compared to those who underwent ultrasound therapy (tongue protrusion: 1.46 mm; burning sensation: 1.4 using VAS). The mouth opening was better in the ultrasound group (6.20 mm) compared to lycopene groups (5.10 mm), but the results were not statistically significant [37]. Singh et al. demonstrated that lycopene capsules were better than intralesional betamethasone injections in improving mouth opening and decreasing burning sensation in their cohort of 44 OSF patients [38]. Arshad et al. compared the efficacy of lycopene with methyl predinisolone as single drug regimen and in combination and found that combination of lycopene and methyl prednisolone yielded favorable results than corticosteroid or antioxidant alone [39]. Bhowmick et al. and Kumar et al. compared the clinical response in patients receiving lycopene and lycopene with intralesional corticosteroids. Combination therapy of lycopene with intralesional corticosteroids was more effective in relieving the clinical symptoms [30, 40].

### 16.5.2 Curcumin (Turmeric)

Curcumin (diferuloylmethane) is a component of turmeric, a rhizomatous plant—Curcuma longa, which is widely used in Asian cooking. It exhibits antioxidant, anti-inflammatory, proapoptotic, and anticancer properties [41, 42]. It suppresses the action of nicotinamide adenine dinucleotide phosphate oxidase, which is responsible for the generation of reactive oxygen species (ROS). Curcumin modulates inflammatory response by reduction of cyclooxygenase-2 (COX-2), lipoxygenase, and inducible nitric oxide synthase (iNOS) enzymes. It also inhibits the synthesis of the inflammatory cytokines, tumor necrosis factor-alpha (TNF-alpha), IL-1, 2, 6, 8, 12, monocyte chemoattractant protein (MCP), and migration inhibitory protein [43]. A comprehensive description of the properties of curcumin is given by Girisa and Kunnumakkara in Chap. 17.

Kopuri et al. compared submucosal layer thickness using ultrasonography in 30 OSF patients treated with oral lycopene and curcumin for 3 months. At the end of 3 months, all patients in both groups showed significant improvement in mouth opening, burning sensation and blanching. The submucosal fibrous bands were reduced in thickness on ultrasonographic examination in both groups. The authors proposed that Lycopene was better than curcumin in the treatment of OSF [44].

Lanjekar et al. compared the efficacy of topical curcumin mucoadhesive semisolid gel, triamcinolone acetonide/hyaluronidase mucoadhesive semisolid gel, and a combination of both in the treatment of 120 OSF patients. The use of three drug combinations showed better improvement in mouth opening (mean increase of 4.05 mm) and change in mucosal color as compared to the other two groups. The triamcinolone and hyaluronidase group reported a better reduction in burning sensation as compared to the other two groups. Curcumin had a synergistic effect when combined with triamcinolone and hyaluronidase [45].

The safety of the administration of turmeric oil was established using nine healthy volunteers [46]. The same group reported a pilot trial in patients with OSF [47]. Rai et al. also reported an increase in local and systemic antioxidative status in OSF by curcumin [48].

The effect of curcumin was compared with submucosal steroid injections in an RCT [49]. The experimental arm ($n$ = 20) received curcumin orally: two tablets of a proprietary preparation film-coated tablet containing 300 mg Curcuma longa and 5 mg piperine) once daily for a period of 3 months. The control group received weekly submucosal injections of 4 mg dexamethasone and 1500 IU of hyaluronidase. Mouth opening improved by 3 mm in the curcumin group compared to control group (1.25 mm), and the burning sensation was significantly reduced in the curcumin group.

In another RCT, a combination of curcumin and turmeric oil was tested by Das et al. [50] Curcumin 1 g per day was given in two divided oral doses in one group, and a second group was given 12 drops of turmeric solution to hold in the mouth and then swallow twice daily. A control group received multivitamins 500 mg twice daily. Patients were followed up monthly for 6 months. Complete relief of pain was reported in both experimental groups after 1 month's treatment. A mean increase in mouth opening of 8.7 mm was noted in both test groups compared to a mean increase of 1.8 mm in the control group.

Pipaliya et al. compared the efficacy of turmeric and black pepper (Piper nigrum) together with black cumin (Nigella sativa) in 40 OSF patients. Turmeric with black pepper formulation showed better improvement than Nigella sativa. There was an improvement in the superoxide dismutase levels post-treatment in both groups [51].

Piyush et al. compared the efficacy of lycopene and curcumin with placebo in 90 OSF patients. Statistically significant improvement in clinical symptoms was observed in both curcumin and lycopene treatment groups in comparison with placebo [51].

Hazarey et al. compared the efficacy of curcumin lozenges with topical clobetasol propionate in 30 OSF patients. The curcumin group showed better improvement in mouth opening and reduction in burning sensation on follow-up of the patients 6 months after treatment [53].

However, Rajbhoj et al. compared the clinical response of 60 OSF patients to aloe vera and curcumin (30 in each group) and found that reduction in burning sensation was statistically significant in the aloe vera group when compared to the curcumin group [54].

### 16.5.3 Tulsi/Holy Basil (Ocimum tenuiflorum/Ocimum sanctum Linn)

Synergistic effects of Tulsi and turmeric paste was reported by Srivastav et al. in 41 OSF patients [55]. Madhulatha et al. evaluated the efficacy of 500 mg of herbal Tulsi paste, twice daily for a duration of 1 month among a cohort of twenty OSF patients [56]. Promising results of tulsi were demonstrated in both studies.

### 16.5.4 Aloe Vera (AV)

Aloe vera is an adaptogen, that helps in enhancing the immune system and is a rich source of vitamins, enzymes, minerals, sugars, lignin, saponins, salicylic acids, and amino acids. The vitamins A, C, and E in AV act as antioxidants and help to neutralize free radicals. AV also contains enzymes: alkaline phosphatase, amylase, bradykinase, carboxypeptidase, catalase, cellulase, lipase, and peroxidase [57, 58]. Bradykinase decreases inflammation on topical application. The gel of the leaves also has polysaccharides that promote wound healing and exhibit anti-inflammatory, anticancer, immunomodulatory, and gastroprotective properties. The anti-inflammatory action of aloe vera is due to the reduction of chemical mediators of inflammation like bradykinin, histamine, leukocyte adhesion, and TNF-α. It stimulates the production of hyaluronic acid and dermatan sulfate in the granulation tissue of a healing wound and imparts elasticity to the skin and mucosa [58].



Anuradha et al. evaluated the efficacy of systemic and topical AV to submucosal injection of hydrocortisone and hyaluronidase in 74 OSF patients for a duration of 6 weeks [59]. A statistically significant improvement in inter-incisal mouth opening was observed in both groups. The improvement in the VAS scale for burning sensation, tongue protrusion, and cheek flexibility were more significant in the AV group. Similar results were obtained by Sudarshan et al. and Singh et al. [60, 61].

Sudarshan et al. compared the effect of topical AV with an oral antioxidant capsule (beta-carotene, Vitamin E, C, zinc, copper, mixed carotenoids, chromium, manganese, selenium). Ten patients with OSF received topical application of aloe vera gel (5 mg applied three times daily to the buccal mucosa for 3 months) and 10 patients received antioxidant capsules twice daily. In the AV group, a 55–65% reduction in burning sensation and an improvement in mouth opening (4.3–7 mm) was observed [61].

Alam et al. studied the effectiveness of aloe vera gel as an adjunct to injection of a mixture of hyaluronidase and dexamethasone and surgical approaches in the treatment of OSF. Sixty patients were randomized to medicinal and surgical groups, and within each group ($n = 30$), half received the gel treatment. Improvements in both mouth opening and burning sensation were found in those treated with aloe vera [62]. However, when Patil et al., compared the efficacy of AV with lycopene in a cohort of 120 OSF patients, lycopene showed better improvement in mouth opening and reduction in burning sensation compared to AV [63].

### 16.5.5 Spirulina

Spirulina is a blue-green alga, with abundant vitamins (A and B12), minerals, carotenoids, and phycocyanin. Spirulina is known to reduce serum cholesterol levels. Spirulina increases IL-2 and decreases IL-6. It has chemopreventive properties due to the abundance of beta carotene and superoxide dismutase [58, 64–66]. Kanjani et al. in their study reported that the patients using a combination of physical exercise (mouth stretching) and spirulina 500 mg fared better than patients using spirulina alone in terms of burning sensation, mouth opening, tongue protrusion, and cheek flexibility [67]. Studies have shown that spirulina significantly improves the mouth opening, ulcers, erosions, and vesicles compared with those receiving topical aloe vera [64]; Spirulina also reduces the burning sensation compared with pentoxifylline [65]; and is more effective in improving both mouth opening and reducing burning sensation compared with a biweekly submucosal steroid injection of betamethasone (4 mg/ml for 3 months) [66].

Kulkarni et al. conducted a systematic review on the efficacy of spirulina in the management of OSF. Five studies were included in this systematic review. All five studies reported that spirulina is an effective herbal medicine in the improvement of mouth opening, reducing burning sensation, ulcers, erosions, or vesicles. In three studies spirulina was compared with lycopene, aloe vera, and oxitard™ When compared with lycopene and oxitard, spirulina was found to be less effective in improving mouth opening; however, spirulina was more effective than AV. The spirulina group also demonstrated better results for reducing oral lesions when compared with these three interventions. All were equally effective, in reducing burning sensation [68].

### 16.5.6 Tea Pigments

Oxidation of Polyphenols in tea leaves produces tea pigments. The tea pigments contain aflavins, which possess antioxidant, antineoplastic, and anti-inflammatory properties. Both polyphenols and flavins reduce the activity of nuclear factor-kappa B (NF-kappa B) and thereby regulate the expression of proinflammatory cytokines. Tea pigments are beneficial in OSF treatment as they augment the actions of superoxide dismutase, reduce blood viscosity and improve microcirculation [4, 69, 70]. Li et al. found tea pigments to be beneficial in patients with early stages of OSF. The authors suggest that in addition to their antioxidant properties, the tea pigments are likely to act by improving microcirculation [71].

### 16.5.7 Salvianolic Acid (Sal-B)

Radix Salviae miltiorrhizae (Danshen), the dried root of Salvia miltiorrhiza Bge is a popular traditional Chinese medicine. Salvianolic acid B (Sal-B) is the most abundant and bioactive member of the hydrophilic components in Danshen. Sal-B contains seven phenolic hydroxyls, which are responsible for its antioxidant activities [72]. Jiang et al. studied the efficacy of salvianolic acid B (Sal-B) combined with triamcinolone acetonide in the treatment of OSF. A net gain of 5.5 mm of mouth opening was reported in the Sal-B group in 20 weeks. However, this relapsed to 3.5 mm in 44 weeks. The exact antifibrosis mechanism of Sal-B is not known [11].

### 16.5.8 Epigallocatechin Gallate (EGCG)

EGCG is a plant-based potent antioxidant that protects the cell against cellular damage caused by free radicals. Hsieh and colleagues noted that EGCG dose-dependently inhibited arecoline-induced transforming growth factor 1 (TGF-β1) activation in Buccal Mucosal Fibroblasts (BMFs). BMFs exposed to arecoline result in the generation of mitochondrial ROS, which activate latent TGF-β1, and, in turn, stimulated Cell Communication Network Factor (CCN2) and early growth response-1 (Egr-1) synthesis. TGF-β1 plays a pivotal role in the pathogenesis of OSF; thus, EGCG may be useful in the prevention and treatment of OSF. Hsieh et al. noted that arecoline induces overexpression of Egr-1, which enhances the profibrotic activity seen in OSF [73]. EGCG was shown to completely block arecoline-induced Egr-1 expression in human BMFs [26].

## 16.6 Vasodilators

The rationale for the use of a peripheral vasodilators is that they relax and dilate the blood vessels in the stromal tissues, ensuring blood supply to the ischemic tissues which help the nutritional and therapeutic agents to reach the affected tissues. The agents that have been used in OSF include pentoxifylline [74, 75]. nylidrin hydrochloride [76], buflomedil hydrochloride [77], Danxuan Koukang [78], Xantinol nicotinate [79] and isoxsuprine [3, 80].

### 16.6.1 Pentoxifylline (PTX)

Pentoxifylline (PTX) is a methylxanthine derivative and a nonspecific type IV phosphodiesterase inhibitor. It is prescribed for intermittent claudication and is known to have properties that alter the course of wound healing. PTX increases fibroblast collagenases and decreases collagen, fibronectin, and glycosaminoglycan production. Fibroblast responsiveness to tumor necrosis factor is also diminished by PTX [81]. PTX enhances red cell deformability, leukocyte chemotaxis, anti-thrombin, and anti-plasmin activities, and suppresses red cell and platelet accretion, granulocyte adhesion, fibrinogen levels, and whole blood viscosity [82]. It enhances the production of prostaglandins (E2 and I2) by vascular epithelium which is critical in preserving cellular integrity and homeostasis after acute phase injury. All these properties are potentially beneficial in the atrophic and ischemic condition of the oral mucosa in OSF.

Rajendran et al. studied 29 OSF patients who were prescribed either oral pentoxifylline or multivitamins. All those enrolled completed the study during a 7-month period [74]. The authors reported statistically significant improvements in the oral pentoxifylline group ($n = 14$) compared with controls with respect to mouth opening, tongue protrusion, and relief from circum-oral fibrotic bands and subjective criteria (intolerance to spices, burning sensations, tinnitus, difficulty in swallowing, and difficulty in speech).

Prabhu et al. assessed the use of PTX on the clinical and histopathologic changes of 30 OSF patients in comparison to conventional therapies [83]. They did not observe any significant clinical and histopathological improvement in the PTX group. Treatment with PTX was not superior to other drug regimens and concluded that their study did not recommend PTX.

Several studies have reported side effects caused by PTX including central nervous system (dizziness, headache, tremor, anxiety, and confusion) and gastrointestinal (dyspepsia, nausea and/or vomiting, bloating, flatus, and bleeding) symptoms [81, 83].

Zwiri et al. conducted a study comparing the efficacy of spirulina (control) and PTX in 112 OSF patients. The maximal mouth opening increased from 21.6 mm at baseline to 27.9 after 3 months in PTX group [84].

Patil et al. in a prospective study compared the efficacy of pentoxifylline with placebo (multivitamin) in 106 OSF subjects. The cohort was divided into two groups: Group A ($n = 53$) was administered 400 mg pentoxifylline twice daily and Group B ($n = 53$) was given multivitamins for 3 months. They reported a significant ($p < 0.05$) improvement in mouth opening, tongue protrusion, speech and swallowing, pain associated with the lesion, and burning sensation in OSF patients [85].

Sadaksharam et al. evaluated the therapeutic efficacy of oral PTX and dexamethasone in the treatment of 30 OSF patients [86]. The width of the submucosal layer and its echogenicity were assessed by ultrasonography, prior to and after treatment. Equivocal improvement was obtained in both groups. Nevertheless, the PTX group exhibited better results than the dexamethasone group. Therefore, the authors proposed, PTX as a safer substitute when intralesional steroids are intolerable or contraindicated.

16

Bhambhal et al. compared the efficacy of oral PTX 400 mg to placebo-multivitamin capsules, in 80 OSF patients [87]. Relief from pain, and burning sensation, was significant. No significant changes were observed with respect to mouth opening, tongue protrusion, cheek flexibility, or blanching of the mucosa in PTX group.

Mehrotra et al. report on 32 patients given pentoxifylline for a period of 7 months (initial 30 days dosage of 400 mg twice daily, increased to 400 mg three times daily for 6 months). The placebo group ($n = 30$) was given multivitamin therapy. They report improved mouth opening by 10 mm with pentoxifylline compared with 6 mm with multivitamins [75]. The improvement in total score (Subjective and Objective) was 25% in placebo and 49% in PTX group. This difference was found to be statistically significant. ($p < 0.05$). Central nervous system side effects such as dizziness, headache, tremor, anxiety, and confusion and gastrointestinal (dyspepsia, nausea and/or vomiting, bloating, flatus, and bleeding) were reported in a few patients [75, 86, 88].

Bishnoi et al. reported that patients on PTX showed a significant increase in mouth opening, decrease in burning sensation, and pain as compared with those on multivitamin capsules [89].

Leelakshi et al. in a cross-sectional study administered 400 mg PTX and two garlic pearls thrice daily for 2 months in 10 OSF patients. Patients exhibited a mean reduction of 95.68% in burning sensation and an increase of 5.37 mm in mouth opening. The cheek flexibility and tongue protrusion also showed significant improvements in the study groups [90].

### 16.6.2 Nylidrin Hydrochloride

Nylidrin hydrochloride marketed in India under the brand name "Arlidin" is available in tablet and injectable forms. "Arlidin" with its active component, nylidrin hydrochloride, is a peripheral vasodilator, that increases blood supply to ischaemic tissues with little or no change in blood pressure or heart rate of the individual. It has been used favorably in Meniere's disease, deafness, dementia, retinopathy, peripheral vascular disease, and premature labor. Sharma et al. in their study on Nylidrin hydrochloride (Arlidine™) in 58 cases of oral submucous fibrosis (6 mg orally), reported clinical improvement in 62% of patients. Side effects included flushing and warm skin in some patients [76].

### 16.6.3 Isoxsuprine

Isoxsuprine, a vasodilator was combined with physiotherapy, and compared with submucosal injections of dexamethasone with hyaluronidase and physiotherapy or physiotherapy alone in OSF patients [91]. Isoxsuprine was given for 6 weeks, with a 4-month follow-up period. Both isoxsuprine and dexamethasone with hyaluronidase treatments significantly alleviated the burning sensation and increased mouth opening by approximately 3 mm.

### 16.6.4 Xantinol Nicotinate

Xantinol nicotinate is a derivative of niacin. It is a vasodilator used to treat peripheral vascular disease. Singh et al. determined the efficacy and safety of intralesional Xantinol nicotinate with a placebo in the treatment of various stages of OSF. The patients had a significant respite from burning sensation and enhancement in the mouth opening, tongue protrusion, and cheek flexibility [79].

### 16.6.5 Buflomedial Hydrochloride

Buflomedial, a peripheral vasodilator, has been found to favourably affect tissues with diffuse fibrosis by improving local ischemia. Lai et al. observed positive treatment outcome for OSF using buflomedial (3 tablets of 450 mg each per day) and topical triamcinolone acetonide 0.1% on mucosal ulcers [77].

## 16.7 Biogenic Stimulation

### 16.7.1 Placental Extract

Intralesional placental extracts act by biogenic stimulation of the metabolic regenerative process of tissue. It was first used by Filatov in 1933. Aqueous extract of human placenta stimulates the pituitary and the adrenal cortex and regulates tissue metabolism [92, 93].

Placentrex™ is available as an injectable aqueous extract of human placenta that contains: (1) Enzymes: alkaline and acid phosphatase, glutamic oxaloacetic acid transaminase, glutamic acid, and pyruvic acid transaminase. (2) Nucleotides: RNA, DNA, and ATP. (3) Vitamins: Vit. E, B1, B2, pantothenic acid, biotin, PABA, folic acid, B12, choline and inositol. (4) Amino acids: Alanine, asparagine, asparagenic acid, cysteine, glyceine, histidine, leucine, lysine, phenylalanin, proline, serine, threonine, tryptophan, tryosine and valine. (5) Steroids: ketosteroids, cholestrin and cholesterol. (6) Fatty acids. (7) Trace elements, Sodium, K, Ca, Mg, Cu, Fe, P and Si [94].

Placental extract is anti-inflammatory and has significant analgesic action. It increases blood circulation and tissue vascularity. Placentrex contains Vitamin E, which has antioxidant properties. Vitamin A plays a major role in the induction and control of epithelial differentiation. Vitamin A slows, delays, arrests, reverses malignant potential and along with Vitamin E improves the mucosal color, mouth opening, and reduces fibrous bands [95].

Ramanjaneyalu and Rao used 2 cc placentrex injection at weekly intervals for 10 weeks in OSF patients. They found it to be superior to intralesional cortisone injections. They reported two cortisone-resistant cases that responded favorably to Placentrex [96].

Katharia et al. in an observational study, injected 2 ml of Placentrex locally in predetermined areas of oral mucosa, once a week for a total duration of 1 month in 22 OSF patients. A significant improvement in the mouth opening (28%) and the color of the oral mucosa (38 %) ($p < 0.01$) with a reduction in the fibrotic bands was observed [94].

Naik et al. reported a better improvement in mouth opening in OSF patients who were given intralesional 2 ml of placentrex at weekly intervals for 8 weeks when compared to OSF patients who received a combination of triamcinolone acetonide (10 mg/ml) + hyaluronidase (1500 IU) at weekly intervals for 8 weeks [97].

Raj et al. in a longitudinal study observed that treatment of OSF with placental extract injection was more effective in moderate fibrosis compared to moderately advanced fibrosis [98]. Significant improvement in mouth opening, color of the mucosa, tongue protrusion, and reduction in burning sensation was observed by Dinesh et al., in a prospective study where 30 OSF patients were administered 2 ml injection placental extract (Inj. Placentrex) submucosally [99]. Priyankar et al. in their cohort of 60 Stage II OSF patients reported maximum improvement in mouth opening with intralesional injection of hyaluronidase (MO = 9.20 mm) followed by placental extract (MO = 8.02 mm) and then dexamethasone (MO = 7.28 mm). They also reported that maximum improvement in burning sensation was observed with intralesional injection of dexamethasone followed by placental extract and the least improvement was seen with hyaluronidase [100].

Singh et al. used 2 ml submucosal injections of placental extract mixed with 2 ml of 2% lignocaine HCL weekly for an interval of 8 weeks and showed an average improvement in mouth opening by 8 mm (average pretreatment mouth opening of 8 mm and average posttreatment mouth opening of 26 mm) with a marked reduction in burning sensation [61].

Shah et al. divided their cohort of 25 patients into two study groups: Group A (placental extract + dexamethasone) and Group B (hyaluronidase + dexamethasone). In Groups A and Group B, the average increase in mouth opening from the baseline record to the eighth week of treatment was $3.53 \pm 1.26$ mm and $3.65 \pm 1.42$ mm respectively and the average decrease in burning sensation, as noted by VAS scale, was $5.13 \pm 1.13$ and $4.90 \pm 1.29$, respectively. The pre- and posttreatment differences were found to be statistically significant for both the groups ($p < 0.001$) and for both treatment outcomes [101].

Shinde et al. conducted a randomized, parallel-group, single-blinded outcome-based study, in a cohort of 40 cases of OSF. The patients were divided into two groups of 20 each: placental extract group and triamcinolone acetonide group, administered intralesionally for 10 weeks. There was a significant improvement in burning sensation, pain, mouth opening, tongue protrusion, and cheek flexibility in both groups. Better and earlier improvement in tongue protrusion and cheek flexibility was achieved in the triamcinolone group as against the placental extract group [102].

Kisave et al. evaluated the efficacy of Placentrex and hydrocortisone injection in two groups: Group A had 30 patients injected with 2 ml of placentrex in the areas where fibrous bands were present, twice a week for 3 months. Group B comprised of 30 patients injected with 2 ml of hydrocortisone twice a week for 3 months. A statistically significant difference in the mean mouth opening (5.19 ± 1.33 in Group A and 11.69 ± 1.26 mm in Group B; $p = 0.0001$) was observed. The authors concluded that hydrocortisone was better in increasing the mouth opening compared to placentrex. However, placentrex reduced the burning sensation more effectively than hydrocortisone [95]. They concluded that local injection of placentrex was safe, cheap, and effective without any significant side effects or contraindications. It has a long-lasting effect and can be administered in the early stages of OSF [95].

Similarly, Kale et al., observed that improvement in mouth opening was better with corticosteroids compared to placental extract; however, in their study, the difference between the study groups were not statistically significant [103].

## 16.8 Micronutrients (Vitamins and minerals)

Vitamins and minerals treat the deficiency states and promote normal cellular processes present in health that help to protect against adverse events, including carcinogenesis. Vitamins (A, B complex, C, D, E) are known to accelerate ulcer healing and relieve symptoms in OSF.

Minerals including zinc and magnesium are essential components for many enzymes and play a crucial role in DNA synthesis and cell division. Zinc controls the complex effects of copper-associated lysyl oxidase upregulation, while magnesium stabilizes excitable membranes. Multivitamins, micronutrients, and antioxidants are effective in controlling the signs and symptoms of OSF [16]. Antioxidants, nutrients, and micronutrients therapy (AONMT) is based on the rationale that reactive oxygen species (ROS) found in areca nut may damage the cellular structure, including lipids and cell membranes, proteins, and nucleic acids resulting in pathological processes. Micronutrient deficiencies impede the healing of inflamed oral mucosa leading to mucosal atrophy which becomes more susceptible to the effects of areca nut.



### 16.8.1 Vitamins

Vitamin A, C, and E are antioxidants that aid in scavenging free radicals. Beta-carotene, an important precursor of vitamin A, when combined with vitamin E has been shown to be effective in increasing mouth opening and tongue protrusion. In one study, treatment with topical vitamin A 50,000 IU in the form of chewable tablets once daily and oral ferrous fumarate tablets in a dose of 200 mg once daily were found to be safe and effective [104]. Vitamin E given concomitantly with submucosal hyaluronidase and betamethasone was better than hyaluronidase and betamethasone alone [105]. The efficacy of vitamin E is attributed to its antioxidant property. Nallapu et al. showed that the addition of vitamin E (400 IU once daily, for a period of 8 weeks) had a significant synergistic effect with the submucosal injections of dexamethasone 2 ml (2 mg/ml) and hyaluronidase (1500 IU) in 0.2 cc lignocaine (2%) [106]. Singh reported that vitamin C given in combination with placentrex and liver extract gave better results than vitamin C alone. It has been suggested that Vitamin C reduces the edema between the collagen bundles and helps in the regeneration of new normal collagen bundles [107]. Nayak et al. conducted a prospective study in 72 OSF patients to compare the clinical outcome of lycopene and lycopene with vitamin E. Lycopene when combined with vitamin E was better in reducing the burning sensation and improving mouth opening [108]. Thakur et al. in a clinical prospective study of 64 OSF patients reported that micronutrients (vitamins, minerals, and omega-three fatty acid) along with physiotherapy substantially improved the mouth opening compared to the use of micronutrients or physiotherapy as sole treatment modality [109].

Raizada et al. conducted an open labeled randomized controlled trial in 48 OSF patients divided into two groups (24 in each group) to study the effectiveness of omega 3 in the treatment of OSF. Group A received a placebo (lactose capsule) for 3 months while group B received 1gm of omega 3 (flaxseed oil) three times daily continuously for 3 months. Patients of both groups were given biweekly intralesional injections of dexamethasone 1.5 ml and hyaluronidase 1500 IU mixed with lignocaine for 6 weeks. After 3 months, statistically significant ($p < 0.05$) improvement among all three clinical parameters, i.e., inter-incisal distance (mean improvement in group $A$ = 3.79 ± 1.07 mm and group $B$ = 6.58 ± 1.24 mm, $p = 0.019$), tongue protrusion (mean improvement in group $A$ = 1.87 ± 1.54 mm and group $B$ = 4.62 ± 1.78 mm, $p = 0.044$), and cheek flexibility (mean improvement in group $A$ = 2.08 ± 1.38 mm and group $B$ = 3.50 ± 1.84 mm, $p = 0.035$) was observed. A significant improvement in burning sensation was observed after 1 month itself in group B when compared to group A (mean drop in group $A$ = 2.5 ± 0.78 points and group $B$ = 6.0 ± 1.144 points, $p < 0.05$). The authors concluded that Omega 3 in conjunction with intralesional injections can be an effective therapy when compared to intralesional injections alone in treating patients with OSF (grade II and III) [110].

### 16.8.2 Minerals

Many studies have shown decreased levels of hemoglobin and serum ferritin in OSF [111]. Iron supplements in patients with anemia can improve the nutritional status of OSF patients and alleviate the burning sensation by correcting epithelial atrophy [4]. Maher et al. reported that micronutrient supplements: vitamins A, B complex, C, D, E; and minerals iron, calcium, copper, zinc, and magnesium were effective ($p < 0.05$) in reduction of signs and symptoms of OSF over a period of 3 years [112].

Dhariwal et al. reported that diet supplementation with zinc acetate along with vitamin A, in a 24-year-old OSF patient, increased mouth opening and reduced burning sensation in the 4 months follow-up period. Histopathologically re-epithelialization was evident along with the appearance of normal rete pegs. The data for mouth opening, collagen content, and epithelial thickness of six other cases similarly treated also showed a significant increase in mouth opening and epithelial thickness and a decrease in collagen content. The authors proposed the use of zinc acetate and vitamin A for the management of OSF [113]. Anil et al. administered Zinc (220 mg) in combination with vitamin A and observed good results in OSF. Zinc plays an essential role in DNA synthesis and cell division [114].

### 16.8.3 Oxitard ™

This is an ayurvedic antioxidant, which contains extracts of "Mangifera indica, Withania somnifera, Daucus carota, Glycyrrhiza glabra, Vitis vinifera, Emblica officinalis and Yashada bhasma, and Triticum sativum." "Mangifera indica" has antibiotic and antiviral action. "Withania somnifera" supresses anxiety, stress, and inflammation. "Daucus carota" is a potent source of vitamin A. "Glycyrrhiza glabra" suppresses the inflammation and is an immunostimulant. "Vitis vinifera" decreases inflammation and burning sensation. "Emblica officinalis" contains vitamin C and "Yashada bhasma" contains zinc which enhances wound healing and cell renewal. "Triticum sativum" contains potent minerals which suppresses oxidative stress [115]. Patil et al. compared the effectiveness of Oxitard capsules with a placebo in the treatment of OSF [116]. The authors concluded that the Oxitard group displayed a significant improvement in the subjective signs and symptoms. Additionally, they also reported improvement in dysphagia and speech articulation.

Oxitard was shown to be the most effective in improving mouth opening [MD, 10.29 (95% CI 6.34–14.25)] followed by a combination therapy of lycopene, hyaluronidase and corticosteroids [MD, 7.07 (95% CI 1.82–12.31)]. Two studies reported abdominal discomfort in eight patients due to Oxitard [75]. Patil et al. in a prospective, randomized single-blinded study observed a significant improvement in mouth opening, tongue protrusion, reduction in burning sensation, difficulty in swallowing and speech, and pain associated with the lesion in oxitard group compared to the aloe vera group [117].

### 16.8.4 Garlic

Garlic (*Allium sativa* L.) is a bulbous flowering plant that belongs to the family of Amaryllidaceae and is a horticultural crop originating from central Asia. Garlic and its products are used for culinary and therapeutic purposes in many countries. Bulbs of raw garlic have been investigated for their role in oral health, which are ascribed to a myriad of biologically active compounds it has such as alliin, allicin, methiin, S-allylcysteine (SAC), diallyl sulfide (DAS), S-ally-mercapto cysteine (SAMC), diallyl disulfide (DADS), diallyl trisulfide (DATS), and methyl allyl disulfide. Garlic has anti-inflammatory, antioxidant, antibacterial, antiviral, antifungal, and antimutagenic properties [118].

Jiang et al., gave submucosal injection of thio-2-propene-1-sulphinic acid S-allyl ester for 16 weeks to their cohort of 26 patients in stage II oral submucous fibrosis. The net gain in mouth opening was 5.16 ± 1.04 mm, burning sensation and the oral health impact profile score improved [119]. In another clinical trial, 15 patients with oral submucosal fibrosis were given pentoxifylline (400 mg) for 3 months with garlic pearls thrice daily. Patients had a 95% reduction in burning sensation and a 5 mm increase in the mouth opening [120].

Jain et al. systemically administered oral Pentoxifylline (400 mg) thrice daily along with garlic pearls, (2 pearls; thrice daily) after food for 3 months, in 15 OSF patients and observed a mean reduction of 95% in the burning sensation and increase of 5 mm in mouth opening. The cheek flexibility and tongue protrusion also showed significant improvements in the study groups [121].

## 16.9 Novel Therapies

### 16.9.1 Colchicine

Colchicine is a natural alkaloid derived from two plants of the lily family: Colchicum autumnale and Gloriosa superba, respectively known as meadow saffron and glory lily. Colchicine is an alternative therapeutic option for idiopathic recurrent aphthous stomatitis (RAS), especially when unresponsive to first-line treatments, such as topical or systemic corticosteroids. Additionally, colchicine might play a role in preventing oral aphthous-like ulcers associated with Bechet disease (BD) or immune-mediated disorders, such as periodic fever, aphthous stomatitis, pharyngitis, and cervical adenitis (PFAPA) syndrome and mouth and genitals ulcers with inflamed cartilage (MAGIC) syndrome [122].

Colchicine reduces collagen synthesis by disrupting microtubule formation and preventing extrusion of collagen from fibroblasts and increasing the activity of collagenase in the underlying submucosa. It neutralizes cytokines that synthesize collagen-like TGF-β, IL-6, and IL-4 [123, 124]. Krishnamoorthy et al. studied the effects of colchicine in two groups of 25 patients each. One group was given 0.5 mg colchicine orally twice daily with 0.5 ml submucosal injection Hyaluronidase 1500 IU into each buccal mucosa once a week. The second group was given 0.5 ml submucosal injection Hyaluronidase 1500 IU and 0.5 ml submucosal injection Hydrocortisone acetate 25 mg/ml in each buccal mucosa once a week alternately [19]. The group that had colchicine had better mouth opening and relief from burning sensation. However, the study by Daga et al. could not find any beneficial effect for systemic colchicine [125] except for improvement in the blanching of the mucosa. The side effects with Colchicine include diarrhea and gastrointestinal adverse events [126]. Colchicine should be used with caution in patients with medical comorbidities. Severe side effects are observed at higher doses and are not advised in subjects with liver disorders. Continuous monitoring of blood count, renal and liver function are required during the entire course of treatment.

16

### 16.9.2 Interferon Gamma (IFN-γ)

Interferon gamma has immuno-regulatory and anti-fibrotic effects and plays an important role in collagen metabolism. *In vitro* Increase in collagen synthesis in response to arecoline is inhibited by IFN-γ (0.01–10.0 U/ml) in a dose-dependent manner [127]. Studies of submucosal injection of 0.01–10.0 U/ml IFN-γ three times a day for 6 months have shown improvement of OSF symptoms. In an open uncontrolled study, submucosal IFN-γ treatment resulted in improvement in the patients' mouth opening: from a pretreatment inter-incisal distance of 21 ± 7 mm, to 30 ± 7 mm immediately after treatment and 30 ± 8 mm 6 months later, giving a net gain of 8 ± 4 mm (42%) (range 4–15 mm). There was also a decrease in burning and dysaesthesia, and increase in suppleness of the buccal mucosa. Post-treatment immunohistochemistry showed a decreased amount of inflammatory cell infiltrate and altered levels of inflammatory cytokines compared with the pre-treatment lesional tissue. However, prohibitive costs of IFN gamma precludes its use in low- and middle-income countries [15, 127].

### 16.9.3 Anti-TGF-β Drugs

Upregulation of TGF-β1, downregulation of bone morphogenic protein (BMP) and remodeling of ECM are characteristic features of the fibrotic process in OSF. The alkaloid and polyphenol components of areca nut induce and activate TGF-β1 in epithelial cells. Exposure to areca nut and stimulation of the TGF-β1 pathway are responsible for overproduction of collagen and decrease in degradation of collagen in OSF. TGF-β1 induces transcription of COL1A1 procollagen gene, increases activity of procollagen proteinases, and promotes the expression of lysyl oxidase (LOX), an enzyme essential for cross-linking collagen fibers. Furthermore, activated TGF-β1 induces myofibroblast transdifferentiation in OSF [128].

Upregulation of TGF-β1 has been described as a key mediator in the pathogenesis of OSF. Activated TGF-β1 induces myofibroblast transdifferentiation in OSF. Several key trials are underway using anti-TGF-β in other fibrotic disorders, e.g., idiopathic lung fibrosis. Drugs that are being developed include Imatinib, Pirfenidone (PFD), and Nintedanib. There have been no trials reported for OSF.

Few agents are discussed below:

- Imatinib

  Imatinib exerts its anti-fibrotic activity by interfering with TGF-β signaling pathways. It has been used successfully as an anti-fibrotic drug in preclinical models for the treatment of scleroderma [129, 130]. Therefore, it has been suggested that it can also be effective in OSF treatment [4].

- Pirfenidone (PFD)

  Pirfenidone (5(1H)-pyridone) is a novel anti-fibrotic agent with anti-inflammatory properties presently used in treating idiopathic lung fibrosis (ILF) which is an inflammatory condition mediated through transforming growth factor beta (TGF-β), like in OSF. PFD is hypothesized to be a novel anti-fibrotic agent beneficial in treating the early stages of OSF as both conditions are mediated through TGF-β. PFD acts by inhibiting tissue inhibitors of metalloproteinases-1 (TIMP1), proinflammatory cytokines TNF-α and fibroblast growth factor (b-FGF), which are upregulated in OSF [4, 128].

It has been hypothesized that PFD could reduce fibrosis in OSF by the following mechanisms:

1. Decreasing the levels of mRNA encoding type I and III collagen and also inhibiting TGF-β1-induced collagen production from fibroblasts [131].
2. Inhibiting tissue inhibitor of metalloproteinases-1 (TIMP1), which is upregulated in OSF [132, 133].
3. Suppressing proinflammatory cytokines TNF-α, which is upregulated in OSF [134, 135].
4. Downregulating fibroblast growth factor (b-FGF), which interacts synergistically with other growth factors enhancing the extracellular matrix deposition in OSF [136, 137].
5. Reducing the level of plasminogen activator inhibitor-1 (PAI-1), which is upregulated by TGF-β1 in OSF [138].

Nintedanib may be beneficial in OSF through the following mechanisms [4, 128]:

1. Directly preventing phosphorylation of TGF-β1 receptor and reducing excessive ECM production, which is a hallmark of OSF [139].
2. Targeting PDGF receptor-α and -β and thus reducing the level of PDGF, which is upregulated in OSF [140].
3. Targeting fibroblast growth factor receptor-1, −2, and − 3 and thereby reducing the level of fibroblast growth factor [141].

### 16.9.4 Valdecoxib

Valdecoxib is a novel selective cyclooxygenase-2 inhibitor used in the management of osteoarthritis, pain, and dysmenorrhea [142, 143]. Averineni et al. developed a mucoadhesive buccal film of valdecoxib for the treatment of OSF. This was a sustained release polymeric film of valdecoxib impregnated in Hydroxypropyl Methylcellulose (HPMC K4M) and chitosan polymers along with sodium taurocholate as a permeation enhancer for local action. Prepared films were thin, flexible, smooth, and transparent. Bioadhesive force and tensile strength of the optimized formulation were found to be $75 \pm 4$ kg $m^{-1}$ $S^{-2}$ and more than 2.5 kg/3 $cm^2$, respectively. The percent drug content was $98.5 \pm 1.3\%$. The *in vitro* drug release from the selected formulation showed that about 69.34% of the drug payload was released for up to 6 hours. Pharmacokinetic studies of the buccal mucoadhesive film showed that the drug was released locally at the target site of action, and very small amount is absorbed systemically.

### 16.9.5 Meta analysis of intervention in OSF

Gopinath et al. conducted a systematic review of randomized controlled trials (RCTs) that compared the efficacy of interventions for OSF [144]. A network meta-analysis was performed, and the interventions were ranked according to their efficacy based on the surface under the cumulative ranking. This systematic review included 32 RCTs comprising 2063 patients. Oxitard, a herbal formulation was ranked as the most efficacious agent in improving mouth opening, [MD, 10.29 (95%CI 6.34–14.25)] followed by combination therapy of Lycopene with corticosteroids and hyaluronidase [MD, 7.07 (95%CI 1.82–12.31)]. Aloe vera ranked first in reducing burning sensation [MD, 6.14 (95%CI 4.58–7.70)] followed by corticosteroids with antioxidants [MD, 6.13 (95%CI 4.12–8.14)] and corticosteroids in combination with hyaluronidase and antioxidants [MD, 5.95 (95%CI 3.79–8.11)].

**Summary and Conclusion**

A wide range of drugs have been used in the medical management of OSF—anti-inflammatory agents, immunomodulatory agents, corticosteroids, antioxidants, vasodilators, biogenic stimulators, fibrinolytic enzymes, vitamins, minerals, micronutrients, and herbal remedies. Many randomized controlled trials have been conducted to study the efficacy of these therapeutic agents as single or combined drug regimens. Most of the studies have short follow-up periods. There is minimal information on cessation of habits. No evidence on reduction in malignant transformation is provided by long-term follow-up studies. Combination of therapeutic agents used makes it difficult to assess the role of individual agents. None of the medical agents studied have yielded a consistent relief of signs and symptoms in OSF. However, the results reported from lycopene and curcumin trials are promising. The medical management of OSF for each patient varies, based on disease stage and individual response to treatment.

## References

1. Tilakaratne WM, Ekanayaka RP, Warnakulasuriya S. Oral submucous fibrosis: a historical perspective and a review on etiology and pathogenesis. Oral Surg Oral Med Oral Pathol Oral Radiol. 2016;122(2):178–91.
2. Kerr AR, Warnakulasuriya S, Mighell AJ, Dietrich T, Nasser M, Rimal J, Jalil A, Bornstein MM, Nagao T, Fortune F, Hazarey VH, Reichart PA, Silverman S, Johnson NW. A systematic review of medical interventions for oral submucous fibrosis and future research opportunities. Oral Dis. 2011;17(Suppl. 1):42–57.

3. Warnakulasuriya S, Kerr AR. Oral submucous fibrosis: a review of the current management and possible directions for novel therapies. Oral Surg Oral Med Oral Pathol Oral Radiol. 2016;122(2):232–41.
4. More CB, Jatti Patil D, Rao NR. Medicinal management of oral submucous fibrosis in the past decade: a systematic review. J Oral Biol Craniofac Res. 2020;10(4):552–68.
5. Awan KH, Patil S, Habib SR, Pejcic A, Zain RB. Evaluation of medicinal interventions for the management of oral submucous fibrosis: a systematic review of the literature. J Contemp Dent Pract. 2014;15(6):812–7.
6. Aishwarya V, Amudhan A, Amudhan A. Management of oral submucous fibrosis – An update. Eur J Mol Clin Med. 2020;7(5):1380–92.
7. Tsai CC, Ma RH, Shieh TY. Deficiency in collagen and fibronectin phagocytosis by human buccal mucosa fibroblasts in vitro as a possible mechanism for oral submucous fibrosis. J Oral Pathol Med. 1999;28(2):59–63.
8. Alora Veedu R, Balan A, Sankar SP. A randomized double-blind, multiple-arm trial comparing the efficacy of submucosal injections of hyaluronidase, dexamethasone, and combination of dexamethasone and hyaluronidase in the management of oral submucous fibrosis. Oral Surg Oral Med Oral Pathol. Oral Radiol. 2015;120(5):588–593 e1.
9. Panigrahi R, Maheshwari A. A prospective, randomized double-blind study comparing intralesional triamcinolone acetonide and hyaluronidase combination versus triamcinolone acetonide alone in the treatment of oral submucosal fibrosis. J Pharm Biomed Sci. 2014;4(4):365–70.
10. Goel S, Ahmed J. A comparative study on efficacy of different treatment modalities of oral submucous fibrosis evaluated by clinical staging in population of Southern Rajasthan. J Canc Res Therapeut. 2015;11(1):113–8.
11. Jiang XW, Zhang Y, Yang SK, Zhang H, Lu K, Sun GL. Efficacy of salvianolic acid B combined with triamcinolone acetonide in the treatment of oral submucous fibrosis. Oral Surg. Oral Med. Oral Pathol. Oral Radiol. 2013;115: 339–44.
12. Jirge V, Ali SM, Anshumalee N. Levamisole and antioxidants in management of oral submucous fibrosis: a comparative study. J Ind Acad Oral Med Radiol. 2009;20:135–9.
13. Shinge AA, Talreja PK, Das D, Navalkar A, Talreja PS, Kakade A. Comparative evaluation of the efficacy of systemic levamisole and antioxidant in the management of oral submucous fibrosis – A randomized control trial. J Adv Clin Res Insights. 2019;6(2):33–8.
14. Tai YS, Liu BY, Wang JT, Sun A, Kwan HW, Chiang CP. Oral administration of milk from cows immunized with human intestinal bacteria leads to significant improvements of symptoms and signs in patients with oral submucous fibrosis. J Oral Pathol Med. 2001;30:618–25.
15. Seema B. Etiopathogenesis and management of oral submucous fibrosis. Qual Primary Care. 2015;23(6):327–32.
16. Arakeri G, Rai KK, Boraks G, Patil SG, Aljabab AS, Merkx MAW, Carrozzo M, Brennan PA. Current protocols in the management of oral submucous fibrosis: an update. J Oral Pathol Med. 2017;46(6):418–23.
17. Chole RH, Gondivkar SM, Gadbail AR, et al. Review of drug treatment of oral submucous fibrosis. Oral Oncol. 2012;48:393–8.
18. Angadi PV, Rao S. Management of oral submucous fibrosis: an overview. Oral Maxillofac Surg. 2010;14:133–42.
19. Krishnamoorthy B, Khan M. Management of oral submucous fibrosis by two different drug regimens: a comparative study. Dent Res J. 2013;10:527–32.
20. Cox S, Zoellner H. Physiotherapeutic treatment improves oral opening in oral submucous fibrosis. J Oral Pathol Med. 2009;38:220–6.
21. James L, Shetty A, Rishi D, Abraham M. Management of oral submucous fibrosis with injection of hyaluronidase and dexamethasone in Grade III oral submucous fibrosis: a retrospective study. J Int Oral Health. 2015;7(8):82–5.
22. Gupta D, Sharma SC. Oral submucous fibrosis--a new treatment regimen. J Oral Maxillofac Surg 1988;46(10):830–833.
23. Ayub S, Siddiqui S, Abrar SK, Atif M, Raheel Allana R, Ahmad M. Effectiveness the combination therapy of chymotrypsin and dexamethasone vs dexamethasone alone in patients with oral sub mucous fibrosis. Rawal Med J. 2021;46(4):932–5.
24. Hurst LC, Badalamente MA, Hentz VR, et al. Injectable collagenase clostridium histolyticum for Dupuytren's contracture. N Engl J Med. 2009;361(10):968–77.
25. Lin HJ, Lin JC. Treatment of oral submucous fibrosis by collagenase: effects on oral opening and eating function. Oral Dis. 2007;13:407–13.
26. Saso L, Reza A, Ng E, Nguyen K, Lin S, Zhang P, Fantozzi PJ, Armagan G, Romeo U, Cirillo N. A comprehensive analysis of the role of oxidative stress in the pathogenesis and chemoprevention of oral submucous fibrosis. Antioxidants (Basel). 2022;11(5):868.
27. Heber D, Lu QY. Overview of mechanisms of action of lycopene. Exp Biol Med (Maywood). 2002;227(10):920–3.
28. Singh M, Krishanappa R, Bagewadi A, Keluskar V. Efficacy of oral lycopene in the treatment of oral leukoplakia. Oral Oncol. 2004;40:591–6.
29. Saawarn N, Shashikanth MC, Saawarn S, Jirge V, Chaitanya NC, Pinakapani R. Lycopene in the management of oral lichen planus: a placebo-controlled study. Indian J Dent Res. 2011;22:639–43.
30. Kumar A, Bagewadi A, Keluskar V, Singh M. Efficacy of lycopene in the management of oral submucous fibrosis. Oral Surg Oral Med Oral Pathol Oral Radiol Endod. 2007;103: 207–13.
31. Karemore TV, Motwani M. Evaluation of the effect of newer antioxidant lycopene in the treatment of oral submucous fibrosis. Indian J Dent Res. 2012;23:524–8.
32. Beenakumary TP, AG T, Varghese M, Raghavan R, Vm MN, Pius A. Evaluation of therapeutic efficacy of different treatment modalities in oral submucous fibrosis: a comparative study. J Contemp Dent Pract. 2019;20(3):390–4.
33. Johny J, Bhagvandas SC, Mohan SP, Punathil S, Moyin S, Bhaskaran MK. Comparison of efficacy of lycopene and lycopene-hyaluronidase combination in the treatment of oral submucous fibrosis. J Pharm Bioallied Sci. 2019;11(2):S260–4.
34. Saran G, Umapathy D, Misra N, et al. A comparative study to evaluate the efficacy of lycopene and curcumin in oral submucous fibrosis patients: a randomized clinical trial. Indian J Dent Res. 2018;29(3):303–12.
35. Selvam NP, Dyanand AA. Lycopene in the management of oral submucous fibrosis. Asian J Pharmaceut Clin Res. 2013;6(3):58–61.
36. Elizabeth N, Gurumani S, Bala AG, Tukalan G. A comparative study between management of oral submucous fibrosis. J Evol Med Dent Sci. 2014;3(47):11344–8.
37. Subramaniam AV, Subramaniam T, Agrawal N. Assessment of the effectiveness of antioxidant therapy(lycopene) and therapeutic ultrasound in the treatment of oral submucous fibrosis. Int J Pharm Therapeut. 2014;5(5):344–50.
38. Singh D, Shashikanth MC, Misra N, Agrawal S. Lycopene and intralesional betamethasone injections in the manage-

ment of oral submucous fibrosis. J Indian Acad Oral Med Radiol. 2014;26:264–8.
39. Arshad O, Siddiqi KM, Rana ZA. Oral submucous fibrosis: comparison of different treatment modalities. Pak Oral Dental J. 2015;35:3.
40. Bhowmick D, Kumar S, Nasreen S, Saba R, Iqbal H, Bhatia LK. Comparative evaluation of Lycopene-Hyaluronidase combination and Lycopene alone in the treatment of OSMF. Int J Health Clin Res. 2021;4(5):102–5.
41. Chainani-Wu N. Safety and anti-inflammatory activity of curcumin: a component of turmeric (Curcuma longa). J Alternat Complement Med. 2003;9:161–8.
42. Epstein J, Sanderson IR, Macdonald TT. Curcumin as a therapeutic agent: the evidence from in vitro, animal and human studies. Br J Nutr. 2010;103:1545–57.
43. Al-Maweri SA. Efficacy of curcumin for management of oral submucous fibrosis: a systematic review of randomized clinical trials. Oral Surg Oral Med Oral Pathol Oral Radiol. 2019;127(4):300–8.
44. Kopuri RKC, Chakravarthy C, Sunder S, et al. A comparative study of the clinical efficacy of lycopene and curcumin in the treatment of oral submucous fibrosis using ultrasonography. J Int Oral Health. 2016;8:687.
45. Lanjekar AB, Bhowate RR, Bakhle S, Narayane A, Pawar V, Gandagule R. Comparison of efficacy of topical curcumin gel with triamcinolone-hyaluronidase gel individually and in combination in the treatment of oral submucous fibrosis. J Contemp Dent Pract. 2020;21(1):83–90.
46. Joshi J, Ghaisas SD, Vaidya A, et al. Early human safety of tumeric oil (Curcuma longa oil) administered orally in healthy volunteers. JAPI. 2003;51:1055–60.
47. Hastak K, Lubri N, Jakhi SD, et al. Therapeutic responses to turmeric oil and turmeric oleoresin in oral submucos fibrosis. Amala Res Bullet. 1998;18:23–8.
48. Rai B, Kaur J, Jacobs R, Singh J. Possible action mechanism for curcumin in pre-cancerous lesions based on serum and salivary markers of oxidative stress. J Oral Sci. 2010;52:251–6.
49. Yadav M, Aravinda K, Saxena VS, et al. Comparison of curcumin with intralesional steroid injections in oral submucous fibrosis—a randomized, open-label interventional study. J Oral Biol Craniofac Res. 2014;4:169–73.
50. Das DA, Balan A, Sreelatha KT. Comparative study of the efficacy of curcumin and turmeric oil as chemopreventive agents in oral submucous fibrosis: a clinical and histopathological evaluation. J Indian Acad Oral Med Radiol. 2010;22:88–92.
51. Pipalia PR, Annigeri RG, Mehta R. Clinicobiochemical evaluation of turmeric with black pepper and nigella sativa in management of oral submucous fibrosis-a double-blind, randomized preliminary study. Oral Surg Oral Med Oral Pathol Oral Radiol. 2016;122(6):705–12.
52. Piyush P, Mahajan A, Singh K, Ghosh S, Gupta S. Comparison of therapeutic response of lycopene and curcumin in oral submucous fibrosis: a randomized controlled trial. Oral Dis. 2019;25(1):73–9.
53. Hazarey VK, Sakrikar AR, Ganvir SM. Efficacy of curcumin in the treatment for oral submucous fibrosis—a randomized clinical trial. J Oral Maxillofac Pathol. 2015;19(2):145–52.
54. Nerkar Rajbhoj A, Kulkarni TM, Shete A, Shete M, Gore R, Sapkal R. A comparative study to evaluate efficacy of curcumin and aloe vera gel along with oral physiotherapy in the management of oral submucous fibrosis: a randomized clinical trial. Asian Pac J Cancer Prev. 2021;22(S1):107–12. https://doi.org/10.31557/APJCP.2021.22.S1.107.
55. Srivastava A, Agarwal R, Chaturvedi TP, Chandra A, Singh OP. Clinical evaluation of the role of tulsi and turmeric in the management of oral submucous fibrosis: a pilot, prospective observational study. J Ayurveda Integr Med. 2015;6(1):45–9.
56. Madhulatha G, Vijayalaxmi N, Harshavardhan T. Tulasi a magical herb and a boon for management of oral submucous fibrosis: a clinical study. Int J Res Med Sci. 2017;5(11):4719–23.
57. Dwivedi N, Agarwal A. Aloe vera: magic or myth. SRM J Res Dent Sci. 2013;4:119.
58. Miranda MS, Cintra RG, Barros SB, Mancini FJ. Antioxidant activity of the microalga Spirulina maxima. Braz J Med Biol Res. 1998;31:1075–9.
59. Anuradha A, Patil B, Asha VR. Evaluation of efficacy of aloe vera in the treatment of oral submucous fibrosis—a clinical study. J Oral Pathol Med. 2017;46(1):50–5.
60. Singh N, Hebbale M, Mhapuskar A, Ul Nisa S, Thopte S, Singh S. Effectiveness of aloe vera and antioxidant along with physiotherapy in the management of oral submucous fibrosis. J Contemp Dent Pract. 2016;17(1):78–84.
61. Sudarshan R, Annigeri RG, Sree VG. Aloe vera in the treatment for oral submucous fibrosis - a preliminary study. J Oral Pathol Med. 2012;41(10):755–61.
62. Alam S, Ali I, Giri KY, et al. Efficacy of aloe vera gel as an adjuvant treatment of oral submucous fibrosis. Oral Surg Oral Med Oral Pathol Oral Radiol. 2013;116:717–24.
63. Patil S, Sghaireen MG, Maheshwari S, Kunsi SR, Sahu R. Comparative study of the efficacy of lycopene and aloe vera in the treatment of oral submucous fibrosis. Int J Health Allied Sci. 2015;4:13–7.
64. Patil S, Al-Zarea BK, Maheshwari S, Sahu R. Comparative evaluation of natural antioxidants spirulina and aloe vera for the treatment of oral submucous fibrosis. J Oral Biol Craniofac Res. 2015;5(1):11–5.
65. Mulk BS, Deshpande P, Velpula N, Chappidi V, Chintamaneni RL, Goyal S. Spirulina and pentoxyfilline: a novel approach for treatment of oral submucous fibrosis. J Clin Diagn Res. 2013;7:3048–50.
66. Shetty P, Shenai P, Chatra L, Rao PK. Efficacy of spirulina as an antioxidant adjuvant to corticosteroid injection in management of oral submucous fibrosis. Indian J Dent Res. 2013;24:347–50.
67. Kanjani V, Annigeri RG, Revanappa MM, Rani A. Efficacy of spirulina along with different physiotherapeutic modalities in the management of oral submucous fibrosis. Ann Maxillofac Surg. 2019;9(1):23–7.
68. Kulkarni R, Kalaskar A, Kalaskar R, Gupta N. Efficacy of spirulina in management of oral submucous fibrosis—a systematic review. J Oral Med Oral Surg. 2022;28:8.
69. More CB, Gavli N, Chen Y, Rao NR. A novel clinical protocol for therapeutic intervention in oral submucous fibrosis: an evidence-based approach. J Oral Maxillofac Pathol. 2018;22(3):382–91.
70. Fedorowicz Z, Chan Shih-Yen E, Dorri M, Nasser M, Newton T, Shi L. Interventions for the management of oral submucous fibrosis. Cochrane Database Syst Rev 2008;8(4):CD007156.
71. Li X, Tang J. Hua Xi, Kou Qiang, Xue Yi, Zhi Za. Clinical treatment observation of tea pigment for oral submucous fibrosis. West China J Stomatol. 1998;16(1):50–2.
72. Zhao Y, Guo Y, Gu X. Salvianolic acid B, a potential chemopreventive agent, for head and neck squamous cell cancer. J Oncol. 2011;2011:534548.
73. Hsieh YP, Wu KJ, Chen HM, Deng YT. Arecoline activates latent transforming growth factor β1 via mitochondrial reactive oxygen species in buccal fibroblasts: suppression by epigallocatechin-3-gallate. J Formos Med. 2018;117:527–34.
74. Rajendran R, Rani V, Shaikh S. Pentoxifylline therapy: a new adjunct in the treatment of oral submucous fibrosis. Indian J Dent Res. 2006;17:190–8.

75. Mehrotra R, Singh HP, Gupta SC, Singh M, Jain S. Pentoxifylline therapy in the management of oral submucous fibrosis. Asian Pac J Cancer Prev. 2011;12:971–4.
76. Sharma JK, Gupta AK, Mukhija RD, Nigam P. Clinical experience with the use of peripheral vasodilator in oral disorders. Int J Oral Maxillofac Surg. 1987;16:695–9.
77. Lai DR, Chen HR, Lin LM, Huang YL, Tsai CC. Clinical evaluation of different treatment methods for oral submucous fibrosis. A 10-year experience with 150 cases. J Oral Pathol Med. 1995;24:402–6.
78. Tan J, Li YC, Chen A, et al. Clinical research of Danxuan Koukang on treatment of oral submucous fibrosis. J Tradit Chin Med. 2006;26:41–3.
79. Singh U. Efficacy and safety of intralesional Xantinol nicotinate in the treatment of various stages of oral submucous fibrosis. J Clin Diagn Res. 2016;10(10):ZC34–ZC37.
80. Liu SF, Shen TH, Tang ZG, Su HP, Luo CF. On treatment of oral submucous fibrosis with glucosidorum tripterygii totorum. Beijing J Stomatol. 1999;7:167–9.
81. Samlaska CP, Winfield EA. Pentoxifylline. J Am Acad Dermatol. 1994;30(4):603–21.
82. Zhou Q, Zheng F, Hou F. Inhibition of tubulointerstitial fibrosis by PTX is associated with improvement of vascular endothelial growth factor expression. Acta Pharmacol Sin. 2009;30(1):98–106.
83. Prabhu N, Rao SS, Kotrashetti SM, et al. PTX in patients with oral submucous fibrosis a randomized clinical trial. J Maxillofac Oral Surg. 2015;14(1):81–9.
84. Zwiri AMA, Patil S, Yadav N. Comparative evaluation of newer drugs pentoxifylline and spirulina in the management of OSMF. Int J Pharmacol Toxicol. 2015;5:141–5.
85. Patil S, Maheshwari S. Efficacy of pentoxifylline in the management of oral submucous fibrosis. J Orofac Sci. 2014;6:94–8.
86. Sadaksharam J, Mahalingam S. Evaluation of oral PTX in the management of oral submucous fibrosis - an ultrasonographic study. Contemp Clin Dent. 2017;8(2):200–4.
87. Bhambal AM, Bhambal A, Shukla US, et al. Effectiveness of Pentoxifylline in the treatment of oral submucous fibrosis patients: a case-control study. Appl Cancer Res. 2019;39:15.
88. Gopinath D, Hui LM, Veettil SK, Nair AB, Maharajan MK. Comparative efficacy of interventions for the management of oral submucous fibrosis: a systematic review and network meta-analysis. J Pers Med. 2022;12:1272.
89. Bishnoi S, Sharma M, Bishnoid S, Sharma Y. Drug pentoxifylline in management of oral submucous fibrosis. Int J Res Rev. 2020;7(4):311–4.
90. Leelakshi NB, Gaurav. Efficacy of garlic in conjunction with pentoxifylline in the management of oral submucous fibrosis—a cross-sectional pilot study. Acta Scientific Dental Sci. 2020;7(4):154–60.
91. Bhadage CJ, Umarji HR, Shah K, Valimaa H. Vasodilator isoxsuprine alleviates symptoms of oral submucous fibrosis. Clin Oral Investig. 2013;17:1375–82.
92. Koneru A, Hunasgi S, Hallikeri K, Surekha R, Nellithady G, Vanishree M, et al. A systematic review of various treatment modalities for oral submucous fibrosis. J Adv Clin Res Insights. 2014;1:64–72.
93. Johar N, Chaurasia S, Phulambrikar T. Management of oral submucous fibrosis: A Review. Int J Oral Health Dent. 2017;3(3):154–7.
94. Katharia SK, Singh SP, Kulshreshtha VK. The effects of placenta extract in management of oral submucous fibrosis. Indian J Pharmacol. 1992;24:181–3.
95. Kisave P, Shekhar V, Babu PS, Hussaini SW, Bhanot R, Kumar A, et al. The study of placentrex and hydrocortisone as an adjunct treatment in oral submucous fibrosis. J Family Med Prim Care. 2020;9:2469–74.
96. Rananjaneyulu P, Rao P. Submucous fibrosis new treatment. J Indian Dent Assoc. 1980;52:379–80.
97. Naik SM, Appaji MK, Ravishankara S, Goutham MK, Devi NP, Mushannavar AS, Naik SS. Comparative Study of intralesional triamcinolone acetonide and hyaluronidase vs placental extract in 60 cases of oral submucous fibrosis. Int J Head Neck Surg. 2012;3(2):59–65.
98. Raj AG, Jayaprasad A, Manasa AM, Darshan DD, Ambili A. A longitudinal study of the effect of placental extract in the treatment of moderate and moderately advanced oral submucous fibrosis. RGUHS J Dent Sci. 2013;5(1):13–6.
99. Dinesh S, Sudhir P, Sara S, Nazima B, Sandeep KV, Aleem AK. Injection placentrex in the management of oral submucous fibrosis. Int J Modern Sci Eng Technol. 2015;2(1):23–30.
100. Priyankar S, Anil P, Ashish S, Tarun A, Sunil S, Sanjay RB, Mridula T. Efficacy of intralesional placental extract, dexamethasone, and hyaluronidase in treatment of oral submucous fibrosis: a comparative study. JK Pract. 2016;21(1–2):29–34.
101. Shah PH, Venkatesh R, More CB, Vassandacoumara V. Comparison of therapeutic efficacy of placental extract with dexamethasone and hyaluronic acid with dexamethasone for oral submucous fibrosis—a retrospective analysis. J Clin Diagn Res 2016;10(10):ZC63–ZC66.
102. Shinde CV, Saawarn N, Kohli S, Khare P, Singh A, Sagar KM. Comparative efficacy of intralesional placental extract and intralesional triamcinolone acetonide in the management of OSMF. J Indian Acad Oral Med Radiol. 2019;31:328–32.
103. Kale MV, Gaikwad NS. Oral submucous fibrosis: a study of qualitative and analytical treatment using intralesional injections: placental extract versus combination of steroid with hyaluronidase. Int J Otorhinolaryngol Head Neck Surg. 2020;6(7):1321–5.
104. Borle RM, Borle SR. Management of oral submucous fibrosis: a conservative approach. J Oral Maxillofac Surg. 1991;49:788–91.
105. Reddi R. Oral Submucous Fibrosis - A recent trend in its treatment. JIAOMR. 1993;4:7–8.
106. Nallapu V, Balasankulu B, Vuppalapati HB, Sambhana S, Mala D, Koppula SK. Efficacy of vitamin E in oral submucous fibrosis: a clinical and histopathologic study. J Indian Acad Oral Med Radiol. 2015;27:387–92.
107. Singh N, Singh J, Singh U. Oral sub mucous fibrosis. A new approach to treatment with combined therapy. J Indian Dent Assoc. 1996;67:168–70.
108. Nayak A, Anitha B, Bhattacharya A, Podder S. Efficacy of lycopene in combination with vitamin E in management of oral submucous fibrosis—a clinical prospective study. J Adv Med Dent Sci Res. 2015;3(3):21–5.
109. Thakur N, Keluskar V, Bagewadi A, Shetti A. Effectiveness of micronutrients and physiotherapy in the management of oral submucous fibrosis. Int Nat Contemp Dentist. 2011;2(1):101–5.
110. Raizada MK, Sable DM. Clinical assessment of efficacy of Omega 3 in oral submucous fibrosis patients—a randomized controlled trial. Asian Pac J Cancer Prev. 2022;23(4):1185–92.
111. Nagaraj T, Santosh HN. Estimation of serum hepcidin in oral submucous fibrosis before and after supplementation with oral iron: a randomized control clinical trial. J Oral Maxillofac Pathol. 2018;22(3):303–6.
112. Maher R, Aga P, Johnson NW, Sankaranarayanan R, Warnakulasuriya S. Evaluation of multiple micronutrient supplementation in the management of oral submucous fibrosis in Karachi. Pakistan Nutr Cancer. 1997;27(1):41–7.

113. Dhariwal R, Mukherjee S, Mohanty S, Chakraborty A, Ray J, Chaudhuri K. Zinc and vitamin A can minimise the severity of oral submucous fibrosis. BMJ Case Rep. 2010:bcr1020092348.
114. Anil K, Sharma SC, Sharma P, Chandra O, Singhal KC, Nagar A. Beneficial role of zinc in the treatement of oral submucous fibrosis. Indian J Pharmac. 1991;23:236–41.
115. Singh BP, Mittal N, Sharma V, Palani. Evaluation of role of Oxitard capsules in the treatment of oral submucous fibrosis. Antiseptic. 2009;106:103–7.
116. Patil S, Santosh BS, Maheshwari S, Deoghare A, Chhugani S, Rajesh PR. Efficacy of oxitard capsules in the treatment of oral submucous fibrosis. J Canc Res Therapeut. 2015;11(2):291–4.
117. Patil S, Halgatti V, Maheshwari S, Santosh BS. Comparative study of the efficacy of herbal antioxdants oxitard and aloe vera in the treatment of oral submucous fibrosis. J Clin Exp Dent. 2014;6(3):e265–70.
118. Sasi M, Kumar S, Kumar M, Thapa S, Prajapati U, Tak Y, et al. Garlic (*Allium sativum* L.) Bioactives and its role in alleviating oral pathologies. Antioxidants (Basel). 2021;10(11):1847.
119. Jiang X, Zhang Y, Li F, Zhu Y, Chen Y, Yang S, Sun G. Allicin as a possible adjunctive therapeutic drug for stage II oral submucous fibrosis: a preliminary clinical trial in a Chinese cohort. Int J Oral Maxillofac Surg. 2015;44:1540–6.
120. Jiang XW, Zhang Y, Song GD, Li FF, Peng HY, Yang SK, Sun GL. Clinical evaluation of allicin oral adhesive tablets in the treatment of recurrent aphthous ulceration. Oral Surg Oral Med Oral Pathol Oral Radiol. 2012;113:500–4.
121. Jain N, Annigeri RG, Pipalia PR. Efficacy of garlic in conjunction with pentoxifylline in the management of oral submucous fibrosis—a preliminary study. Int J Pharm Sci Res. 2016;7:5017.
122. Cabras M, Carrozzo M, Gambino A, Broccoletti R, Sciascia S, Baldovino S, Arduino PG. Value of colchicine as treatment for recurrent oral ulcers: a systematic review. J Oral Pathol Med. 2020;49(8):731–40.
123. Segovia A, Niembro RF, Ibanez KG, Alcocer G, Tamayo P. Long term evaluation of colchicine in the treatment of scleroderma. J Rheumatol. 1979;6:705–12.
124. Diegelmann RF, Peterkofsky B. Inhibition of collagen secretion from bone and cultured fibroblasts by microtubular descriptive drugs. Proc Natl Acad Sci U S A. 1972;69: 892–6.
125. Daga D, Singh RK, Pal US, Gurung T, Gangwar S. Efficacy of oral colchicine with intralesional hyaluronidase or triamcinolone acetonide in the Grade II oral submucous fibrosis. Natl J Maxillofac Surg. 2017;8(1):50–4.
126. Stewart S, Yang KCK, Atkins K, et al. Adverse events during oral colchicine use: a systematic review and meta-analysis of randomised controlled trials. Arthritis Res Ther. 2020;22:28.
127. Haque MF, Meghji S, Nazir R, Harris M. Interferon-gamma (IFN-gamma) may reverse oral submucous fibrosis. J Oral Pathol Med. 2001;30:12–21.
128. Sheshaprasad R, Pai A. Oral sub mucous fibrosis: exploring therapeutic strategies using -anti TGF β drugs. Asian Pac J Cancer Care. 2018;3(2):21–7.
129. Moinzadeh P, Hunzelmann N, Krieg T. Pharmacology and rationale for imatinib in the treatment of scleroderma. J Exp Pharmacol. 2013;5:15–22.
130. Akhmetshina A, Venalis P, Dees C, et al. Treatment with imatinib prevents fibrosis in different preclinical models of systemic sclerosis and induces regression of established fibrosis. Arthritis Rheum. 2009;60(1):219–24.
131. Gan Y, Herzog EL, Gomer RH. Pirfenidone treatment of idiopathic pulmonary fibrosis. Therap Clin Risk Manage. 2011;7:39–47.
132. Garcia L, Hernandez I, Sandoval A, Salazar A, Garcia J, Vera J, et al. Pirfenidone effectively reverses experimental liver fibrosis. J Hepatol. 2002;37(6):797–805.
133. Yu CC, Tsai CH, Hsu HI, Chang YC. Elevation of S100A4 expression in buccal mucosal fibroblasts by arecoline: involvement in the pathogenesis of oral sub mucous fibrosis. PLoS One. 2013;8(1):e55122.
134. Nakazato H, Oku H, Yamane S, Tsuruta Y, Suzuki R. A novel anti-fibrotic agent pirfenidone suppresses tumor necrosis factor-alpha at the translational level. Eur J Pharmacol. 2002;446(1–3):177–85.
135. Kaur J, Jacobs R. Proinflammatory cytokine levels in oral lichen planus, oral leukoplakia, and oral sub mucous fibrosis. J Korean Assoc Oral Maxillofac Surg. 2015;41(4):171–5.
136. Bishen KA, Radhakrishnan R, Satyamoorthy K. The role of basic fibroblast growth factor in oral submucous fibrosis pathogenesis. J Oral Pathol Med. 2008;37(7):402–11.
137. Tsai CH, Lee SS, Chang YC. Hypoxic regulation of plasminogen activator inhibitor-1 expression in human buccal mucosa fibroblasts stimulated with arecoline. J Oral Pathol Med. 2015;44(9):669–73.
138. Hilberg F, Roth GJ, Krssak M, Kautschitsch S, Sommergruber W, Tontsch-Grunt U, et al. BIBF 1120: triple angiokinase inhibitor with sustained receptor blockade and good antitumor efficacy. Cancer Res. 2008;68(12):4774–82.
139. Seema Nayak MMG, Makker A, Bhatia V, Chandra S, Sandeep Kumar SP, Agarwal. Fibroblast Growth Factor (FGF-2) and its receptors FGFR-2 and FGFR-3 may be putative biomarkers of malignant transformation of potentially malignant oral lesions into oral squamous cell carcinoma. PLoS One. 2015;
140. Haque MF, Meghji S, Khitab U, Harris M. Oral submucous fibrosis patients have altered levels of cytokine production. J Oral Pathol Med. 2000;29(3):123–8.
141. Hajari Case A, Johnson P. Clinical use of nintedanib in patients with idiopathic pulmonary fibrosis. BMJ Open. Respir Res. 2017;4(1)
142. Joshi M, Patravale V. Formulation and evaluation of nanostructured lipid carrier (NLC)-based gel of valdecoxib. Drug Dev Ind Pharmacy. 2006;32:911–8.
143. Averineni RK, Sunderajan SG, Mutalik S, et al. Development of mucoadhesive buccal films for the treatment of oral submucous fibrosis: a preliminary study. Pharm Dev Technol. 2009;14:199–207.
144. Gopinath D, Hui LM, Veettil SK, Balakrishnan Nair A, Maharajan MK. Comparative efficacy of interventions for the management of oral submucous fibrosis: a systematic review and network meta-analysis. J Pers Med. 2022;12(8):1272.

# Curcumin as a Chemopreventive Agent for Oral Submucous Fibrosis

*Sosmitha Girisa, Aviral Kumar, and Ajaikumar B. Kunnumakkara*

## Contents



© The Author(s), under exclusive license to Springer Nature Switzerland AG 2023
S. Warnakulasuriya, K. Ranganathan (eds.), *Oral Submucous Fibrosis*, Textbooks in Contemporary Dentistry,
https://doi.org/10.1007/978-3-031-12855-4_17

## 17.1 Introduction

As OSF is a serious disease that hampers the quality of life of patients, efficacious treatment modalities are imperative for its management. An expert group who met at Fifth World Workshop on Oral Medicine conducted a systematic review on medical (i.e., non-surgical) interventions available for the management of oral submucous fibrosis (OSF) [1]. This systematic review explored and updated the medical (i.e., non-surgical) interventions for OSF and reported on 27 published medical interventions that were reviewed by the expert group, which included four randomized controlled trials (RCTs). The rest were observational or retrospective studies. The review identified significant limitations of the reported studies and none of the pharmacological treatments that had been tried were found to be effective in treating OSF except for some limited improvement in mouth opening. An earlier reported Cochrane review by Fedorowicz et al. [2] had the objective to assess the effectiveness of interventions in the management of pain and restricted jaw opening or movement occurring as a result of oral submucous fibrosis. In two RCTs identified in their searches the data were considered of insufficient quality to draw any conclusions. A further update on the evidence on the medical interventions used for the management of OSF is given in ▶ Chap. 16 [3]. Based on the evidence presented in these reviews it is clear that the established pharmacological agents do not provide any significant clinical improvement for OSF sufferers. Therefore, alternate modalities for the prevention and treatment of OSF are need of the hour. Interestingly, various pre-clinical and clinical studies have enumerated the role of the Indian spice turmeric and its active component curcumin for the prevention and treatment of OSF. Hence, in this chapter we focus on the potential of this agent in the prevention and treatment of OSF and present the underlying mechanisms of action.



**Learning Goals**

- What is turmeric and curcumin?
- The effect of turmeric and curcumin on various hallmarks of OSF.
- Mechanism of action of turmeric and curcumin on OSF.
- The pre-clinical and clinical studies of turmeric and curcumin on OSF.

## 17.2 Turmeric, Curcumin and OSF

Since ancient times, plants, herbs, and spices have been utilized for their outstanding medicinal and biological properties against various human ailments [4–6]. They have been reported with a plethora of bioactive components that contribute to their broad pharmacological activities. Turmeric, which is botanically known as *Curcuma longa,* belongs to Zingiberaceae family is one such plant consisting of various bioactive compounds [7, 8]. It is extensively employed as a medicinal plant in various traditional medicine systems of Ayurveda, Unani, and Sidha, used for the treatment of various human diseases due to its anti-cancer, anti-inflammatory, anti-microbial, anti-mutagenic and anti-oxidant activities [7, 8]. Turmeric has been widely employed for centuries to cure inflammatory and other diseases where it's medicinal and pharmacological activities could be attributed to the group of compounds like curcuminoids and other compounds contained in its rhizomes [9]. Curcumin, also known as diferuloylmethane, is a major active curcuminoid that represents approximately 2 percent by weight of the rhizomes of turmeric [10–13]. Curcumin has been widely reported for its various pharmacological properties such as anti-arthritic, anti-atherosclerotic, anti-depressant, anti-diabetic, anti-growth, anti-inflammatory, anti-microbial, anti-oxidant, and anti-tumor effects. It is also effective against various chronic diseases such as autoimmune, cardiovascular, pulmonary, and neurological disorders [14–17]. Thus, curcumin is a highly potent medicinal compound in treating various human ailments. Various studies have shown the efficacy of curcumin to target multiple signaling cascades, transcription factors and its downstream effector molecules [18–20]. In line with this, curcumin has been reported to modulate various signaling pathways such as phosphoinositide 3-kinases (PI3K)/Akt, β-catenin, adenosine monophosphate-activated protein kinase (AMPK), Janus kinase (JAK)/signal transducer and activator of transcription protein (STAT), mitogen-activated protein kinase (MAPK), and nuclear factor *kappa B* (NF-κB) [21]. It also regulates various transcription factors and proteins associated with these pathways to exert its therapeutic effect against different diseases [22]. Further, curcumin inhibits nitric oxide synthases (NOS), nitric oxide (NO) oxidation, and reactive oxygen species (ROS) generation, and the modulation of NOS results in the activation of NF-κB and activating protein 1 (AP-1) levels [23].

It is well-established that inflammation plays a significant role in the development and malignant transformation of OSF. Accumulating evidence has implicated the efficacy of curcumin as a potent anti-inflammatory agent. Curcumin inhibits both acute and chronic inflammation via suppressing the levels of tumor necrosis factor α (TNF-α) and NF-κB [24, 25]. In addition, curcumin has also been shown to suppress acute vascular inflammation by activating heme oxygenase-1 (HO-1) and nuclear factor-E2-related factor 2 (Nrf2) through the p38 MAPK signaling pathway [26]. Further, curcumin represses the inflammatory processes in periodontal disease by suppressing the levels of interleukin (IL)-6, TNF-α, osteoprotegerin (OPG), receptor activator of nuclear factor-κB (RANK), and receptor activator of nuclear factor-κB ligand (RANKL) in *in vivo* models [27]. Moreover, treatment with curcumin was also found to help in the resolution of oral leukoplakia [28]. In this chapter we present and discuss the potential role of curcumin in the prevention and treatment of OSF through a critical appraisal of different pre-clinical and clinical studies.

**Definition**

**Turmeric** (*Curcuma longa* L.) is a perennial plant that belongs to the Zingiberaceae family with short stems and large leaves and branched yellow or brownish rhizomes. This plant is native to Southeast Asia, and its dried rhizomes are used as a spice in different cuisines of Indian, Chinese, and Thai origin. **Curcumin** is a phenolic compound present in the rhizomes of turmeric spice. It is the principal curcuminoid (polyphenolic compounds) that contributes to the yellow color and biological activity of the turmeric spice.

## 17.3 Mechanism of Curcumin on Inflammation and Inflammatory Pathways

Inflammation may be defined as the response of the body's immune system to the damage caused by pathogens or chemical and physical agents to repair the damaged tissues [29]. Studies over the past couple of decades have elucidated that inflammation alters the signaling pathways, which lead to the generation of excess free radicals, inflammatory markers, and lipid peroxides. It is also associated with wound healing and fighting against infection in the body [30]. Two types of inflammation are observed where acute inflammation forms a part of the innate immune system protecting the body from pathogens, while chronic inflammation is often associated with several chronic diseases such as arthritis, cancer, cardiovascular, diabetes, metabolic disorders, obesity, and neurodegenerative diseases [30]. It is now well established that cytokines play an important role in inflammation and inflammation-mediated diseases. The cytokine response is mediated through various signaling pathways that are associated with cell survival and proliferation. Cytokines are also known to activate NF-κB and STAT3, which further activate various signaling cascades associated with inflammation, cell survival, proliferation, and differentiation. Thus, suggesting the importance of cytokines in mediating the inflammatory responses [25]. TNF-α is a major mediator of inflammation and exhibits its activity through the activation of NF-κB signaling pathway. TNF-α has been reported as the potent activator of NF-κB; however, the latter also regulates the expression of the former protein [31, 32]. NF-κB plays a major role in modulating genes involved in inflammatory and immune responses. It is now well established that TNF-α plays a multifunctional role in OSF by regulating the inflammation and degradation of collagen type I. The expression of TNF-α was also associated with the increased risk of OSF [33]. Interestingly, curcumin has been reported to mediate anti-inflammatory activity by suppressing various cytokines, inflammatory transcription factors, enzymes, protein kinases, and redox species [21, 34]. A study evaluating the anti-inflammatory activity of curcumin showed that it suppressed the TNF-α-mediated activation of NF-κB, intracellular ROS, monocyte adhesion, phosphorylated c-Jun N-terminal kinases (p-JNK), p38, and STAT-3 levels in HUVEC cells. It also attenuated the expression of intracellular cell adhesion molecule (ICAM)-1, IL-8 and monocyte chemoattractant protein (MCP)-1 [25]. Further, curcumin was shown to inhibit the activity of NF-κB via targeting IκB kinase (IKK) in head and neck cancers [35]. Various studies have shown that the cytokines mediate their effect via the JAK/STAT pathway [36–38]. Curcumin has been demonstrated to significantly inhibit JAK/STAT pathway and downregulate various pro-inflammatory cytokines such as IL-1, IL-2, IL-6, IL-8, and IL-12, as well as MCP-1 [39, 40]. In addition, curcumin was found to induce anti-inflammatory cytokines by targeting the JAK/STAT pathway [41]. Moreover, in an experimental animal model of psoriasis-like inflammation, the treatment with curcumin decreased the expression of TNF-α, IL-17A, IL-17F, IL-22, and IL-1β [42].

The anti-inflammatory properties of curcumin are also exhibited through the inhibition of cyclooxygenase (COX)-1 and COX-2 to prevent the production of the eicosanoid's prostaglandin $E_2$ ($PGE_2$) and 5- hydroxyeicosatetraenoic acid [43]. COX-2 also plays an important role in regulating inflammation by inducing vascular permeability and stimulating inflammatory cell infiltration in OSF and oral cancer [44]. Moreover, a study has reported the induction of inflammatory proteins such as COX-2 and $PGE_2$ by areca nut (AN) extracts in gingival keratinocytes and oral cancer cells [45]. While an *in vitro* study has shown that the treatment of oral potentially malignant (AMOL) and malignant (AMOS-III) cell lines with curcumin inhibited the expression of tobacco-induced NF-κB and COX-2 [35, 46]. Additionally, the administration of curcumin complexed with zinc inhibited inflammatory factors such as TNF-α and IL-6 and modulated the oxidative enzymes like glutathione peroxidase (GPx), malondialdehyde (MDA), and superoxide dismutase (SOD) [47]. Further, the administration of 0.1 percent curcumin (0.01%) (Curcuma-P®) in combination with white pepper in subcutaneous models in rat significantly decreased pro-inflammatory cytokines IL-6 and TNF-α [48]. According to recent research, curcumin's anti-inflammatory activity appears to be mediated through NLR family pyrin domain containing 3 (NLRP3) in multiple cell systems [49–51]. In line with this, curcumin treatment have shown to suppress NLRP3 inflammasome level, caspase-1 activation, and IL-1 secretion in a dose-dependent manner in THP-1 macrophages treated with phorbol myristate acetate (PMA), an activator of the NLRP3 inflammasome, via down-regulating the toll-like receptor 4 (TLR4)/NF-κB signal transduction pathway [52]. Thus, curcumin could potentially inhibit inflammation and its associated molecules, due to which it might be helpful in abrogating the symptoms of OSF.

**Important**

Curcumin has been reported to mediate anti-inflammatory activity by suppressing various cytokines, inflammatory transcription factors, enzymes, protein kinases, and redox species.

## 17.4 Turmeric and Curcumin Against the Hallmarks of OSF

Various studies have evinced the potential role of turmeric and curcumin in abrogating different hallmarks of OSF such as cytokine storm, inflammation, ECM remodeling, oxidative stress, matrix metalloproteinase (MMP) deregulation and excessive deposition of fibrotic tissues. Thus, in the next part of this chapter, we describe the role of these hallmarks in OSF and their suppression by turmeric and curcumin (Fig. 17.1).

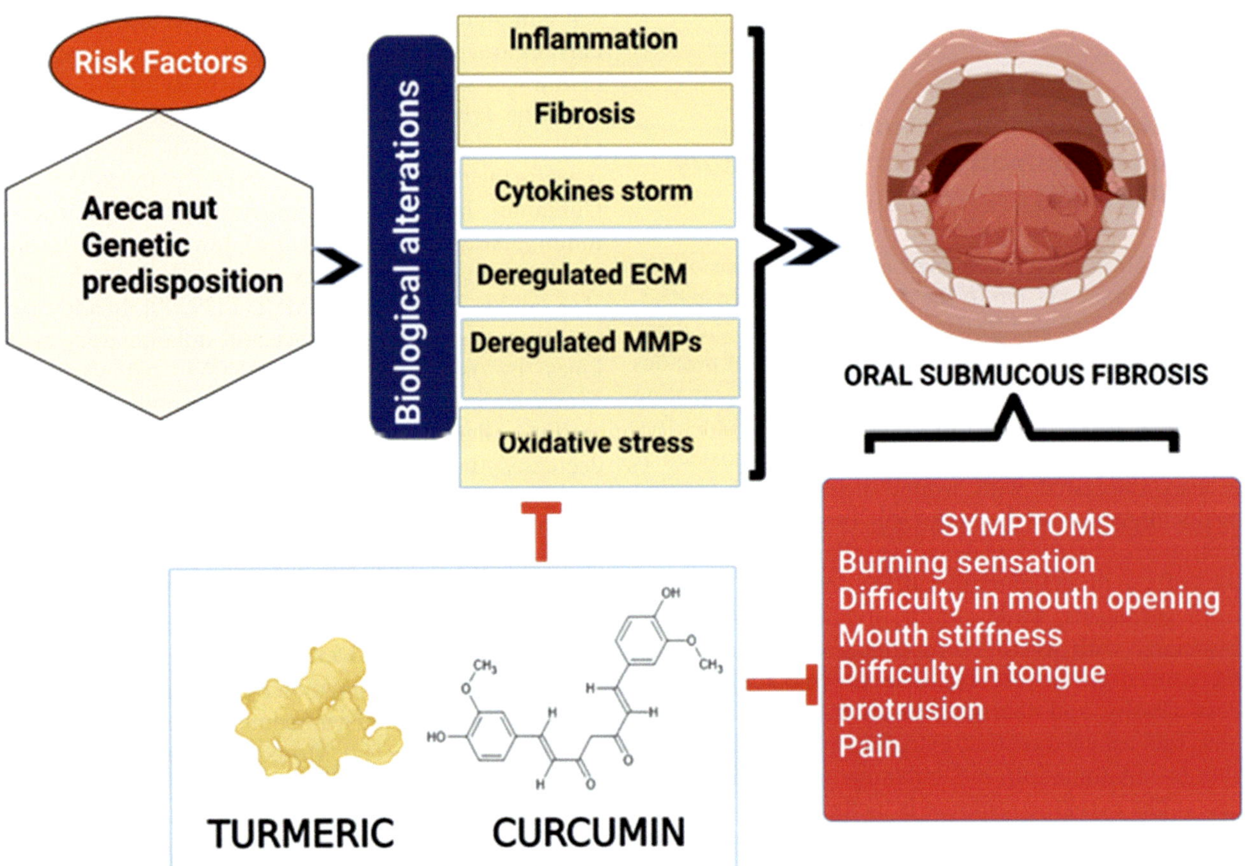


Fig. 17.1 Effect of turmeric/curcumin against OSF

17

### 17.4.1 Cytokines/Interleukins in OSF and Its Inhibition by Turmeric/Curcumin

Increased pro-inflammatory cytokines are associated with the induction of inflammatory processes leading to the onset of OSF [53, 54]. The elevation of the cytokines in OSF is attributed to many factors [53]. The excessive chewing of AN initiates inflammation through the activation of macrophages, leading to the secretion of cytokines. The altered levels of cytokines and growth factors in the damaged tissues initiate the proliferation of fibroblasts and collagen synthesis, resulting in fibrosis. Transforming growth factor-β (TGF-β) is one of the major cytokines that modulate the expression of alpha-smooth muscle actin (α-SMA) and collagen type I in myofibroblast [55]. Various studies have shown that the patients suffering from OSF express elevated levels of cytokines like IL-1β, IL-6, IL-8, and TNF-α and decreased level of interferon-gamma (IFN-γ) [56–58]. Interestingly, studies have reported the efficacy of curcumin in suppressing the pro-inflammatory cytokines. In line with this, curcumin was shown to inhibit the levels of IL-1β, IL-6, IL-8, and TNF-α in various inflammatory settings [18, 59, 60]. Similarly, turmeric was also found to reduce the levels of cytokines, IL-1 and IL-6 through the suppression of nitrous oxide that might induce the flexibility of collagen in OSF patients [61].

As OSF patients are reported with down regulation of IFN-γ, the treatment with IFN-γ or its induction could improve the symptoms of OSF in the patients by reducing the synthesis of collagen and inflammatory cell infiltrates and cytokines [62]. In accordance with this, studies have shown the efficacy of curcumin in inducing IFN-γ in various inflammatory models [63–65]. Moreover studies have shown that the pro-inflammatory cytokines could induce COX-2 at the site of inflammation, and the overexpression of COX-2 could lead to malignant transformation in OSF [66]. However, in a study, it was shown that curcumin could inhibit the expression of smokeless tobacco-induced COX-2 in oral potentially malignant and malignant cell lines which shows the potential of curcumin in preventing malignant transformation [46]. Taken together, these studies advocate the immense potential of curcumin in abrogating various inflammatory cytokines related to OSF.

### 17.4.2 ECM/Collagen Synthesis in OSF and Its Inhibition by Turmeric/Curcumin

Regulation of ECM and its components like collagen is an important factor in the management of OSF [67]. The ECM consists of collagens and elastic fibers present in the viscoelastic gel of proteoglycans, hyaluronan, and assorted glycoproteins where they form a bioactive polymer by crosslinking and charge-dependent interactions [68]. The fibrosis of the buccal mucosa in OSF is associated with the excessive deposition of collagen and other components of the extracellular matrix [68]. The disturbance of the homeostasis between MMPs and tissue inhibitors of matrix metalloproteinases (TIMPs) increases the accumulation of ECM [69, 70]. In line with this, MMP-2 and TIMP-2 were found to be overexpressed in advanced stages of OSF [69]. One of the studies reported that OSF development involves ECM remodeling by varying the synthesis of its components in different phases. For instance, the early stage was reported with the excessive synthesis of collagen type III, fibronectin, perlecan, and tenascin in the connective tissue (lamina propria) and buccal mucosa. While in the intermediate stage of OSF, elastin and these molecules were deposited excessively and irregularly adjacent to muscle fibers. However, the synthesis of these ECM molecules was decreased and replaced by collagen type I in the advanced stages. Thus, the loss of various ECM molecules and elastin and the entire replacement of muscle fibers by collagen type I results in the rigidity in mouth opening of OSF patients [71]. The molecular mechanisms behind the unstable ECM synthesis were caused by cystatin, lysyl oxidase, plasminogen activator inhibitor-1 (PAI-1), TGF-β1, and TIMPS. These molecules and factors reduce the degradation of ECM and increased deposition and stability of collagen and its crosslinking, which ultimately results in tissue fibrosis and OSF [67]. The degradation of ECM is initiated by a family of proteases known as MMPs [72]. The potential of curcumin in regulating ECM components in OSF has been investigated. For example, in an *in vitro* study, the treatment of myofibroblasts with curcumin suppressed the expression of collagen type I and type III in a dose-dependent manner. It also caused G0/G1 cell cycle arrest and apoptosis and inhibited proliferation in myofibroblasts, which suggests the therapeutic potential of curcumin in inhibiting the deposition of ECM, which is one of the important targets to suppress OSF [73]. Another *in vitro* study also confirmed the efficacy of curcumin in inhibiting the expression of molecules induced by arecoline such as collagen type I alpha 1 (COL1A1), collagen type III alpha 1 chain (COL3A1), and tissue inhibitor of metalloproteinases 2 (TIMP2) in oral mucosal fibroblasts [74]. Thus, curcumin has high potential in modulating ECM and its components that might be helpful in the prevention and management of OSF.

level of inducible nitric oxide synthase (iNOS) ; while curcumin treatment inhibited its expression [87]. Furthermore, the overexpression of hypoxia-inducible factor 1-alpha (HIF-1α) (induce oxidative stress) was found to induce fibrosis through the increased expression of COL1A1 and COL3A1. However, curcumin treatment inhibited the expression of HIF-1α as well as COL1A1 and COL3A1. Thus, these studies suggest the potential of curcumin in modulating oxidative stress and molecules associated with fibrosis leading to better management of OSF [74].

### 17.4.3 Oxidative Stress in OSF and Its Inhibition by Turmeric/Curcumin

Oxidative stress is defined as a condition with an imbalance in ROS and antioxidant response [75, 76]. The consumption of AN causes auto-oxidation in the saliva or activation of intracellular metabolites which lead to the synthesis of ROS. The ROS generation in turn activates several signaling pathways such as JAK, MAPK, Ras signaling, Src Kinase, PI3K/ Akt, and NF-κB [77]. In a study, it was shown that the levels of antioxidant enzymes such as SOD and GPx were down regulated in OSF patients compared to normal subjects. The high ROS synthesis initiates oxidative stress in the tissues, which have been suggested to play a role in OSF pathogenesis [78]. The DNA damage (in guanine bases) caused by ROS produces 8-hydroxydeoxyguanosine (8-OHdG), which could be used as a biomarker for oxidative stress in OSF patients [79]. Lipid peroxidation is another process associated with oxidative damage that leads to the disruption of the lipid membrane through the production of lipid peroxides and aldehydes (by-products). MDA one of the end products of this process, is generated through the breakdown of polyunsaturated fatty acids and its associated esters [80]. Studies have evaluated the levels of serum and salivary MDA in OSF patients which showed its elevated expression and were positively correlated with the advanced stages of OSF [81–84].

Various studies have evaluated the potential of turmeric and curcumin in inhibiting lipid peroxidation in OSF. In a clinical study, it was shown that the treatment with curcumin inhibited the by-products of lipid peroxidation, i.e., 8-OHdG and MDA, in OSF patients with significant improvements in the signs and symptoms of the disease [85]. In addition, the treatment with turmeric in OSF patients showed a reduction in MDA level and lipid peroxidation, which led to the improvement of OSF symptoms [86]. Further, in a study, the immunohistochemical analysis of OSF tissues showed an elevated

### 17.4.4 MMPs in OSF and Its Modulation by Turmeric/Curcumin

MMPs are an important group of molecules regulating the components of ECM. They are a family of enzymes that can degrade the protein molecules of ECM [88]. They are usually down regulated under normal conditions; however, they are promptly synthesized and activated during tissue remodeling [88, 89]. The activities of MMPs are inhibited by their natural inhibitors, such as TIMPs and macroglobulin [88]. As discussed, MMPs induce the degradation of ECM and the major MMPs involved in these processes include MMP-1 (known as collagenases), MMP-2 and -9 (known as gelatinases), MMP-3 (also known as stromelysin), and other membrane-associated MMPs [89, 90]. Besides its role in ECM degradation, MMPs also induce tissue fibrosis through the excessive production of cell surface proteins, chemokines, cytokines, TGF-β1, and other inflammatory molecules [72]. Analysis of the polymorphism of the MMP-3 gene revealed that 5A/5A and 6A/6A alleles were significantly expressed in OSF patients [91]. In another study, it was reported that the expression of MMP-1 (collagenase-1) was down regulated in OSF patients as compared to a control group [92]. However, the level of serum MMP-2 was upregulated in OSF patients compared to control, and was positively associated with interincisal opening, with no effect on burning sensation. In the same study, it was also shown that the level of serum MMP-2 was associated with different histopathological grades of OSF [93]. While in a study, it was shown that the treatment of oral mucosal fibroblasts with curcumin modulated the expression of MMP-2 that was earlier induced by arecoline [74]. As previously mentioned, OSF has a high potential to transform into OSCC; studies have also shown the efficacy of curcumin against OSCC. In line with this, Zhen et al. evaluated the therapeutic potential of curcumin in inhibiting OSCC where curcumin treatment decreased the invasive property of SCC-25 cells by reducing the expression of MMP-2 and MMP-9 [94]. Another study by Lee and his group aimed to study the effect of curcumin treatment on the invasive properties of the SCC-25 OSCC cell line. It was reported that the treatment with curcumin downregulated MMP-2 and MMP-9 levels along with the regulation of various epithelial-mesenchymal-transition (EMT) markers [95]. Thus, curcumin might be beneficial in regulating MMPs in OSF patients; however, further studies are required to understand the mechanism of curcumin in inhibiting these molecules.

### 17.4.5 Fibrosis in OSF and Its Inhibition by Turmeric/Curcumin

It is well known that OSF is associated with tissue fibrosis due to the excessive deposition of collagen [96]. The prevalence of tissue fibrosis in patients with this disease causes stiffness of the oral cavity, which reduces the flexibility of mouth opening and movement of the tongue. These symptoms results in poor quality of life in patients with symptoms such as difficulty in consuming and swallowing food, with impaired signs of communication [70, 97]. Studies have reported that chemical agents in AN induce fibrosis of oral tissues in the OSF patients [98]. It was reported that the expression of fibrosis associated genes such as *HIF-1α, TGF-β*, and connective tissue growth factor (*CTGF* or *CCN2*) were induced by arecoline; however, the treatment with curcumin significantly suppressed these genes. In addition, treatment with curcumin inhibited the expression of fibrosis-associated protein molecules like COL1A1, COL3A1, TIMP2 and MMP-2 induced by arecoline in oral mucosal fibroblasts [74]. In another study, the expression of CTGF, a downstream target of TGF-β that regulates the production of ECM and contributes to the sustenance of fibrosis in OSF was shown to be enhanced in fibroblasts, epithelial and endothelial cells. Interestingly, the same study also showed that curcumin inhibited arecoline-induced CTGF in human buccal mucosa fibroblasts (BMFs) and reverted them to a 'normal like' phenotype [99]. Thus, suppressing this factor represent a novel prospect in improving the conditions of OSF patients. While curcumin shows great promise in the prevention of fibrosis by modulating various molecular mediators in OSF, it can be used as a potential therapeutic agent for the management of this disease.

### 17.4.6 TGF-β Signaling in OSF and Its Inhibition by Turmeric/Curcumin

TGF-β has been found to play an important role in the progression of OSF [100]. In line with this, a study was undertaken to determine the gene expression profile of ten OSF tissues. It was found that these tissues highly expressed the proteins associated with the TGF-β signaling such as TGF-β1, transforming growth factor-β-induced *protein* (TGFβIp), thrombospondin 1 (THBS1) (activator of TGF-β), transglutaminase 2 (TGM2), secreted phosphoprotein 1 (SPP1), tazarotene-induced gene-1 (TIG1) and Smad and down regulated expression of bone morphogenic protein 7 (BMP7) (a negative regulator of fibrosis). Thus, this study suggests that the suppression of BMP7 and activation of TGF-β signaling majorly contribute to the progression of OSF [101]. Another study found that AN activated JNK through the muscarinic acid receptor/$Ca^{2+}$/calcium/calmodulin-dependent protein kinase II (CAMKII), which later phosphorylates activating transcription factor 2 (ATF2), subsequently initiating TGF-β signaling cascades. This activation induces the progression of OSF via upregulating genes involved in fibrosis [102]. In another study, Khan et al. reported the activation of TGF-β signaling by the alkaloids (arecoline, arecaidine, and guvacine) and polyphenols (catechin and tannin) of AN in OSF patients. It was shown that water extracts of AN containing various alkaloids and polyphenols activated TGF-β signaling through the activation of TGF-β2 and THBS1, which also led to phosphorylation of Smad-2 protein. Moreover, it was also shown that TGF-β activated by AN induces fibrogenic activity on fibroblasts cells through matrix components like collagen [103].

Turmeric and curcumin have shown high efficacy in suppressing TGF-β in OSF. In one study, curcumin was found to inhibit the expression of TGF-β in tissue samples obtained from the OSF patients [87]. Zhang et al. suggested the regulation of fibrosis in OSF through the HIF-1α/TGF-β/CTGF signaling axis. The overexpression of HIF-1α and TGF-β induced the expression of fibrosis-related molecules such as COL1A1 and COL3A1. While curcumin treatment resulted in the inhibition of COL1A1 and COL3A1, however, the action of curcumin was reversed via overexpression of HIF-1α and TGF-β. Moreover, the activity of curcumin on MMP-2 was reversed by the overexpression of HIF-1α and TGF-β, which leads to tissue fibrosis. Thus, this study suggested the importance of the HIF-1α/TGF-β/CTGF signaling axis in modulating fibrosis in OSF and also the action of curcumin against fibrotic molecules [74]. Another study showed that curcumin treatment inhibited the arecoline-induced CTGF in BMFs, one of the downstream targets of TGF-β that contribute to synergistic induction of fibrosis in OSF [99]. Further, the treatment of patient samples with curcumin showed decreased expression of TGF-β, suggesting the chemopreventive potential of curcumin in the management of OSF [87]. Therefore, targeting TGF-β signaling and its related molecules by curcumin could be helpful in the management of OSF, as evident from the above studies. In addition, various pre-clinical and clinical studies have explored the efficacy of curcumin against this disease. Therefore, the next part of the chapter highlights the pre-clinical and clinical studies of curcumin against OSF.

## 17.5 Experimental Laboratory Studies

Various pre-clinical studies have evaluated the prospective impact of curcumin against OSF (◘ Table 17.1) [73, 99]. In one of these studies, the treatment of myofibroblasts with curcumin decreased proliferation and induced cell cycle arrest and apoptosis. Curcumin was shown to elevate the expression of Bcl-2-associated X protein (Bax) and suppress B-cell lymphoma 2 (Bcl-2), in a dose dependent manner, as compared to the untreated control. It also inhibited the deposition of collagen type I and type III, one of the causative factors in OSF [73]. In another study, Deng et al., showed that the treatment of fibroblasts, endothelial cells treated with curcumin and also tissue samples examined by immunohistochemistry showed decreased the levels of arecoline-induced CTGF [99]. A further study has also demonstrated that curcumin inhibited the expression of CTGF, HIF-1α, TGF-β and ECM components such as collagens and TIMP2 and also modulated MMPs in arecoline-treated normal oral mucosal fibroblasts, suggesting the therapeutic potential of curcumin for the treatment of OSF [74].

**◘ Table 17.1** Pre-clinical studies of curcumin against OSF

| In vitro/ In vivo | Cell lines/ models | Mechanism | References |
|---|---|---|---|
| In vitro | BMFs | ↓CTGF | [99] |
| In vivo | Parrafin-embedded tissues | ↓CTGF | [99] |
| In vitro | Fibroblasts, myofibroblasts | ↓proliferation, ↑apoptosis, ↓Bcl-2/Bax, ↓collagen (type I and III) | [73] |

*Bax* Bcl-2-associated X protein, *Bcl-2* B-cell lymphoma 2, *BMFs* Buccal mucosa fibroblasts, *CTGF* connective tissue growth factor

## 17.6 Clinical Studies

Several clinical studies have shown the efficacy of turmeric and curcumin in the management and treatment of OSF (◘ Table 17.2) [61, 85, 87, 104–117]. For example, in a RCT, one hundred and nineteen patients were assigned into three groups (group I as control, and groups II and III received curcumin in systemic and topical form, respectively) and this study showed that curcumin could improve the symptoms associated with OSF by improving mouth opening and tongue protrusion, and by inhibiting burning sensation. The application of systemic and topical form of curcumin together showed a better outcome in controlling the symptoms of OSF compared to systemic application alone [113]. Another clinical study by Lanjekar et al., involving one hundred and twenty patients showed that the application of curcumin gel, three times per day for six weeks could reduce the burning sensation of the mouth and also showed improvement in the color change of mucosa [109]. Further, the administration of 600 mg curcumin tablet per day for six months in ninety patients showed improvement in mouth opening, tongue protrusion and cheek flexibility, and decreased oral burning sensation [112]. In another clinical trial, the consumption of 1000 mg curcumin tablet (in combination with piperine and lycopene) per day for three months also showed improvement in mouth opening, tongue protrusion, and mucosal flexibility, and reduction in burning sensation. Moreover, the curcumin treatment increased oral reepithelization and decreased collagen deposition in OSF patients [110]. In addition, in a study involving sixty patients, the application of curcumin gel for six weeks showed that it could increase interincisal distance and tongue protrusion, and decrease the burning sensation [114]. Similarly, other studies have also shown that adminstration of curcumin tablets, gel, lozenges and mucoadhesive patches could reduce the burning sensation and increase the mouth opening in OSF patients [105–107, 111, 115]. Further, Yadav et al. studied the efficacy of curcumin's treatment in forty patients with a dose of 600 mg tablets per day for three months. It was observed to be beneficial and effective in reducing burning sensation, and increased the interincisal distance between the incisors by 1.25 mm [116]. Another study demonstrated the effect of curcumin caplets in one hun-

**Table 17.2** Clinical studies of turmeric/curcumin against OSF

| No of subjects | Dose & period | Form | Mechanism/outcome | References |
|---|---|---|---|---|
| 60 | 2 times/d, 8 weeks 2% curcumin gel | Curcumin gel and mucoadhesive patches | ↑mouth opening, ↓burning sensation, ↓LDH | [105] |
| 30 | 500 mg, 3 months | Curcumin tablet | ↑mouth opening, ↓burning sensation | [106] |
| 60 | 6 weeks 5 mg of gel /d | Curcumin gel | ↑mouth opening, ↓burning sensation | [111] |
| 120 | 3 times/d, 6 weeks | Curcumin gel | ↓burning sensation, improved mucosal color | [109] |
| 40 | 500 mg 2/d, 3 months | Curcumin tablet | ↑mouth opening, ↑MF, ↑TP, ↑epithelial thickness, ↓burning sensation, ↓collagen deposition | [110] |
| 90 | 300 mg 2/d, 6 months | Curcumin tablet | ↑mouth opening, ↑TP, ↑cheek flexibility, ↓burning sensation | [112] |
| 119 | Curcumin 300 mg and piperine 5 mg | Curcumin | ↑mouth opening, ↑TP, ↓burning sensation | [113] |
| 60 | 5 mg 2/d, 6 weeks | Curcumin gel | ↑interincisal distance, ↑TP, ↓burning sensation | [114] |
| 40 | 10 ml 4/d, 2 months | Turmeric | ↑mouth opening, ↓blanched mucosa, ↓pain | [104] |
| 80 | 3 times/d, 1 month | Turmeric gel | ↑mouth opening, ↑TP, ↑cheek flexibility, ↓burning sensation, safe and effective | [61] |
| 60 | 300 mg 3/d, 3 months | Curcumin | ↑mouth opening, ↓burning sensation | [115] |
| 28 | – | Curcumin | ↓p53, TGF-β, ↓ iNOS | [87] |
| 30 | 800 mg/d, 3 months | Curcumin | ↑mouth opening, ↓burning sensation, ↓blanching, ↓fibrous band thickness | [108] |
| 30 | 2 g/d, 3 months | Curcumin lozenges | ↑mouth opening, ↓burning sensation | [107] |
| 40 | 300 mg 2, 3 months | Curcumin tablet | ↓burning sensation, ↑interincisal distance, ↑TP, beneficial and effective | [116] |
| 48 | 1 g/d (curcumin), 600 mg/d (turmeric oil), 3 months | Curcumin capsules, turmeric oil | ↓burning sensation, ↓pain, ↑spicy food tolerance, ↑mouth opening, ↑TP, beneficial and well tolerated | [117] |
| 100 | 1 g | Curcumin caplets | ↑Vitamin C & E, ↑mouth opening, ↓MDA, ↓8-OHdG, ↓pain, ↓DNA damage, ↓lipid peroxidation | [85] |

*8-OHdG* 8-hydroxydeoxyguanosine, *iNOS* inducible nitric oxide synthase, *LDH* lactate dehydrogenase, *MDA* malonaldehyde, *MF* mucosal flexibility, *TP* tongue protrusion

dred patients who were divided into four groups (each with twenty five patients), consisting of healthy patients, patients with oral leukoplakia, OSF and lichen planus. In this study, the administration of curcumin increased mouth opening in OSF patients and also prevented DNA damage and lipid peroxidation. It was also shown to increase vitamins (C and E) in both serum and saliva, and decrease pain, and suppress MDA and 8-OHdG levels [85]. In another study, curcumin treatment was shown to inhibit the overexpressed TGF-β and iNOS levels in OSF patients [87]. Another study evaluated the effect of curcumin and turmeric oil compared to multinal tablets in 48 OSF patients for 3 months which showed a reduction in burning sensation and improvement in tolerance to spicy food. This treatment also relieved pain and increased mouth opening and tongue protrusion in these patients [117]. Histopathological changes in the epithelium were observed along with decreased inflammatory cells and mitotic cell count, and suppressed hyaliniced connective tissues with the curcumin or turmeric oil treatment. In addition, the turmeric oil improved blanched mucosal color to normal (pinker) appearance, which could be correlated to increased vascular supply following treatment [117]. Further, the administration of 800 mg per day (divided into two doses) of curcumin in OSF patients for 3 months enhanced mouth opening and relieved severe burning sensation and mucosal blanching, and decreased oral mucosal fibrous band thickness [108]. Furthermore, the application of a mouth rinse solution containing turmeric in 40 patients (12 females and 28 males) showed improvement in mouth opening and oral blanched mucosa and decreased pain in OSF patients [104]. In another study with 80 OSF patients, where the patients were divided into four groups and treated with ultrasound therapy, aloe vera, turmeric gel, and a combination of turmeric gel and aloe vera respectively, the turmeric group showed significant improvement in mucosal blanching and fibrosis, cheek flexibility, jaw opening and tongue protrusion and inhibition in burning sensation without causing any side effects. Thus, these studies suggest the efficacy of turmeric gel in improving the symptoms of OSF, which might be potentially due to the presence of active flavonoids, including curcumin [61].

## 17.7 Conclusion

Relentless approaches are needed to find a suitable therapy for the clinical management and treatment of OSF. The common treatment modalities for this disease include the application of a wide range of medications i.e. anti-inflammatory, anti-cytokines, and anti-fibrotic agents, immunomodulators, and vasodilators. The treatment modalities also include the consumption of dietary supplements like anti-oxidants and vitamins. However, most of the therapies have limited efficacy and is also associated with relapse of the disease. Therefore, there is an urgent need to develop an alternate, safe and efficacious strategy for the management and treatment of OSF. Curcumin, a polyphenol, also known as diferuloylmethane, is a potential compound isolated from *C. longa* L. (turmeric) and it is reported for its pleiotropic anti-inflammatory properties and immunomodulatory activities. Turmeric and its compound, curcumin, have been studied in various experimental settings for its anti-inflammatory and anti-fibrotic activities in various chronic diseases, including OSF. Pre-clinical studies with curcumin have shown its high efficacy in inhibiting the molecules involved in the pathogenesis of OSF. It has been demonstrated that curcumin could inhibit inflammatory factors like TNF-α, interleukins, and interferons; COX-2, MMPs, collagens, and TIMP-2. Curcumin was also found to inhibit several signaling pathways such as TGF-β, HIF-1 α, Akt, and NF-κB pathway in OSF.

Further, it was shown that curcumin could inhibit oxidative stress and lipid peroxidation by suppressing ROS generation and DNA damage and the by-products of lipid peroxidation like 8-OHdG and MDA. Various clinical studies with curcumin have also shown that this compound could ameliorate the symptoms associated with OSF such as pain and burning sensation, while improving mouth opening, cheek flexibility and tongue protrusion in patients leading to improvement in quality of life. Further, curcumin was also found to be safe and nontoxic in the OSF patients during or after the treatment. Thus, with all these properties of curcumin in suppressing the molecules associated with OSF pathogenesis, and its signs and symptoms, it could be considered as a potential agent for the management and treatment of OSF.

**Summary**

Overall, considering various studies of curcumin used in treating OSF, it could be a highly potent agent in the management by its property in regulating various biomolecules associated with this disease. Following these impressive pilot studies, it is clear that randomized, well-controlled clinical trials are now required to fully evaluate the potential of turmeric and curcumin in terms of the optimal dose, route of administration, targets, and possible drug interactions.

**Conflicts of Interest** The authors express no conflict of interest.

## References


1. Kerr AR, Warnakulasuriya S, Mighell A, Dietrich T, Nasser M, Rimal J, et al. A systematic review of medical interventions for oral submucous fibrosis and future research opportunities. Oral Dis. 2011;17:42–57.
2. Fedorowicz Z, Chan Shih-Yen E, Dorri M, Nasser M, Newton T, Shi L. Interventions for the management of oral submucous fibrosis. Cochrane Database Syst Rev. 2008;(4):CD007156.
3. Ranganathan K, Logendran K In: Warnakulasuriya S, Ranganathan K, editors. Medical management of oral submucous fibrosis. Switzerland: Springer; 2022.
4. Girisa S, Parama D, Harsha C, Banik K, Kunnumakkara A. Potential of guggulsterone, a farnesoid X receptor antagonist, in the prevention and treatment of cancer. Explor Target Anti-tumor Ther. 2020;1(5):313–42.
5. Henamayee S, Banik K, Sailo BL, Shabnam B, Harsha C, Srilakshmi S, et al. Therapeutic emergence of rhein as a potential anticancer drug: a review of its molecular targets and anticancer properties. Molecules. 2020;25(10):2278.
6. Parama D, Rana V, Girisa S, Verma E, Daimary UD, Thakur KK, et al. The promising potential of piperlongumine as an emerging therapeutics for cancer. Explor Target Anti-tumor Ther. 2021;2:323–54.
7. Chattopadhyay I, Biswas K, Bandyopadhyay U, Banerjee RK. Turmeric and curcumin: biological actions and medicinal applications. Curr Sci. 2004:44–53.
8. Hewlings SJ, Kalman DS. Curcumin: a review of its' effects on human health. Foods. 2017;6(10):92–8.
9. Maheshwari RK, Singh AK, Gaddipati J, Srimal RC. Multiple biological activities of curcumin: a short review. Life Sci. 2006;78(18):2081–7.

10. Akram M, Shahab-Uddin AA, Usmanghani K, Hannan A, Mohiuddin E, Asif M. Curcuma longa and curcumin: a review article. Rom J Biol Plant Biol. 2010;55(2):65–70.
11. Anderson AM, Mitchell MS, Mohan RS. Isolation of curcumin from turmeric. J Chem Educ. 2000;77(3):359.
12. Nisar T, Iqbal M, Raza A, Safdar M, Iftikhar F, Waheed M. Turmeric: a promising spice for phytochemical and antimicrobial activities. Am Eur J Agric Environ Sci. 2015;15(7):1278–88.
13. Soleimani V, Sahebkar A, Hosseinzadeh H. Turmeric (Curcuma longa) and its major constituent (curcumin) as nontoxic and safe substances. Phytother Res. 2018;32(6):985–95.
14. Alsamydai A, Jaber N. Pharmacological aspects of curcumin. Int J Pharm. 2018;5(6):313–26.
15. Fu Y-S, Chen T-H, Weng L, Huang L, Lai D, Weng C-F. Pharmacological properties and underlying mechanisms of curcumin and prospects in medicinal potential. Biomed Pharmacother. 2021;141:111888.
16. Girisa S, Kumar A, Rana V, Parama D, Daimary UD, Warnakulasuriya S, et al. From simple mouth cavities to complex Oral mucosal disorders—curcuminoids as a promising therapeutic approach. ACS Pharmacol Transl Sci. 2021;4(2):647–65.
17. Rathaur P, Raja W, Ramteke P, John SA. Turmeric: the golden spice of life. Int J Pharm Sci Res. 2012;3(7):1987.
18. Aggarwal BB, Gupta SC, Sung B. Curcumin: an orally bioavailable blocker of TNF and other pro-inflammatory biomarkers. Br J Pharmacol. 2013;169(8):1672–92.
19. Kumar A, Harsha C, Parama D, Girisa S, Daimary UD, Mao X, et al. Current clinical developments in curcumin-based therapeutics for cancer and chronic diseases. Phytother Res. 2021;35:6768.
20. Kunnumakkara AB, Harsha C, Banik K, Vikkurthi R, Sailo BL, Bordoloi D, et al. Is curcumin bioavailability a problem in humans: lessons from clinical trials. Expert Opin Drug Metab Toxicol. 2019;15(9):705–33.
21. Shehzad A, Lee YS. Molecular mechanisms of curcumin action: signal transduction. Biofactors. 2013;39(1):27–36.
22. Patel SS, Acharya A, Ray R, Agrawal R, Raghuwanshi R, Jain P. Cellular and molecular mechanisms of curcumin in prevention and treatment of disease. Crit Rev Food Sci Nutr. 2020;60(6):887–939.
23. Wongcharoen W, Phrommintikul A. The protective role of curcumin in cardiovascular diseases. Int J Cardiol. 2009;133(2):145–51.
24. Baum L, Ng A. Curcumin interaction with copper and iron suggests one possible mechanism of action in Alzheimer's disease animal models. J Alzheimers Dis. 2004;6(4):367–77.
25. Kim YS, Ahn Y, Hong MH, Joo SY, Kim KH, Sohn IS, et al. Curcumin attenuates inflammatory responses of TNF-α-stimulated human endothelial cells. J Cardiovasc Pharmacol. 2007;50(1):41–9.
26. Xiao Y, Xia J, Wu S, Lv Z, Huang S, Huang H, et al. Curcumin inhibits acute vascular inflammation through the activation of heme oxygenase-1. Oxid Med Cell Longev. 2018;2018:1.
27. Zhou T, Chen D, Li Q, Sun X, Song Y, Wang C. Curcumin inhibits inflammatory response and bone loss during experimental periodontitis in rats. Acta Odontol Scand. 2013;71(2):349–56.
28. Hsieh C. Phase I clinical trial of curcumin, a chemopreventive agent, in patients with high-risk or pre-malignant lesions. Anticancer Res. 2001;21(2895):e2900.
29. Landskron G, De la Fuente M, Thuwajit P, Thuwajit C, Hermoso MA. Chronic inflammation and cytokines in the tumor microenvironment. J Immunol Res. 2014;2014:1.
30. He Y, Yue Y, Zheng X, Zhang K, Chen S, Du Z. Curcumin, inflammation, and chronic diseases: how are they linked? Molecules. 2015;20(5):9183–213.
31. Aggarwal BB. Signalling pathways of the TNF superfamily: a double-edged sword. Nat Rev Immunol. 2003;3(9):745–56.
32. Aggarwal BB, Harikumar KB. Potential therapeutic effects of curcumin, the anti-inflammatory agent, against neurodegenerative, cardiovascular, pulmonary, metabolic, autoimmune and neoplastic diseases. Int J Biochem Cell Biol. 2009;41(1):40–59.
33. Lee Y-H, Yu C-C, Hsieh P-L, Liao Y-W, Yu C-H, Su T-R. Inhibition of lncRNA HOTTIP ameliorated myofibroblast activities and inflammatory cytokines in oral submucous fibrosis. J Formos Med Assoc. 2021;120(5):1188–93.
34. Kujundžić RN, Stepanić V, Milković L, Gašparović AČ, Tomljanović M, Trošelj KG. Curcumin and its potential for systemic targeting of inflamm-aging and metabolic reprogramming in cancer. Int J Mol Sci. 2019;20(5):1180.
35. Vander Broek R, Snow GE, Chen Z, Van Waes C. Chemoprevention of head and neck squamous cell carcinoma through inhibition of NF-κB signaling. Oral Oncol. 2014;50(10):930–41.
36. Catanzaro M, Fagiani F, Racchi M, Corsini E, Govoni S, Lanni C. Immune response in COVID-19: addressing a pharmacological challenge by targeting pathways triggered by SARS-CoV-2. Signal Transduct Target Ther. 2020;5(1):1–10.
37. Mohammadi A, Blesso CN, Barreto GE, Banach M, Majeed M, Sahebkar A. Macrophage plasticity, polarization and function in response to curcumin, a diet-derived polyphenol, as an immunomodulatory agent. J Nutr Biochem. 2019;66:1–16.
38. Zeinali M, Rezaee SA, Hosseinzadeh H. An overview on immunoregulatory and anti-inflammatory properties of chrysin and flavonoids substances. Biomed Pharmacother. 2017;92:998–1009.
39. Lashgari N-A, Roudsari NM, Momtaz S, Sathyapalan T, Abdolghaffari AH, Sahebkar A. The involvement of JAK/STAT signaling pathway in the treatment of Parkinson's disease. J Neuroimmunol. 2021;361:577758.
40. Shehzad A, Qureshi M, Anwar MN, Lee YS. Multifunctional curcumin mediate multitherapeutic effects. J Food Sci. 2017;82(9):2006–15.
41. Ashrafizadeh M, Rafiei H, Mohammadinejad R, Afshar EG, Farkhondeh T, Samarghandian S. Potential therapeutic effects of curcumin mediated by JAK/STAT signaling pathway: a review. Phytother Res. 2020;34(8):1745–60.
42. Sun J, Zhao Y, Hu J. Curcumin inhibits imiquimod-induced psoriasis-like inflammation by inhibiting IL-1beta and IL-6 production in mice. PLoS One. 2013;8(6):e67078.
43. Huang M-T, Lysz T, Ferraro T, Abidi TF, Laskin JD, Conney AH. Inhibitory effects of curcumin on in vitro lipoxygenase and cyclooxygenase activities in mouse epidermis. Cancer Res. 1991;51(3):813–9.
44. Chang M-C, Chen Y-J, Chang H-H, Chan C-P, Yeh C-Y, Wang Y-L, et al. Areca nut components affect COX-2, cyclin B1/cdc25C and keratin expression, PGE2 production in keratinocyte is related to reactive oxygen species, CYP1A1, Src, EGFR and Ras signaling. PLoS One. 2014;9(7):e101959.
45. Chang M-C, Wu H-L, Lee J-J, Lee P-H, Chang H-H, Hahn L-J, et al. The induction of prostaglandin E2 production, interleukin-6 production, cell cycle arrest, and cytotoxicity in primary oral keratinocytes and KB cancer cells by areca nut ingredients is differentially regulated by MEK/ERK activation. J Biol Chem. 2004;279(49):50676–83.

46. Sharma C, Kaur J, Shishodia S, Aggarwal BB, Ralhan R. Curcumin down regulates smokeless tobacco-induced NF-kappaB activation and COX-2 expression in human oral premalignant and cancer cells. Toxicology. 2006;228(1):1–15.
47. Mei X, Xu D, Xu S, Zheng Y, Xu S. Novel role of Zn (II)–curcumin in enhancing cell proliferation and adjusting proinflammatory cytokine-mediated oxidative damage of ethanol-induced acute gastric ulcers. Chem Biol Interact. 2012;197(1):31–9.
48. Neyrinck AM, Alligier M, Memvanga PB, Névraumont E, Larondelle Y, Préat V, et al. Curcuma longa extract associated with white pepper lessens high fat diet-induced inflammation in subcutaneous adipose tissue. PLoS One. 2013;8(11):e81252.
49. Gong Z, Zhao S, Zhou J, Yan J, Wang L, Du X, et al. Curcumin alleviates DSS-induced colitis via inhibiting NLRP3 inflammsome activation and IL-1β production. Mol Immunol. 2018;104:11–9.
50. Yin H, Guo Q, Li X, Tang T, Li C, Wang H, et al. Curcumin suppresses IL-1β secretion and prevents inflammation through inhibition of the NLRP3 inflammasome. J Immunol. 2018;200(8):2835–46.
51. Zhao J, Wang J, Zhou M, Li M, Li M, Tan H. Curcumin attenuates murine lupus via inhibiting NLRP3 inflammasome. Int Immunopharmacol. 2019;69:213–6.
52. Kong F, Ye B, Cao J, Cai X, Lin L, Huang S, et al. Curcumin represses NLRP3 inflammasome activation via TLR4/MyD88/NF-κB and P2X7R signaling in PMA-induced macrophages. Front Pharmacol. 2016;7:369.
53. Hande AH, Chaudhary MS, Gawande MN, Gadbail AR, Zade PR, Bajaj S, et al. Oral submucous fibrosis: An enigmatic morpho-insight. J Cancer Res Ther. 2019;15(3):463.
54. Zhang JM, An J. Cytokines, inflammation, and pain. Int Anesthesiol Clin. 2007;45(2):27–37.
55. Shih Y-H, Wang T-H, Shieh T-M, Tseng Y-H. Oral submucous fibrosis: a review on etiopathogenesis, diagnosis, and therapy. Int J Mol Sci. 2019;20(12):2940.
56. Haque M, Harris M, Meghji S, Barrett A. Immunolocalization of cytokines and growth factors in oral submucous fibrosis. Cytokine. 1998;10(9):713–9.
57. Haque M, Meghji S, Khitab U, Harris M. Oral submucous fibrosis patients have altered levels of cytokine production. J Oral Pathol Med. 2000;29(3):123–8.
58. Kamath VV, Satelur K, Komali Y. Biochemical markers in oral submucous fibrosis: a review and update. Dent Res J (Isfahan). 2013;10(5):576–84.
59. Cho J-W, Lee K-S, Kim C-W. Curcumin attenuates the expression of IL-1β, IL-6, and TNF-α as well as cyclin E in TNF-α-treated HaCaT cells, NF-κB and MAPKs as potential upstream targets. Int J Mol Med. 2007;19(3):469–74.
60. Jain SK, Rains J, Croad J, Larson B, Jones K. Curcumin supplementation lowers TNF-α, IL-6, IL-8, and MCP-1 secretion in high glucose-treated cultured monocytes and blood levels of TNF-α, IL-6, MCP-1, glucose, and glycosylated hemoglobin in diabetic rats. Antioxid Redox Signal. 2009;11(2):241–9.
61. Meshram M, Bhowate RR, Madke B, Sune R. Evaluation of the effect of ultrasound physiotherapy interventions in combination with local application of aloe-vera and turmeric gel in the management of oral submucous fibrosis. J Dent Invest. 2018;1(1):16–33.
62. Haque M, Meghji S, Nazir R, Harris M. Interferon gamma (IFN-γ) may reverse oral submucous fibrosis. J Oral Pathol Med. 2001;30(1):12–21.
63. Bhattacharyya S, Hossain DMS, Mohanty S, Sen GS, Chattopadhyay S, Banerjee S, et al. Curcumin reverses T cell-mediated adaptive immune dysfunctions in tumor-bearing hosts. Cell Mol Immunol. 2010;7(4):306–15.
64. Chen H, Yang R, Tang Y, Fu X. Effects of curcumin on artery blood gas index of rats with pulmonary fibrosis caused by paraquat poisoning and the expression of Smad 4, Smurf 2, interleukin-4 and interferon-γ. Exp Ther Med. 2019;17(5):3664–70.
65. Gertsch J, Güttinger M, Heilmann J, Sticher O. Curcumin differentially modulates mRNA profiles in Jurkat T and human peripheral blood mononuclear cells. Bioorg Med Chem. 2003;11(6):1057–63.
66. Basnet P, Skalko-Basnet N. Curcumin: an anti-inflammatory molecule from a curry spice on the path to cancer treatment. Molecules. 2011;16(6):4567–98.
67. Cheng R-H, Wang Y-P, Chang JY-F, Pan Y-H, Chang M-C, Jeng J-H. Genetic susceptibility and protein expression of extracellular matrix turnover-related genes in oral submucous fibrosis. Int J Mol Sci 2020;21(21):8104.
68. Wight TN, Potter-Perigo S. The extracellular matrix: an active or passive player in fibrosis? American journal of physiology-gastrointestinal and liver. Phys Ther. 2011;301(6):G950–G5.
69. Ekanayaka RP, Tilakaratne WM. Oral submucous fibrosis: review on mechanisms of malignant transformation. Oral Surg Oral Med Oral Pathol Oral Radiol. 2016;122(2):192–9.
70. Tilakaratne W, Klinikowski M, Saku T, Peters T, Warnakulasuriya S. Oral submucous fibrosis: review on aetiology and pathogenesis. Oral Oncol. 2006;42(6):561–8.
71. Utsunomiya H, Tilakaratne WM, Oshiro K, Maruyama S, Suzuki M, Ida-Yonemochi H, et al. Extracellular matrix remodeling in oral submucous fibrosis: its stage-specific modes revealed by immunohistochemistry and in situ hybridization. J Oral Pathol Med. 2005;34(8):498–507.
72. Arpino V, Brock M, Gill SE. The role of TIMPs in regulation of extracellular matrix proteolysis. Matrix Biol. 2015;44:247–54.
73. Zhang S-S, Gong Z-J, Li W-H, Wang X, Ling T-Y. Antifibrotic effect of curcumin in TGF-β1-induced myofibroblasts from human oral mucosa. Asian Pac J Cancer Prev. 2012;13(1):289–94.
74. Zhang L, Tan J, Liu Y-P, Liu X, Luo M. Curcumin relieves the arecoline-induced fibrosis of oral mucosal fibroblasts via inhibiting HIF-1α/TGF-β/CTGF signaling pathway: an in vitro study. Toxicol Res. 2021;10(3):631–8.
75. Betteridge DJ. What is oxidative stress? Metabolism. 2000;49(2):3–8.
76. Rana V, Parama D, Girisa S, Harsha C, Kunnumakkara AB. Oxidative stress and inflammation. Antioxidants and functional foods for neurodegenerative disorders. CRC Press; 2021. p. 21–36.
77. Rai A, Siddiqui M, Parveen S, Parveen S, Rasheed A, Ali S. Molecular pathogenesis of oral submucous fibrosis: a critical appraisal. Biomed Pharmacol J. 2019;12(04):2027–36.
78. Agrawal S, Ambad R. Evaluation of antioxidant status in Oral submucous fibrosis: a hospital based study. Int J Innov Res Med Sci. 2017;2(07):903–7.
79. Chandramohan Kulasekaran MD, Dhivya K, Vijayalakshmi D, Sathishkumar M, Madhanmohan A. Immunohistochemical detection of 8-hydroxydeoxyguanosine: a biomarker of oxidative DNA damage in oral submucous fibrosis. J Oral Maxillofac Pathol. 2020;24(3):536.
80. Leutner S, Eckert A, Müller W. ROS generation, lipid peroxidation and antioxidant enzyme activities in the aging brain. J Neural Transm. 2001;108(8–9):955–67.

81. Avinash Tejasvi ML, Bangi BB, Geetha P, Anulekha Avinash CK, Chittaranjan B, Bhayya H, et al. Estimation of serum superoxide dismutase and serum malondialdehyde in oral submucous fibrosis: a clinical and biochemical study. J Cancer Res Ther. 2014;10(3):722–5.
82. Bale R, Kattappagari KK, Vidya D, Vuddandi S, Gummalla C, Baddam VRR. Oral submucous fibrosis: a quantitative assessment of serum malondialdehyde, superoxide dismutase and correlation with clinical staging. J Oral Maxillofac Pathol. 2017;21(1):41–5.
83. Ganta SR, Chittemsetti S, Sravya T, Guttikonda VR. Salivary malondialdehyde in oral submucous fibrosis - a marker for oxidative damage. J Oral Maxillofac Pathol. 2021;25(1):82–7.
84. Shetty SR, Babu SG, Kumari S, Rao V, Vijay R, Karikal A. Malondialdehyde levels in oral sub mucous fibrosis: a clinicopathological and biochemical study. N Am J Med Sci. 2012;4(3):125–8.
85. Rai B, Kaur J, Jacobs R, Singh J. Possible action mechanism for curcumin in pre-cancerous lesions based on serum and salivary markers of oxidative stress. J Oral Sci. 2010;52(2):251–6.
86. Kapgate TD. Effect of turmeric on serum malondialdehyde levels in oral submucous fibrosis. Int J Dent Res. 2020;5:29.
87. Gupta S, Ghosh S, Gupta S, Sakhuja P. Effect of curcumin on the expression of p53, transforming growth factor-β, and inducible nitric oxide synthase in oral submucous fibrosis: a pilot study. J Investig Clin Dent. 2017;8(4):e12252.
88. Rajendran R, Mohammed PR, Shaikh S, Pillai M. Expression of matrix metalloproteinases (MMP-1, MMP-2 and MMP-9) and their inhibitors (TIMP-1 and TIMP-2) in oral submucous fibrosis. Indian J Dent Res. 2006;17(4):161.
89. Johansson N, Ahonen M, Kähäri V-M. Matrix metalloproteinases in tumor invasion. Cell Mol Life Sci. 2000;57(1):5–15.
90. Roeb E. Matrix metalloproteinases and liver fibrosis (translational aspects). Matrix Biol. 2018;68:463–73.
91. Chaudhary AK, Singh M, Bharti AC, Singh M, Shukla S, Singh AK, et al. Synergistic effect of stromelysin-1 (matrix metalloproteinase-3) promoter (−1171 5A-> 6A) polymorphism in oral submucous fibrosis and head and neck lesions. BMC Cancer. 2010;10(1):1–9.
92. Mishra G, Ranganathan K. Matrix metalloproteinase-1 expression in oral submucous fibrosis: an immunohistochemical study. Indian J Dent Res. 2010;21(3):320.
93. Kherde P, Gosavi S. Serum levels of matrix metalloproteinase-2 in patients with oral submucous fibrosis and oral squamous cell carcinoma. Int J Res Med Sci. 2020;8:636.
94. Zhen L, Fan D, Yi X, Cao X, Chen D, Wang L. Curcumin inhibits oral squamous cell carcinoma proliferation and invasion via EGFR signaling pathways. Int J Clin Exp Pathol. 2014;7(10):6438–46.
95. Lee AY-L, Fan C-C, Chen Y-A, Cheng C-W, Sung Y-J, Hsu C-P, et al. Curcumin inhibits invasiveness and epithelial-mesenchymal transition in oral squamous cell carcinoma through reducing matrix metalloproteinase 2, 9 and modulating p53-E-cadherin pathway. Integr Cancer Ther. 2015;14(5):484–90.
96. Warnakulasuriya S, Kujan O, Aguirre-Urizar JM, Bagan JV, González-Moles MÁ, Kerr AR, et al. Oral potentially malignant disorders: a consensus report from an international seminar on nomenclature and classification, convened by the WHO collaborating Centre for Oral Cancer. Oral Dis. 2021;27(8):1862–80.
97. Al-Maweri SA. Efficacy of curcumin for management of oral submucous fibrosis: a systematic review of randomized clinical trials. Oral Surg Oral Med Oral Pathol Oral Radiol. 2019;127(4):300–8.
98. Thakur N. Effectiveness of micronutrients and physiotherapy in the management of oral submucous fibrosis. International journal of contemporary. Dentistry. 2011;2(1)
99. Deng Y-T, Chen H-M, Cheng S-J, Chiang C-P, Kuo MY-P. Arecoline-stimulated connective tissue growth factor production in human buccal mucosal fibroblasts: modulation by curcumin. Oral Oncol. 2009;45(9):e99–e105.
100. Liu J, Li F, Liu B, Yao Z, Li L, Liu G, et al. Adipose-derived mesenchymal stem cell exosomes inhibit transforming growth factor-β1-induced collagen synthesis in oral mucosal fibroblasts. Exp Ther Med. 2021;22(6):1–10.
101. Khan I, Agarwal P, Thangjam GS, Radhesh R, Rao SG, Kondaiah P. Role of TGF-β and BMP7 in the pathogenesis of oral submucous fibrosis. Growth Factors. 2011;29(4):119–27.
102. Pant I, Rao SG, Kondaiah P. Role of areca nut induced JNK/ATF2/Jun axis in the activation of TGF-β pathway in precancerous Oral submucous fibrosis. Sci Rep. 2016;6(1):1–15.
103. Khan I, Kumar N, Pant I, Narra S, Kondaiah P. Activation of TGF-β pathway by areca nut constituents: a possible cause of oral submucous fibrosis. PLoS One. 2012;7(12):e51806.
104. Aich R, Ghanta S, Das A, Giri D, Majumdar M, Bhattacharjee S. Evaluation of the role of a mouth rinse containing turmeric, triphala, and honey in the treatment of oral submucous fibrosis: An open label clinical study. J Indian Acad Oral Med Radiol. 2018;30(4):376.
105. Chandrashekar A, Annigeri RG, Usha V, Thimmasetty J. A clinicobiochemical evaluation of curcumin as gel and as buccal mucoadhesive patches in the management of oral submucous fibrosis. Oral Surg Oral Med Oral Pathol Oral Radiol. 2021;131(4):428–34.
106. Deepak T, Manjunath M, Thakur H. Efficacy of curcumin and topical steroids in the treatment for oral submucous fibrosis: a comparative study. J Pharm Bioallied Sci. 2021;13(5):542.
107. Hazarey VK, Sakrikar AR, Ganvir SM. Efficacy of curcumin in the treatment for oral submucous fibrosis: a randomized clinical trial. J Oral Maxillofac Pathol. 2015;19(2):145.
108. Kopuri RKC, Chakravarthy C, Sunder S, Patil RS, Shivaraj W, Arakeri G. A comparative study of the clinical efficacy of lycopene and curcumin in the treatment of oral submucous fibrosis using ultrasonography. J Int Oral Health. 2016;8(6):687.
109. Lanjekar AB, Bhowate RR, Bakhle S, Narayane A, Pawar V, Gandagule R. Comparison of efficacy of topical curcumin gel with triamcinolone-hyaluronidase gel individually and in combination in the treatment of oral submucous fibrosis. J Contemp Dent Pract. 2020;21(1):83–90.
110. Mahato B, Prodhan C, Mandal S, Dutta A, Kumar P, Deb T, et al. Evaluation of efficacy of curcumin along with lycopene and piperine in the management of oral submucous fibrosis. Contemp Clin Dent. 2019;10(3):531.
111. Nerkar Rajbhoj A, Kulkarni TM, Shete A, Shete M, Gore R, Sapkal R. A comparative study to evaluate efficacy of curcumin and aloe Vera gel along with oral physiotherapy in the management of oral submucous fibrosis: a randomized clinical trial. Asian Pac J Cancer Prev. 2021;22(S1):107–12.
112. Piyush P, Mahajan A, Singh K, Ghosh S, Gupta S. Comparison of therapeutic response of lycopene and curcumin in oral submucous fibrosis: a randomized controlled trial. Oral Dis. 2019;25(1):73–9.
113. Rai A, Kaur M, Gombra V, Hasan S, Kumar N. Comparative evaluation of curcumin and antioxidants in the management

of oral submucous fibrosis. J Investig Clin Dent. 2019;10(4):e12464.
114. Rizvi D, Abidi A, Faiz SM, Hasan R, Thadani A. Efficacy of curcumin gel and tulsi gel in oral submucous fibrosis. Natl J Physiol Pharmacy Pharmacol. 2019;9(4):343–8.
115. Saran G, Umapathy D, Misra N, Channaiah SG, Singh P, Srivastava S, et al. A comparative study to evaluate the efficacy of lycopene and curcumin in oral submucous fibrosis patients: a randomized clinical trial. Indian J Dent Res. 2018;29(3):303–12.
116. Yadav M, Aravinda K, Saxena VS, Srinivas K, Ratnakar P, Gupta J, et al. Comparison of curcumin with intralesional steroid injections in Oral submucous fibrosis–a randomized, open-label interventional study. J Oral Biol Craniofacial Res. 2014;4(3):169–73.
117. Das DA, Balan A, Sreelatha K. Comparative study of the efficacy of curcumin and turmeric oil as chemopreventive agents in oral submucous fibrosis: a clinical and histopathological evaluation. J Indian Acad Oral Med Radiol. 2010;22(2):88.

# Surgical Management of Oral Submucous Fibrosis

*Moni Abraham Kuriakose, Vijay Pillai, and Pallavi Priyadarshini*

**Contents**



© The Author(s), under exclusive license to Springer Nature Switzerland AG 2023
S. Warnakulasuriya, K. Ranganathan (eds.), *Oral Submucous Fibrosis*, Textbooks in Contemporary Dentistry,
https://doi.org/10.1007/978-3-031-12855-4_18

## 18.1 Introduction

Oral submucous fibrosis (OSF) is one of the oral potentially malignant disorders (OPMD). Along with its malignant transformation potential, the progressive nature of the disease causes significant disability, especially trismus, which needs to be addressed both to improve the function as well as surveillance of the oral cavity. A recent meta-analysis showed a prevalence of 4.47% OPMD (95%CI-2.43–7.08), the most common OPMD being OSF [1]. OSF is common among the population of the South East Asia. Clinicians are commonly challenged with deciding the treatment modalities for patients presenting with OSF. There are numerous interventions designed to reduce the severity of the disease, reverse the fibrosis and alleviate the symptom complex that develops with it.

Broadly classified as medical and surgical, the interventions would be based on the extent of pain, burning sensation and fibrosis present in the patient [2]. Treatment modalities in OSF are generally centered on providing relief of symptoms like burning sensation and reduced mouth opening. These symptoms in the initial stage can be medically managed [3, 4]. This is detailed in the previous chapter on medical management of submucous fibrosis. However, in advanced OSF when there is significant restriction of mouth opening, surgical intervention needs to be considered. It not only relieves the trismus but also facilitates examination and surveillance of the oral cavity to detect early any malignant transformation.

Surgical management is indicated in patients who have established trismus with inter-incisal mouth opening of less than 25 mm [5]. The primary aim of surgery is to improve mouth opening in an attempt to restore articulation, mastication, and oral hygiene [6]. Various surgical procedures have been proposed by different authors, with variable success rates. In this chapter we present the indications and the surgical techniques.



**Learning Goals**

- Understand the indications for surgical intervention in OSF.
- Learn details of surgical steps in managing OSF.
- Understand limitations and usefulness of various resurfacing techniques.
- Appreciate potential complications and measures to prevent and manage them.

## 18.2 Indications of Surgery

Given the variable spectrum of the signs and symptoms of OSF, interventions can be tailored based on the severity of the disease. Various grading systems are in vogue to help the clinician to decide between medical or surgical interventions (Chap. 6). Decision regarding the treatment would be based on the clinical findings especially the interincisal distance.

Pindborg and Sirsat were the first to classify OSF depending only on histopathological features [7]. Based on this grading, medical intervention is indicated for early inflammatory phase (grade 1–2) and surgical intervention for fibrosis phase (grade 3 and above).

Khanna et al. in a series of 100 patients, categorised them into four groups based on presenting symptoms, site of involvement, interincisal opening, distribution of fibrous bands, clinical alterations in the mucosa, presence of malignant transformation with histopathological features. Surgical treatment was considered for patients in group III (interincisal opening of 15–25 mm) and group IV (interincisal opening of 2–15 mm and also for cases with premalignant and malignant changes [5]. Mehrotra et al. in their study of 100 cases of OSF also suggested surgical intervention for grade III and above. Based on their study they have even come up with a classification that suggests surgical management based on the severity of the disease [8].

| Grading | Signs and symptoms |
|---|---|
| Grade I: | Stomatitis and burning sensation in the buccal mucosa with no detection of fibres. Suggested treatment for this group is abstinence from habit and medicinal management |
| Grade II: | Symptoms of grade I, plus palpable fibrous bands, involvement of soft palate, and maximum mouth opening 26–35 mm. Suggested treatment: Abstinence from habit and medicinal management |
| Grade III: | Symptoms of grade II, plus blanched oral mucosa, involvement of the tongue, and maximal mouth opening 6–25 mm. Suggested treatment: Abstinence from habit and surgical management |
| Grade IV: | Symptoms of grade III, plus fibrosis of lips, and mouth opening 5 mm. Suggested treatment: Abstinence from habit and surgical management |

A proposed algorithm for the management of OSF is given in Fig. 18.1.

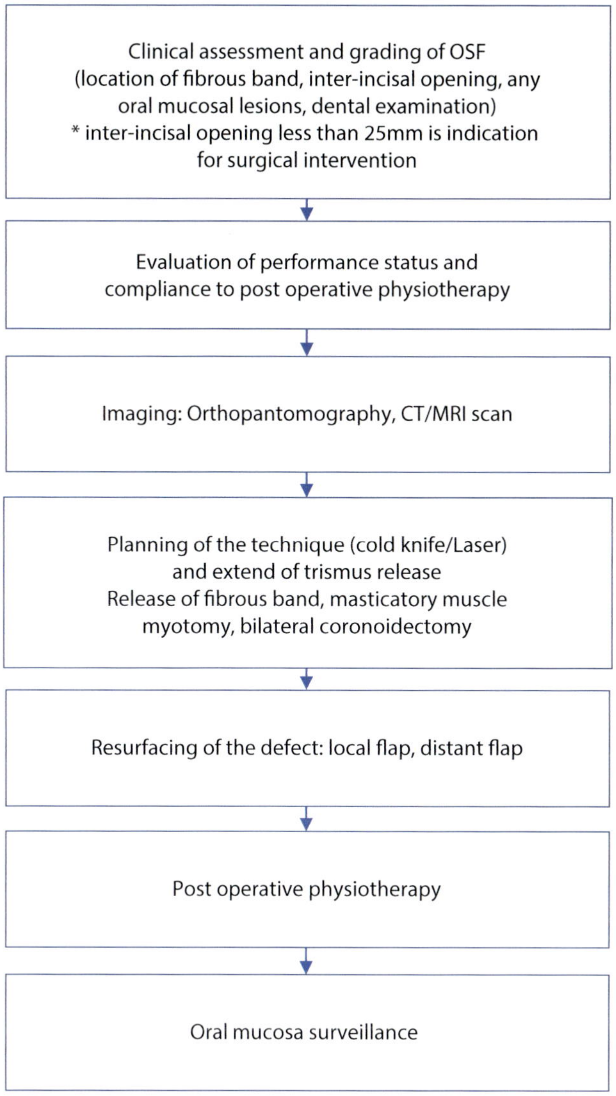


**Fig. 18.1** Algorithmic approach to management of OSF

## 18.3 Principles of Surgery and Surgical Steps

The broad principles of surgery include (▶ Box 18.1):
(a) Release of the fibrous bands.
(b) Adjunctive procedures such as coronoidectomies and masticatory muscle myotomy.
(c) Resurfacing the defects with grafts, biological membranes or flaps.
(d) Post operative physiotherapy.

Physical division of fibrosed tissue with postoperative maintenance of the mouth opening created by fibrous band release is the basis for surgical intervention [2, 9, 10]. Although submucous fibrosis is primarily a mucosal disease, gradual restriction of mouth opening leads to shortening and contraction of muscles of mastication, particularly the elevators of mandible- masseter, medial pterygoid and temporalis. The goal of muscle release is the detachment of muscles from its bony attachment so that the muscles could be repositioned to a longer position and rehabilitated by the post-operative muscle stretching exercises. To facilitate this, the muscle attachments need to be separated in a subperiosteal plane, so that the periosteum along with the muscles will be reattached to a newer position.

Limited myotomy is done for those muscles that cannot be easily repositioned (temporalis) or in severe cases with almost no mouth opening to gain access to muscle release (insertion of masseter to the zygomatic bone). The surgical interventions follow a standard protocol:

**Box 18.1 Steps in the Surgical Management of OSF**
- Fibrous band release or fibrotomy
- Coronoidectomy and masticator muscle myotomy
- Resurfacing the defect
- Physiotherapy

### 18.3.1 Preoperative Evaluation

Preoperative clinical and radiological examination needs to be carried out. A careful assessment of the mouth opening with a documentation of the interincisal distance, examination of the buccal mucosa, labial mucosa, tongue, soft palate, faucial pillars and oropharynx for fibrotic bands is mandatory. In addition examination and screening for any suspicious lesion that would need biopsy before proceeding with a definitive surgical plan. This can be facilitated with the aid of a flexible endoscope to inspect all the oral mucosal surfaces to identify and map any oral ulceration or erosions, which are signs of malignant transformation. These early lesions cannot be appreciated in imaging studies, especially since puffed cheek technique could not be readily performed in OSF.

Imaging is generally not indicated for soft tissue assessment [11]. An orthopantomogram is indicated if planning coronoidectomy. MRI is recommended if mouth opening is severely restricted. Alternatively CT scan with contrast may be recommended to evaluate any oral lesions identified during clinical examination.

### 18.3.2 Anesthesia, Preparation of the Patient and Intraoperative Evaluation

General anesthesia with nasal endotracheal intubation is required. As the patients indicated for surgical intervention to release trismus (grade 3 or 4) will have less than 2.5 cm mouth opening; awake fiberoptic nasal intubation would be required. Although blind nasal intubation with regional anesthesia could be attempted, the anesthetist should be adept with fibreoptic intubation and the necessary equipment should be available.

After inducing the anesthesia, bilateral temporary tarsorrhaphy may be performed to protect the eyes and to expose the paranasal areas for possible nasolabial or temporalis flap harvesting. A shoulder roll is recommended to allow forward thrusting of the mandible and to make the occlusal plane 90 degrees to horizontal plane. Bilateral face, neck, oral cavity and anterior half of scalp needs to be prepped and draped. A self-retained plastic lip retractor may be inserted and secured using sutures placed on upper and lower lips away from the commissure of the mouth.

Because of the trismus, visualization of the oral cavity may be limited. To improve visualization, a metallic Heister-mouth-opening device may be placed on the contralateral molar region and stretch the mouth to open as much as possible. The surgeons may wear headlight or use fibreoptic light source to illuminate the oral cavity.

The initial step would be examination of all the oral mucosa to look for any advanced oral potentially malignant or malignant lesions and if required, biopsy needs to be performed. In addition, with the assistance of a dental surgeon, examination of dentition may be carried out. In severe cases this oral evaluation may be possible only after release of trismus.

### 18.3.3 Incision of Fibrous Bands Followed by Adequate Muscular Release

A horizontal incision of the mucosa is made using monopolar cautery starting at the junction of hard and soft palate behind the tuberosity of maxilla, extending anteriorly towards the commissure of the mouth. The incision should be made about 7.0 mm inferior to the parotid duct. Anteriorly the incision is extended to a point about 1 cm posterior to the commissure, protecting the modiolus. Depending on the fibrosis of upper and lower lip sulci, the incision may be extended to these regions in a 'Y' shaped fashion. A similar incision is made on the contralateral side (Fig. 18.2).



The mucosal incision is deepened to release the fibrous band which would be most prominent around the anterior pillar of fauces. This would include the release of pterygomandibular raphe and the fibrous band underneath the anterior pillar of fauces. This can be assisted by the gradual activation of the Heister's mouth opening device.

**Laser in OSF fibrous band release**: The literature reports the use of laser other than cold knife for the excision of the fibrous bands [12–18]. The ErYCCG laser, KTP 532, and diode lasers are the most often utilized lasers [13–18]. The principle of laser for surgical fibrotomy in OSF is by photothermal action, which causes tissue disruption by deposition of enough heat to evaporate the tissue. The laser energy is preferentially absorbed in the target tissues, resulting in a direct tissue cut (cold cut) or tissue rupture due to water vaporization within a cell (thermo-mechanical tissue ablation). This process protects the extracellular collagen matrix by limiting collagen damage to 5 μm (about 2 cell widths). Characteristics such as laser type, wavelength, energy employed, and exposure period all play a role in ensuring the laser's desired effects. Furthermore, the optical qualities of the target tissue, as well as its absorptive nature, determine the amount of laser energy required to achieve good clinical results. Laser therapy may produce less postoperative pain and hasten the healing as reported by Kameshwaran et al. and Nayak et al. [14, 15].

The majority of the studies have used diode lasers [16–18]. It is a semiconductor laser, with a wavelength range of 800–980 nm. It emanates through a fiber-optic cable and has a good cutting efficacy without causing damage to dental hard tissues. The KTP-532 laser uses a 532 nm wavelength that is specifically absorbed by blood vessels, resulting in superior hemostatic properties. The wavelength of an ErCr:YSGG laser is 2780 μm. Water absorbs this wavelength effectively, therefore it can be used on oral soft tissue without inflicting thermal injury. Choudhary et al. have reported efficacy of ErCr:YSGG laser in OSF.

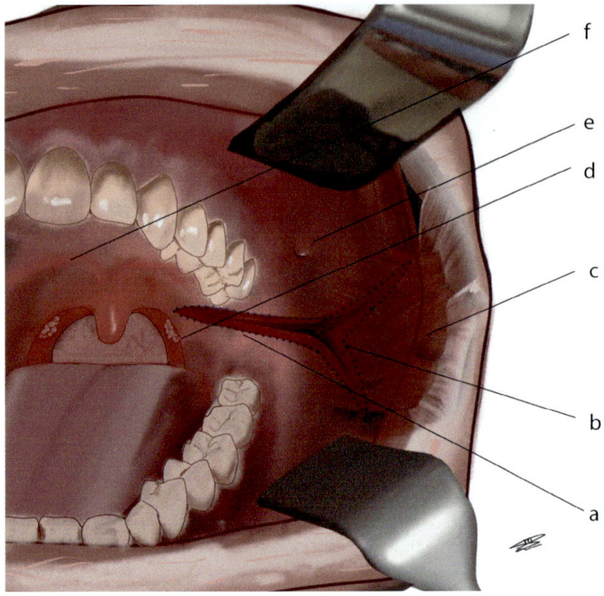


Fig. 18.2 Incision design. **a.** Proposed incision for buccal and perioral fibrous bands, **b**. Anterior limit of incision 1 cm behind modiolus **c**, **d**. Anterior faucial pillar, **e**. Parotid papilla, **f**. Junction of hard and soft palate

The outcomes of laser therapy in oral submucous fibrosis have been reviewed by Gondivkar et al. [19]. The authors have suggested laser fibrotomy as a cost effective tool in the surgical armamentarium for fibrous band release under local anesthesia, and can be performed with a short or minimal hospital stay and gives good control of the depth of release. Incisions for laser fibrotomy such as multiple parallel and inverted Y have been employed to give better release of trismus. The other significant benefit is the perceived improvement in quality of life (QoL) with patient reported outcomes better with regard to pain, increased cheek flexibility and tongue protrusion.

A very comprehensive review of the reported use of lasers in OSF by Jawanda et al. has analysed the outcomes of lasers in OSF, compare the different available lasers, the role of adjunctive therapy with lasers, the patient outcomes and the comparison of surgery with a non-invasive technique such as lasers. The reported studies are summarised in ◘ Table 18.1.

The lasers used in OSF are soft tissue lasers such as $C0_{2,}$ KTP-532, Diode and Nd: YAG, soft and hard tissue

**◘ Table 18.1** Results of use of lasers in OSF [20]

| S. No | Authors | Laser used | Number of patients | GA/LA | Treatment done | Follow up period | Results | | | Complications |
|---|---|---|---|---|---|---|---|---|---|---|
| | | | | | | | MO | Pain | Epitheliali-sation | |
| 1. | Shah et al | Diode | 10 | GA | Fibrotomy | 3 Mos | Y | | | None |
| 2. | Kamesh-waran et al | KTP-532 | 15 | GA | Fibrotomy | 12–18 Mos | Y | | Y | None |
| 3. | Talsania et al | Diode | 8 | GA | Fibrotomy | 3 Mos-3y | Y | Y | | None |
| 4. | Nayak et al | KTP-532 | 9 | GA | Fibrotomy | 1y | Y | | | None |
| 5. | Chaaya et al | C02 | 16 | LA | Fibrotomy | 1y | Y | | | None |
| 6. | Cheng et al | KTP-532 | 4 | LA | Fibrotomy | NA | Y | | | None |
| 7. | Chaudhary et al | Er Cr: YSGG | 1 | LA | Fibrotomy | 6 Mos | Y | | | None |
| 8. | Garde et al | Diode | 9 | GA | Fibrotomy | 1 yr | Y | | Y | None |
| 9. | Chaudhary et al | Er Cr: YSGG | 16 | LA | Fibrotomy | 1 yr | Y | | | None |
| 10. | Lokesh et al | Diode | 50 | LA | Fibrotomy | 6 Mos | Y | | | None |
| 11. | Asnani et al | Diode | 1 | LA | Fibrotomy | 6 Mos | Y | Y | | None |
| 12. | Tripathy et al | Diode | 5 | GA | Fibrotomy | 3 Mos | Y | | | None |
| 13. | Agarwal et al | Diode | 30 | GA | Fibrotomy | 6 Mos | Y | | | None |
| 14. | Devgan et al | CO2 | 20 | LA | Fibrotomy | 6 Mos | Y | Y | | None |
| 15. | Mudigonda et al | Diode | 12 | LA | Fibrotomy | 6mos | Y | Y | | None |
| 16. | Singh et al | Diode | 20 | LA | Laser biostimulation | 15 days | Y | Y | | None |
| 17. | Kunusoth et al | Diode | 1 | LA | Fibrotomy | 6 Mos | Y | Y | | None |
| 18. | Farista et al | Diode | 2 | LA | Fibrotomy, LLLT | 1 y | Y | | | None |
| 19. | Gupta et al | Diode | 30 | LA | Fibrotomy | 9 Mos | Y | Y | Y | None |
| 20. | Chandra et al | Diode | 1 | LA | Photobiostimulation | 1 mo | Y | Y | | None |

*GA* General anesthesia, *LA* local anesthesia, *LLT* low level laser therapy, *mos* months, *yr* year, *Y* yes, *NA* not available, *MO* mouth opening lasers: Er: YAG and ErCr: YSGG.The reported advantages include the shortened duration, ability to perform the procedure under local anesthesia, better hemostasis, retarding the inflammationand pain mediators such as $K^+$, $H^+$, ATP, histamine with better healing, inhibition of TGF-ß, CCN2 thus reducing collagen deposition, fibrosis, scarring and trismus; better wound healing and reepithelialisation. The monochromatism, coherence and collimation affects only the target field without affecting other tissues. The marked disadvantages are the need for special safety measures, need for special training, high cost and maintenance.

The published literature cited above supports that lasers have a definitive role in the management of OSF and needs further studies to make it a part of the standard armamentarium [20].

### 18.3.4 Masticator Muscle Myotomy

The procedure starts by exposing the anterior border of the ascending ramus. This is to be followed by the release of insertion of anterior fibres of temporalis muscle from the coronoid process. The release of lateral and medial fibers inserted to the coronoid process to be followed. As there will be poor access to the superior and posterior fibers of temporalis muscle attached to the tip of coronoid process, this can be performed after obtaining sufficient mouth opening. It is to be noted that because of prolonged pull of temporalis muscle, one may encounter longer coronoid process especially in long-standing OSF. A long curved Kocher's clamp turned upwards may be used to grab the coronoid process, which may serve as a retractor of soft tissue (◻ Figs. 18.3 and 18.4).

Following the release of temporalis tendon, attention is focused on detaching the masseter from the lateral border of ascending ramus of mandible. The muscle is primarily attached at the region of the lateral aspect of angle of mandible. The separation of the muscle needs to carried out on a subperiosteal plane to minimize intra-muscular bleeding, post-operative swelling and scarring. This may be aided by a gauze and a Howarth periosteal elevator. Turning the sharp end of Howarth's periosteal elevator medially the pterygomasseteric sling is then separated from the lower border of the mandible.

The next step is to release the insertion of medial pterygoid from the medial aspect of angle of mandible. The process starts at the retromolar trigone. Dissect the lingual mucosa off the medial aspect the ramus of the mandible in a subperiosteal plane. Care is taken to identify and protect the lingual nerve running close the periosteum at the medial aspect of retromolar trigone region. Further dissection in the subperiosteal plane is directed to the angle of the mandible on the medial side, hugging the bone throughout this step. This medial dis-



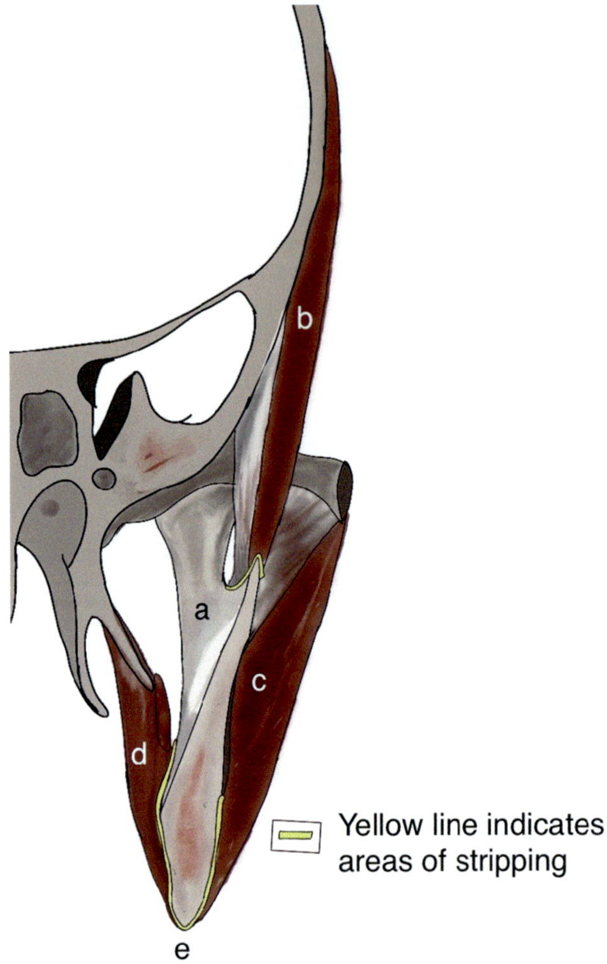


◻ **Fig. 18.3** Coronal section through Mandible showing areas of stripping of muscles of mastication (yellow lines), **a**. Mandible, **b**. Temporalis muscle, **c**. Masseter muscle, **d**. Medial pterygoid muscle, **e**. Pterygomasseteric sling

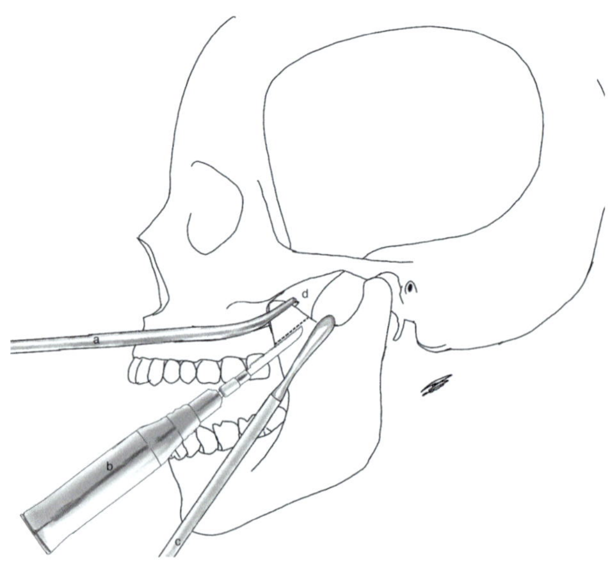

◻ **Fig. 18.4** Coronoidectomy. **a**. Kocher's clamp grabbing coronoid process, **b**. Reciprocating saw, **c**. Periosteal elevator placed in sigmoid notch area to limit cut to coronoid process. **d**. Temporalis muscle

section would require at least 3 cm mouth opening. If this cannot be achieved, the procedure is carried out after completing the planned procedure on the contralateral side of releasing temporalis tendon, masseter and medial pterygoid insertions on the mandible (◘ Fig. 18.3).

### 18.3.5 Bilateral Coronoidectomy

The jaw is opened as wide as possible by activating the Heister jaw opening device on the contralateral molar region. This allows exposure of the tip of the coronoid process. Kocher's forceps is then used to grab the coronoid process. A periosteal elevator is used to detach temporalis tendon from the medial aspect of coronoid process and extended towards sigmoid notch. Similarly another periosteal elevator is used to expose the sigmoid notch laterally. The masseteric branches of maxillary artery exit through sigmoid notch which needs to be cauterized. As the mandible would have come forward with the opening of the mouth, care should be taken to not to confuse the posterior border of mandible as the sigmoid notch. This can be ensured by the fact that the breadth of coronoid process at the base is not longer than 2.0 cm. The coronoid process is then divided using a reciprocating saw. The bone is then removed. If the Kocher's forceps slips, the coronoid process may get retracted into the infratemporal fossa. It's safe to leave the retracted coronoid process as attempt to remove it blindly, can injure maxillary artery traversing medial to the mandibular condyle. The procedure of coronoidectomy is then repeated on the contralateral side.

This manoeuvre allows mouth opening of around 4.0 cm. If there are still restriction of mouth opening, completeness of the release of masseter, medial pterygoid insertions may be carried out. If the opening still remains limited, the anterior one third of masseter origin from the zygomatic bone on one side may be detached. (◘ Fig. 18.4).

Occasionally the condyle may get dislocated anteriorly during the vigorous jaw opening manures. This needs to be identified and the dislocated condyle needs to be reduced. Coronoidectomy is usually done when the mouth opening is less than 3.5 cm after surgical myotomy. and the contralateral coronoidectomy is carried out if the desired mouth opening is not achieved [21]. The chance for condylar dislocation is higher when bilateral coronoidectomy along with muscle stripping are carried out.

### 18.3.6 Resurfacing of the Surgical Defect

The ideal resurfacing option is a thin local skin flap. Since most of the patients are relatively young, local skin flap will have aesthetic impact. The resurfacing options are- buccal pad of fat, bilateral naso-labial flap, temporalis fascia flap, bilateral supraclavicular flap, and radial forearm flap.

The most common surgical intervention in OSF has been the use of interpositional flaps in areas of band excision. For the ease of understanding we will broadly divide the grafts into local, distant flaps and others (Summarised in ◘ Table 18.2).

**Local Flaps:** subdivided into intraoral and extraoral flaps:

(A) Intraoral flaps
- (a) Tongue flaps
- (b) Palatal island flaps
- (c) Buccal fat pad

(B) Extraoral flaps
- (a) Nasolabial flap
- (b) Tempero-parietal fascia flap

**Distant Flaps:** Most commonly used Radial forearm free flap and Anterolateral thigh free flap.

**Coverage with grafts and membranes:** Split skin graft (SSG), and allografts (collagen membrane and alloderm).

#### 18.3.6.1 Intraoral Flaps

(a) **Tongue flap**

Interpositional tongue flaps have been described in the literature [8, 22–25]. Most of the case series are from the early 2000. The use of a tongue flap as an interpositional graft was employed because of accessibility, good vasculature and arc of rotation. However it cannot be considered as a tool in the surgical armamentarium in the present era due to the associated speech and swallowing difficulties,

◘ **Table 18.2** Surgical Options for resurfacing the fibrotomy defect

| Local flaps | | Distant flaps | Others (grafts/membranes) |
|---|---|---|---|
| Intraoral | Extraoral | | |
| Tongue flap | Nasolabial | Radial forearm flap<br>Anterolateral thigh | Split skin graft<br>Allografts: collagen membrane, alloderm |
| Palatal island flap | Temporalis | | |
| Buccal flap | Platysma Myocutaneous | | |

need for a secondary procedure and with the availability of better reconstructive options. The associated dysphagia, need for secondary procedure and also for the fact that the tongue is often involved by submucous fibrosis.

**Technique**: A brief description of the procedure is given below:

(a) Release of fibrous band to be carried out as described before.
(b) Fergusson's mouth gag is then used to forcefully open the mouth.
(c) On either side of the tongue, a tongue flap is marked, the size of which is determined by the size of the raw region to be covered. Its base should be on the posterior one-third of the tongue, towards the anterior pillar, and it should be able to cover the retromolar region without tension.
(d) The flap is then rotated 90 degrees before being sutured to the raw area using 3–0 vicryl.
(e) Dental props are placed on either side of the sutured flaps to keep the mouth open.

Bleeding during the operation can be stopped by applying pressure and ligation.

(b) **Palatal island flaps**

There are two series in the literature which describe the use of the palatal island flap to resurface the defect following fibrotomy. Based on the greater palatine vessels, these flaps are primarily used to resurface the buccal defects. Golhar et al. and Khanna et al. have described the use of this flap [5, 25]. The purported advantages of this flap are the transfer of tissue from a site of low incidence of submucous fibrosis (6–7%). The reported incidence of flap loss and contracture is also low beause of the absence of any muscle in the flap.

**Technique**: Most commonly used in case of buccal mucosal defects, the incision is made 3–4 mm distant from the gingival edge and a mucoperisosteal flap is raised along the midline posteriorly. The flap is sutured to cover the bare areas and rotated buccally, posterior to the second molar. The second molar may need to be extracted where the greater palatine foramen is anterior to its normal anatomic position. The greater palatine foramen can be enlarged to allow the flaps to move more freely. The defect on the palate can be covered with betadine ointment dressings and acrylic plates and allowed for secondary healing.

(c) **Buccal Fat Pad (BFP)** (Fig. 18.5a–c)

In the treatment of OSF, the buccal fat pad was the second most preferred interpositional flap [26]. Being in the vicinity of the surgical site, the buccal fat pad can be easily accessed through the same incision. The volume of fat is generally not affected by the disease but can be reduced based on the body habitus [20, 25–40].

**Technique:** After the primary excision of bands, with blunt dissection the BFP is mobilised out until adequate tissue is obtained to cover the defect without excessive strain After haemostasis, bilateral buccal defects of 3–4 cm can be filled with BFP flap with no visible donor defects in the cheek. The BFP is then sutured in place with vicryl 3–0 sutures around the perimeter and some quilting sutures.

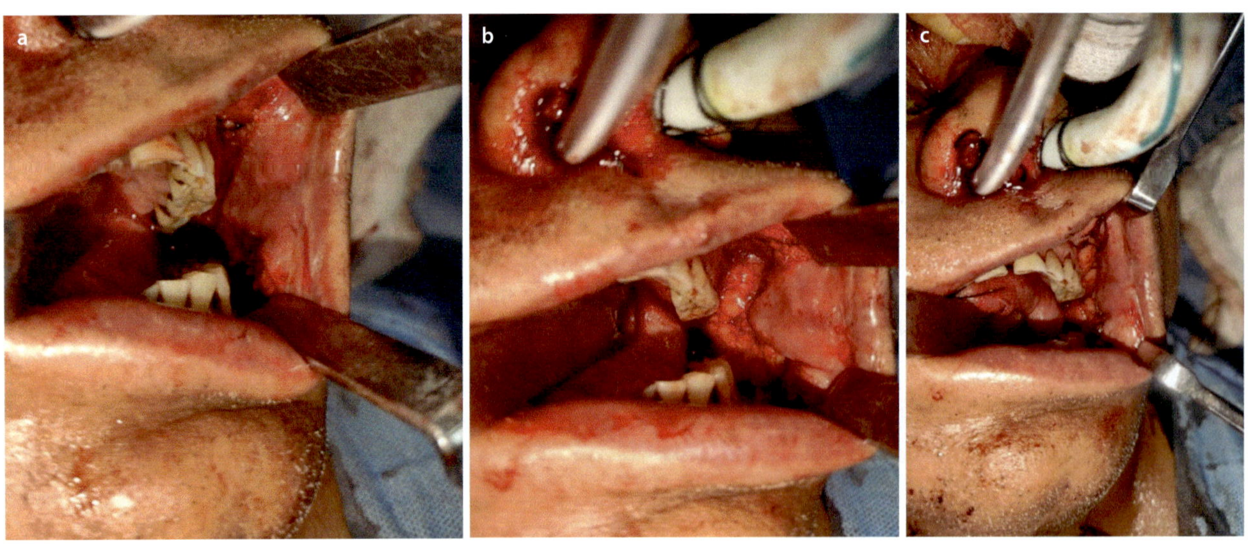

**Fig. 18.5** **a**. Release of fibrous band. **b**. Exposing the Buccal fat pad. **c** BFP in situ

#### 18.3.6.2 Extraoral Flaps

(a) **Nasolabial flap**

The nasolabial flap has proven to be the most versatile surgical method for reconstructing surgical defects in OSF. This could be attributed to the ease of harvest, and availability of adequate tissue adjacent to the surgical defect. The technique of harvest is reasonably straightforward with minimal complications. It is a viable modality of reconstruction in centres which do not have the facility for microvascular reconstruction [6, 28, 32, 41–49]. Aside from the standard harvesting approach, modifications such as an expanded incision down to the lower lip to permit flap tissue with a longer reach have been used. Being a random pattern axial flap deriving its blood supply from the facial artery the flap has the potential to cover the regions of the oral cavity defects created for trismus release, making it a good option for OSF.

At the end of follow-up periods ranging from 1 to 36 months, majority of studies using the nasolabial flap revealed stable interincisal opening of over 35 mm. Tauro reported an acceptable mouth opening of 40 mm post-operatively in his series of 85 cases in the single largest study using nasolabial flaps [48]. Scars in the facial region, a reduction or accentuation of the nasolabial fold, and the development of hair on the flap tissue in the intraoral region are all common issues of using this flap. The flap's narrow breadth precludes its use in wide band excision of extensive OSF.

**Technique:** The flap is designed along the nasolabial crease to ensure the final scar line is well concealed in the nasolabial fold. A pinch test would give a fair approximation of the laxity of the skin before designing the flap. The length and width of the flap are based on the extent of the defect and designing it from the pivot of rotation. The flap's base is left intact while the incision is carried out up to the subdermal tissues. The flap is raised by blunt dissection, which is done with care to avoid disturbing the facial muscles. Ensure that the flap does not shear off from the subdermal plexus. Attempt should be made to incorporate facial artery within the flap. After elevating the flap, a wide tunnel is created towards the base of the flap to allow the flap to enter the oral cavity uncompressed. The flap is then de-epithelialized at the base and along the section that will rest in the myomucosal tunnel, rotated intraorally and sutured. The skin edges are undermined and closed in two layers with subcuticular sutures.

It has been noted that nasolabial flaps provide adequate covering while releasing trismus and maintaining the mouth opening.

(b) **Temporoparietal fascial flap**

The temporoparietal fascial flap has been used in a few reported cases [44, 50]. The primary disadvantage is the limited reach of the flap to resurface anterior defects of the oral cavity.

**Technique**: In most cases, a zigzag incision is performed, starting at the preauricular region and extending to the superior temporal line. To avoid unintended damage to the hair follicles, the anterior and posterior scalp flaps are lifted in the subfollicular plane immediately deep to the hair follicles using loupe magnification. A flap of the appropriate size is marked when adequate exposure has been obtained with a height of 14–17 cm and a width of 10 cm. The traditional fascial flap can be stretched up to 3–4 cm above the temporal muscle's origin. The temporoparietal fascial flap is then raised from superior to inferior by dissecting between the two layers of fascia in the loose areolar tissue plane. The flap base is shortened to 2.0–2.5 cm for ease of transfer, and the pedicle carrying the superficial temporal artery and vein is identified. The flap is placed in the recipient area. Because of its pliability, it's ideal for draping over irregular surfaces. Suction drains are placed in the donor site area and it is closed in two layers.

The morbidity of temporal hollowing and scarring of the muscle on mucosalization of the muscle leading to further fibrosis and relapse of trismus are common complications. The flap appears to be the least popular of all the local flaps.

#### 18.3.6.3 Distant Flaps

The advent of microvascular surgery has expanded the armamentarium for the surgeon for resurfacing defects in OSF. The requisites of the ideal tissue are thin, pliable with an adequate length of vascular pedicle to be able to perform anastomosis. With the current available fasciocutaneous flaps the radial forearm free flap is probably the gold standard for the reconstruction of defects. There are reports of the usage of the anterolateral thigh flap however the thick skin paddle and unpredicatability of the subcutaneous tissues based on the body habitus preclude it from becoming the first choice for reconstruction. Huang et al. reported a series on the use of the anterolateral thigh flap with two skin paddles being designed on the descending branch of the lateral circumflex femoral artery. The authors reported an increase in the mean interincisal opening but half the series of flaps needed secondary debulking [51].

#### 18.3.6.4 Radial Forearm Free Flap

The usage of the radial forearm free flap for resurfacing the submucous fibrosis defect ensures coverage of the mucosal defect with thin and pliable tissue [52–54]. The

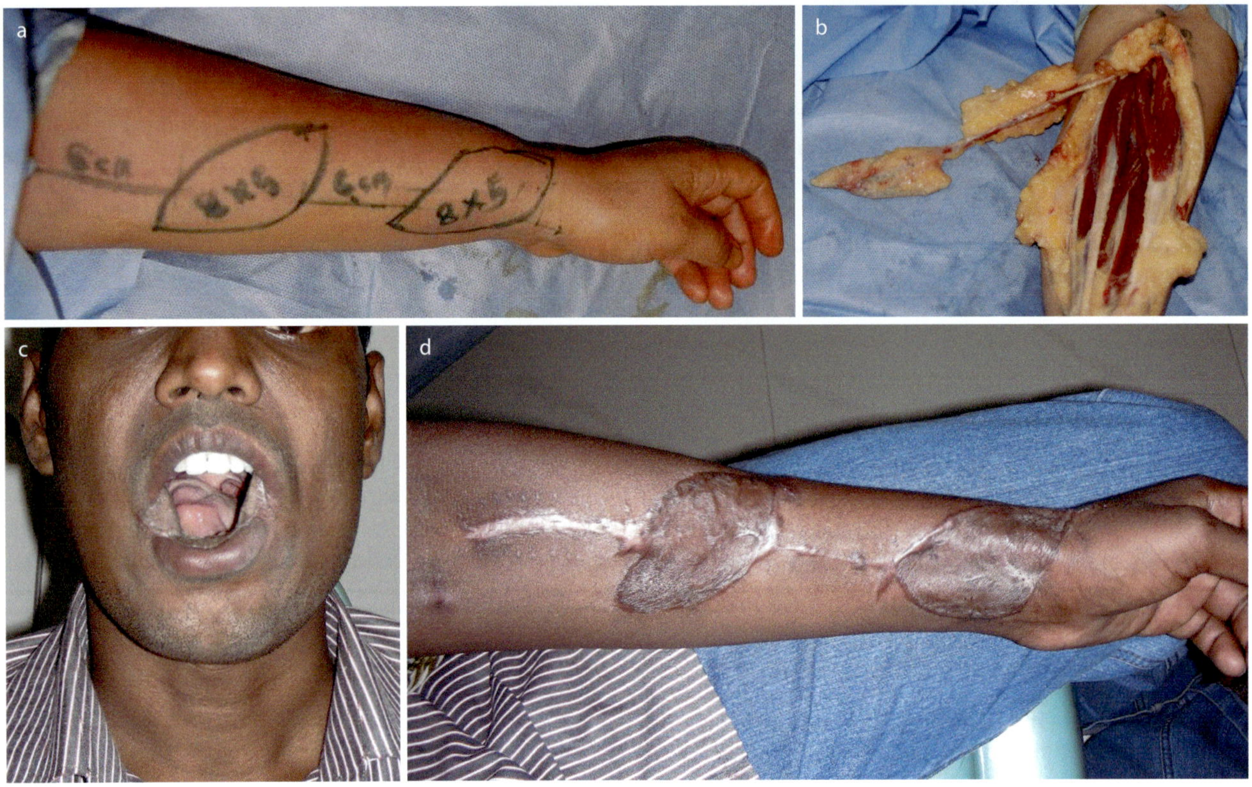


**Fig. 18.6** **a.** Outline and design of the bipaddled Radial artery forearm flap. **b.** Flap Harvest complete. **c.** Post operative mouth opening at 1 month. **d.** Healed donor site

design of the flap can be customised to the defect. The authors have described a single bi-paddled flap at their institution with the intervening tissue placed in the mandibular anterior sulcus (Fig. 18.6a–d). The bi-paddled radial forearm flap with its long vascular pedicle ensures a single flap with ease of reconstruction, a single anastomosis and a simultaneous two team approach makes this the free flap of choice for OSF defects. The main drawbacks are the expertise needed for microvascular reconstruction, the associated costs, the need for secondary debulking procedures for the flap as the volume of tissue in the anterior vestibule may interfere with mastication and the small risk of kinking of vessels [55]. The description of harvest of the flap is as mentioned in the literature. There have been modifications reported in the literature of the bipaddled radial forearm flap with two separately designed skin paddles which avoid the need for two separate anastomosis [56, 57].



#### 18.3.6.5 Coverage with Grafts and Membranes

Split skin grafts, collagen membranes, artificial dermis, and human placenta have been used to graft the surgical bed. None of these materials have been compared with the use of flaps. They primarily serve to reduce the pain, minimise blleding and to not leave a raw surface during healing. Loss of the material, wound dehiscence, fibrosis and scar tissue formation are the common complications. Many centres tend to use this when the expertise or facilities to resurface the defect are unavailable. Commercially available dermis and collagen are readily available and overcome the donor site morbidity, however its effectiveness needs to be proven. Placental grafts and human amnion were previously reported but are not current accepted standard of care [9].

## 18.4 Pitfalls and Solutions of Resurfacing Techniques

Intraoral flaps should not be a preferred modality for the resurfacing of defects as better options are available. It could be still indicated for small defects or if patients desire and have a poor performance status contraindicating other techniques.

**Tongue flap:** They are prone to secondary haemorrhage due to the raw surface, torsion of the flap may cause dehiscence and necrosis. It needs a secondary procedure delayed by at least 4 weeks to detach the flap during which oral hygiene, speech and oral intake would have to be addressed. There have been few case reports of malignant lesions developing in the resurfaced defect when a tongue flap has been used.

**Palatal island flap:** Being a mucoperiosteal flap based on the greater palatine vessels, the arc of rotation is limited to small buccal mucosal defects. It would need extraction of the last maxillary molar (mostly the second or third) to allow it to be brought to the surgical defects. It leaves behind a raw surface that needs to heal by secondary intention. The bulk of the flap along the arc of rotation may be a hindrance to patients when they masticate.

**Buccal fat pad:** The buccal fat pad is associated with minimal morbidity, however in certain patients inadequate tissue may be present and difficult to resurface defects beyond the premolars. The graft mucosalises rapidly without any additional cover but may devascularize and slough off if excessively manipulated. Vigorous postoperative physiotherapy is needed as it has a tendency to develop fibrosis similar to the native tissues, especially if partial necrosis develops.

The common complications associated with extra-oral flaps are summarised below:

(a) **Nasolabial flap:** Extraoral scar, wound dehiscence, pincushioning effect, orocutaneous fistula, loss of nasomaxillary crease, partial or complete loss of flap, intraoral hair growth [58].
(b) **Temporoparietal fascial flap:** Alopecia and a visible scar, rarely temporal hollowing, flap necrosis and dehiscence.
(c) **Radial Forearm free flap:** The common complications associated with radial forearm flap would include the donor site scar due to the skin graft, paresthesia of the forearm, loss of graft and tendon exposure, complications related to a microvascular procedure such as vascular insufficiency and the need for reexploration, partial flap loss, hair growth on the flap.

A recent head on comparison study demonstrated better mouth opening when reconstruction was done with a radial forearm flap versus a nasolabial flap [59, 61].

## 18.5 Postoperative Physiotherapy

The key to stabilise the mouth opening and prevent a recurrence of trismus is early initiation of physiotherapy. The ideal time is arbitrary with some surgical centers advocating a soft to hard splint placement intraorally at the time of surgery carried into the initial postoperative phase till such time the patient is comfortable to start physiotherapy. Recommendations are to start physiotherapy by the third post-operative day. Patient compliance is the key to success with exercises being performed at least 3 times daily for a minimum 3 minute period for minimum 3 months [6, 60–62]. It is recommended to have an initial supervised regimen to educate the patients regarding the technique of placement of the device and activation of the device. This can be done either by the surgeon or therapists. Mouth opening can be done with a variety of devices. Initial splints fabricated from dental impression or putty, mouth opening devices such as Heister's, Therabite Jaw motion rehabilitation system or simple ice-cream sticks or wooden spatulas with a gradual increase in the daily number to guide the extent of mouth opening achieved can be used [63]. A comparative study between wooden tongue depressors versus Heister's jaw opener has not established the superiority of any one device in physiotherapeutic regimens. The importance of physiotherapy was demonstrated by Cox and Zoellner who assigned patients into three groups: Graded physiotherapy regimen, intralesional hyaluronidase with steroids, no active treatment. The results showed that physiotherapy improved the mouth opening [64].

## 18.6 Results of Surgical Intervention

There have been no randomised trials to demonstrate the benefit of one surgical modality over the other. The available literature essentially comprises small cohorts of patients treated based on the institutional and operator preference.

With the current available armamentarium resurfacing with microvascular flaps would be the gold standard. Aggressive postoperative physiotherapy is recommended to maintain the mouth opening.

Table 18.3 summarises the various options that have been used in the available literature and the reported follow up. The most common flap utilised at centres is the nasolabial flap which probably is due to the ease of harvest, reliable and pliable tissue available and the advantage of it being away from the fibrotic site.

The other options in descending frequency are artificial membranes followed by tongue flap and buccal fat pad. The lesser number of microvascular flaps can be probably be attributed to the fact that centres across the subcontinent are slowly developing the expertise and thus the reported numbers are not high.

**Table 18.3** Results of surgical options in OSF [26]

| S. No. | Treatment modality | No of cases reported | Average follow up |
|---|---|---|---|
| 1. | Tongue flap | 138 | 1–84 months |
| 2. | Palatal flap | 33 | 48 months |
| 3. | Buccal fat pad | 139 | 2 weeks–36 months |
| 4. | Nasolabial flap | 227 | 6–66 months |
| 5. | Temporalis fascia | 5 | NA |
| 6. | Radial forearm free flap | 65 | 3–48 months |
| 7. | Anterolateral thigh flap | 9 | 16.2 months |
| 8. | Split skin graft | 96 | 10 weeks–48 months |
| 9. | Collagen membrane | 107 | 3–24 months |
| 10. | Artificial dermis | 39 | 3–6 months |
| 11. | Human placenta/ amnion grafts | 39 | NA |

*NA* not available

The series with the buccal fat pad have reported good mucosalisation and an average mouth opening of around 30–35 mm over a period of 6 months. Additional procedures mentioned include bilateral coronoidectomy and the use of a nasolabial flap.

In the series of nasolabial flaps the average interincisal opening reported is 38 mm, bilateral nasolabial flaps have been harvested in the majority of series and also with adjunct procedures such as coronoidectomies.

The palatal island flaps have been always described with adjuncts such as temporalis myotomy and coronoidectomy.

The radial forearm literature mentions the use of adjunct procedures in almost all series, the average mouth opening of around 38 mm measured interincisally and the need for secondary debulking procedures.

The authors recommend that the interpretation of these surgical series needs to be done carefully. The series are heterogenous and across many decades. The earlier use of local flaps reflects the expertise and resources available at that point of time. No technique can be shown superior to the other in terms of the final outcome with respect to the mouth opening. The common parameter irrespective of any flap is the early initiation of postoperative physiotherapy. With the advent of free flaps the use of adjunct procedures to improve the mouth opening is also more common.

**Key Points**

- Assess the interincisal opening and location of fibrotic bands: Decide on surgical vs non surgical management.
- Ensure patient's compliance with regard to length of treatment and aggressive post operative physiotherapy, educate them about the aids and regimen.
- Rule out any foci of malignancy.
- Assess the need for adjunct procedures such as coronoidectomy and myotomy.
- Plan the reconstruction based on the volume of defect that needs to be resurfaced.
- Assess esthetic concerns and microvascular facilities and expertise availablility.
- Armamentarium ladder and selection of modality based on the above(descending order of preference).

- Microvascular free flaps.
- Nasolabial flaps.
- Buccal fat pad.
- Skin grafts, membranes.

## 18.7 Post Surgery Surveillance

Pindborg and Sirsat have described the malignant transformation of OSF in 1966, an annual transformation rate of 0.5% [7]. In 2006, OSF has been categorized as a potentially malignant disorder [60]. In spite of this there is no characterised natural history for OSF and thus it is difficult to predict which cases may progress to malignancy. This implies the need for close surveillance with regular clinical examinations post the surgical treatment for the fibrosis.The temporal span for the risk of malignant transformation would be 10–15 years and thus the need for long term close surveillance [65]. Warning signs and symptoms include redness, ulceration and presence of pain. It is a good practice to educate the patients on mouth self-examination techniques and the early warning sings and symptoms.

Unlike other OPMDs, malignant lesions in OSF can develop in any areas of the oral mucosa, including dorsum of tongue and buccal mucosa. As the advanced OSF mucosae are atrophic and depapillation is commonly seen on the tongue it is difficult to delineate early malignant transformation. Oral visual examination with palpation and examination of the neck would still be the recommended tool on surveillance.The use of adjuncts such as autofluorescence imaging, chemiluminescence and vital staining are still being investigational. The gold standard would be a representative biopsy. Frequent biopsy can lead to scarring and induce trismus, therefore judicious use of biopsy is necessary. Histopathologic confirmation of dysplasia in OSF needs to be carefully interpreted. The conventional three tier reporting system as given by WHO guidelines as mild, moderate or severe has only a fair interobserver agreement among head and neck pathologists. The use of the two grade system is recommended to avoid the variation in decision making. Characterisation of the lesion based on architectural and cytologic criteria are the hall mark of the two tier system [66]. Suspicious lesions based on the clinical morphology need biopsy and close surveillance [67].

Malignant transformations rates reported for OSF are different across the SE Asian region. Yang et al. in the population based series from Taiwan showed a high malignant transformation rate of 9.13% for OSF with a mean duration of malignant transformation in 2.5 years. Concomitant presence of leukoplakia increased the transformation rate to 15.1% [68, 69]. The study from India also supports the hypothesis that OSF related oral squamous cell carcinoma (OSCC) is a clinicopathologically distinct entity. Its hallmarks are an earlier age of presentation, male predilection, better differentiation, earlier tumor stage, lower neck metastasis and lesser incidence of extracapsular spread. Oral tongue is more commonly involved in OSF. The blockage of the submucosal lymphatics is speculated to explain the lower propensity for nodal metastasis [70].

- **Pearls in Surveillance**
  - Rates of malignant transformation vary; 0.5–9.1%.
  - Risk factors; younger age, males, concomitant leukoplakia, tongue.
  - Close surveillance for 2 years and long-term intermitted surveillance.
  - Altered mucosa makes interpretation difficult.
  - Adjuncts to visual examination are investigational.
  - Hallmark for diagnosis: Biopsy.
  - Dysplasia: 3 tier and 2 tier grading.
  - OSCC in OSF is a distinct entity with better prognosis.

## 18.8 Summary and Future Perspectives

Surgery is recommended for advanced cases to improve mouth opening and oral mucosal surveillance. A skin lined local flap is the preferred reconstructive option. Laser fibrous band release is increasingly being used to minimize the post-operative fibrosis. Irrespective of the technique, the success of the surgical intervention is dependent on the intensity and compliance to post surgery physiotherapy. Therefore a structured physiotherapy regimen must be introduced.

With the advent of regenerative medicine, the role of stem cells has been studied which would likely lead to new advancements in the treatment of OSF. The mechanism of release of cytokines and growth factors (paracrine effects) and increasing antioxidant (naturally occurring or exogenous) capabilities to scavenge free radicals, can enhance blood vessel development It may also aid in the transition of resident tissue stem cells into new fibroblasts, hence assisting in the removal of biochemically and morphologically disrupted collagen fibres. In OSF laboratory-purified pluripotent stem cells have shown promising benefits. Stem cells are predicted to restore oral mucosa and become an effective way for treating OSF in the future, giving breakthrough in OSF research [71].

It is possible to reduce the incidence, recurrence rate, and malignant transformation rate of OSF through through habit cessation and better understanding of OSF pathogenesis and related carcinogenesis, as well as the advancement of scientific research. The future of these biologic modifiers to minimize post-operative fibrosis needs to be intensively evaluated to improve the results. In addition, development of appropriate chemopreventive interventions are necessary to reverse the malignant transformation potential.

## 18.9 Conclusions

- Surgery for improving mouth opening, pain, trismus, QOL.
- Gold standard for resurfacing defects: skin lined flaps.
- Laser fibrotomy is emerging as a good alternative.
- Aggressive physiotherapy is the cornerstone to success.
- Biologic modifiers, stem cells, chemopreventive agents are investigational.

**Acknowledgement** The diagrams of this chapter were drawn by Dr. Manish Tiwari, the authors acknowledge Dr. Naveen Chandrashekar, Dr. Sachin Chavre, Dr. Naveen BS for the clinical photos.

## References

1. Mello FW, Miguel AFP, Dutra KL, Porporatti AL, Warnakulasuriya S, Guerra ENS, Rivero ERC. Prevalence of oral potentially malignant disorders: a systematic review and meta-analysis. J Oral Pathol Med. 2018;47(7):633–40.
2. Arakeri G, Brennan PA. Oral submucous fibrosis: an overview of the aetiology, pathogenesis, classification, and principles of management. Br J Oral Maxillofac Surg. 2013;51:587–93.
3. Federowicz Z, Chan Shih-Yen E, Dorri M, Nasser M, Newton T, Shi L. Interventions for the management of oral submucous fibrosis. Cochrane Database Syst Rev 2008;(4): CD007156.
4. Kerr AR, Warnakulasuriya S, Mighell AJ, et al. A systematic review of medical interventions for oral submucous fibrosis and future research opportunities. Oral Dis. 2011;17(Suppl. 1):42–57.
5. Khanna J, Andrade N. Oral submucous fibrosis: a new concept in surgical management. Int J Oral Maxillofac Surg. 1995;24(6):433–9.
6. Chang YM, Tsai CY, Kildal M, Wei FC. Importance of coronoidotomy and masticatory muscle myotomy in surgical release of trismus caused by submucous fibrosis. Plast Reconstr Surg. 2004;113(7):1949–54.
7. Pindborg JJ, Sirasat SM. Oral submucous fibrosis. Oral Surg Oral Med Oral Pathol. 1966;22:746–79.
8. Mehrotra D, Pradhan R, Gupta S. Retrospective comparison of surgical treatment modalities in 100 patients with oral submucous fibrosis. Oral Surgery, Oral Medicine, Oral Pathology, Oral Radiology, and Endodontology. 2009;107(3):e1–e10.
9. Kamath VV. Surgical Interventions in oral submucous fibrosis: a systematic analysis of the literature. J. Maxillofac. Oral Surg.14(3): 521–531.
10. Arakeri G, Rai KK, Boraks G, Patil SG, Aljabab AS, Merkx MAW, Carrozzo M, Brennan PA. Current protocols in the management of oral submucous fibrosis: an update. J Oral Pathol Med. 2017;46(6):418–23.
11. Sandu K, Makharia SM. Unusual experience in OSF. Indian J Otolaryngol Head Neck Surg. 2004;56(1):65–6.
12. Chaaya VA, Sinha V, Rathor R, Modi N, Rashmi GS, Parmar V, et al. Oral submucous fibrosis surgical treatment with $CO_2$ laser. World Arctic Ear Nose Throat. 2010;3:1–2.
13. Chaudhary Z, Verma M, Tandon S. Treatment of oral submucous fibrosis with ErCr: YSGG laser. Indian J Dent Res. 2011;22:472–4.
14. Kameshwaran M, Raghavan D, Anand Kumar RS, Murali S. Surgical management of trismus due to oral submucous fibrosis-lysis of fibrotic bands with the KTP-532 laser. Indian J Otolaryngol Head Neck Surg. 2007;58:229–31.
15. Nayak DR, Mahesh SG, Agrawal D, Pavithran P, Pujary K, Pillai S. Role of KTP-532 laser in management of oral submucous fibrosis. J Laryngol Otol. 2009;123:418–21.
16. Shah A, Raj S, Rasaniya V, Patel S, Vakade M. Surgical management of oral submucous fibrosis using "opus 5" diode laser. J Oral Laser Appl. 2005;5:37–43.
17. Murugavel C, Gnanam T, Roopesh. A modified approach using diode laser to reduce trismus in oral submucous fibrosis. Kerala state. Dent J. 2012;35:224–8.
18. Talsania JR, Shah UB, Shah AI, Singh NK. Use of diode laser in oral submucous fibrosis with trismus. Prospective study. Ind. J Otolaryngol Head Neck Surg. 2009;61:22–5.
19. Gondivkar SM, Gadbail AR, Sarode SC, Gondivkar RS, Patil S, Gaikwad RN, Chu DT, Yuwanti M. Treatment outcomes of laser therapy in oral submucous fibrosis: a systematic review. J Oral Biol Craniofac Res. 2020;10:315–20.
20. Gupta S. Jawanda MK laser as a promising non-invasive technique to treat oral submucous fibrosis: a systematic review of the literature. Saudi Dental J. 2021;33:413. https://doi.org/10.1016/j.sdentj.2020.11.005.
21. Suresh A, Anehosur V, Hallikeri K. Role of coronoidectomy and temporalis myotomy in surgical management of oral submucous fibrosis. Oral Maxillofac Surg. 2021;26:131. https://doi.org/10.1007/s10006-021-00971-x.
22. Bhrany AD, Izzard M, Wood AJ, Futran ND. Coronoidectomy for the treatment of patients in head and neck cancer. Laryngoscope. 2007;117:1952–6.
23. Tepan MG, Saigal GS, Tilak SB. Use of tongue flap in submucous palatal fibrosis. J Laryngol Otol. 1986;100:455–60.
24. Ramadass T, Manokaran G, Pushpala SM, Narayanan N, Kulkarni GN. Oral submucous fibrosis- new dimensions in surgery. Indian J Otolaryngol Head Neck Surg. 2005;57:99–102.
25. Golhar S, Mahore MN, Narkhede S. Tongue flap in oral submucous fibrosis. Indian J Otolaryngol Head Neck Surg. 1989;41:104–7.
26. Kamath VV. Surgical interventions in oral submucous fibrosis: a systematic analysis of the literature. J Maxillofac Oral Surg. 2015;14:521–31.
27. Adeyemo WL, Ladeinde AL, Ogunlewe MO, Bambgbose BO. The use of buccal fat pad in oral reconstruction. Niger Postgrad Med J. 2004;11:207–11.
28. Girotra C, Padhye M, Desai R. Versatility of buccal fat pads in closure of oral defects. Sci J. 2008;8:1–3.
29. Jeevan Kumar KA, Brahmaji RJ. Versatility of pedicled buccal fat pad in surgical management of oral submucous fibrosis: a study in 20 cases. Indian J Dent Adv. 2009;1:5–11.
30. Chao C-K, Chang L-C, Liu S-Y, Wang J-J. Histologic examination of pedicled buccal fat pad graft in oral submucous fibrosis. J Oral Maxillofac Surg. 2002;60:1131–4.
31. Yeh CJ. Application of buccal fat pad to the surgical treatment of oral submucous fibrosis. Int J Oral Maxillofac Surg. 1996;25:130–3.
32. Pandya H, Patel H, Dewan H, Babaria U, Bhavsar B, Thakkar D, et al. Comparison of nasolabial flap versus buccal fat pad graft for management of submucous fibrosis. J Dent Sci. 2011;1:6–7.
33. Sharma R, Thapliyal GK, Sinha R, Menon PS. Use of buccal fat pad graft in the treatment of oral submucous fibrosis. J Oral Maxillofac Surg. 2011;70:228.
34. Lai DR, Chen HR, Lin LM, Huang YL, Tsai CC. Clinical evolution of different treatment methods for oral submucous fibrosis. A 10-year experience with 150 cases. J Oral Pathol Med. 1995;24:402–6.
35. Nataraj S, Guruprasad Y, Shetty JN. A comparative clinical evaluation of buccal fat pad and collagen in surgical management of oral submucous fibrosis. Arch Dent Sci. 2011;2:15–22.
36. Krishna Prasad L, Chakravarthy PS, Sridhar M, Ramkumar S, Krishan S, Vivekanand SK. An evaluation of various treatment modalities in the management of oral submucous fibrosis. A clinical study J Orofac Sci. 2009;1:17–20.
37. Gupta LC, Kohli M, Punn K, Abhishek. Use of buccal fat pad in oral submucous fibrosis. A case report. Asian J Oral Health Allied Sci. 2011;1:51–2.

38. Mehta AK, Panwar SS, Verma RK, Pal AK. Buccal fat pad reconstruction in oral submucous fibrosis. Med J Armed Forces Inst. 2003;59:340–1.
39. Surej Kumar LK, Kurien NM, Sakir N. Buccal fat pad reconstruction for oral submucous fibrosis. Nat J Maxillofac Surg. 2010;1:164–7.
40. Saravanan K, Narayanan V. The use of buccal fat pad in the treatment of oral submucous fibrosis: a newer method. Int J Dent.
41. Borle RM, Nimonkar PV, Rajan R. Extended nasolabial flaps in the management of oral submucous fibrosis. Br J Oral Maxillofac Surg. 2009;47:382–5.
42. Maria A, Sharma Y, Kaur P. Use of nasolabial flap in the management of of oral submucous fibrosis- a clinical study. People's J Sci Res. 2011;4:28–30.
43. Cunha-Gomes D, Kavarana NM, Choudhari C, Rajendraprasad JS, Bhathena HM, Desai PB, et al. Total oral reconstruction for cancers associated with advanced oral submucous fibrosis. Ann Plast Surg. 2003;51:283–9.
44. Januja OS, Bukhari SGA, Ibrahim MW, Mehmood S, Sarfraz T. Oral submucous fibrosis- reconstruction with nasolabial flap 2011. Pak Armed Forces Med J. 2011;2:1–3.
45. Patel SG, Deshmukh S, Savant DN. Squamous cell carcinoma arising in a nasolabaial flap used in the treatment of oral submucous fibrosis. Br J Plast Surg. 1994;47:388–9.
46. Kavarana NM, Bhathena HM, Griffiths RW. Surgery for severe trismus in submucous fibrosis. Plast Reconstr Surg. 1989;83:401–3.
47. Agrawal M, Gupta DK, Tiwari AD. Extended nasolabial flaps in the treatment of oral submucous fibrosis. J Oral Maxillofac Surg. 2011;10:216–9.
48. Tauro DP. A unique melolabial flap in the surgical management of oral submucous fibrosis-"the sea gull flap"- an experience with 85 cases. A clinical study. Int J Oral Maxillofac Surg. 2009;38:508–12.
49. Kshirsagar R, Chugh A, Rai A. Bilateral inferiorly based nasolabial flaps for the management of advanced oral submucous fibrosis. J Maxillofac Oral Surg. 2010;9:22–6.
50. Mokal NJ, Raje RS, Ranade SV, Rajendra Prasad JS, Thatte RL. Release of oral submucous fibrosis and reconstruction using superficial temporal fascia flap and split skin graft—a new technique. Br J Plast Surg. 2006;58:1055–60.
51. Huang J-J, Wallace C, Lin J-Y, Tsao C-K, Huang W-C, Cheng M-S. Two small flaps from one anterolateral thigh donor site for bilateral buccal mucosa reconstruction after release of submucous fibrosis and/or contracture. J Plast Reconstr Aesthet Surg. 2010;63:440–5.
52. Wei FC, Chang YM, Kildal M, Tsang WS, Chen HC. Bilateral small radial forearm flaps for the reconstruction of buccal mucosa after surgical release of submucosal fibrosis: a new, reliable approach. Plast Reconstr Surg. 2001;107:1679–83.
53. Lee J-T, Cheng LF, Chen P-R, Wang C-H, Hsu H, Chien SH, et al. Bipaddled radial forearm flap for the reconstruction of bilateral buccal defects in oral submucous fibrosis. Int J Oral Maxillofac Surg. 2007;36:615–9.
54. Tsao CK, Wei FC, Chang YM, Cheng MH, Chwei-Chin Chuang D, Kao HK, Dayan JH. Reconstruction of the buccal mucosa following release for submucous fibrosis using two radial forearm flaps from a single donor site. J Plast Reconstr Aesthet Surg. 2010;63:1117–23.
55. Shivanand NB, Chavre S, Chandrashekar NH, Chauhan S. Bipaddled radial forearm free flap in the reconstruction of bilateral buccal mucosal defects-a case series. Oral Surg Oral Med Oral Pathol Oral Radiol. 2016;122:e107–9.
56. Hallock GG. Simultaneous bilateral foot reconstruction using a single radial forearm flap. Plast Reconstr Surg. 1987;80:836–8.
57. Safak T, Kayikcioglu A, Ozcan G, et al. Sharing the radial forearm flap in reconstruction of two separate defects in the same patient. Ann Palst Surg. 1996;36:313–5.
58. Kshirsagar R, Mohite A, Gupta S, Patankar A, Sane V, Raut P. Complications in the use of bilateral inferiorly based nasolabial flaps for advanced oral submucous fibrosis. Natl J Maxillofac Surg. 2016;7:115–21.
59. Faisal M, Rana M, Shaheen A, Warraich R, Kokemueller H, Eckardt AM, et al. Reconstructive management of the rare bilateral oral submucous fibrosis using nasolabial flap in comparison with free radial forearm flap—a randomised prospective trial. Orphanet J Rare Dis. 2013;8:56.
60. Tilakaratne WM, Klinikowski MF, Takashi S, Peters TJ, Warnakulasuriya S. Oral submucous fibrosis: review on etiology and pathogenesis. Oral Oncol. 2006;42:561–8.
61. Warnakulasuriya S, Kerr AR. Oral submucous fibrosis: a review of the current management and possible directions for novel therapies. Oral Surg Oral Med Oral Pathol Oral Radiol. 2016;122(2):232–41.
62. Huang IY, Wu CF, Shen YS, Yang CF, Shieh TY, Hsu HJ, Chen CH, Chen CM. Importance of patient's cooperation in surgical treatment for oral submucous fibrosis. J Oral Maxillofac Surg. 2008;66:699–703.
63. Vadepally AK, Salavadi RK, Sinha R. A comparative clinical study on physiotherapy outcomes with wooden tongue depressors versus heister jaw opener in oral submucous fibrosis patients. J Oral Biol Craniofac Res. 2019;9:263–7.
64. Cox S, Zoellner H. Physiotherapeutic treatment improves oral opening in oral submucous fibrosis. J Oral Pathol Med. 2009;38:220–6.
65. Warnakulasuriya S, Kovacevic T, Madden P, Coupland VH, Sperandio M, Odell E, et al. Factors predicting malignant transformation in oral potentially malignant disorders among patients accrued over a 10-year period in south East England. J Oral Pathol Med. 2011;40:677–83.
66. Kujan O, Oliver RJ, Khattab A, Roberts SA, Thakker N, Sloan P. Evaluation of a new binary system of grading oral epithelial dysplasia for prediction of malignant transformation. Oral Oncol. 2006;42:987–93.
67. Warnakulasuriya S. Oral potentially malignant disorders: a comprehensive review on clinical aspects and management. Oral Oncol. 2020;102:104550.
68. Yang PY, Chen YT, Wang YH, Su NY, Yu HC, Chang YC. Malignant transformation of oral submucous fibrosis in Taiwan: a nationwide population-based retrospective cohort study. J Oral Pathol Med. 2017;46:1040–5.
69. Speight PM, Khurram SA, Kujan O. Oral potentially malignant disorders: risk of progression to malignancy. Oral Surg Oral Med Oral Pathol Oral Radiol. 2018;125:612–27.
70. Chaturvedi PP, Vaishampayan SS, Nair S, et al. Oral squamous cell carcinoma arising in background of oral submucous fibrosis: a clinicopathologically distinct disease. Head Neck. 2013;35:1401–9.
71. Suma GN, Arora MP, Lakhanpal M. Stem cell therapy: a novel treatment approach for oral mucosal lesions. J Pharm Bioallied Sci. 2015;7:2–8.

# Areca Nut Addiction and Treatment

## Contents

# Areca Nut Addiction: Tools to Assess Addiction

*K. A. L. A. Kuruppuarachchi and A. Hapangama*

## Contents



© The Author(s), under exclusive license to Springer Nature Switzerland AG 2023
S. Warnakulasuriya, K. Ranganathan (eds.), *Oral Submucous Fibrosis*, Textbooks in Contemporary Dentistry,
https://doi.org/10.1007/978-3-031-12855-4_19

## 19.1 Introduction

Arecanut (AN) otherwise known as betel nut has been reported as the world's fourth most commonly used psychoactive substance after tobacco, alcohol, and caffeine [1] and it is reported to be used by one fifth of the world's population [2].

The use of areca nut is widely prevalent and considered acceptable culturally and socially in Asian countries such as India, Sri Lanka, Maldives, Bangladesh, Myanmar, and Taiwan [3] .

Its use is also reported among people of South Pacific islands [3] as well as in parts of Thailand, Indonesia, Malaysia, Cambodia, Vietnam, Philippines, Laos, and China and migrants from the above countries living in the United Kingdom, the United States of America, South and East Africa, and Australia [2, 4].

Researchers have tried to highlight its dependence potential and the fact that it fulfils the criteria for a dependence syndrome during the last few decades [5].

An historical account citing colloquial Anglo-Indian words and phrases reports that *"They are always chewing Arecca, a certaine Fruit like a Peare, cut in quarters and rolled up in leaves of a Tree called Bettre (or Vettele), like Bay leaves, which having chewed they spit forth. It makes the mouth red. They say they do it to comfort the heart, nor could live without it"* [6].

In this chapter we would be looking into the concepts of addiction, dependence, assessment, and measurement of addiction/dependence. We examine the evidence on whether there is addiction to AN and if so how to assess it.

**Learning Goals**

- Goals of this chapter are to review the concepts of addiction and dependence, and to outline the methods of measurement/assessment of addiction/dependence. We propose to explore the evidence supporting an addiction or dependence to arecanut (AN) and if there is confirmed evidence how to assess such behaviours in clinical practice.

19

## 19.2 Dependence or Addiction to a Substance

The concept of substance dependence syndrome appears largely to have developed from the seminal work of Edwards and Gross in the mid-1970s s [7]. Their paper highlighted a group of features which they called a syndrome which included craving, impaired control over substance use, stereotyping of use, and prioritizing of substance use, and physiological features of tolerance and withdrawal. Saunders reports that prior to this, such behaviours were termed either as "abuse" and or "addiction" due to the mental and social complications, externalizing behaviours and denial of the problem [8].

The term substance dependence and its psychometric properties have been supported by numerous studies [8]. In a memorandum published in 1981, the World Health Organization proposed a classification system in the field of drug- and alcohol-related problems [9]. The *Diagnostic and Statistical Manual* also included the term "dependence "in its version III (DSM-III) [10] and this terminology was continued in to its next revision, i.e., DSM IV [11].

**Definition**

Addiction has been defined as the development of tolerance and withdrawal upon discontinuation of a substance or refer to compulsive use of a substance known by the user to be physically, psychologically, or socially harmful [12].

Dependence on the other hand is defined as a `cluster of physiological, behavioural and cognitive phenomena in which the use of a substance or a class of substances takes on a much higher priority for a given individual than other behaviours that once had greater value'.

Key concepts such as loss of control, tolerance, withdrawal and craving are central but not essential components to the diagnosis of dependence to any substance [8].

Howver, O'Brien argues that the word 'dependence' was already in use for many years prior to DSM-III-R to describe the adaptations that occur when medications that act on the central nervous system are ingested with rebound if the medication is discontinued abruptly. He argues that it is addiction rather than dependence which describes the collection that stands for compulsive, uncontrolled, drug-seeking behaviour [13].

It appears that the DSM and ICD classification preferred the word dependence over addiction as it was less stigmatizing [14].

In order to address these problems, DSM-5 has included certain changes including elimination of a diagnoses of substance dependence and amalgamated all those criteria (abuse and dependence) together under a single category called "substance use disorder" [15].

However, ICD-11, beta draft has chosen a somewhat different approach. It retains the diagnosis of substance dependence and describes substance dependence as, "a disorder of regulation of the use of a psychoactive substance arising from repeated or continuous use of the substance. Its central feature is a strong internal drive to use the substance, manifested by impaired ability to control use, increasing priority given to use of the substance over other activities, and persistence of use despite harm and adverse consequences." [16].

For the purpose of this chapter, we will use the term dependence to describe a diagnosis of intense craving, tolerance, withdrawal symptoms, to areca nut..

## 19.3 Methods of Assessment of Addiction/ Dependence

### 19.3.1 Diagnostic Criteria and Screening Tools

In clinical practice and more specifically as per Samel et al. research, the instrument used for substance use assessment could make the difference between null and significant findings [17].

In addition to the clinician led interviews several screening tools have been utilized to assess/ screen for and or measure dependence over the years. Some of these are clinical diagnostic criteria such as the Diagnostic and Statistical Manual fifth version (DSM 5) developed by the American Psychiatric Association and the International classification of diseases tenth version (ICD 10) developed by the World Health Organization [15, 18]. These are mostly used in the day-to-day clinical practice.

ICD 10 has a set of criteria developed specifically for the research setting (ICD 10 research diagnostic criteria). In addition there are several structured tools such as the (Addiction Severity Index (ASI); Composite International Diagnostic Interview (CIDI); Structured Clinical Interview for DSM-IV (SCID); Psychiatric Research Interview for Substance and Mental Disorders (PRISM); and Semi-Structured Assessment for Drug Dependence and Alcoholism (SSADDA) [19–23].

All the above instruments have been shown to have good reliability, validity, and acceptance in clinical research settings as well as in the community setting [16].

All of the above are clinician administered tools. However, there are several self-administered tools developed to screen for substance dependence, such as the adult substance use survey (ASUS), drug abuse screening test (DAST), the drug Use Screening Inventory-Revised (DUSI-R) or the "Drinksmeter". The self-reported instruments are available in paper-and-pencil questionnaires, computer assisted self-interviews or interactive voice recordings [24, 25].

These scales (either self - administered or interviewer administered) are most of the time specific for one particular substance. e,g CAGE and the alcohol use disorders identification test (AUDIT) was developed to screen for alcohol misuse while some are more generalizable. Some of these scales have additional items to detect associated disabilities (Alcohol Use Disorders and Associated Disabilities Interview Schedule (AUDADIS); [26–28].

Such structured interviews provide more robust and reliable information regarding substance use especially for a research purpose by providing diagnostic consistency and avoiding misclassification.

### 19.3.2 Biological Assessment Techniques

In addition, biological measures of substance use have been used at times as an alternative or an adjunct to screening tools especially in medico-legal settings such as analysing of hair, saliva or urine samples.

### 19.3.3 Limitations of Existing Instruments for Measuring and or Screening for Dependence

As per Conway et al. [29] despite most of the instruments having proven utility, reliability, and validity, they appear to have certain limitations [29]. The authors mention that the instruments which are currently available are based on a variety of related but different constructs of addiction severity such as behavioural and social consequences, quantity or type of DSM symptoms that are fulfilled, use patterns within and across substances, and number of different DSM diagnoses. In addition, they report that the content of existing measures does not fully reflect the full range of addiction severity.

In addition, most of the scales have been developed in the Western countries to reflect the substances that are prevalent in those settings. To our knowledge, even though these scales and diagnostic criteria have been used to assess/screen or measure substance dependence prevalent in other parts of the world none are validated in measuring dependence to areca nut or related substances.

## 19.4 Pharmacology of Areca Nut

The primary route of areca nut administration is oral and it is systemically absorbed through the buccal and sublingual mucosa [5]. The onset of effect in the majority of areca chewers is reported to be within 5 min of ingestion and it is reported to last for about 2–3 h [5].

During the last few decades, areca nut and related substances have been available around the globe in preparations called "pan masala" which may have areca in a more refined form which might have different absorption times to the ones mentioned above [30].

Areca nut is also reported to have a stimulant effect through several psychoactive alkaloids which it contains

[31]. Out of these, arecoline has been reported as the chemical that is predominantly present [5].

Studies report that betel quid (primary ingredient areca nut) has both the sympathetic and parasympathetic effects such as changes in the size of the pupil, heart rate and blood pressure [32–34]. These effects on the autonomic nervous system are thought to be possibly dose-dependent, with the parasympathetic activity enhanced at higher doses [35].

The reported effects of areca nut in the central nervous system include a sense of well-being and euphoria [36]. In addition Atukorala et al. report, that areca nut chewing produces a warm sensations of the body, sweating, salivation, palpitation and heightened alertness, and tolerance to hunger [37].

Electroencephalographic studies suggest an increase in both alpha, and particularly beta, rhythms which may explain the so called "stimulant effect" [38].

Some researchers suggest that areca nut increases relaxant qualities through arecaidine which appears to act on GABA uptake inhibitors [39]. Winstock had suggested that areca nut has stimulant and anxiolytic effects similar to tobacco [5].

## 19.5 Does Areca Nut Fulfil the Operational Criteria for a Dependence Syndrome?

Winstock has highlighted that the potential for abuse of any substance could be modified by its preparation, route of use, as well as by the sociocultural factors [5].

In countries in which the areca nut use is prevalent, existing cultural and ritualistic associations with areca could influence its dependence through the conditioning and reinforcement of its use [5].

Even though most psychoactive drugs have complex pharmacological effects on the brain, the final common pathway of pharmacological effects of dependence is accepted as mediated through release of dopamine at the nucleus accumbens of the ventero-tegmental dopa minergic limbic pathway [40] .

Winstock describes tolerance and withdrawal as the core biological components of a dependence syndrome and that areca nut use would strongly support the existence of a dependence syndrome [5].

A study done among Cambodian women suggests that areca nut has an addictive potential as strong as cigarettes [41].

The UK study on areca nut users has suggested that tolerance to the above-mentioned stimulant effects may occur in regular users [42].

In the first ever study which investigated the psychological profile of areca use Winstock et al. [42] report that participants had used areca nut for an average of 35 years with the mean age of first use at 13 years. They also report that most participants reported beneficial psychosocial effects including ten out of the eleven reporting cessation withdrawal effects. Their study reported the mean Severity of Dependence Score of 7.3 in the Severity of Dependence Scale (SDS) [42].

A study by Bhat et al. in India found that about 44% met at least one of the following symptoms: continued use despite illness or mouth wounds, difficulty in refraining from chewing in forbidden places, or craving during periods of abstinence [43]. They also report that the dependence scores were positively correlated with frequency of chews per day [43]. This study had used the modified versions of several scales; namely the Fagerström Tolerance Questionnaire, Cigarette Dependence Scale (CDS-5) and the Smokeless Tobacco Dependence Scale (STDS) [44–46].

In another study Benegal et al. report that 38.8% of persons using areca nut preparations without tobacco additives met diagnostic criteria for dependence as per the DSM-IV as well as the ICD-10 criteria respectively [47]. Interestingly none of the above had met the "giving up activities to use the substance" criteria as per DSM IV and or ICD 10. "According to Benegal et al. the areca nut users were significantly older, more likely to be women, from rural backgrounds and from lower socio- economic levels than non -users [47].

In the above study Benegal et al. also had found that the participants who used only areca were significantly younger and more educated than those who used both areca and tobacco [47].

In a relatively larger study conducted in 2011 Mirza et al. reported that individuals using areca nut with tobacco additives were significantly more likely to have a dependency syndrome (OR = 2.17, 95% CI 1.39–3.40) as assessed with DSM IV diagnostic criteria [3].

In addition, there are also a couple of case reports that have documented neonatal withdrawal syndromes in children prenatally exposed to areca [48, 49].

However, there are only a couple of studies which have looked into the reasons for areca nut chewing [50–52]. Kuo et al. in their study which was conducted among Taiwanese taxi cab drivers [52], suggest that individuals chew betel-quid for some of the same reasons that individuals smoke tobacco. A large cross-sectional school-based survey conducted among 2200 participants in Karachi, Pakistan [51] has reported that those participants who believed that BQ chewing relaxed them were twice as likely to be dependent on BQ (OR = 2.36, 95% CI (1.20–4.65) as compared with others [51].

Sullivan et al. in a cross-sectional study of 70 people with schizophrenia report that betel quid chewers (areca nut) with schizophrenia scored significantly lower on the positive ($P = 0.001$) and negative ($P = 0.002$) sub-scales of the PANSS than did non-chewers, indicating that areca nut chewing is associated with milder symptomatology

19

and avoidance of more harmful recreational drugs [53]. A study conducted in India among 988 patients treated for major psychiatric disorders found that about 24% of the sample reported recent areca nut use, and 10% reported severe use suggesting dependence [54]. It also mentions that common reasons for use included to improve mood (31% of users), socialization (31%), digestion (22%), or performance (7%) and to decrease aches and pains (6%). In addition predictors for areca nut use among the participants of this study included lower education levels, diagnosis of bipolar disorder, and current tobacco use.

In a subsequent study among patients with schizophrenia, Sullivan et al. reported that high-consumption betel quid had significantly milder positive symptoms than low-consumption chewers over 1 year as measured by the PANNS. In addition, the use of betel quid was associated with tobacco use but not with cannabis or alcohol in this population [55].

In a large community based study conducted in northern Taiwan, Lin et al. found that areca nut chewing had an odds ratio (OR) of 1.828 (95% CI: 1.165–2.869) with common mental illnesses [56].

In a hospital-based study conducted among 1000 patients with mental health issues in Sri Lanka, 20.9% participants were found to chew betel quid (95% CI: 18.4–23.4%) [59]. The rates of betel quid chewing among patients with and without a mental illness in this study had been 20.7% (95% CI: 17.0–24.4%) and 21.0% (95% CI: 17.6–24.5%) [57]. The authors did not find a statistically significant difference between the occurrence of positive or negative symptoms and or extrapyramidal side effects in patients with schizophrenia with betel quid use [57].

Hung et al. reports that the frequency of betel quid chewing is higher among patients with depression and that patients who chewed betel-quid showed more severe depressive symptoms [58]. In addition, they mentioned that, following antidepressant therapy, the addictiveness to betel quid was significantly reduced by 4 times [58].

## 19.6 Development of Scales to Measure Betel Quid Depeendence/Use

We briefly outline the studies that have so far used different scales to measure dependancy to areca nut.

### 19.6.1 Betel Quid Dependence Scale (BQDS)

Lee et al. were the first to develop an instrument designed specifically for measuring betel quid dependence—the Betel Quid Dependence Scale (BQDS) [59]. The items of BQDS were originally developed in Chinese, It consists of three factors: "physical and psychological urgent need," "increasing dose," and "maladaptive use." It was found to have good internal consistency ($\alpha = 0.92$) and construct validity. However, there are some limitations in its development, such as it was developed and evaluated depending on retropspective information. Not being validated among females and the psychometric properties of the original scale had not been evaluated in English [59] (see ▶ Box 19.1 below) .

**Box 19.1: The Items of Betel Quid Dependence Scale (BQDS)**

1. Have you ever felt that you can not go on without betel quid?
2. Have you found yourself having trouble stopping chewing betel quid once you start?
3. Have you ever chewed betel quid non stop?
4. Have you experienced strong craving for betel quid after you reduce or completely stop chewing betel.
5. quid?
6. Whenever you want to chew betel quid but not available, would you spend a lot of time to find it?
7. Whenever you want to chew betel quid but not available, would you take extra steps and travel a great.
8. distance trying to buy it? For example, even suffer from fatigue by long journey.
9. Have you felt agitated, irritated or anxious after you reduce or completely stop chewing betel quid?
10. Have you experienced difficulty in concentrating or focusing after you reduce or completely stop chewing.
11. betel quid?
12. Have you experienced depression or drowsiness after you reduce or completely stop chewing betel quid?
13. Do you have a situation that amount of betel quid is gradually increased every time you chew it from the first time you experienced it?
14. Have you felt the need to increase the amount of betel quid chewing periodically in order to achieve a pleasant or refreshing effect?
15. Have you often found yourself chewing more betel quid than expected and/or spending more time in chewing betel quid than expected?
16. Would you continue chewing betel quid if you find your teeth loosened or wiggled?
17. Would you continue chewing betel quid if you have sensitive teeth (to hot or cold food)?
18. Would you continue chewing betel quid if you experience canker sores or mouth ulcers?
19. Have you reduced or given up any of your social, work or leisure activities because of betel quid chewing?

In order to overcome this, Herzog et al. had validated the BQDS among a sample of English-speaking male and female betel quid chewers living in Guam [60]. They report that confirmatory factor analysis revealed an adequate fit with the hypothesized three-factor measurement model and also that the BQDS is valid for current English-speaking male and female chewers in Guam. They also found that the overall levels of betel quid dependence were high among the study population and that measures using the BQDS are similar to those observed for nicotine dependence.

### 19.6.2 Reasons for Betel-Quid Chewing Scale (RBCS)

The Reasons for Betel-quid Chewing Scale (RBCS) is a 10-item measure adapted from several existing "reasons for smoking" scales. The confirmatory factor analysis of this measure revealed a three-factor structure: reinforcement, social/cultural, and stimulation. Further tests revealed strong support for the internal consistency and convergent validity of this three-factor measure [61] (◘ Box 19.2).

**Box 19.2: Individual Items in the Reasons for Betel-Quid Chewing Scale (RBCS)**

**Reinforcement Construct**

1. I like the taste.
2. I like to have something in my mouth at all times.
3. Social/cultural construct.
4. All of my friends chew.
5. My family members chew.
6. It's rude not to chew.
7. People will not respect me if I don't chew.
8. Stimulation construct.
9. It relaxes me.
10. It gives me energy.
11. It helps me make decisions.
12. I like the way it makes me feel.

19

### 19.6.3 DSM-5 Betel-Quid Use Disorder

Lee at al from the Asian Betel-quid Consortium defines DSM −5 betel quid use disorder (BUD) as follows [62].

> Users of betel quid (BQ) who met all the DSM-5 substance use disorder (SUD) diagnostic criteria are considered as having a BUD [62].

Lee et al. conducted six cross-sectional studies concurrently across East Asia (Taiwan and mainland China), Southeast Asia (Malaysia and Indonesia), and South Asia (Nepal and Sri Lanka) to test for this concept [62].

The authors used eleven DSM-5 symptoms to assess BUD for current users [62] (see ▶ Box 19.3 below).

**Box 19.3: DSM-5 Betel-Quid Use Disorder**

1. Larger amount or longer history of betel-quid use.
2. Unsuccessful cutdown.
3. Time spent using betel-quid.
4. Craving.
5. Neglected major roles.
6. Social or interpersonal problems.
7. Given up activities.
8. Hazardous use.
9. Continued use despite knowing problems.
10. Tolerance.
11. Withdrawal.

Lee et al. reported that a positive diagnosis of BUD required the presence of at least 2 of the 11 symptoms within the 12 months before they conducted the interviews with the participants. Further, current users of BQ with 0 to 1 symptom was classified as having no BUD, those with 2 to 3 symptoms as having mild BUD, those with 4 to 5 symptoms as having moderate BUD, and those with 6 or more symptoms as having severe BUD. The above study had been conducted under a single framework using an identical protocol, measuring tools, and diagnostic instruments across all the study sites . However, the above study was conducted in a cross-sectional manner which precluded any causal interpretations which is a major limitation.

### 19.6.4 Self-Report Screening Test for Areca Quid Abuser (SSTAA)

Areca nut is generally consumed with tobacco and betel leaves. Chen et al. developed the Self-report Screening Test for Areca quid Abuser (SSTAA) to identify whether an areca quid chewer has reached the level of substance abuse [63]. The authors developed a specific self-reporting questionnaire modified from the SCAN system (65), DSM-IV [11] and ICD-10 [18]. The authors screened 125 areca quid users. The final self-report measure has 11 questions (▶ Box 19.4) where a person filing the form answers with a score of 4 or more in these 11 questions would be considered an areca quid abuser. The authors developed this for use in Taiwan and therefore further studies will be needed for its generalizability in other countries.

**Box 19.4: SSTAA Self-reporting questionnaire**

1. Do you like chewing betel quid?
2. Have you ever found that once you start chewing, you are unable to stop?
3. When you cut down on or completely quit chewing betel quid, do you have the desire for them?
4. Do you feel cheerful and spiritual when you have betel quid?
5. Have you ever felt that you have to chew betel quid?
6. When you feel your teeth are sensitive to hot or cold food do you still chew betel quid?
7. When you cut down on or completely quit chewing betel quid, do you find it hard to concentrate?
8. Are you able to give up the habit of betel quid chewing at any time you want?
9. Have you ever tried to quit or cut down on betel quid but didn't succeed?
10. When you feel your teeth are loose, do you still chew betel quid?
11. When you suffer from oral cavity ulcer pains, do you still keep on chewing betel-nuts?

## 19.7 Conclusions and Future Perspectives

Current evidence indicates of the existence of an areca nut dependence disorder. Further longitudinal prospective studies on areca nut use and its correlates will enhance the knowledge of this substance and formal inclusion of the substance in currently accepted diagnostic guidelines of SUDS .

**Summary**

Chewing of areca nut either on its own or in a quid is a socially acceptable practice in the Indo-Asia-Pacific region. In fact a large proportion of people living in this region and Asian migrant communities in Western countries are reported to use areca nut. Arecoline is the principal active agent in the areca nut and has been found to have effects on the prevailing mood and alertness. Tolerance and withdrawal symptoms have been observed in long-term areca nut users. Studies undertaken in several countries indicate that areca nut use in certain people amounts to dependence and meet formal diagnostic criteria.

## References

1. Boucher BJ. Paan without tobacco: an independent risk factor for oral cancer. I J Cancer. 2001;91:592–3. https://doi.org/10.1002/1097-0215).
2. Gupta P, Warnakulasuriya S. Global epidemiology of areca nut usage. Addict Biol. 2002;7(1):77–83.
3. Mirza SS, Shafique K, Vart P, Arain MI. Areca nut chewing and dependency syndrome: is the dependence comparable to smoking? Across sectional study. Subst Abuse Treat Prev Policy. 2011;6:23. https://doi.org/10.1186/1747-597X-6-23.
4. Auluck A., Hislop G., Poh C., Zhang L., Rosin M.P. Areca nut and betel quid chewing among south Asian immigrants to Western countries and its implications for oral cancer screening. Rural Remote Health 2009; 9:1118–1.
5. Winstock A. Areca nut-abuse liability, dependence and public health. Addict Biol. 2002;7:133–8. https://doi.org/10.1080/13556210120091509.
6. Yule H, Burnell AC. Hobson-Jobson: A glossary of colloquial Anglo-Indian words and phrases, and of kindred terms, etymological, historical, geographical and discursive, vol. 2. J. Murrey; 1903.
7. Edwards G, Gross MM. Alcohol dependence: provisional description of a clinical syndrome. Br Med J. 1976;1(6017):1058–61. https://doi.org/10.1136/bmj.1.6017.1058.
8. Saunders JB. Substance use and addictive disorders in DSM-5 and ICD 10 and the draft ICD 11. Curr Opin Psychiatry. 2017;30(4):227–37. https://doi.org/10.1097/YCO.0000000000000332.
9. Edwards G, Arif A, Hodgson R. Nomenclature and classification of drug and alcohol-related problems: a WHO memorandum. Bull World Health Org. 1981;59:225–42.
10. American Psychiatric Association. Diagnostic and statistical manual of mental disorders. 3rd ed; 1980.
11. American Psychiatric Association. Diagnostic and statistical manual of mental disorders. 4th ed; 1994.
12. Maddux JF, Desmond DP. Addiction or dependence? Addiction. 2000;95(5):661–5.
13. O'Brien C. Addiction and dependence in DSM-V. Addiction. 2011;106(5):866–7. https://doi.org/10.1111/j.1360-0443.2010.03144.x.
14. Debasish B, Ghosh A. Substance use and other addictive disorders in international classification of diseases-and their relationship with diagnostic and statistical Manual-5 and international classification of diseases. Indian J Soc Psychiatry. 2019;34(5):54–62.
15. American Psychiatric Association. Diagnostic and statistical manual of mental disorders. 5th ed; 2013. https://doi.org/10.1176/appi.books.9780890425596.
16. World Health Organization. International classification of diseases for mortality and morbidity statistics (11th Revision); 2018. Retrieved from https://icd.who.int/browse11/l-m/en
17. Samet S, Waxman R, Hatzenbuehler M, Hasin DS. Assessing addiction: concepts and instruments. Addict Sci Clin Pract. 2007;4(1):19–31. https://doi.org/10.1151/ascp074119.
18. World Health Organization. International classification of diseases for mortality and morbidity statistics 10th Revision; 1993.

19. McLellan AT, Luborsky L, Cacciola J, Griffith J, Evans F, Barr HL, et al. New data from the addiction severity index: reliability and validity in three centers. J Nerv Ment Dis. 1985;173(7):412–23. https://doi.org/10.1097/00005053-198507000-00005.
20. Robins LN, Wing J, Wittchen HU, Helzer JE, Babor TF, Burke J, et al. The composite international diagnostic interview. An epidemiologic instrument suitable for use in conjunction with different diagnostic systems and in different cultures. Arch Gen Psychiatry. 1988;45(12):1069–77. https://doi.org/10.1001/archpsyc.1988.01800360017003.
21. First M.B., Spitzer R.L., Gibbon M., Williams J.B. Structured clinical interview for the DSM-IV Axis I disorders (SCID PTSD module); 1996.
22. Hasin DS, Trautman KD, Miele GM, Samet S, Smith M, Endicott J. Psychiatric research interview for substance and mental disorders (PRISM): reliability for substance abusers. Am J Psychiatry. 1996;153(9):1195–201. https://doi.org/10.1176/ajp.153.9.1195.
23. Yang BZ, Wang LJ, Huang MC, Wang SC, Tsai MC, Huang YC, et al. Diagnostic reliability and validity of the semi-structured assessment for drug dependence and alcoholism (SSADDA). Chinese Version. 2020;6:62–7. https://doi.org/10.1159/000511606.
24. Jonasson U, Jonasson B, Wickstrom L, Andersson E, Saldeen T. Analgesic use disorders among orthopedic and chronic pain patients at a rehabilitation clinic. Subst Use Misuse. 1998;33:1375–85.
25. Skinner HA. The drug abuse screening test. Addict Behav. 1982;7(4):363–71. https://doi.org/10.1016/0306-4603(82)90005-3.
26. Fidalgo TM, Tarter R, da Silveira ED, Kirisci L, da Silveira DX. Validation of a short version of the revised drug use screening inventory in a Brazilian sample of adolescents. Am J Addict. 2010;19(4):364–7. https://doi.org/10.1111/j.1521--0391.2010.00058.x.
27. Hasin DS, Greenstein E, Aivadyan C, Stohl M, Aharonovich E, Saha T, et al. The alcohol use disorder and associated disabilities interview Schedule-5 (AUDADIS-5): procedural validity of substance use disorders modules through clinical re-appraisal in a general population sample. Drug Alcohol Depend. 2015;148:40–6. https://doi.org/10.1016/j.drugalcdep.2014.12.011.
28. Grant BF, Goldstein RB, Smith SM, Jung J, Zhang H, Chou SP, et al. The alcohol use disorder and associated disabilities interview Schedule-5 (AUDADIS-5): reliability of substance use and psychiatric disorder modules in a general population sample. Drug Alcohol Depend. 2015;148:27–33. https://doi.org/10.1016/j.drugalcdep.2014.11.026.
29. Conway K, Levy J, Vanyukov M, Chandler R, Rutter J, Swan G, et al. Measuring addiction propensity and severity: the need for a new instrument☆. Drug Alcohol Depend. 2010;111(1–2):4–12. https://doi.org/10.1016/j.drugalcdep.2010.03.011.
30. Trivedy C, Johnson NW. Oral cancer in South Asia [letter]. Br Dent J. 1997;182:206.
31. Chu NS. Neurological aspects of betel chewing. Addict Biol. 2002;7:111–4.
32. Huang LS, Wang CK, Sheu MJ, Kao LS. Phenolic compounds of piper betel flower as flavouring and neuronal activity modulating agents. In: Ho CT, Lee CY, Huang MT, editors. Phenolic compounds in food and their effects on health, vol. 506. Am Chem Soc Ser; 1992. p. 200–13.
33. Leyko E. CA. 1929;23:1440.
34. Chu NS. Cardiovascular responses to betel nut chewing. J Formos Med Assoc. 1993;92:835.
35. Chu NS. Effects of betel chewing on RR interval variation. J Formos Med Assoc. 1995;94:106–1.
36. Sharan RN, Mehrotra R, Choudhury Y, Asotra K. Association of Betel nut with carcinogenesis: revisit with a clinical perspective. PLoS One. 2012;7(8):e42759. https://doi.org/10.1371/journal.pone.0042759.
37. Athukora IA, Tilakaratne WM, Jayasinghe RD. Areca nut chewing: initiation, addiction, and harmful effects emphasizing the barriers and importance of cessation. J Addict 2021, 9967097, 2021. doi: https://doi.org/10.1155/2021/9967097.
38. Chu NS. The effects of betel chewing on electroencephagraphic activity: spectral analysis and topographic mapping. J Formos Med Assoc. 1994;93:167–9.
39. Johnston CA, Krogsgaard-Larsen P, Stephanson A. Betel nut constituents as inhibitors of gamma aminobutyric acid uptake. Nature. 1975;258:627–8.
40. Wise RA. Action of drugs of abuse on brain reward mechanisms. Pharmacol Biochem Behav. 1980;13(1):213–23.
41. Pickwell SM, Schimelpfening S, Palinkas LA. 'Betelmania'. Betel quid chewing by Cambodian women in the United States and its potential health effects. West J Med. 1994;160:326–30.
42. Bhat SJ, Blank MD, Balster RL, Nichter M, Nichter M. Areca nut dependence among chewers in a south Indian community who do not also use tobacco. Addiction. 2010;105(7):1303–10. https://doi.org/10.1111/j.1360-0443.2010.02952.x.
43. Heatherton TF, Kozlowski LT, Frecker RC, Fagerstrom KO. The Fagerstrom test for nicotine Dependance: a revision of the Fagerstrom tolerance Questionnire. Br J Addict. 1991;86(9):1119–27. https://doi.org/10.1111/j.1360-0443.1991.tb01879.x.
44. Huang CL, Cheng CP, Lu CC. Using the short-form cigarette dependence questionnaire in a busy clinical practice. Clin Nurs Res. 2017;26(4):451–63. https://doi.org/10.1177/1054773815625468.
45. Ferketich AK, Wee AG, Shultz J, Wewers ME. A measure of nicotine dependence for smokeless tobacco users. Addict Behav. 2007;32(9):1970–5. https://doi.org/10.1016/j.addbeh.2007.01.005.
46. Benegal V, Rajkumar RP, Muralidharan K. Does areca nut use lead to dependence? Drug Alcohol Depend. 2008;97(1–2):114–21. https://doi.org/10.1016/j.drugalcdep.2008.03.016.
47. Garcia-Algar O, Vall O, Alameda F, Puig C, Pellegrini M, Pacifici R, et al. Prenatal exposure to arecoline (areca nut alkaloid) and birth outcomes. Arch Dis Child Fetal Neonatal Ed. 2005;90:F276–7.
48. Lopez-Vilchez MA, Seidel V, Farré M, García-Algar O, Pichini S, Mur A, et al. Areca-nut abuse and neonatal withdrawal syndrome. Pediatrics. 2006;117(1):129–31.
49. Wen CP, Tsai SP, Cheng TY, Chen CJ, Levy DT, Yang HJ, et al. Uncovering the relation between betel quid chewing and cigarette smoking in Taiwan. Tob Control. 2005;14((I1)):i16–22. https://doi.org/10.1136/tc.2004.008003.
50. Hussain A, Zaheer S, Shafique K. Reasons for betel quid chewing amongst dependent and non-dependent betel quid chewing adolescents: a school-based cross-sectional survey. Subst Abuse Treat Prev Policy. 2018;13:16. https://doi.org/10.1186/s13011-018-0154-5.
51. Kuo S, Lew-Ting C. The health lifestyles of areca quid-chewing taxi drivers-an exploratory study from the viewpoint of social context. Taiwan J Public Health. 2008;27(1):67–80.
52. Sullivan R, Allen J, Otto C, Tiobech J, Nero K. Effects of chewing betel nut (Areca catechu) on the symptoms of people with schizophrenia in Palau, Micronesia. BJPsych. 2000;177(2):174–8. https://doi.org/10.1192/bjp.177.2.174.
53. Chandra PS, Carey MP, Carey KB, Jairam KR. (2003). Prevalence and correlates of areca nut use among psychiatric patients in India. Drug Alcohol Depend. 2003;69(3):311–6. https://doi.org/10.1016/S0376-8716(02)00329-0.

54. Sullivan RJ, Andres S, Otto C, Miles W, Kydd R. The effects of an indigenous muscarinic drug, betel nut (Areca catechu), on the symptoms of schizophrenia: a longitudinal study in Palau. Micronesia Am J Psychiatry. 2007;164(4):670–3. https://doi.org/10.1176/ajp.2007.164.4.670.
55. Lin TY, Chang HC, Hsu KH. Areca nut chewing is associated with common mental disorders: a population-based study. Soc Psychiatry Psychiatr Epidemiol. 2018;53(4):393–401. https://doi.org/10.1007/s00127-017-1460-3.
56. Isuru A, Ediriweera D, Pathmeswaran A, Embuldeniya A, Narammalage H, Warnakulasuriya S, et al. Betel-quid use and its effects on symptoms of schizophrenia and extrapyramidal symptoms among a group of patients in a tertiary care hospital in Sri Lanka. SLJP. 2020;11(1):32–8. https://doi.org/10.4038/sljpsyc.v11i1.8244.
57. Hung CC, Lee CH, Chung CM, Nithiyanantham S, Lane HY, Ko YC. Antidepressant-induced reduction in betel-quid use in patients with depression: a pioneer clinical study. Medicine. 2020;99(1):e18672. https://doi.org/10.1097/MD.0000000000018672.
58. Lee CY, Chang CS, Shieh TY, Chang YY. Development and validation of a self-rating scale for betel quid chewers based on a male-prisoner population in Taiwan: the betel quid dependence scale. Drug Alcohol Depend. 2012;121:18–22.
59. Herzog TA, Murphy KL, Little MA, Suguitan GS, Pokhrel P, Kawamoto CT. The betel quid dependence scale: replication and extension in a Guamanian sample. Drug Alcohol Depend. 2014;138:154–60. https://doi.org/10.1016/j.drugalcdep.2014.02.022.
60. Little MA, Pokhrel P, Murphy KL, et al. The reasons for betel-quid chewing scale: assessment of factor structure, reliability, and validity. BMC Oral Health. 2014;14:62. https://doi.org/10.1186/1472-6831-14-62.
61. Lee CH, Ko AM, Yang FM, et al. Association of DSM-5 betel-quid use disorder with Oral potentially malignant disorder in 6 betel-quid endemic Asian populations. JAMA Psychiat. 2018;75(3):261–9. https://doi.org/10.1001/jamapsychiatry.2017.4307.
62. Chen MJ, Yang YH, Shieh TY. Evaluation of a self-rating screening test for areca quid abusers in Taiwan. Public Health. 2002 Jul;116(4):195–200. https://doi.org/10.1038/sj.ph.1900861.
63. Wing JK, Babor T, Brugha T, Burke J, Cooper JE, Giel R, Jablenski A, Regier D, Sartorius N. SCAN. Schedules for clinical assessment in neuropsychiatry. Arch Gen Psychiatry 1990;47(6):589–593. doi: https://doi.org/10.1001/archpsyc.1990.01810180089012.

# Behavioural Interventions for Areca Nut Cessation in the Prevention and Management of Oral Submucous Fibrosis

*Thaddeus A. Herzog and Neal A. Palafox*

## Contents



© The Author(s), under exclusive license to Springer Nature Switzerland AG 2023
S. Warnakulasuriya, K. Ranganathan (eds.), *Oral Submucous Fibrosis*, Textbooks in Contemporary Dentistry,
https://doi.org/10.1007/978-3-031-12855-4_20

## 20.1 Introduction

Areca nut, the drupe fruit of the Areca palm (Areca catechu), contains psychoactive alkaloids that have stimulating effects on the autonomic nervous system [1]. Areca nut is widely consumed across several regions of the world, including South Asia, Southeast Asia, and the western Pacific islands. Although the manner and mode of areca nut consumption varies by culture, region, and personal preference, areca nut often is chewed wrapped in the leaf of a pepper plant (Piper betle), along with slaked lime (calcium hydroxide), tobacco, and other spices [2, 3]. The areca nut combined with other ingredients is often referred to as betel quid (BQ), though the names for various areca preparations vary by country. In some scientific publications, particularly those describing research conducted on chewers from South Asian cultures, commercially manufactured products containing areca nut and tobacco are often referred to as "Gutkha".

Areca nut and betel quid (ANBQ) is the fourth most consumed psychoactive substance in the world, followed only by alcohol, tobacco, and caffeine. ANBQ is consumed by an estimated 600 million people worldwide, which is approximately 8% of the world's population [2]. Its use has social, cultural, and religious importance in various parts of the world. However, ANBQ is also associated with a variety of health problems, including oral submucous fibrosis and other oral diseases [4]. Despite the global prominence of ANBQ and the health risks associated with its use, ANBQ remains an understudied research topic, and an unappreciated global public health issue [5]. In addition, there is no established framework for ANBQ control, and evidence-based practices regarding prevention and cessation of ANBQ chewing are in their nascent stages of development [6].

**Learning Goals**

- The primary learning goal of this chapter is to familiarize the reader with the international research literature on behavioral areca nut and betel quid (ANBQ) cessation programs.
- A second goal of the current chapter is to encourage future researchers to further develop and disseminate behavioral cessation programs for ANBQ.

20

## 20.2 The Scope of Behavioral Interventions

Behavioral interventions for ANBQ cessation may be targeted at the individual or population level. Individual level cessation programs focus on changing the chewing behavior of individuals, whereas population and public health level interventions include programs aimed at influencing social, cultural, and political norms associated with ANBQ use. Population level approaches affect access to areca nut by pricing, age restrictions, use restrictions at particular sites (worksites, schools, institutions), and availability. Interventions using policies, systems, and environmental approaches are population-based strategies applied in public health practice. This chapter focuses on behavioral interventions for ANBQ cessation that target individual behavior or small-scale community changes through education initiatives. Larger population-based behavior change strategies will not be the primary focus of this chapter.

The rationale for developing ANBQ cessation interventions parallels the rationale for cigarette smoking cessation interventions as a means to reduce the prevalence of lung cancer and other diseases caused by cigarette smoking. By quitting ANBQ use, a person can reduce the likelihood of developing oral submucous fibrosis, oral cancer, and other oral diseases. Whereas the research literature on behavioral cigarette smoking cessation interventions is large, the research literature on behavioral cessation programs for ANBQ is small and underdeveloped. Thus, one goal of the current chapter is to encourage researchers to further develop and disseminate behavioral ANBQ cessation programs in an effort to curb the global impact of ANBQ consumption on oral submucous fibrosis and other oral diseases.

Intervention studies on ANBQ chewing vary along a number of dimensions. One dimension regards the distinction between cessation (a current chewer ceasing ANBQ use) and prevention (preventing a person from chewing ANBQ in the first instance; i.e., initiation). Some interventions combine cessation and prevention. Hussain et al. [7], for example, conducted an intervention in a large sample of Pakistani adolescents. The intervention was designed to both encourage quitting among current chewers and to discourage chewing among non-chewers. Whereas the intervention succeeded in bringing about attitudinal changes in favor of quitting ANBQ and against chewing ANBQ as a general proposition, cessation was not assessed as an outcome. Thus, the Hussain et al. paper is an example of a study that contained an aspect of ANBQ cessation, but the intervention was more general in its orientation and did not focus exclusively on the issue of ANBQ cessation.

Another dimension of ANBQ intervention studies relates to the range of substances targeted by an intervention. This issue is complicated by the large variety of ANBQ and tobacco products chewed in the global context [8]. Further, a plethora of terms are used to describe products containing areca nut and tobacco throughout the world. Some authors employ the term "smokeless tobacco" to refer to a variety of areca-containing products. Croucher et al. [9], for example, conducted a cessation intervention study with Bangladeshi women chewers of "paan-with-tobacco" in the UK. (Paan is an ANBQ product that contains areca nut and other ingredients.) The title of the Croucher paper referenced "tobacco" but not areca nut even though paan includes areca nut as the primary ingredient. Another cessation intervention study by Raja et al. [10], included participants who smoked and chewed a variety of tobacco products, including cigarettes, beedis, paan, and others. In that study, many participants used areca nut mostly in the form of paan. Siddiqi et al. [11], to describe another example, developed and feasibility-tested a cessation program designed for smokeless tobacco users in Pakistan and the UK. Although their program generally focused on smokeless tobacco, most participants consumed some form of areca-containing preparation. Their results revealed that the program was feasible and acceptable. These studies and others illustrate how complex and variegated tobacco and ANBQ products are, even within a given study. Parsing these distinctions among various international intervention studies in the research literature is a complicated task. Here we wish only to draw attention to the complexity of the issue, and to place the review into this complex international context.

One particularly neglected area of ANBQ research is randomized cessation intervention trials for ANBQ-specific chewers who are currently trying to quit [12]. Whereas randomized cessation trials focused on cigarette smoking cessation for smokers who want to quit are plentiful (see [13]), behavioral studies focused specifically on ANBQ cessation for chewers who want to quit are rare. Recently, researchers have identified this gap in the research literature and have begun to address the issue. Lee, Wu, Chen, and Chang [14], for example, conducted a qualitative study of ANBQ cessation among oral cancer patients in Taiwan. They found that motivation to quit chewing among ANBQ chewers varied among patients much in the way that motivation to quit smoking varies among smokers [15]. Tami-Maury et al. [16] explored, qualitatively, the potential for ANBQ cessation strategies to be administered in Taiwanese dental settings. The authors concluded that dental settings could provide a promising venue for behavioral intervention. Papke, Hatsukami, and Herzog [17] hypothesized that ANBQ cessation programs ultimately should include both behavioral and pharmaceutical components. Hung et al. [18] recently conducted a randomized trial of anti-depressant medications for ANBQ cessation. Although this trial was relatively small and did not include a behavioral intervention, the results suggested that antidepressant medications could be helpful for ANBQ cessation. The authors further recommended that future research should test the potential of treatments that combine behavioral and pharmacological components (See ► Chap. 21). Finally, Paulino et al. [19] described a randomized clinical trial to test the efficacy of an intensive behavioral ANBQ cessation program on the western Pacific islands of Guam and Saipan. The results of the trial, aptly named the "Betel Nut Intervention Trial" (BENIT), showed that 34 out of 88 (38.6%) participants in the intervention condition self-reported ANBQ cessation. This compared to 8 out of 88 (9.1%) participants in the control condition, thereby yielding a significant outcome for ANBQ cessation ($p = 0.0058$). Thus, it appears that intensive ANBQ cessation programs can be effective, at least among defined populations.

## 20.3 Review of the Relevant Intervention Studies

We conducted a literature search that focused on ANBQ behavioral cessation intervention studies published between 1980 and 2021. We searched PubMed, Scopus, and Google Scholar databases for research articles using terms for ANBQ and related items including: betel quid, betel nut, smokeless tobacco, Paan, Gutka, Pan Masala, Khilli Paan, Dohra, Mawa, Mainpuri and Tombol. The following inclusion criteria were used: (1) the study must have at least some participants who chew ANBQ, Paan, or smokeless tobacco with areca nut, and (2) the study must have a behavioral cessation intervention component or be of direct relevance to the development of ANBQ cessation interventions. We list here the studies meeting the criteria alphabetically according to country.

### 20.3.1 Bangladesh

Bangladeshi women, including those who live in the UK, are among the South Asian populations who chew paan, which is comprised of betel leaf, lime, areca nut, and with tobacco as an optional ingredient [20]. Studies have confirmed that there is a relationship between chewing paan and potentially malignant oral conditions, including oral submucous fibrosis [21]. Authors of two studies hypothesized that nicotine replacement therapy (NRT) would improve cessation rates among Bangladeshi women in the UK who chew paan or smokeless tobacco. The first study was conducted by Croucher et al. in 2003 [20]. The intervention condition consisted of four counseling sessions plus access to NRT gum, whereas the control condition was comprised of only one session that included advice and encouragement on quitting. The intervention condition yielded slightly better short-term results compared to the control condition, but these differences were not statistically significant. The second study was conducted by

Croucher et al. in 2012 [9] and assessed predictors of paan cessation among Bangladeshi women in the UK in the context of a tobacco cessation clinic. The results revealed that a four-week course of NRT (gum, lozenge, microtab, inhaler, patch, or combination NRT) plus behavioral support led to superior self-reported cessation outcomes compared to the control group, who received only behavioral support (adjusted odds ratio = 4.93, $p = 0.001$). However, the authors cautioned that participants were self-selected to treatment groups, rather than being randomly allocated.

### 20.3.2 Guam

A study by Moss et al. in 2015 [22] reported the feasibility of the first ANBQ behavioral cessation program in the island of Guam of the Mariana Islands of the western Pacific. This ANBQ cessation program was modeled after an intensive behavioral treatment program for smoking cessation [23]. The group-based cognitive-behavioral ANBQ cessation program comprised of groups of five to ten people who met for five one-hour sessions over a period of 22 days. The intervention covered topics such as the negative health effects of ANBQ chewing, self-monitoring, social support, and relapse prevention. The study also assessed issues related to social and cultural challenges encountered during the recruitment and implementation of the program. Moss's study was the precursor for the BENIT, a randomized ANBQ-specific trial in Guam and Saipan [19] described earlier in this chapter.

### 20.3.3 India

Behavioral and educational intervention studies of tobacco cessation have been conducted in India for several decades. Most of these studies do not focus exclusively on ANBQ, but rather refer to the broader category of "smokeless tobacco." Nonetheless, these studies are clearly relevant to the topic of ANBQ cessation interventions.

Intervention studies conducted in India have employed community education programs for tobacco control [24, 25], broad-based worksite interventions [26], and school-based interventions [27]. These studies have demonstrated generally positive effects as measured by substantial reductions in tobacco consumption. Gupta et al. [28] also reported that their intervention resulted in the resolution of oral leukoplakia in some subjects who quit the ANBQ products.

Additional studies in India have employed cognitive and behavioral intervention approaches. Raja et al. [10] conducted a tobacco cessation intervention that compared cognitive behavioral therapy to a basic health education condition in a sample of 40 smokeless tobacco users. The study revealed the cognitive behavioral therapy to be more successful in helping tobacco users quit as compared to the basic health education intervention. Mall and Bhagyalaxmi [29] studied the effects of a peer-led anti-tobacco intervention on users of chewing tobacco products (including pan masala) in a sample of Indian adolescents. The authors concluded that the peer-led intervention was effective in reducing the consumption of chewing tobacco in its various forms. A recent small randomized clinical trial by Haokip et al. [30] compared a video-assisted nurse-led NRT intervention to a control group of standard NRT advice. The results revealed a significant decrease in smokeless tobacco intake among participants in the intervention condition compared to the control condition. The LifeFirst organization has recently developed a large tobacco and ANBQ cessation program for children ages 13–15. According to the organization's website, the cessation rates for this program are strikingly high. In summary, India has produced many impressive intervention studies related to ANBQ, and recent years has seen additional progress. However, randomized trials of intensive behavioral interventions for ANBQ chewers who want to quit remain rare.

### 20.3.4 Pakistan

Siddiqi et al. [11] designed a behavioral intervention to help South Asians in Pakistan and the UK quit chewing smokeless tobacco (including ANBQ). The intervention was feasibility-tested among 32 chewers. The intervention was comprised of activities such as raising awareness about the health risks of chewing smokeless tobacco (including ANBQ) as well as the benefits of quitting. Other aspects of the intervention included increasing a client's motivation and self-efficacy to quit chewing and developing strategies to manage temptations to chew. Intervention participants received information on the products' health risks. However, most participants only reported reductions in smokeless tobacco consumption rather than full cessation. Hussain et al. [7] also employed a smokeless tobacco (including ANBQ) intervention study among 1185 high-risk youths in Pakistan. The study combined elements of both cessation and prevention, as previously discussed in this chapter. This intervention had a positive effect, but did not include cessation as an outcome measure.

### 20.3.5 Sri Lanka

Researchers in Sri Lanka recently reported on a successful workshop targeted at building capacity for smokeless tobacco and ANBQ cessation among dental surgeons [31]. Although no evidence-based cessation program has been formally tested in Sri Lanka at this time, progress towards capacity building is apparent. The authors note that efforts are needed to tailor current tobacco cessation protocols to the specific needs of Sri Lankan ANBQ chewers.

### 20.3.6 Taiwan

Taiwan is known for its extensive public health efforts geared toward ANBQ control, and has been very active in ANBQ research [32]. Government efforts include an annual "Areca Prevention Day" and ANBQ cessation services on a large scale. To date, more than 7000 chewers have participated in the cessation services, efforts which have contributed to a decline in ANBQ chewing in Taiwan in recent years.

Researchers in Taiwan also have conducted several studies designed to inform the development of ANBQ cessation interventions. Lai et al. [33], for example, conducted a cross-sectional survey study of psychological factors and substance-use behaviors among 326 participants. The results revealed that betel quid chewers who were older and less educated are less likely to attempt quitting compared to younger and more educated chewers. Although the report is not an intervention study, it has clear relevance to the goal of developing cessation interventions.

Yang and Lin [34] conducted a qualitative interview study with 25 Taiwanese taxi drivers and their successful experiences with quitting areca nut chewing. The authors found that the negative health effects of chewing, and how that could affect family obligations, were chief motivators for successful cessation. They also found that addiction (dependence) and social situations that involved ANBQ chewing were significant challenges to their efforts to quit. These findings suggest that behavioral cessation interventions should address health risks, addiction, and social support from friends and family during and after ANBQ cessation.

Tamí-Maury et al. [16] conducted a study using surveys and interviews of 41 adult ANBQ chewers in Taiwan. The authors observed that dental settings are often where early signs of oral disease are first detected and concluded that brief behavioral cessation interventions in dental settings may be a promising way to reduce ANBQ consumption in Taiwan.

Lee et al. [14] conducted a qualitative study of betel quid cessation among 25 oral cancer patients in Taiwan. This analysis described psychological stages that some patients experience on their way to cessation, and sometimes back to a relapse to ANBQ chewing. The authors revealed that patients who quit chewing ANBQ because of oral cancer usually also quit alcohol and tobacco. These poly-substance quitters were found to have a low likelihood of relapse to the use of any of the substances that they previously consumed.

As mentioned previously, Hung et al. [18] conducted a randomized trial of anti-depressant medications (escitalopram and moclobemide) for ANBQ cessation. Although the trial did not include a behavioral intervention, the results suggested that antidepressant medications for ANBQ cessation should be further evaluated. Ko et al. [35] also examined potential cessation therapeutic drugs in BQ chewers in Taiwan. These two studies provide data for future research aimed at identifying pharmaceutical aids for ANBQ cessation.

**Tips**

Approaches and methods commonly used for smoking cessation, properly adjusted, are likely also to be helpful for ANBQ cessation.

## 20.4 Discussion

Areca nut cessation programs targeting individual behavior change through intensive behavioral interventions are promising. Translating the individual cessation programs to additional populations will require further study and additional resources, including randomized clinical trials. Cultural differences will need to be considered and respected when adapting cessation programs to diverse cultures. Challenges to program design may include levels of educational attainment and health literacy, access to program sites, and designing educational content for specific subgroups (e.g., culture, age, gender, social position). There are also limitations with regards to the evaluation, reinforcement, and efficacy of individual cessation programs. Evaluation may depend on the availability of accurate biomarkers, methods involving the use of direct observation, surveys, or self-reporting tools that accurately estimate cessation and decreases in amount of ANBQ use. Principles of implementation science, such as feasibility, acceptability, and sustainability can be used to develop successful cessation programs within communities.

## 20.5 Conclusion

International research efforts conducted in South Asia, some Pacific islands, and among migrant communities in the UK have identified the essential elements of behavioral ANBQ cessation. Not surprisingly, these programs are similar, though not identical, to tobacco cessation programs, most of which have been developed and applied to cigarette smokers. In some countries, such as Taiwan, behavioral cessation services are already available. Researchers are also currently exploring several potential pharmaceutical cessation aids, including nicotine replacement products, varenicline, pilocarpine [17], and antidepressant medications [18, 35]. What is most needed at this time is more carefully controlled and fully statistically powered randomized trials of behavioral cessation programs to determine how these programs can be refined and improved in order to provide the evidence needed to develop national guidelines and polices for ANBQ control.

**Important**

Behavioral ANBQ cessation programs have shown promise towards the objective of helping ANBQ chewers to quit.

**Summary**

This chapter reviews the current international research literature on behavioral interventions for areca nut and betel quid (ANBQ) cessation. The research literature is small but growing, and reveals encouraging results. Studies have shown that behavioral programs can help chewers to quit ANBQ. Additional development of ANBQ cessation programs through population specific translational research and randomized clinical trials is needed.



## References

1. Chu NS. Effects of Betel chewing on the central and autonomic nervous systems. J Biomed Sci. 2001;8(3):229–36.
2. Gupta PC, Warnakulasuriya S. Global epidemiology of areca nut usage. Addict Biol. 2002;7(1):77–83.
3. Paulino YC, Novotny R, Miller MJ, Murphy SP. Areca (Betel) Nut chewing practices in micronesian populations. Hawaii J Public Health. 2011;3(1):19–29.
4. IARC. Betel-quid and areca-nut chewing and some areca-nut derived nitrosamines. IARC Monogr Eval Carcinog Risks Hum. 2004;85:1–334.
5. Warnakulasuriya S, Chaturvedi P, Gupta PC. Addictive behaviours need to include Areca nut use. Addiction. 2015;110(9):1533.
6. Mehrtash H, Duncan K, Parascandola M, David A, Gritz ER, Gupta PC, et al. Defining a global research and policy agenda for betel quid and areca nut. Lancet Oncol. 2017;18(12):e767–e75.
7. Hussain A, Zaheer S, Shafique K. School-based behavioral intervention to reduce the habit of smokeless tobacco and betel quid use in high-risk youth in Karachi: a randomized controlled trial. PLoS One. 2018;13(11):e0206919.
8. Niaz K, Maqbool F, Khan F, Bahadar H, Ismail Hassan F, Abdollahi M. Smokeless tobacco (paan and gutkha) consumption, prevalence, and contribution to oral cancer. Epidemiol Health. 2017;39:e2017009.
9. Croucher R, Shanbhag S, Dahiya M, Kassim S, McNeill A. Predictors of successful short-term tobacco cessation in UK resident female Bangladeshi tobacco chewers. Addiction. 2012;107(7):1354–8.
10. Raja M, Saha S, Mohd S, Narang R, Reddy LV, Kumari M. Cognitive behavioural therapy versus basic health education for tobacco cessation among Tobacco users: a randomized clinical trail. J Clin Diagn Res. 2014;8(4):Zc47–9.
11. Siddiqi K, Dogar O, Rashid R, Jackson C, Kellar I, O'Neill N, et al. Behaviour change intervention for smokeless tobacco cessation: its development, feasibility and fidelity testing in Pakistan and in the UK. BMC Public Health. 2016;16:501.
12. Herzog TA, Pokhrel P. Introduction to the special issue: International research on areca nut and betel quid use. Subst Use Misuse. 2020;55(9):1383–4.
13. Fiore M. Treating tobacco use and dependence: 2008 update: clinical practice guideline. Department of Health and Human Services. Rockville, MD: Diane Publishing; 2008.
14. Lee CY, Wu CF, Chen CM, Chang YY. Qualitative study for betel quid cessation among oral cancer patients. PLoS One. 2018;13(7):e0199503.
15. Herzog TA. Analyzing the transtheoretical model using the framework of Weinstein, Rothman, and Sutton (1998): the example of smoking cessation. Health Psychol. 2008;27(5):548–56.
16. Tamí-Maury I, Ma WF, Lin MT, Lin CC, Tsai MH, Li CI, et al. A qualitative study of attitudes to and perceptions of betel quid consumption and its oral health implications in Taiwan. Community Dent Oral Epidemiol. 2019;47(1):58–64.
17. Papke RL, Hatsukami DK, Herzog TA. Betel Quid, health, and addiction. Subst Use Misuse. 2020;55(9):1528–32.
18. Hung CC, Lee CH, Ko AM, Lane HY, Lee CP, Ko YC. Effect of antidepressants for cessation therapy in betel-quid use disorder: a randomised, double-blind, placebo-controlled trial. Epidemiol Psychiatr Sci. 2020;29:e125.
19. Paulino YC, Wilkens LR, Sotto PP, Franke AA, Kawamoto CT, Chennaux JSN, et al. Rationale and design of a randomized, controlled, superiority trial on areca nut/betel quid cessation: The Betel Nut Intervention Trial (BENIT). Contemp Clin Trials Commun. 2020;17:100544.
20. Croucher R, Islam S, Jarvis MJ, Garrett M, Rahman R, Shajahan S, et al. Oral tobacco cessation with UK resident Bangladeshi women: a community pilot investigation. Health Educ Res. 2003;18(2):216–23.
21. Pearson N, Croucher R, Marcenes W, O'Farrell M. Prevalence of oral lesions among a sample of Bangladeshi medical users aged 40 years and over living in Tower Hamlets, UK. Int Dent J. 2001;51(1):30–4.
22. Moss J, Kawamoto C, Pokhrel P, Paulino Y, Herzog T. Developing a Betel Quid cessation program on the Island of Guam. Pac Asia Inq. 2015;6(1):144–50.
23. Brown R. Intensive behavioral treatment. The tobacco dependence treatment handbook: a guide to best practices. Guilford Press. 2003, pp. 118–77.
24. Gupta PC, Mehta FS, Pindborg JJ, Aghi MB, Bhonsle RB, Daftary DK, et al. Intervention study for primary prevention of oral cancer among 36,000 Indian tobacco users. Lancet. 1986;1(8492):1235–9.

25. Anantha N, Nandakumar A, Vishwanath N, Venkatesh T, Pallad YG, Manjunath P, et al. Efficacy of an anti-tobacco community education program in India. Cancer Causes Control. 1995;6(2):119–29.
26. Sorensen G, Pednekar M, Cordeira LS, Pawar P, Nagler EM, Stoddard AM, et al. Effects of a worksite tobacco control intervention in India: the Mumbai worksite tobacco control study, a cluster-randomised trial. Tob Control. 2017;26(2):210–6.
27. Sorensen G, Pednekar MS, Sinha DN, Stoddard AM, Nagler E, Aghi MB, et al. Effects of a tobacco control intervention for teachers in India: results of the Bihar school teachers study. Am J Public Health. 2013;103(11):2035–40.
28. Gupta PC, Murti PR, Bhonsle RB, Mehta FS, Pindborg JJ. Effect of cessation of tobacco use on the incidence of oral mucosal lesions in a 10-yr follow-up study of 12,212 users. Oral Dis. 1995;1(1):54–8.
29. Mall ASK, Bhagyalaxmi A. An informal school-based, peer-led intervention for prevention of Tobacco consumption in adolescence: a cluster randomized trial in rural Gandhinagar. Indian J Commun Med. 2017;42(3):143–6.
30. Haokip HR, Kumar R, Rawat VS, Sharma SK. Efficacy of standard nicotine replacement therapy (NRT) versus video-assisted nurse-led NRT on tobacco cessation: a randomized controlled pilot trial. Clin Epidemiol Global Health. 2021;9:141–6.
31. Jayasinghe RD, Jayasooriya PR, Amarasinghe H, Hettiarachchi P, Siriwardena B, Wijerathne U, et al. Evaluation of successfulness of capacity building programmes on smokeless Tobacco and Areca Nut Cessation. Asian Pacific J Cancer Prev. 2021;22(4):1287–93.
32. Yang YH, Warnakulasuriya S, Yang HF, Lin LJ, Wang YW. Public health measures to reduce areca nut and betel quid use for control of oral cancer in Taiwan. Oral Oncol. 2020;108:104915.
33. Lai CS, Shieh TY, Yang YH, Chong MY, Hung HC, Tsai CC. Factors associated with quitting areca (betel) quid chewing. Community Dent Oral Epidemiol. 2006;34(6):467–74.
34. Yang TY, Lin HR. Taking actions to quit chewing betel nuts and starting a new life: taxi drivers' successful experiences of quitting betel nut chewing. J Clin Nurs. 2017;26(7–8):1031–41.
35. Ko AM, Lee CH, Ko AM, Ko YC. Betel quid dependence mechanism and potential cessation therapy. Prog Neuro-Psychopharmacol Biol Psychiatry. 2020;103:109982.

# Pharmaceutical Agents for Areca Nut Cessation

*Sumali Sumithrarachchi and Ruwan Jayasinghe*

**Contents**



© The Author(s), under exclusive license to Springer Nature Switzerland AG 2023
S. Warnakulasuriya, K. Ranganathan (eds.), *Oral Submucous Fibrosis*, Textbooks in Contemporary Dentistry,
https://doi.org/10.1007/978-3-031-12855-4_21

## 21.1 Introduction

Areca nut is considered as the fourth most commonly used psycho-active substance in the world after nicotine, alcohol and caffeine use. The term "betel nut" as a synonym for areca nut, is frequently used in the literature even though not scientifically correct. This is primarily due to the practice of betel quid chewing which includes areca nut with or without smokeless tobacco (SLT) wrapped with a betel leaf. This habit of betel quid chewing is an ancient practice and tradition in the Indian subcontinent and is still widely prevalent in many parts of Asia, the western Pacific region [1] and among migrant communities arising there from such as in South and East Africa, Australia, Europe and North America [2].

Additionally, numerous commercially produced areca nut preparations with or without added tobacco such as gutka, thul, supari, sweet supari, pan masala, mawa, red tooth powder, khaini and zarda are also widely available [3]. Some Indian State Governments have banned marketing of some of these products but the implementation of the ban needs further ascertainment (◘ Fig. 21.1).

Pharmaceutical agents for cessation of areca nut addiction needs scientific investigation and should move one step beyond, to include pharmacotherapy for betel quid addiction which includes both the addictive elements of areca nut as well as SLT which is often added to the quid.

This chapter mainly focuses on prevention of Oral Potentially Malignant Disorders (OPMDs) and Oral cancer in those who have severe addiction to the habit of areca nut use with or without SLT added betel quid, beyond behavioural therapy. The addiction to areca nut is described in detail in Chap. 19 and this Chapter provides an overview on the cessation of areca nut addiction through the use of pharmaco-therapeutic agents in those identified as betel quid/ areca nut dependent.

**Learning Goals**

1. To examine the necessity for pharmacotherapy to assist areca nut cessation.
2. To describe added smokeless tobacco in the betel quid and its addictive nature.
3. To discuss addictive mechanisms in areca nut.
4. To explore various pharmaceutical agents for areca nut and betel quid cessation.

## 21.2 Betel Quid Addiction Beyond Behavioural Therapy

There are many situations in which behavioural therapy alone has not been successful for cessation of betel quid chewing. It is mainly due to dependence on various chemical substances in areca nut and SLT.

Addiction to areca nut leading to dependence liability, tolerance and withdrawal symptoms that strongly support a dependency syndrome have been suggested, which appear to be similar to nicotine addiction and dependence [2, 4, 5].

Hence, professional support and proven cessation medications can more than double the chance of successful quitting in areca nut dependent users. It is important to address this global menace of areca nut addiction

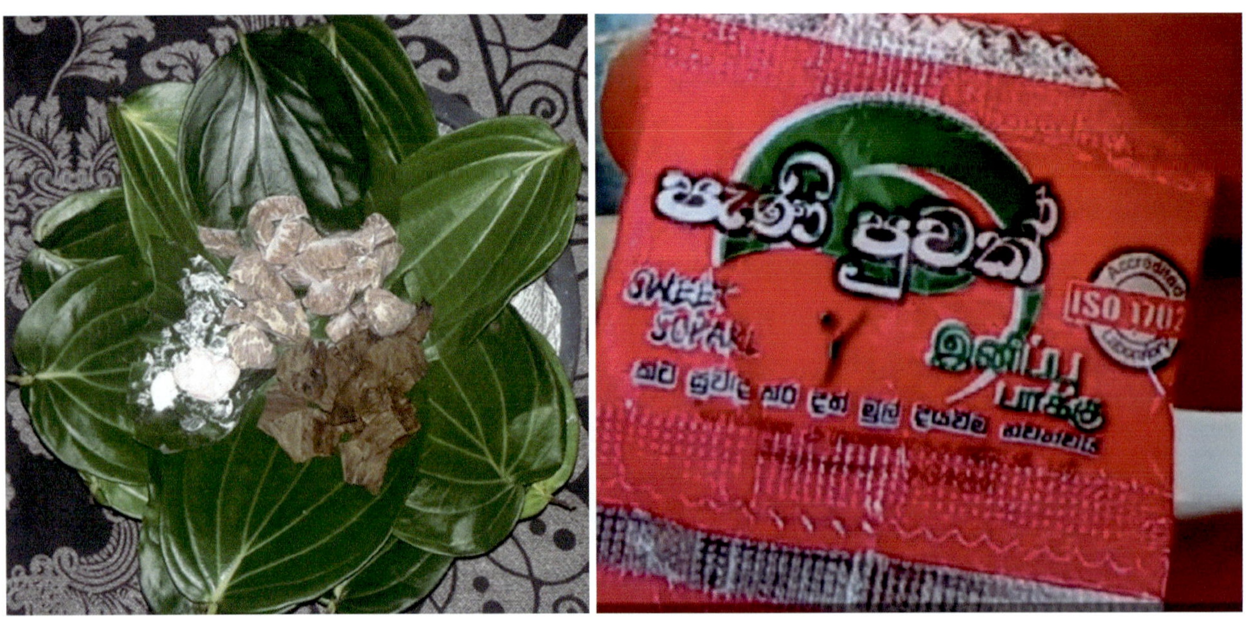

◘ **Fig. 21.1** Areca nut in the betel quid and as a commercially available product

with prime concern, due to presence of active addictive constituents.

In order to clearly understand the mechanism of dependence and hence possible cessation therapy, a systematic review revealed that neurological mechanisms link the brain reward, cognitive, and impulsive systems in areca nut/betel quid users [6].

The use of areca nut increases both brain serotonin and noradrenaline levels, in which arecoline, a potentially addictive component, has monoamine oxidase-A (MAO-A) inhibitor like properties. MAO-A inhibitors prevent neurotransmitter breakdown and increase dopamine and serotonin concentrations in the brain [4]. Additionally, added tobacco in the betel quid of areca nut users with betel quid chewing, has a higher addictive nature due to the presence of nicotine in SLT.

Hence, there is an interest towards the pharmacological management for areca nut/betel quid users who do not respond positively to behavioural therapy alone.

Even though pharmacological management for tobacco smoking cessation is well established with Food and Drug Administration (FDA) of USA approved medications such as Nicotine Replacement Therapy (NRT) including trans-dermal patch, gum, nasal spray, inhaler and lozenges; Bupropion and Varenicline [7], the use of pharmacotherapy in betel quid cessation (which includes both areca nut and SLT) is still at the phase of clinical trials. So far, several clinical trials for SLT cessation have been carried out with varying levels of success with the use of NRT, Varenicline and anti-depressants such as Bupropion [8]. However, studies solely based on pharmacotherapy for areca nut cessation are limited to a very few initial trials [9].

### 21.2.1 Smokeless Tobacco; Addictive Mechanism

The primary addictive component in chewing tobacco is nicotine. Nicotine which enters the circulation is carried to the brain, where it binds to nicotinic cholinergic receptors (ligand-gated ion channels that normally bind acetylcholine). The nicotinic cholinergic receptor consists of five subunits out of which the $\alpha4\beta2$ receptor is the principal mediator for nicotine dependence. Stimulation of nicotinic cholinergic receptors releases various neurotransmitters in the brain including dopamine which signals a pleasurable experience and is necessary for the reinforcing effects of self-administration as well as for irresistible drives such as eating. Nicotine also elevates both glutamate release, which facilitates the release of dopamine, and γ-aminobutyric acid (GABA) release, which inhibits dopamine release [10].

Hence cessation of addiction to nicotine in SLT through pharmacotherapy is studied in great detail with the available scientifically proven addictive nicotinic mechanisms.

### 21.2.2 Areca nut; Addictive Mechanisms

Even though nicotine is reported as the main tobacco extract alkaloid (15,454 μg/g) relatively minute amounts of nicotine have also been identified in the areca nut extracts (0.1 and 1.4 μg/g respectively) [11]. Though this may propose that addiction in areca nut chewers may also be due to nicotine, other addictive chemicals have also been detected such as major alkaloids (arecoline, arecaidine, guavacine, and guavacoline), which comprise approximately 2% of the areca nut composition by dry weight [12]. Among the areca nut alkaloids, arecoline has been detected at concentrations of approximately 5.5 mg/g [12], which is 55,000 times higher than the detected nicotine (0.1 μg/g). Hence it is crucial to understand the addictive mechanisms of these alkaloids prior to finding targeted pharmacotherapy for areca nut cessation.

Papke et al. [13], states that arecoline has activity on selected nicotinic acetylcholine receptor (nAChR) subtypes, including the two classes of nAChR mostly related to the addictive properties of nicotine: receptors containing $\alpha4$ and $\beta2$ subunits and those which also contain $\alpha6$ and $\beta3$ subunits. Arecoline's activity on nAChR associated with addiction may account for the habitual use of areca nut by regular chewers, but requires further study. Hence it is crucial to understand the addictive mechanisms of these alkaloids prior to finding targeted pharmacotherapy for areca nut cessation.

Arecoline is a tertiary amine with good brain penetration, as manifested by its numerous central nervous system effects [14]. Studies have shown that arecoline is taken up through the buccal mucosa, inducing neurobiological effects within 5 min of delivery [14]. Lime through alkalization of the masticate increases the fraction of the alkaloids that are in an uncharged form and therefore can be more readily absorbed into the blood. Arecoline is suggestive as an active compound of dependence. It behaves as a partial agonist with approximately 6–10% potency for the $\alpha4^*$ and $\alpha6^*$ nicotinic acetylcholine receptors (nAChR) demonstrated in Xenopus oocytes [13]. Studies propose that areca nut elevates brain serotonin levels via Mono Amine Oxidase-A (MAO-A) inhibitors [15, 16]. MAO-A is required in the common degradation pathway of both dopamine and serotonin. Therefore, MAO-A inhibitors block neurotransmitter breakdown and holds potential antidepressant effects through stimulation of dopamine, serotonin and noradrenaline concentrations in the brain. Guavacoline as a muscarinic agonist acts at 1/15 of the arecoline activity [17].

There are two stages to the process of drug taking behavior leading to addiction [13]. The first stage involves short-term "reinforcing" effects which stimulates the continuous use in naive chewers. The second stage involves the development of dependence which leads to craving and eventually withdrawal. It is not likely that arecoline has reinforcing effects mediated by the low level of nAChR activation produced. It is more probable that short-term reinforcement of areca nut use is associated with the muscarinic "high" or intoxication. However, the habitual use of areca nut will also work on the same receptors as nicotine. This may lead to dependence and promote craving and withdrawal if areca nut use is discontinued. Hence, areca nut chewers attempting to quit their habit manifest withdrawal symptoms similar to those of tobacco smokers [18].

The above evidence indicates that α4* nAChR are the main receptors which leads to nicotine addiction and may also be the case for areca nut addiction. Nevertheless, arecoline is 20–250 times less efficacious than equimolar nicotine, depending on the analysis type [19]. Thus, trace nicotine amounts may also be of clinical significance and should be accurately considered for areca nut dependence and treatment effects.

## 21.3 Pharmacotherapy for Areca Nut Cessation

As addictive constituents in areca nut addiction are still under research for both the presence of nicotine as well as the addictive nature of alkaloids such as arecoline, current pharmaceutical agents suggested for areca nut cessation may target nicotine addiction, arecoline addiction or both constituents when considering the mechanism of action.

The first part of this section will focus on pharmaceutical agents against nicotine addiction. According to Papke et al. [13] the nut's active ingredient, arecoline, acts on the same receptor proteins in the brain as nicotine. This raises the possibility that prescription drugs now used to break nicotine dependence could also be effective against areca nut addiction. In addition to it, as betel quid chewing is the commonest habit of areca nut use, pharmacotherapy for nicotine addiction is suitable in betel quid chewers, especially with added tobacco in their quid.

21

### 21.3.1 Pharmaco-Therapy for Nicotine Addiction

Nicotine Replacement Therapy for betel quid cessation has been reported in several studies in which the main focus has been on the smokeless tobacco (SLT) addiction. However, these studies on pharmacotherapy for SLT addiction may provide evidence for the nicotinic pathway of areca nut addiction. Hence pharmaceutical agents against nicotine addiction are highlighted in this section.

The nicotine gum and lozenges have been commonly used, as these have the advantage of providing an oral substitute as well as having a similar pharmacokinetic pattern to that of areca nut/ betel quid. Furthermore, the amount of nicotine content from the nicotine gum is less than from a usual dose of chewing tobacco [20]. A study was conducted in Minnesota, USA with a group of 30 participants having SLT habits which included snuff and chewing tobacco. It was an open-label, one-arm, phase II clinical trial to evaluate the efficacy of the 4-mg nicotine lozenge for the treatment of withdrawal and craving associated with tobacco abstinence among SLT users. It revealed that at 12 weeks (end of treatment) and at 6 months, the biochemically confirmed 7-day point-prevalence tobacco abstinence rate was 53% (95% CI = 34%–72%) and 47% (95% CI = 28%–66%) respectively. Due to small sample size and absence of a placebo controlled group, the results cannot be validated accurately [21]. A further, placebo controlled trial conducted in USA with use of nicotine gum as pharmacotherapy revealed that the biochemically verified abstinence rate at end of 6 months was 40% and 36% for the intervention and control groups respectively. In addition, the self-reported abstinence rate at the end of 12 months was 20% and 24% for the intervention and control groups respectively showing that in this study there was no therapeutic effect of nicotine when compared with the placebo [22].

Varenicline, an anti-smoking agent against nicotine is also another medication which can be suggested for SLT addiction. A double blind, placebo controlled, parallel group, multicentre, randomised controlled trial in medical clinics of Norway and Sweden were provided with Varenicline 1 mg twice daily (titrated during the first week) or placebo for 12 weeks, with 14 weeks' follow-up after treatment. Continuous abstinence rate at week 9–12 was higher in the Varenicline group than the placebo group (59% (125) v 39% (85); relative risk 1.60, 95% confidence interval 1.32 to 1.87, $p < 0.001$; risk difference 20%) [23]. A systematic review and meta-analysis [24] on the effectiveness and safety of Varenicline in SLT cessation revealed that subjects in the Varenicline arm had a significantly higher 7-day point prevalence of SLT abstinence at 12 weeks (48% vs. 33%; RR = 1.45, 95% CI = 1.22–1.72, $p < 0.0001$, I2 = 0%; RD = 13%, 95% CI = 4–23%, $p = 0.008$).

In addition to NRT and Varenicline, the use of anti-depressants have also been suggested for nicotine addiction. A double-blind, placebo controlled trial for sustained-release (SR) Bupropion in SLT cessation revealed that Bupropion 300 mg/day (150 bd) produced significantly higher quit rates at the end of treatment (7 weeks) than placebo ($p = 0.04$) with an OR (CI) of 2.73 (1.07, 7.72) [25]. Similarly, another multicenter, randomized, double-blind, placebo-controlled, clinical trial to assess the efficacy and safety of bupropion SR for tobacco abstinence among SLT users revealed that a time-by-treatment interaction was observed in craving over time with greater decreases in the bupropion SR group [26]. However, 7-day point-prevalence of abstinence rates did not differ between bupropion SR and placebo at the end treatment significantly (53.1% vs. 46.4%; odds ratio (OR) 1.3; $p = 0.301$). A pilot study of bupropion SR or placebo for 12 weeks showed that at the end of 12 weeks of therapy, the point-prevalence of SLT abstinence rate was 44% in the bupropion group and 26% in the placebo group ($p = 0.064$) providing benefits [27]. Some of these studies show promising, positive outcomes for the use of antidepressants for nicotine addiction.

**Pharmaceutical agents for nicotine addiction**
- Nicotine Replacement therapy (eg; nicotine lozenges/gum)
- Varenicline
- Bupropion

## 21.3.2 Pharmaceutical Agents for Arecoline Addiction

Since the composition of alkaloids is higher in areca nut, pharmacotherapy targeting the addiction due to alkaloids such as arecoline are also currently under research. Use of anti-depressants in the pharmacological management of betel quid/ areca nut cessation has recently been reported in the literature.

MAO-A Inhibitors and Selective Serotonin Receptor Inhibitors (SSRI) are suggested as primary alternatives for betel quid cessation, while other antidepressants or monoamine neurotransmitters are viewed as second-line alternatives [4]. Phenelzine and St. John's Wort may also be considered as acceptable for clinical use [4]. Phenelzine is a non-SSRI with higher side effects, while St. John's Wort is an antidepressant with a less effectiveness compared with areca nut and other antidepressants [15]. Varenicline's pharmacological mechanism is through α4* nAChR-binding and hence suggested for areca nut cessation treatment [13]. Similarly, Bupropion may prove to be having a therapeutic effect for betel quid/ areca nut dependence through higher dopamine levels [28] similar to the action of arecoline through MAO-A pathway, but need to be tested with clinical trials.

A randomized, double-blinded, placebo controlled trial on the effect of antidepressants (Escitalopram-MAO-A inhibitor and Moclobemide- SSRI) for cessation therapy in betel quid use disorder was conducted as a pioneer clinical study at the psychiatric outpatient department of China Medical University Hospital in Taichung, Taiwan. A total of eligible 111 male patients with betel quid dependence were randomized into 03 groups; placebo (n=37), Escitalopram 10mg/tab daily (n=38) and Moclobemide 150mg/tab daily (n=36). The primary outcome was defined as betel quid dependent users who continuously stopped chewing for ≥6 weeks. Drug treatment phase was 4-6 weeks while follow-ups were carried at 2, 4, 6 and 8 weeks for betel quid use and other disorder related outcomes such as dependence, side effects and withdrawal symptoms. The statistical analysis revealed that the Escitalopram and Moclobemide groups respectively, had a 28.7% and 31.2% higher proportion of betel quid abstinence than that for the placebo group (◘ Table 21.1). It also revealed that after antidepressant therapy with, Escitalopram and Moclobemide the mean level of areca nut use significantly fell from 39 ± 43 to 4 ± 6 quids/day and the frequency of areca nut consumption fell from 5.3 ± 3 to 0.7 ± 1.1 days/week. The novel findings of this study were that antidepressants could potentially be a therapeutic agent for patients with areca nut addiction, mainly via the MAO-A pathway [29] (◘ Table 21.1). More trials with larger sample

◘ **Table 21.1** Percentage, percentage difference and ratio of cessation of betel chewing for 6–8 weeks associated with drug treatment among male betel quid dependent users [29]

| Group | No. of participants | Cessation of betel chewing | | | [a]Adjusted % | Adjusted % difference (95% CI) | Adjusted % ratio (95% CI) |
|---|---|---|---|---|---|---|---|
| | | No | Yes | % | | | |
| Placebo | 37 | 35 | 2 | 5.4% | 5.4% | Ref. | 1.0 (Ref) |
| Escitalopram | 38 | 25 | 13 | 34.2% | 34.1% | 28.7% (11.8%–45.6%) | 6.3 (1.5–26.1) |
| Moclobemide | 36 | 24 | 12 | 33.3% | 36.6% | 31.2% (13.4%–49.1%) | 6.8 (1.6–28.0) |

[a]Adjusted % was obtained from the logistic regression model adjusted for age, educational level, cigarette smoking and the level of betel quid dependence

sizes need to be conducted to further validate these findings.

**Pharmaceutical agents for arecoline addiction**

- MAO-A inhibitors (eg; Escitalopram)
- SSR-I (eg; Moclobemide)
- Bupropion
- Phenelzine
- St. John's wort

## 21.4 Conclusion

Pharmaceutical agents for areca nut cessation are still under research and mainly considered together with SLT addiction as betel quid chewing with tobacco is the more popular habit of areca nut use particularly in India as mentioned earlier. Hence, smokeless tobacco (nicotine) and areca nut (arecoline + trace amounts of nicotine) cessation therapy go hand in hand. However, due to commercial preparations of areca nut now becoming more popular specially among the youth, more clinical trials targeting on pharmaceutical interventions against arecoline addiction should be conducted.

**Summary**

Nicotinic cholinergic receptor activation in the brain by constituents in areca nut releases dopamine. Areca nut also augments brain serotonin levels via MAO-A Inhibitors. This could be due to the presence of nicotine in areca nut as minute quantities, or other alkaloids including arecoline. Increased dopamine and serotonin levels possess potential antidepressant effects resulting in initial short-term "reinforcing" effects which promote the continuous use and later development of dependence with craving and withdrawal. Hence cessation through behavioural therapy for areca nut dependent users may not always be successful. Adjunct pharmacotherapy for nicotinic addiction includes Nicotine Replacement Therapy and Varenicline. Mono Amine Oxidase-Inhibitors, Selective Serotonin Re-uptake Inhibitors and Norepinephrine Dopamine Re-uptake Inhibitors have been suggested to show positive results against arecoline addiction, but requires further research.



## References

1. Gupta PC, Warnakulasuriya S. Global epidemiology of areca nut usage. Addict Biol. 2002;7(1):77–83. https://doi.org/10.1080/13556210020091437.
2. Warnakulasuriya S, Peters T. Introduction: biology, medical and socio-economic aspects of areca nut use. Addict Biol. 2002;7(1):75–6.
3. Sinha D, Galapatti K, Rinchen S, Kahandaliyanage A, Mehta F, Jayasuriya-Dissanayake N, Somatunga L, Sumanasekera P. Smokeless tobacco use in Sri Lanka. Indian J Cancer. 2012;49(4):357. https://doi.org/10.4103/0019-509x.107729.
4. Ko AMS, Lee CH, Ko AMJ, Ko YC. Betel quid dependence mechanism and potential cessation therapy. Prog Neuro-Psychopharmacol Biol Psychiatry. 2020;103:109982.
5. Winstock AR, Trivedy CR, Warnakulasuriya KA, Peters TJ. A dependency syndrome related to areca nut use: some medical and psychological aspects among areca nut users in the Gujarat community in the UK. Addict Biol. 2000;5(2):173–9.
6. Sariah A, Liu Z, Pu W, Liu H, Xue Z, Huang X. Structural and functional alterations in Betel-Quid Chewers: a systematic review of neuroimaging findings. Front Psychiatr. 2019; https://doi.org/10.3389/fpsyt.2019.00016.
7. Tønnesen P, Tonstad S, Hjalmarson A, Lebargy F, Van Spiegel PI, Hider A, Sweet R, Townsend J. A multicentre, randomized, double-blind, placebo-controlled, 1-year study of bupropion SR for smoking cessation. J Intern Med. 2003;254:184–92.
8. Ebbert J, Montori VM, Erwin PJ, Stead LF. Interventions for smokeless tobacco use cessation. Cochrane Database Syst Rev. 2011;16(2):CD004306.
9. Sumithrarachchi SR, Jayasinghe R, Warnakulasuriya S. betel quid addiction: a review of its addiction mechanisms and pharmacological management as an emerging modality for habit cessation. Subst Use Misuse. 2021; https://doi.org/10.1080/10826084.2021.1963990.
10. Benowitz NL. Nicotine addiction. N Engl J Med. 2010;362(24):2295–303. https://doi.org/10.1056/NEJMra0809890.
11. Franke AA, Mendez AJ, Lai JF, Arat-Cabading C, Li X, Custer LJ. Composition of betel specific chemicals in saliva during betel chewing for the identification of biomarkers. Food Chem Toxicol. 2015;80:241–6. https://doi.org/10.1016/j.fct.2015.03.012.
12. Wang CK, Su HY, Lii CK. Chemical composition and toxicity of Taiwanese betel quid extract. Food Chem Toxicol. 1999;37(2-3):135–44.
13. Papke RL, Horenstein NA, Stokes C. Nicotinic activity of arecoline, the psychoactive element of "Betel Nuts", suggests a basis for habitual use and anti-inflammatory activity. PLoS ONE. 2015;10(10):e0140907. https://doi.org/10.1371/journal.pone.0140907.
14. Chu NS. Neurological aspects of areca and betel chewing. Addict Biol. 2002;7:111–4. Pmid: 11900630
15. Abbas G, Naqvi S, Erum S, Ahmed S, Attaur R, Dar A. Potential antidepressant activity of Areca catechu nut via elevation of serotonin and noradrenaline in the hippocampus of rats. Phytother Res. 2013;27(1):39–45.
16. Chen PH, Tu HP, Wang SJ, Ko AM, Lee CP, Chiang TA, Tsai YS, Lee CH, Shieh TY, Ko CH, Chiang SL, Ko YC. Monoamine oxidase A variants are associated with heavy betel quid use. Addict Biol. 2012;17:786–97.
17. Horenstein NA, Quadri M, Stokes C, Shoaib M, Papke RL. Cracking the betel nut: cholinergic activity of areca alkaloids and related compounds. Nicotine Tob Res. 2019;21(6):805–12. https://doi.org/10.1093/ntr/ntx187.
18. Garg, A., Chaturvedi, P., & Gupta, P. C. (2014). A review of the systemic adverse effects of areca nut or betel nut Indian J Med Paediatr Oncol 35: 3–9. pmid:25006276.
19. Whiteaker P, Garcha HS, Wonnacott S, Stolerman IP. Locomotor activation and dopamine release produced by nicotine and isoarecolone in rats. Br J Pharmacol. 1995;116(3):2097–105.
20. Hatsukami DK, Severson HH. Oral spit tobacco: addiction, prevention and treatment. Nicotine Tob Res. 1999;1:21–44.
21. Ebbert JO, Dale LC, Severson H, Croghan IT, Rasmussen DF, Schroeder DR, VanderWeg MW, Hurt RD. Nicotine lozenges for the treatment of smokeless tobacco use. Nicotine Tob Res. 2007;9(2):233–40.

22. Boyle, R., Severson, H., Lichtenstein, E., & Gordon, J. (1993). Smokeless tobacco cessation with nicotine reduction: a placebo controlled trial. Paper presented at the 21st Annual Meeting of the American Public Health Association, San Franciso, CA.
23. Fagerström K, Gilljam H, Metcalfe M, Tonstad S, Messig M. Stopping smokeless tobacco with varenicline: randomised double blind placebo controlled trial. BMJ. 2010;341:c6549. Published 2010 Dec 6. https://doi.org/10.1136/bmj.c6549.
24. Schwartz J, Fadahunsi O, Hingorani R, Mainali NR, Oluwasanjo A, Aryal MR, Donato A. Use of varenicline in smokeless tobacco cessation: a systematic review and meta-analysis. Nicotine Tob Res. 2016;18(1):10–6. https://doi.org/10.1093/ntr/ntv010. Epub 2015 Feb 2
25. Glover ED, Glover PN, Sullivan R, Cerullo CL, Hobbs G. A comparison of sustained-release bupropion and placebo for smokeless tobacco cessation. Am J Health Behav. 2002;26(5):386–93.
26. Dale LC, Ebbert JO, Glover ED, Croghan IT, Schroeder DR, Severson HH, Hurt RD. Bupropion SR for the treatment of smokeless tobacco use. Drug Alcohol Depend. 2007;90(1):56–63. https://doi.org/10.1016/j.drugalcdep.
27. Dale LC, Ebbert JO, Schroeder DR, Croghan IT, Rasmussen DF, Trautman JA, Cox LS, Hurt RD. Bupropion for the treatment of nicotine dependence in spit tobacco users: a pilot study. Nicotine Tob Res. 2002;4(3):267–74. https://doi.org/10.1080/14622200210153821.
28. Stahl SM, Pradko JF, Haight BR, Modell JG, Rockett CB, Learned-Coughlin S. A review of the neuropharmacology of bupropion, a dual norepinephrine and dopamine reuptake inhibitor. Prim Care Companion J Clin Psychiatry. 2004;6(4):159–66. https://doi.org/10.4088/pcc.v06n0403.
29. Hung CC, Lee CH, Ko AM-S, Lane HY, Lee CP, Ko YC. Effect of antidepressants for cessation therapy in betel quid use disorder: a randomised, double blind, placebo-controlled trial. Epidemiol Psychiatr Sci. 2020:1–10. https://doi.org/10.1017/S2045796020000384.

# World Literature: Bibliography

*Radhika Manoj Bavle and P Sharada*

## Contents



© The Author(s), under exclusive license to Springer Nature Switzerland AG 2023
S. Warnakulasuriya, K. Ranganathan (eds.), *Oral Submucous Fibrosis*, Textbooks in Contemporary Dentistry,
https://doi.org/10.1007/978-3-031-12855-4_22

## 22.1 Bibliography

### 22.1.1 Reviews


1. Chaudhry K, Khatana S, Bali R, Kaur A, Dutt N. Quality of life in oral submucous fibrosis: a systematic review. J Maxillofac Oral Surg. 2022;21(1):14–24.
2. Sarode SC, Sarode GS, Yuwanati M, Gadbail A, Gondivkar S. A brief overview of 100 best-cited papers on oral submucous fibrosis in Oral Oncology. Oral Oncol. 2022;126:105769.
3. Xu H, Lyu FY, Song JY, Xu YM, Jiang EH, Shang ZJ, et al. Research achievements of oral submucous fibrosis: progress and prospect. Biomed Res Int. 2021;2021:1–10.
4. Gupta S, Jawanda MK. Oral submucous fibrosis: an overview of a challenging entity. Indian J Dermatol Venereol Leprol. 2021;87(6):768–77.
5. Rao NR, Villa A, More CB, Jayasinghe RD, Kerr AR, Johnson NW. Oral submucous fibrosis: a contemporary narrative review with a proposed interprofessional approach for an early diagnosis and clinical management. J Otolaryngol Head Neck Surg. 2020;49(1):1–11.
6. More CB, Patila DJ, Rao NR. Medicinal management of oral submucous fibrosis in the past decade - a systematic review. J Oral Biol Craniofac Res. 2020;10:552–68.
7. Shen YW, Shih YH, Fuh LJ, Shieh TM. Oral submucous fibrosis: a review on biomarkers, pathogenic mechanisms, and treatments. Int J Mol Sci. 2020;21(19):1–19.
8. Hande AH, Chaudhary MS, Gawande MN, Gadbail AR, Zade PR, Bajaj S, et al. Oral submucous fibrosis: an enigmatic morpho-insight. J Can Res Ther. 2019;15:463–9.
9. Ray JG, Chatterjee R, Chaudhuri K. Oral submucous fibrosis: A global challenge. Rising incidence, risk factors, management, and research priorities. Periodontol 2000. 2019;80(1):200–12. ► https://doi.org/10.1111/prd.12277.
10. Shih YH, Wang TH, Shieh TM, Tseng YH. Oral submucous fibrosis: a review on etiopathogenesis, diagnosis, and therapy. Int J Mol Sci. 2019;20:1–22.
11. Bari S, Metgud R, Vyas Z, Tak A. An update on studies on etiological factors, disease progression, and malignant transformation in oral submucous fibrosis. J Cancer Res Ther. 2017;13(3):399–405.
12. Ekanayaka RP, Tilakaratne WM. Oral submucous fibrosis: review on mechanisms of malignant transformation. Oral Surg Oral Med Oral Pathol Oral Radiol. 2016;122(2):192–9.
13. Dionne KR, Warnakulasuriya S, Zain RB, Cheong SC. Potentially malignant disorders of the oral cavity: current practice and future directions in the clinic and laboratory. Int J Cancer. 2015;136:503–15.
14. Arakeri G, Brennan PA. Oral submucous fibrosis: an overview of the aetiology, pathogenesis, classification, and principles of management. Br J Oral Maxillofac Surg. 2013;51:587–93.
15. Kerr AR, Warnakulasuriya S, Mighell AJ, Dietrich T, Nasser M, Rimal J, et al. A systematic review of medical interventions for oral submucous fibrosis and future research opportunities. Oral Dis. 2011;17(1):42–57.
16. Zhang X, Reichart PA. A review of betel quid chewing, oral cancer and precancer in Mainland China. Oral Oncol. 2007;43:424–30.
17. Tilakaratne WM, Klinikowski MF, Saku T, Peters TJ, Warnakulasuriya S. Oral submucous fibrosis: review on aetiology and pathogenesis. Oral Oncol. 2006;42(6):561–8.
18. Gupta PC, Sinor PN, Bhonsle RB, Pawar VS, Mehta HC. Oral submucous fibrosis in India: a new epidemic? Natl Med J India. 1998;11(3):113–6.
19. VanWyk CW. Oral submucous fibrosis. The South African experience. Indian J Dent Res. 1997;8(2):39–45.
20. Cox SC, Walker DM. Oral submucous fibrosis. A review. Aust Dent J. 1996;41:294–9.
21. Rajendran R. Oral submucous fibrosis: etiology, pathogenesis, and future research. Bull World Health Organ. 1994;72(6):985–96.
22. Paissat DK. Oral submucous fibrosis. Int J Oral Surg. 1981;10:307–12.
23. Pindborg JJ, Sirsat SM. Oral submucous fibrosis. Oral Surg Oral Med Oral Pathol. 1966;22(6):764–79.


### 22.1.2 Epidemiology of OSF Worldwide


1. Peng Q, Li H, Chen J, Wang Y, Tang Z. Oral submucous fibrosis in Asian countries. J Oral Pathol Med. 2020;49(4):294–304.
2. Yang SF, Wang YH, Su NY, Yu HC, Wei CY, Yu CH, et al. Changes in prevalence of precancerous oral submucous fibrosis from 1996 to 2013 in Taiwan: a nationwide population-based retrospective study. J Med Assoc. 2018;117:147–52.
3. Aishwarya KM, Reddy MP, Kulkarni S, Doshi D, Reddy BS, Satyanarayana D. Effect of frequency and duration of tobacco use on oral mucosal lesions—a cross-sectional study among tobacco

users in Hyderabad, India. Asian Pac J Cancer Prev. 2017;18(8):2233–8.
4. Yang PY, Chen YT, Wang YH, Su NY, Yu HC, Chang YC. Malignant transformation of oral submucous fibrosis in Taiwan: a nationwide population-based retrospective cohort study. J Oral Pathol Med. 2017;46:1040–5.
5. Aishwarya KM, Reddy MP, Kulkarni S, Doshi D, Reddy BS, Satyanarayana D. Effect of frequency and duration of tobacco use on oral mucosal lesions—a cross-sectional study among tobacco users in Hyderabad, India. Asian Pac J Cancer Prev. 2017;18(8):2233–8.
6. Singhvi A, Joshi A, Bagul N, Bhatia S, Singh G, Gupta R. The insight for initiation and maintenance of areca nut chewing habit and its effects on oral health status among school age population in Western Rajasthan, India. J Clin Diagn Res. 2016;10(11):ZC15–8.
7. Yongxiu D, Dongye S, Xinchun J, Qiuhua M, Yanan C, Pu X. Epidemiological investigation of chewing fresh or dried betel nut and oral mucosal disease. Hua Xi Kou Qiang Yi Xue Za Zhi. 2016;34(4):391–4.
8. Holla VA, Chatra LK, Shenai P, Shetty D, Baliga A. A study to analyze different patterns of quid usage among subjects with oral submucous fibrosis in mangalore population. Adv Med. 2016;2016:1–6. ► https://doi.org/10.1155/2016/6124059.
9. Wang YY, Tail YH, Wang WC, Chen CY, Kao YH, et al. Malignant transformation in 5071 southern Taiwanese patients with potentially malignant oral mucosal disorders. BMC Oral Health. 2014;14:1–9.
10. Lian Ie B, Tseng YT, Su CC, Tsai KY. Progression of precancerous lesions to oral cancer: results based on the Taiwan National Health Insurance Database. Oral Oncol. 2013;49:427–30.
11. Heck JE, Marcotte EL, Argos M, Parvez F, Ahmed A, Islam T, et al. Betel quid chewing in rural Bangladesh: prevalence, predictors and relationship to blood pressure. Int J Epidemiol. 2012;41(2):462–71.
12. Angadi PV, Rekha KP. Oral submucous fibrosis: a clinicopathologic review of 205 cases in Indians. Oral Maxillofac Surg. 2011;15(1):15–9.
13. Jalouli J, Ibrahim SO, Mehrotra R, Jalouli MM, Sapkota D, Larsson PA, et al. Prevalence of viral (HPV, EBV, HSV) infections in oral submucous fibrosis and oral cancer from India. Acta Otolaryngol. 2010;130:1306–11.
14. Auluck A, Hislop G, Poh C, Zhang L, Rosin MP. Areca nut and betel quid chewing among South Asian immigrants to Western countries and its implications for oral cancer screening. Rural Remote Health. 2009;9(2):1–8.
15. Mathew AL, Pai KM, Sholapurkar AA, Vengal M. The prevalence of oral mucosal lesions in patients visiting a dental school in Southern India. Indian J Dent Res. 2008;19(2):99–103.
16. Lee CH, Ko YC, Huang HL, Chao YY, Tsai CC, Shieh TY, et al. The precancer risk of betel quid chewing, tobacco use and alcohol consumption in oral leukoplakia and oral submucous fibrosis in Southern Taiwan. Br J Cancer. 2003;88:366–72.
17. Yang YH, Lee HY, Tung S, Shieh TY. Epidemiological survey of oral submucous fibrosis and leukoplakia in aborigines of Taiwan. J Oral Pathol Med. 2001;30(4):213–9.
18. Tang JG, Jian XF, Gao ML, Ling TY, Zhang KH. Epidemiological survey of oral submucous fibrosis in Xiangtan City, Hunan Province, China. Community Dent Oral Epidemiol. 1997;25:177–80.
19. Babu S, Bhat RV, Kumar PU, Sesikaran B, Rao KV, Aruna P, et al. A comparative clinico-pathological study of oral submucous fibrosis in habitual chewers of pan masala and betelquid. J Toxicol Clin Toxicol. 1996;34(3):317–22.

### 22.1.3 Clinical Presentation and Evaluation: Paediatric and Adult Patients of OSF

1. Rai A, Jain A, Arora A, Motiwale T. Oral submucous fibrosis in children: an alarming condition and challenges in management. BMJ Case Rep. 2021;14(3):1–4.
2. Sachdev R, Garg K, Shwetam S, Srivastava A. Nonspecific chief complaints among oral submucous fibrosis patients at outpatient department and pan shop at rural region in India. J Int Soc Prev Community Dent. 2021;11(4):382–8.
3. Kariya P, Khobragade V, Sura S, Singh S. No age predilection for a disease like OSMF. A case report of 5-year-old child. J Oral Biol Craniofac Res. 2020;10(2):153–7.
4. Shah JS, Lunagariya N. Hearing efficiency in oral submucous fibrosis: a clinical study. Indian J Otolaryngol Head Neck Surg. 2020;1:1–5.
5. Tripathy M, Anekar J, Raj AC, Sandeepa NC, Napplli D, Lokanath P, et al. Cephalometric study on the morphometric evaluation of soft palate in oral submucous fibrosis. Asian Pac J Cancer Prev. 2020;21(7):2169–76.
6. Cai X, Yao Z, Liu G, Cui L, Li H, Huang J. Oral submucous fibrosis: a clinicopathological study of 674 cases in China. J Oral Pathol Med. 2019;48(4):321–5.

7. Chaudhry K, Bali R, Patnana AK, Bindra S, Jain G, Sharma PP. Impact of oral submucous fibrosis on quality of life: a cross-sectional study. J Maxillofac Oral Surg. 2019;18(2):260–5.
8. Gondivkar SM, Bhowate RR, Gadbail AR, Sarode SC, Gondivkar RS. Assessment of oral health-related quality of life instruments for oral submucous fibrosis: a systematic review using the COnsensus-based Standards for the selection of health Measurement Instruments (COSMIN) checklist. Oral Oncol. 2019 Jun;93:39–45.
9. Talla H, Reddy PR, Mudavath M, Bathina T. Oral submucous fibrosis in a 5 year old child. Contemp Clin Dent. 2019;10:679–81.
10. Jain A, Taneja S. Oral submucous fibrosis in pediatric patients: a systematic review and protocol for management. Int J Surg Oncol. 2019;2019:1–6. ► https://doi.org/10.1155/2019/3497136.
11. Bangi BB, Ginjupally U, Nadendla LK, Mekala MR. Evaluation of gustatory function in oral submucous fibrosis patients and Gutka chewers. Asian Pac J Cancer Prev. 2019;20(2):569–73.
12. Domir SK, Gargava A, Deoghare A, Agrawal R. Morphometric evaluation of soft palate in OSMF patients using cephalometrics. Indian J Otolaryngol Head Neck Surg. 2019;71(Suppl. 1):1018–102.
13. Gondivkar SM, Bhowate RR, Gadbail AR, Gaikwad RN, Gondivkar RS, Sarode SC, Sarode GS. Development and validation of oral health-related quality of life measure in oral submucous fibrosis. Oral Dis. 2018 Sep;24(6):1020–8.
14. Tadakamadla J, Kumar S, Lalloo R, Gandhi Babu DB, Johnson NW. Impact of oral potentially malignant disorders on quality of life. J Oral Pathol Med. 2018;47(1):60–5.
15. Kanodia S, Giri VP, Giri OP, Devi MP, Garima Y. Assessment of anxiety, depression, and serum cortisol level in oral submucous fibrosis patients: a controlled clinical trial. Eur J Dent. 2017;11(3):293–8.
16. Chandran A, Aswath N. Assessment of function of eustachian tube in oral submucous fibrosis—a tympanometric study. J Clin Diagn Res. 2016;10(9):ZC13–5.
17. Wollina U, Verma SB, Ali FM, Patil K. Oral submucous fibrosis: an update. Clin Cosmetic Investig Dermatol. 2015;8:193–204.
18. Ankita C, Panat SR, Sangamesh NC, Aggarwal A, Jha PC. Evaluation of masseter muscle hypertrophy in OSF patients: an ultrasonographic study. J Clin Diagn Res. 2014;8(9):ZC45–7.
19. Siddiqui SN, Saawarn N, Nair PP, Singh P, Gharote HP, Hegde K. Eustachian tube dysfunction in OSMF-often present seldom discovered. J Clin Exp Dent. 2014;6(4):e369–73.
20. Ali FM, Patil A, Patil K, Prasant MC. Oral submucous fibrosis and its dermatological relation. Indian Dermatol Online J. 2014;5(3):260–5.
21. Gupta VK, Malhotra S, Patil R, Tripathi A. Oral submucous fibrosis at pediatric age, now time to think: series of two cases. Indian J Med Paediatr Oncol. 2013;34(2):107–10.
22. Deshpande A, Kiran S, Dhillon S, Mallikarjuna R. Oral submucous fibrosis: a premalignant condition in a 14-year-old Indian girl. BMJ Case Rep. 2013;2013:1–4. ► https://doi.org/10.1136/bcr-2013-200786.
23. Agrawal A, Sarkar PA, Shigli A. Oral submucous fibrosis in a 9-year-old Indian girl. BMJ Case Rep. 2011;2011:1–3. ► https://doi.org/10.1136/bcr.08.2011.4588.
24. Chaturvedi P. Uvular abnormalities in patients with submucous fibrosis. Oral Dis. 2009;15(7):516.
25. Aziz SR. Oral submucous fibrosis: case report and review of diagnosis and treatment. J Oral MaxillofacSurg. 2008;66:2386–9.
26. Auluck A, Rosin MP, Zhang L, Sumanth KN. Oral submucous fibrosis, a clinically benign but potentially malignant disease: report of 3 cases and review of the literature. J Can Dent Assoc. 2008;74(8):735–40.
27. Rajendra R, George B, Sivakaran S, Narendranathan N. Visceral organ involvement is infrequent in oral submucous fibrosis (OSF). Indian J Dent Res. 2001;12(1):7–20.
28. Misra SP, Misra V, Dwivedi M, Gupta SC. Oesophageal subepithelial fibrosis: an extension of oral submucosal fibrosis. Postgrad Med J. 1998;74(878):733–6.
29. Maher R, Sankaranarayanan R, Johnson NW, Warnakulasuriya KA. Evaluation of inter-incisor distance as an objective criterion of the severity of oral submucous fibrosis in Karachi, Pakistan. Eur J Cancer B Oral Oncol. 1996;32B(5):362–4.
30. Warnakulasuriya S. Semi-quantitative clinical description of oral submucous fibrosis. Ann Dent. 1987;46:18–21.

### 22.1.4 Classification, Grading and Staging Systems Used in OSF

1. Ingle Y, Sarode GS, Sarode SC. A novel histological grading system for minor salivary gland involvement in oral submucous fibrosis patients with clin-

ico-pathological validation. J Oral BiolCraniofac Res. 2021;11(4):596–600.
2. Ramadoss R, Krishnan R, Vasanthi V, Bose D, Vijayalakshmi R, Padmanabhan R, et al. New insights for consummate diagnosis and management of oral submucous fibrosis using reactive and reparative fibrotic parameter derived algorithm. J Pharm Bioali Sci. 2021;13(5):323–32.
3. More CB, Rao NR. Proposed clinical definition for oral submucous fibrosis. J Oral BiolCraniofac Res. 2019;9(4):311–4.
4. Hameed S, Chatra L, Shenai P. Establishing a new staging system for oral submucous fibrosis and correlation of the proposed staging system to traditional histopathological grading: a clinico-histopathological study. Saudi Dent J. 2019;31(4):445–50.
5. Zhou S, Zhu Y, He Z, Zhang D, Guo F, Jian X, Zhang C. Long non-coding RNA expression profile associated with malignant progression of oral submucous fibrosis. J Oncol. 2019;2019:1–12. ► https://doi.org/10.1155/2019/6835176.
6. Arakeri G, Thomas D, Aljabab AS, Hunasgi S, Rai KK, Hale B, et al. TFM classification and staging of oral submucous fibrosis: a new proposal. J Oral Pathol Med. 2018;47(4):403–9.
7. Gupta H, Grover N, Tyagi N, Misra A. Classification systems in oral submucous fibrosis patients: a review. TMU J Dent. 2018;5(2):13–9.
8. Divyambika CV, Sathasivasubramanian S, Vani G, Vanishree AJ, Malathi N. Correlation of clinical and histopathological grades in oral submucous fibrosis patients with oxidative stress markers in saliva. Indian J Clin Biochem. 2018;33:348–55.
9. Passi D, Bhanot P, Kacker D, Chahal D, Atri M, Panwar Y. Oral submucous fibrosis: newer proposed classification with critical updates in pathogenesis and management strategies. Natl J Maxillofac Surg. 2017;8(2):89–94.
10. Lakshmi CR, Thabusum DA, Bhavana SM. An innovative approach to evaluate the morphological patterns of soft palate in oral submucous fibrosis patients: a digital cephalometric study. Int J Chronic Dis. 2016;2016:1–6. ► https://doi.org/10.1155/2016/5428581.
11. Patil S, Maheshwari S. Proposed new grading of oral submucous fibrosis based on cheek flexibility. J Clin Exp Dent. 2014;6(3):e255–8.
12. More CB, Das S, Patel H, Adalja C, Kamatchi V, Venkatesh R. Proposed clinical classification for oral submucous fibrosis. Oral Oncol. 2012;48(3):200–2.
13. Shivakumar GC, Sahana S. Clinical staging of oral submucous fibrosis: a review. Int J Oral-Med Sci. 2011;10(3):216–9.
14. Krishnan MMR, Pal M, Bomminayuni SK, Chakraborty C, Paul RR, Chatterjee J, Ray AK. Automated classification of cells in sub-epithelial connective tissue of oral sub-mucous fibrosis-an SVM based approach. Comput Biol Med. 2009;39(12):1096–104.
15. Ceena DE, Bastian TS, Ashok L, Annigeri RG. Comparative study of clinicofunctional staging of oral submucous fibrosis with qualitative analysis of collagen fibers under polarizing microscopy. Indian J Dent Res. 2009;20(3):271–6.
16. Ranganathan K, Mishra G. An overview of classification schemes for oral submucous fibrosis. J Oral MaxFac Pathol. 2006;10:55–8.
17. Paul RR, Mukherjee A, Dutta PK, Banerjee S, Pal M, Chatterjee J, et al. A novel wavelet neural network based pathological stage detection technique for an oral precancerous condition. J Clin Pathol. 2005;58:932–8.
18. Haider SM, Merchant AT, Fikree FF, Rahbar MH. Clinical and functional staging of oral submucous fibrosis. Br J Oral Maxillofac Surg. 2000;38(1):12–5.

### 22.1.5 Etiopathogenesis of OSF as an OPMD

1. Venkatesh D, Puranik RS, Vanaki SS, Puranik SR. Study of salivary arecoline in areca nut chewers. J Oral Maxillofac Pathol. 2018;22(3):446. Coletta RD and Salo T. Myofibroblasts in oral potentially malignant disorders: Is it related to malignant transformation? Oral Dis 2018;24(1–2):84–88
2. Hsieh YP, Wu KJ, Chen HM, Deng YT. Arecoline activates latent transforming growth factor beta1 via mitochondrial reactive oxygen species in buccal fibroblasts: suppression by epigallocatechin-3-gallate. J Formos Med Assoc. 2018;117:527–34.
3. Ekanayaka RP, Tilakaratne WM. Oral submucous fibrosis: review on mechanisms of pathogenesis and malignant transformation. Oral Surg Oral Med Oral Pathol Oral Radiol. 2018;125(6):612–27.
4. Arakeri G, Rai KK, Hunasgi S, Merkx MA, Gao S, Brennan PA. Oral submucous fibrosis: an update on current theories of pathogenesis. J Oral Pathol Med. 2017;46(6):406–12.
5. Gandhi P, Prasad UC. Evaluation of myofibroblasts in oral submucous fibrosis and oral squamous cell carcinoma: the pathogenesis and correlation. Dent Res J (Isfahan). 2017;14(5):314–20.
6. Ho YC, Yang SF, Lee SS, Chang YC. Regulation of hypoxia-inducible factor-1alpha in human buccal

mucosal fibroblasts stimulated with arecoline. J Formos Med Assoc. 2017;116:484–7.
7. Bari S, Metgud R, Vyas Z, Tak A. An update on studies on etiological factors, disease progression, and malignant transformation in oral submucous fibrosis. J Cancer Res Ther. 2017;13(3):399–405.
8. Patel JB, Shah FD, Joshi GM, Patel PS. Clinical significance of inflammatory mediators in the pathogenesis of oral cancer. J Cancer Res Ther. 2016;12(2):447–57.
9. Tilakaratne WM, Ekanayaka RP, Warnakulasuriya S. Oral submucous fibrosis: a historical perspective and a review on etiology and pathogenesis. Oral Surg Oral Med Oral Pathol Oral Radiol. 2016;122(2):178–91.
10. Lee YH, Yang LC, Hu FW, Peng CY, Yu CH, Yu CC. Elevation of Twist expression by arecoline contributes to the pathogenesis of oral submucous fibrosis. J Formos Med Assoc. 2016;115(5):311–7.
11. Wang YP, Wu YC, Cheng SJ, Chen H, Sun A, Chang JY. High frequencies of vitamin B12 and folic acid deficiencies and gastric parietal cell antibody positivity in oral submucous fibrosis patients. J Formos Med Assoc. 2015;114(9):813–9.
12. Ratheesh AV, Kumar B, Mehta H, Sujatha GP, Shankarmurthy SP. Etiopathogenesis of oral submucous fibrosis. J Med Radiol Pathol Surg. 2015;1:16–21.
13. Shakunthala GK, Annigeri RG, Arunkumar S. Role of oxidative stress in the pathogenesis of oral submucous fibrosis: a preliminary prospective study. Contemp Clin Dent. 2015;6:S172–4.
14. Illeperuma RP, Kim DK, Park YJ, Son HK, Kim JY, Kim J, et al. Areca nut exposure increases secretion of tumor-promoting cytokines in gingival fibroblasts that trigger DNA damage in oral keratinocytes. Int J Cancer. 2015;137:2545–57.
15. Liu B, Shen M, Xiong J, Yuan Y, Wu X, Gao X, et al. Synergistic effects of betel quid chewing, tobacco use (in the form of cigarette smoking), and alcohol consumption on the risk of malignant transformation of oral submucous fibrosis (OSF): a case-control study in Hunan Province, China. Oral Surg Oral Med Oral Pathol Oral Radiol. 2015;120:337–45.
16. Pant I, Kumar N, Khan I, Rao SG, Kondaiah P. Role of areca nut induced TGF-beta and epithelial-mesenchymal interaction in the pathogenesis of oral submucous fibrosis. PLoS ONE. 2015;10(6):e0129252. ► https://doi.org/10.1371/journal.pone.0129252.
17. Namboodiripad PA. Cystatin C: its role in pathogenesis of OSMF. J Oral Biol Craniofac Res. 2014;4(1):42–6.
18. Arakeri G, Patil SG, Ramesh DN, Hunasgi S, Brennan PA. Evaluation of the possible role of copper ions in drinking water in the pathogenesis of oral submucous fibrosis: a pilot study. Br J Oral MaxillofacSurg. 2014;52(1):24–8.
19. Prasad AS. Zinc is an antioxidant and anti-inflammatory agent: its role in human health. Front Nutr. 2014;1:14.
20. Nigam NK, Aravinda K, Dhillon M, Gupta S, Reddy S, Srinivas RM. Prevalence of oral submucous fibrosis among habitual gutkha and areca nut chewers in Moradabad district. J Oral BiolCraniofac Res. 2014;4:8–13.
21. Prabhu RV, Prabhu V, Chatra L, Shenai P, Suvarna N, Dandekeri S. Areca nut and its role in oral submucous fibrosis. J Clin Exp Dent. 2014;6:e569–75.
22. Ullah M, Cox S, Kelly E, Boadle R, Zoellner H. Arecoline is cytotoxic for human endothelial cells. J Oral Pathol Med. 2014;43:761–9.
23. Kiran G, Sekhar MM, Hunasgi S, Ahmed SA, Suri C, Krishna A. Plasma fibrinogen degradation products in betel nut chewers-with and without oral submucous fibrosis. J Oral Maxillofac Pathol. 2013;17(3):324–8.
24. Das RK, Anura A, Pal M, Bag S, Majumdar S, Barui A, et al. Epithelio-mesenchymal transitional attributes in oral sub-mucous fibrosis. Exp Mol Pathol. 2013;95:259–69.
25. Chang MC, Lin LD, Wu HL, Ho YS, Hsien HC, Wang TM, et al. Areca nut-induced buccal mucosa fibroblast contraction and its signaling: a potential role in oral submucous fibrosis—a precancer condition. Carcinogenesis. 2013;34:1096–104.
26. Chang JZ, Yang WH, Deng YT, Chen HM, Kuo MY. EGCG blocks TGFÎ²1-induced CCN2 by suppressing JNK and p38 in buccal fibroblasts. Clin Oral Investig. 2013;17(2):455–61.
27. Zhang SS, Li WH, Gao YJ, Liu ZW, Liu L, Tang JQ, et al. Betel-quid and oral submucous fibrosis: a cross-sectional study in Hunan Province, China. J Oral Pathol Med. 2012;41:748–54.
28. Lipson KE, Wong C, Teng Y, Spong S. CTGF is a central mediator of tissue remodeling and fibrosis and its inhibition can reverse the process of fibrosis. Fibrogenesis Tissue Repair. 2012;5:1–8.
29. Hu CW, Chao MR. Direct-acting DNA alkylating agents present in aqueous extracts of arecanut and its products. Chem Res Toxicol. 2012;25:2386–92.
30. Khan I, Kumar N, Pant I, Narra S, Kondaiah P. Activation of TGF-Î² pathway by areca nut constituents: a possible cause of oral submucous fibrosis. PLoS ONE. 2012;7(12):1–12.
31. Shafique K, Mirza SS, Vart P, Memon AR, Arain MI, Tareen MF, et al. Areca nut chewing and sys-

temic inflammation: evidence of a common pathway for systemic diseases. J Inflamm (Lond). 2012;9(1):1–8.
32. Tsai WC, Wu MT, Wang GJ, Lee KT, Lee CH, Lu YH, et al. Chewing areca nut increases the risk of coronary artery disease in Taiwanese men: a case-control study. BMC Public Health. 2012;12:1–7.
33. Javed F, Al-Hezaimi K, Warnakulasuriya S. Areca-nut chewing habit is a significant risk factor for metabolic syndrome: a systematic review. J Nutr Health Aging. 2012;16(5):445–8.
34. Reichart PA, Warnakulasuriya S. Oral lichenoid contact lesions induced by areca nut and betel quid chewing: a mini review. J Investig Clin Dent. 2012;3(3):163–6.
35. Tseng SK, Chang MC, Su CY, Chi LY, Chang JZ, Tsang WY, et al. Arecoline induced cell cycle arrest, apoptosis, and cytotoxicity to human endothelial cells. Clin Oral Investig. 2012;16(4):1267–73.
36. Pitiyage GN, Lim KP, Gemenitzidis E, Teh MT, Waseem A, Prime SS, et al. Increased secretion of tissue inhibitors of metalloproteinases 1 and 2 (TIMPs-1and -2) in fibroblasts are early indicators of oral sub-mucous fibrosis and ageing. J Oral Pathol Med. 2012;41(6):454–62.
37. Khan S, Chatra L, Prashanth SK, Veena KM, Rao PK. Pathogenesis oforal submucous fibrosis. J Cancer Res Ther. 2012;8(2):199–203.
38. Angadi PV, Rao SS. Areca nut in pathogenesis of oral submucous fibrosis: revisited. Oral Maxillofac Surg. 2011;15:1–9.
39. Al-Rmalli SW, Jenkins RO, Haris PI. Betel quid chewing elevated human exposure to arsenic, cadmium and lead. J Hazard Mater. 2011;190(1–3):69–74.
40. Moutasim Karwan A, Veronika J, Karen S, Daniel M, Weinreb Paul H, et al. Betel-derived alkaloid up-regulates keratinocyte alphavbeta6 integrin expression and promotes oral submucous fibrosis. J Pathol. 2011;223(3):366–77.
41. Campisi J, Andersen JK, Kapahi P, Melov S. Cellular senescence: a link between cancer and age-related degenerative disease? Semin Cancer Biol. 2011;21:354–9.
42. Pitiyage GN, Slijepcevic P, Gabrni A, Chianea YG, Lim KP, Prime SS, et al. Senescent mesenchymal cells accumulate in human fibrosis by a telomere—independent mechanism and ameliorate fibrosis through matrix metalloproteinases. J Pathol. 2011;223:604–17.
43. Anila K, Hallikeri K, Shubhada C, Naikmasur VG, Kulkarni RD. Comparative study of Candida in oral submucous fibrosis and healthy individuals. Rev OdontoCiencia. 2010;26(1):71–6.
44. Zhang LN, Yang YM, Xu ZR, Gui QF, Hu QQ. Chewing substances with or without tobacco and risk of cardiovascular disease in Asia: a meta-analysis. J Zhejiang Univ Sci B. 2010;11(9):681–9.
45. Raja KB, Hazarey VK, Peters TJ, Warnakulasuriya S. Effect of areca nut on salivary copper concentration in chronic chewers. Biometals. 2007;20:43–7.
46. Hazarey VK, Erlewad DM, Mundhe KA, Ughade SN. Oral submucous fibrosis: study of 1000 cases from central India. J Oral Pathol Med. 2007;36(1):12–7. ► https://doi.org/10.1111/j.1600-0714.2006.00485.x.
47. Luo CW, Roan CH, Liu CJ. Human papillomaviruses in oral squamous cell carcinoma and pre-cancerous lesions detected by PCR-based gene-chip array. Int J Oral Maxillofac Surg. 2007;36:153–8.
48. Rajalalitha P, Vali S. Molecular pathogenesis of oral submucous fibrosis—a collagen metabolic disorder. Oral Pathol Med. 2005;34:321–8.
49. Chang MC, Chiang CP, Lin CL, Lee JJ, Hahn LJ, Jeng JH. Cell-mediated immunity and head and neck cancer: with special emphasis on betel quid chewing habit. Oral Oncol. 2005;41:757–75.
50. IARC Working Group on the Evaluation of Carcinogenic Risks to Humans. Betel-quid and areca-nut chewing and some areca-nut derived nitrosamines. IARC Monogr Eval Carcinog Risks Hum No 85. Lyon: International Agency for Research on Cancer; 2004, pp:1–334.
51. Jacob BJ, Straif K, Thomas G, Ramadas K, Mathew B, Zhang ZF, et al. Betel quid without tobacco as a risk factor for oral precancers. Oral Oncol. 2004;40(7):697–704.
52. Nair U, Bartsch H, Nair J. Alert for an epidemic of oral cancer due to use of the betel quid substitutes gutkha and pan masala: a review of agents and causative mechanisms. Mutagenesis. 2004;19(4):251–62.
53. Jeng JH, Wang YJ, Chiang BL, Lee PH, Chan CP, Ho YS, et al. Roles of keratinocyte inflammation in oral cancer: regulating the prostaglandin E2, interleukin-6 and TNF-alpha production of oral epithelial cells by areca nut extract and arecoline. Carcinogenesis. 2003;24:1301–15.
54. Wollina U, Verma S, Parikh D, Parikh A. Oral and extraoral disease due to betel nut chewing. Hautarzt. 2002;53(12):795–7.
55. Trivedy CR, Warnakulasuriya KA, Peters TJ, Senkus R, Hazarey VK, Johnson NW. Raised tissue copper levels in oral submucous fibrosis. J Oral Pathol Med. 2000;29(6):241–8.
56. Kaur J, Rao M, Chakravarti N, Shukla NK, Mathur M, Sanwal BD, et al. Co-expression of colligin and

collagen in oral submucous fibrosis: plausible role in pathogenesis. Oral Oncol. 2001;37(3):282–7.
57. Trivedy C, Meghji S, Warnakulasuriya KA, Johnson NW, Harris M. Copper stimulates human oral fibroblasts in vitro: a role in the pathogenesis of oral submucous fibrosis. J Oral Pathol Med. 2001;30(8):465–70.
58. Tsai CC, Ma RH, Shieh TY. Deficiency in collagen and fibronectin phagocytosis by human buccal mucosa fibroblasts in vitro as a possible mechanism for oral submucous fibrosis. J Oral Pathol Med. 1999;28(2):59–63.
59. Jeng JH, Tsai CL, Hahn LJ, Yang PJ, Kuo YS, Kuo MY. Arecoline cytotoxicity on human oral mucosal fibroblasts related to cellular thiol and esterase activities. Food Chem Toxicol. 1999;37(7):751–6.
60. Norton SA. Betel: consumption and consequences. J Am Acad Dermatol. 1998;38(1):81–8.
61. Hazare VK, Goel RR, Gupta PC. Oral submucous fibrosis, areca nut and pan masala use: a case-control study. Natl Med J India. 1998;11(6):299.
62. Shah N, Sharma PP. Role of chewing and smoking habits in the etiology of oral submucous fibrosis (OSF): a case-control study. J Oral Pathol Med. 1998;27(10):475–9.
63. Murti PR, Bhonsle RB, Gupta PC, Daftary DK, Pindborg JJ, Mehta FS. Etiology of oral submucous fibrosis with special reference to the role of areca nut chewing. J Oral Pathol Med. 1995;24(4):145–52.

### 22.1.6 Histopathology and Special Stains in OSF, as OPMD

1. Abdul SN. Oral submucous fibrosis and its relation with stromal vascularity: a systematic review. Eur J Med Health Sci. 2020;2(2):1–3.
2. Kumar LB, Mathew P, Madhavan N, Siddique S, Kshetrimayum N, Iyer K. Evaluation of mast cells and burning sensation in various stages of Oral Submucous Fibrosis. J Oral Biol Craniofac Res. 2020;10(4):430–4.
3. Tamgadge S, Tamgadge A. Histopathology of oral submucous fibrosis in third dimension with an additional note on hypothesis of epithelial atrophy. J Microsc Ultrastruct. 2019;8(1):31–4.
4. Bhatt P, Manjunath M, Khakhla D, Gubrellay P, Bhargava R, Guruprasad L. Assessment and correlation between functional and histological staging of oral submucous fibrosis: a clinicohistopathologic study. Natl J Maxillofac Surg. 2019;10:27–32.
5. Gupta N, Rakshit A, Srivastava S, Suryawanshi H, Kumar P, Naik R. Comparative evaluation of micronuclei in exfoliated oral epithelial cells in potentially malignant disorders and malignant lesions using special stains. J Oral Maxillofac Pathol. 2019;23:157–62.
6. Pammar C, Nayak RS, Kotrashetti VS, Hosmani J. Comparison of microvessel density using CD34 and CD105 in oral submucous fibrosis and its correlation with clinicopathological features: an immunohistochemical study. J Cancer Res. 2018;14:983–8.
7. Rathod YG, Kulkarni SP, Khairnar MR, Joshi PN, Patle BK, Pagare JS. Estimation of serum beta-carotene level in patients suffering from oral submucous fibrosis. J Exp Oncol. 2018;2:267–71.
8. Tekade SA, Chaudhary MS, Tekade SS, Sarode SC, Wanjari SP, Gadbail AR, et al. Early stage oral submucous fibrosis is characterized by increased vascularity as opposed to advanced stages. J Clin Diagn Res. 2017;11(5):ZC92–6.
9. Reshma V, Varsha BK, Rakesh P, Radhika MB, Soumya M, D'Mello S. Aggrandizing oral submucous fibrosis grading using an adjunct special stain: a pilot study. J Oral Maxillofac Pathol. 2016;20(1):36–46.
10. Radhika T, Sekaran P, Narasimhan M. Qualitative analysis of collagen fibers in oral submucous fibrosis using picrosirius red stain and polarising microscope. J Clin Diagn Res. 2016;10(2):ZC04–ZC7.
11. Ray JG, Ranganathan K, Chattopadhyay A. Malignant transformation of oral submucous fibrosis: overview of histopathological aspects. Oral Surg Oral Med Oral Pathol Oral Radiol. 2016;122(2):200–9.
12. Chawla H, Urs AB, Augustine J, Kumar P. Characterization of muscle alteration in oral submucous fibrosis-seeking new evidence. Med Oral Patol Oral Cir Bucal. 2015;20(6):670–7.
13. Murgod VV, Kale AD, Angadi PV, Hallikerimath S. Morphometric analysis of the mucosal vasculature in oral submucous fibrosis and its comparison with oral squamous cell carcinoma. J Oral Sci. 2014;56:173–8.
14. Jayasooriya PR, Nadeeka Jayasinghe KA, Tilakaratne WM. Relationship between thickness of fibrosis and epithelial dysplasia in oral submucous fibrosis. J Investig Clin Dent. 2011;2:171–5.
15. Pandya S, Chaudhary AK, Singh M, Singh M, Mehrotra R. Correlation of histopathological diagnosis with habits and clinical findings in oral submucous fibrosis. Head Neck Oncol. 2009;1:1–10.
16. Rajendran R, Paul S, Mathews PP, Raghul J, Mohanty M. Characterization and quantification of mucosal vasculature in oral submucous fibrosis. Ind J Dent Res. 2005;16:83–91.
17. Haque MF, Harris M, Meghji S, Speight PM. An immunohistochemical study of oral submucous fibrosis. J Oral Pathol Med. 1997;26(2):75–82.

### 22.1.7 Molecular Biology and Genetics of OSF, and Malignant Transformation


1. James A, Jayan L, Ramadoss R, Arunachalam P. Leaving no stone unturned: role of profibrotic genes in oral submucous fibrosis - a systematic review. J Oral Maxillofac Pathol. 2022;26(2):228–35.
2. Singh AG, Roy S, Oza S, Singhavi H, Chatterjee K, Chaturvedi P. A contemporary narrative review to guide molecular epidemiology of oral submucous fibrosis. Int J Mol Epidemiol Genet. 2021;12(4):61–70.
3. Jian X, Jian Y, Wu X, Guo F, Hu Y, Gao X, Jiang C, Li N, Wu Y, Liu D. Oral submucous fibrosis transforming into squamous cell carcinoma: a prospective study over 31 years in mainland China. Clin Oral Investig. 2021;25(4):2249–56.
4. Kundu P, Pant JR, Rao SG, Kondaiah P. Genome-wide DNA methylation changes in oral submucous fibrosis. Oral Dis. 2021;00:1–10.
5. Zhang L, Tan J, Liu YP, Liu X, Luo M. Curcumin relieves the arecoline-induced fibrosis of oral mucosal fibroblasts via inhibiting HIF-1α/TGF-β/CTGF signaling pathway: an in vitro study. Toxicol Res (Camb). 2021;10(3):631–8.
6. Gupta SR, Sharma A, Gupta N, Mani K. Single nucleotide polymorphisms and serologic levels of hypoxia-inducible factor1 α and vascular endothelial growth factor are associated with increased risk of oral submucous fibrosis in gutka users among a North Indian population. Oral Surg Oral Med Oral Pathol Oral Radiol. 2020;130(5):557–64.
7. Fang CY, Yu CC, Liao YW, Hsieh PL, Ohiro Y, Chu PM, et al. miR-10b regulated by Twist maintains myofibroblasts activities in oral submucous fibrosis. J Formos Med Assoc. 2020;119:1167–73.
8. Li J, Yao M, Zhu X, Li Q, He J, Chen L, et al. YAP-Induced endothelial-mesenchymal transition in oral submucous fibrosis. J Dent Res. 2019;98:920–9.
9. Tu HF, Chen MY, Lai JC, Chen YL, Wong YW, Yang CC, et al. Arecoline-regulated ataxia telangiectasia mutated expression level in oral cancer progression. Head Neck. 2019;41:2525–37.
10. Yuan Y, Li N, Zeng L, Shen Z, Jiang C. Pathogenesis investigation of miR-199-5p in oral submucous fibrosis based on bioinformatics analysis. Oral Dis. 2019;25:456–65.
11. Liu CM, Liao YW, Hsieh PL, Yu CH, Chueh PJ, Lin T, et al. miR-1246 as a therapeutic target in oral submucosa fibrosis pathogenesis. J Formos Med Assoc. 2019;118:1093–8.
12. Liao YW, Yu CC, Hsieh PL, Chang YC. miR-200b ameliorates myofibroblast transdifferentiation in precancerous oral submucous fibrosis through targeting ZEB2. J Cell Mol Med. 2018;22:4130–8.
13. Lu MY, Yu CC, Chen PY, Hsieh PL, Peng CY, Liao YW, et al. miR-200c inhibits the arecoline-associated myofibroblastictransdifferentiation in buccal mucosal fibroblasts. J Med Assoc. 2018;117:791–7.
14. Lin CY, Liao YW, Hsieh PL, Lu MY, Peng CY, Chu PM, et al. LncRNA GAS5-AS1 inhibits myofibroblasts activities in oral submucous fibrosis. J Formos Med Assoc. 2018;117:727–33.
15. Zade PR, Gosavi SR, Hazarey VK, Ganvir SM. Matrix metalloproteinases-3 gene-promoter polymorphism as a risk factor in oral submucous fibrosis in an Indian population: a pilot study. J Investig Clin Dent. 2017;8(3):1–6.
16. Bazarsad S, Zhang X, Kim KY, Illeperuma R, Jayasinghe RD, Tilakaratne WM, et al. Identification of a combined biomarker for malignant transformation in oral submucous fibrosis. J Oral Pathol Med. 2017;46:431–8.
17. Tang D, Tao D, Fang Y, Deng C, Xu Q, Zhou J. TNF-Alpha promotes invasion and metastasis via NF-Kappa B pathway in oral squamous cell carcinoma. Med Sci Monit Basic Res. 2017;23:141–9.
18. Hou X, Liu R, Huang C, Jiang L, Zhou Y, Chen Q. Cyclophilin A was revealed as a candidate marker for human oral submucous fibrosis by proteomic analysis. Cancer Biomark. 2017;20:345–56.
19. Jayasinghe RD, Manoja KGD, Gunasinghe MS, Gurusinghe SKB, Sitheeque MAM, Hettiarachchi RM, Kularathne MSM. An analysis of rate and factors affecting malignant transformation of oral submucous fibrosis in patients attending the Oral Medicine Clinic, Dental Hospital Peradeniya, Sri Lanka - a retrospective study. SLJM. 2016;24
20. Dalmia A, Hazarey V, Talkal R, Ganvir S, Purohit HJ, Gupta S, Pimpale A. Role of Hypoxia Inducible Factor-1α messenger RNA expression in malignant transformation of oral submucous fibrosis: a RT-PCR study. Transl Res Oral Oncol. 2016;1:1–5.
21. Chattopadhyay A, Ray JG. Molecular pathology of malignant transformation of oral submucous fibrosis. J Environ Pathol Toxicol Oncol. 2016;35(3):193–205.
22. Kallalli BN, Rawson K, Singh AM, Awati MA, Shivhare P. Lactate dehydrogenase as a biomarker in oral cancer and oral submucous fibrosis. J Oral Pathol Med. 2016;45:687–90.
23. Languino LR, Singh A, Prisco M, Inman GJ, Luginbuhi A, Curry JM, et al. Exosome-mediated transfer from the tumor microenvironment increases

TGFβ signaling in squamous cell carcinoma. Am J Transl Res. 2016;15;8(5):2432-2437
24. Kaliyaperumal S, Sankarapandian S. Evaluation of p16 hypermethylation in oral submucous fibrosis: a quantitative and comparative analysis in buccal cells and saliva using real-time methylation-specific polymerase chain reaction. South Asian J Cancer. 2016;5:73–9.
25. Wang TH, Hsia SM, Shieh TM. Lysyl oxidase and the tumor microenvironment. Int J Mol Sci. 2016;18:1–12.
26. Shridhar K, Walia GK, Aggarwal A, Gulati S, Geetha AV, Prabhakaran D, et al. DNA methylation markers for oral pre-cancer progression: a critical review. Oral Oncol. 2016;53:1–9.
27. Chen J, Liu BJ, Du C, Cao Q, Li M, Feng H. Target regulation of micro-RNA-203 to the expression of collagen type alpha 4 and its role in oral submucous fibrosis. Chin J Stomatol. 2016;51:526–31.
28. Yuan Y, Hou X, Feng H, Liu R, Xu H, Gong W, et al. Proteomic identification of cyclophilin A as a potential biomarker and therapeutic target in oral submucous fibrosis. Oncotarget. 2016;7:60348–65.
29. Xie X, Jiang Y, Yuan Y, Wang P, Li X, Chen F, et al. MALDI imaging reveals NCOA7 as a potential biomarker in oral squamous cell carcinoma arising from oral submucous fibrosis. Oncotarget. 2016;7:59987–60004.
30. Kallalli BN, Rawson K, Singh AM, Awati MA, Shivhare P. Lactate dehydrogenase as a biomarker in oral cancer and oral submucous fibrosis. J Oral Pathol Med. 2016;45:687–90.
31. Davalli P, Mitic T, Caporali A, Lauriola A, D'Arca D. ROS, cell senescence, and novel molecular mechanisms in aging and age-related diseases. Oxid MedCell Longev 2016; 2016.1-19.
32. Bautista-Nino PK, Portilla-Fernandez E, Vaughan DE, Danser AH, Roks AJ. DNA damage: a main determinant of vascular aging. Int J Mol Sci. 2016;17(5):1–26.
33. Yuan Y, Hou X, Feng H, Liu R, Xu H, Gong W, et al. Proteomic identification of cyclophilin A as a potential biomarker and therapeutic target in oral submucous fibrosis. Oncotarget. 2016;7:60348–65.
34. Anura A, Conjeti S, Das RK, Pal M, Paul RR, Bag S, et al. Computer-aided molecular pathology interpretation in exploring prospective markers for oral sub-mucous fibrosis progression. Head Neck. 2016;38(5):653–69.
35. Zhou S, Chen L, Mashrah M, Zhu Y, Liu J, Yang X, et al. Deregulation of secreted frizzled-related proteins is associated with aberrant beta-catenin activation in the carcinogenesis of oral submucous fibrosis. Onco Targets. 2015;8:2923–31.
36. Tsai CH, Lee SS, Chang YC. Hypoxic regulation of plasminogen activator inhibitor-1 expression in human buccal mucosa fibroblasts stimulated with arecoline. J Oral Pathol Med. 2015;44:669–73.
37. Gupta S, Ghosh S, Gupta S, Sakhuja P. Effect of curcumin on the expression of p53, transforming growth factor-β, and inducible nitric oxide synthase in oral submucous fibrosis: a pilot study. J Investig Clin Dent. 2017;8(4):1–6.
38. Chang YC, Tsai CH, Lai YL, Yu CC, Chi WY, Li JJ, et al. Arecolineinduced myofibroblast transdifferentiation from human buccal mucosal fibroblasts is mediated by ZEB 1. J Cell Mol Med. 2014;18(4):698–708.
39. Udupa R, Hallikeri K, Trivedi DJ. The comet assay a method to measure DNA damage in oral submucous fibrosis patients: a case-control study. Clin Cancer Investig J. 2014;3:299–304.
40. Chaudhuri SR, Mukherjee S, Paul RR, Haldar A, Chaudhuri K. CYP1AI and CYP2E1 gene polymorphisms may increase susceptibility to Oral Submucous Fibrosis among betel quid chewers of Eastern India. Gene. 2013;513:268–71.
41. Leight JL, Wozniak MA, Chen S, Lynch ML, Chen CS. Matrix rigidity regulates a switch between TGF-beta1-induced apoptosis and epithelial-mesenchymal transition. Mol Biol Cell. 2012;23:781–91.
42. Ji WT, Yang SR, Chen JY, Chen YP, Lee YR, Chiang MK, et al. Arecoline downregulates levels of p21 and p27 through the reactive oxygen species/mTOR complex 1 pathway and may contribute to oral squamous cell carcinoma. Cancer Sci. 2012;103(7):1221–9.
43. Ghosh T, Gupta S, Bajpai P, Agarwal D, Agarwal M, Gupta OP, et al. Association of CYP1A1, GSTM1, and GSTT1 gene polymorphism with risk of oral submucous fibrosis in a section of North Indian population. Mol Biol Rep2012; 39: 9383-9389.
44. Xie H, Liu J, Ling TY. Expression of cytochrome P450 related genes in oral submucous fibrosis tissue. Zhonghua Kou Qiang Yi Xue Za Zhi. 2012;47:743–7.
45. Mukherjee S, Bhowmik AD, Roychoudhury P, Mukhopadhyay K, Ray JG, Chaudhuri K. Association of XRCC1, XRCC3, and NAT2 polymorphisms with the risk of oral submucous fibrosis among eastern Indian population. J Oral Pathol Med. 2012;41:292–302.
46. Hu CW, Chao MR. Direct-acting DNA alkylating agents present in aqueous extracts of arecanut and its products. Chem Res Toxicol. 2012;25:2386–92.
47. Xu C, Zhao J, Loo WT, Hao L, Wang M, Cheung MNB, et al. Correlation of epigenetic change and

identification of risk factors for oral submucous fibrosis. Int J Biol Markers. 2012;27:e314–21.
48. Jeyapradha D, Saraswathi T, Ranganathan K, Wilson K. Comparison of the frequency of sister chromatid exchange in pan chewers and oral submucous fibrosis patients. J Oral MaxillofacPathol. 2011;15:278–82.
49. Joshi MS, Verma Y, Gautam AK, Parmar G, Lakkad BC, Kumar S. Cytogenetic alterations in buccal mucosa cells of chewers of areca nut and tobacco. Arch Oral Biol. 2011;56(1):63–7.
50. Pitiyage GN, Slijepcevic P, Gabrni A, Chianea YG, Lim KP, Prime SS, et al. Senescent mesenchymal cells accumulate in human fibrosis by a telomere—independent mechanism and ameliorate fibrosis through matrix metalloproteinases. J Pathol. 2011;223:604–17.
51. Li N, Hu Q, Jiang C, Hu Y, Yuan Y, Jian X, et al. Novel genetic biomarkers for susceptibility to oral submucous fibrosis: cytochrome P450 3A. Med Hypotheses. 2011;77:834–6.
52. Choudhury Y, Sharan RN. Altered BRCA1 and BRCA2 responses and mutation of BRCA1 gene in mice exposed chronically and transgenerationallyto aqueous extract of betel nut (AEBN). Environ Toxicol Pharmacol. 2011;31:57–69.
53. Lee IT, Lin CC, Wu YC, Yang CM. TNF-alpha induces matrix metalloproteinase-9 expression in A549 cells: role of TNFR1/TRAF2/PKCalpha-dependent signaling pathways. J Cell Physiol. 2010;224:454–64.
54. Yin X, Wen C, Han Y, Gao Y, Tang Z. Expression of FHIT and MDM2 in oral submucous fibrosis and canceration tissues. Zhong Nan Da XueXue Bao Yi Xue Ban. 2010;35:572–5.
55. Rajendran R, Harish RK, Anil S, Vidyadharan R, Banerjee M. Transforming growth factor-β-1 polymorphisms are infrequent but exist at selected loci in oral submucous fibrosis. Indian J Dent Res. 2010;21:413–9.
56. Chaudhary AK, Singh M, Bharti AC, Singh M, Shukla S, Singh AK, et al. Synergistic effect of stromelysin-1 (matrix metalloproteinase-3) promoter (-1171 5A->6A) polymorphism in oral submucous fibrosis and head and neck lesions. BMC Cancer. 2010;10:1–9. ► https://doi.org/10.1186/1471-2407-10-369.
57. Shieh TM, Tu HF, Ku TH, Chang SS, Chang KW, Liu CJ. Association between lysyl oxidase polymorphisms and oral submucous fibrosis in older male areca chewers. J Oral Pathol Med. 2009;38: 109–13.
58. Li N, Jian XC, Xu CJ. Expression of loricrin and cytochrome P450 3A5 in oral submucous fibrosis and their significance. Hua Xi Kou Qiang Yi Xue Za Zhi. 2009;27:29–33.
59. Teh MT, Tilakaratne WM, Chaplin T, Young BD, Ariyawardana A, Pitiyage G, et al. Fingerprinting genomic instability in oral submucous fibrosis. J Oral Pathol Med. 2008;37:430–6.
60. Zhou S, Li L, Jian X, Ou X, Jiang H, Yao Z, et al. The phosphorylation of survivin Thr34 by p34cdc2 incarcinogenesis of oral submucous fibrosis. Oncol Rep. 2008;20:1085–91.
61. Lin YC, Huang HI, Wang LH, Tsai CC, Lung O, Dai CY, et al. Polymorphisms of COX-2 -765G>C and p53 codon 72 and risks of oral squamous cell carcinoma in a Taiwan population. Oral Oncol. 2008;44:798–804.
62. Lalli A, Tilakaratne WM, Ariyawardana A, FitchettC LIM, Hagi-Pavli E, et al. An altered keratinocyte phenotype in oral submucous fibrosis: correlation of keratin K17 expression with disease severity. J Oral Pathol Med. 2008;37:211–20.
63. Hu Y, Jian X, Peng J, Jiang X, Li N, Zhou S. Gene expression profiling of oral submucous fibrosis using oligonucleotide microarray. Oncol Rep. 2008;20(2):287–94.
64. Shieh TM, Lin SC, Liu J, Chang SS, Ku TH, Chang KW. Association of expression aberrances and genetic polymorphisms of lysyl oxidase with areca-associated oral tumorigenesis. Clin Cancer Res. 2007;13:4378–85.
65. Shieh DH, Chiang LC, Shieh TY. Augmented mRNA expression of tissue inhibitor of metalloproteinase-1in buccal mucosal fibroblasts by arecoline and safrole as a possible pathogenesis for oral submucous fibrosis. Oral Oncol. 2003;39:728–35.
66. Chiu CJ, Chiang CP, Chang ML, Chen HM, Hahn LJ, Hsieh LL, et al. Association between genetic polymorphism of tumor necrosis factor-alpha and risk of oral submucous fibrosis, a pre-cancerous condition of oral cancer. J Dent Res. 2001;80:2055–9.
67. Chang MC, Ho YS, Lee PH, Chan CP, Lee JJ, Hahn LJ, et al. Areca nut extract and arecoline induced the cell cycle arrest but not apoptosis of cultured oral KB epithelial cells: association of glutathione, reactive oxygen species and mitochondrial membrane potential. Carcinogenesis. 2001;22(9):1527–35.
68. Hsieh LL, Wang PF, Chen IH, Liao CT, Wang HM, Chen MC, et al. Characteristics of mutations in the p53 gene in oral squamous cell carcinoma associated with betel quid chewing and cigarette smoking in Taiwanese. Carcinogenesis. 2001;22(9):1497–503.
69. Jeng JH, Ho YS, Chan CP, Wang YJ, Hahn LJ, Lei D, et al. Areca nut extract up-regulates prostaglan-

din production, cyclooxygenase-2 mRNA and protein expression of human oral keratinocytes. Carcinogenesis. 2000;21:1365–70.

### 22.1.8 Immunohistochemistry in OSF

1. Kholakiya Y, Jose A, Rawat A, Nagori S.A, Jacob S, Roychoudhury A. Surgical management of oral submucous fibrosis with "Seagull-nasolabial flap" combined with short-term oral pentoxifylline for preventing relapse. J Stomatol Oral Maxillofac Surg 2020;121(5):512-516.
2. Singh I, Juneja S, Tandon A, Jain A, Shetty DC, Sethi A. Immunoexpression of alpha smooth muscle actin correlates with serum transforming growth factor-β1 levels in oral submucous fibrosis. J Investig Clin Dent 2019;10(4):1-8.
3. Lin CY, Hsieh PL, Liao YW, Peng CY, Yu CC, Lu MY. Arctigenin reduces myofibroblast activities in Oral Submucous Fibrosis by LINC00974 inhibition. Int J Mol Sci 2019; 20:1328-1339.
4. Fang CY, Yu CC, Liao YW, Hsieh PL, Lu MY, Lin KC et al. LncRNA LINC00974 activates TGF-beta/Smadsignaling to promote oral fibrogenesis. J Oral Pathol Med 2019; 48: 151–158.
5. Raffat MA, Hadi NI, Hosein M, Zubairi AM, Ikram S, Akram Z. Differential expression of salivary S100A7 in oral submucous fibrosis. Saudi Dent J 2019; 31:39–44.
6. Gadbail AR, Chaudhary M, Sarode SC, Gondivkar S, Tekade SA, Zade P, et al. Ki67, CD105, and α-SMA expression supports the transformation relevant dysplastic features in the atrophic epithelium of oral submucous fibrosis. PLoS One 2018;13(7):1-12.
7. Malik SN, Vyas Z, KotariH, Prabhu VD, Alam MK, Kumar BSK. Association of Histological Grading of Oral Submucous Fibrosis to Cytokeratin 19 Immunohistochemical Staining. World J Dent 2018; 9(2):117-121.
8. Gottipamula S, Sundarrajan S, Moorthy A, Padmanabhan S, Sridhar KN. Buccal mucosal epithelial cells downregulate CTGF expression in buccal submucosal fibrosis fibroblasts. J Maxillofac Oral Surg 2018;17(2):254-259.
9. Shinde AV, Humeres C, Frangogiannis NG. The role of alpha-smooth muscle actin in fibroblast-mediated matrix contraction and remodeling. Biochim Biophys Acta Mol Basis Dis 2017;1863(1):298–309.
10. Daga D, Singh RK, Pal US, Gurung T, Gangwar S. Efficacy of oral colchicine with intralesional hyaluronidase or triamcinolone acetonide in the grade II oral submucous fibrosis. Natl J MaxillofacSurg 2017;8(1):50-54.
11. Keshav R, Narayanappa U. Expression of Proliferating Cell Nuclear Antigen (PCNA) in Oral Submucous Fibrosis: an immunohistochemical study. J Clin Diagn Res 2015;9: ZC20–ZC23.
12. Kaur J, Matta A,Kak I, Srivastava G,Assi J, Leong I, et al. S100A7 overexpression is a predictive marker for high risk of malignant transformation in oral dysplasia. Int J Cancer 2014;134: 1379–1388.
13. Krishnamurthy V.K.P.S.R. Transforming growth factor beta 1 in oral submucous fibrosis: an immunohistochemical study—understanding the pathogenesis. J Dent Res Rev 2014;1:75 -80.
14. Pandiar D, Shameena P. Immunohistochemical expression of CD34 and basic fibroblast growth factor(bFGF) in oral submucous fibrosis. J Oral Maxillofac Pathol 2014; 18:155–161.
15. Varun B.R, Ranganathan K, Rao UK, Joshua E. Immunohistochemical detection of p53 and p63 in oral squamous cell carcinoma, oral leukoplakia, and oral submucous fibrosis. J InvestigClinl Dent 2014; 5:214–219.
16. Anura A, Das RK, Pal M, Paul RR, Ray AK, Chatterjee J. Correlated analysis of semiquantitative immunohistochemical features of E-cadherin, VEGF and CD105 in assessing malignant potentiality of oral submucous fibrosis. Pathol Res Pract 2014; 210:1054-1063.
17. Shrestha A, Carnelio S. Evaluation of matrix metalloproteinases-2 (MMP-2) and tissue inhibitors of metalloproteinases-2 (TIMP-2) in oral submucous fibrosis and their correlation with disease severity. Kathmandu Univ Med J (Kumj) 2013; 11:274–281.
18. Bag S, Conjeti S, Das RK, Pal M, Anura A, Paul RR, et al. Computational analysis of p63(+) nuclei distribution pattern by graph theoretic approach in an oral pre-cancer (sub-mucous fibrosis). J Pathol Inform 2013; 4:1-17.
19. Kale AD, Mane DR, Shukla D. Expression of transforming growth factor β and its correlation with lipodystrophy in oral submucous fibrosis: an immunohistochemical study. Med Oral Patol Oral Cir Bucal 2013;18(1):1-7.
20. Angadi PV, Krishnapillai R. Evaluation of PTEN immunoexpression in oral submucous fibrosis: role in pathogenesis and malignant transformation. Head Neck Pathol 2012; 6:314-321.
21. Sabarinath B, Sriram G, Saraswathi TR, Sivapathasundharam B. Immunohistochemical evaluation of mast cells and vascular endothelial proliferation in oral submucous fibrosis. Indian J Dent Res 2011;22:116-121.

22. Ranganathan K and Kavitha R. Proliferation and apoptosis markers in oral submucous fibrosis. J Oral MaxillofacPathol 2011;15(2):148-53.
23. Khan I, Agarwal P, Thangjam GS, Radhesh R, Rao SG, Kondaiah P. Role of TGF-Î2 and BMP7 in the pathogenesis of oral submucous fibrosis. Growth Factors 2011;29(4):119-27.
24. Desai RS, Mamatha GS, Khatri MJ, Shetty SJ. Immunohistochemical expression of CD34 for characterization and quantification of mucosal vasculature and its probable role in malignant transformation of atrophic epithelium in oral submucous fibrosis. Oral Oncol 2010; 46:553–558.
25. Illeperuma RP, Ryu MH, Kim KY, Tilakaratne WM, Kim J. Relationship of fibrosis and the expression of TGF-β1, MMP-1, and TIMP-1 with epithelial dysplasia in oral submucous fibrosis. Oral Med Pathol 2010; 15: 21-28.
26. Mishra G, Ranganathan K. Matrix metalloproteinase-1 expression inoral submucous fibrosis: an immunohistochemical study. Indian J Dent Res 2010;21(3):320-325.
27. Rajendran R, Rajeesh MP, Shaikh S, Pillai SMR. Expression of matrix metalloproteinases (MMP-1, MMP-2 and MMP-9) and their inhibitors (TIMP-1 and TIMP-2) in oral submucous fibrosis. Indian J Dent Res 2006; 17:161–166.
28. Utsunomiya H, Tilakaratne WM, Oshiro K, Maruyama S, Suzuki M, Ida-Yonemochi H, et al. Extracellular matrix remodeling in oral submucous fibrosis: its stagespecific modes revealed by immunohistochemistry and in situ hybridization. J Oral Pathol Med 2005;34(8):498-507.
29. Tsai CH, Yang SF, Chen YJ, Chou MY, Chang YC. Raised keratinocyte growth factor-1 expression in oral submucous fibrosis in vivo and upregulated by arecoline in human buccal mucosal fibroblasts in vitro. J Oral Pathol Med 2005;34(2):100–105.
30. Srinivasan M, Jewell SD. Evaluation of TGF-alpha and EGFR expression in oral leukoplakia and oral submucous fibrosis by quantitative immunohistochemistry. Oncology 2001;61(4):284–292.
31. Haque MF, Harris M, Meghji S, Barrett AW. Immunolocalization of cytokines and growth factors in oral submucous fibrosis. Cytokine 1998; 10:713–719.
32. Haque MF, Harris M, Meghji S, Speight PM. An immunohistochemical study of oral submucous fibrosis. J Oral Pathol Med. 1997;26(2):75-82
33. Reichart PA, Van Wyk CW, Becker J, Schuppan D. Distribution of procollagen type III, collagen type VI and tenascin in oral submucous fibrosis (OSF). J Oral Pathol Med 1994;23(9):394-8.

### 22.1.9 Diagnostic, Serology and Prognostic evaluation

1. Hande A, Bansod AV, Agrawal AG, Gadbail A, Reche AM. Estimation of serum copper and zinc in patients of oral submucous fibrosis in rural population. World J Dent 2020;11(6):478–481.
2. Mukul SK, Kumar S, Pandey S, Mokhtar EA, Kumar A. Ultrasound elastography as a potential diagnostic aid in oral submucous fibrosis. Natl J Maxillofac Surg 2019;10(2):129-133.
3. Alexander AJ, Ramani P, Sherlin HJ, Gheena S. Quantitative analysis of copper levels in areca nut plantation area—a role in increasing prevalence of oral submucous fibrosis: an in vitro study. Indian J Dent Res 2019;30(2):261-266.
4. Sachdev PK, Freeland-Graves J, Beretvas SN, Sanjeevi N. Zinc, copper, and iron in oral submucous fibrosis: a meta-analysis. Int J Dent 2018;2018:1-15.
5. Bag S, Dutta D, Chaudhary A, Sing BC, Pal M, Ray AK, et al. Identification of alpha-enolase as a prognostic and diagnostic precancer biomarker in oral submucous fibrosis. J Clin Pathol 2018;71:228–238.
6. Mishra S, Kritika C, Bajoria AA, Choudhury P, Sahoo SK, Sangamesh NC. Estimation of salivary and serum lactate dehydrogenase in oral submucous fibrosis. J Int Soc Prev Community Dent 2018; 8:289–295.
7. Rathod YG, Kulkarni SP, Khairnar MR, Joshi PN, Patle BK, Pagare JS. Estimation of serum beta-carotene level in patients suffering from oral submucous fibrosis. J Exp Oncol 2018; 2:267–271.
8. Jani YV, Chaudhary AR, Dudhia BB, Bhatia PV, Soni NC, Patel PS. Evaluation of role of trace elements in oral submucous fibrosis patients: a study on Gujarati population. J Oral MaxillofacPathol 2017;21(3):455.
9. Thakur M, Guttikonda VR. Estimation of hemoglobin, serum iron, total iron-binding capacity and serum ferritin levels in oral submucous fibrosis: a clinicopathological study. J Oral MaxillofacPathol 2017;21(1):30-35.
10. More CB, Shah PH, Venkatesh R. Estimation of Serum protein in oral potentially malignant disorders and oral malignancy—a cross-sectional study. J Clin Diagn Res 2017;11: ZC17–ZC19.
11. Prajapati KJ, Chawda JG. Estimation of major immunoglobulins in smokers and gutkha chewers. J Oral MaxillofacPathol 2016;20(2):219-23.
12. Kandasamy M, Jaisanghar N, Austin RD, Srivastava KC, Anusuya GS, Anisa N. Comparative evaluation

of serum and salivary immunoglobulin G and A levels with total serum protein in oral submucous fibrosis patients: a case control study. J Pharm Bioallied Sci 2016;8(Suppl. 1):S126-S132.
13. Paulose S, Rangdhol V, Ramesh R, Jeelani SA, Brooklyin S. Estimation of serum malondialdehyde and assessment of DNA damage using comet assay in patients with oral submucous fibrosis. J Investig Clin Dent 2016; 7:286–293.
14. Kaur J, Politis C, Jacobs R. Salivary 8-hydroxy-2-deoxyguanosine, malondialdehyde, vitamin C, and vitamin E in oral pre-cancer and cancer: diagnostic value and free radical mechanism of action. Clin Oral Investig 2016;20:315–319.
15. Balakrishnan C, Aswath N. Estimation of serum, salivary immunoglobulin G, immunoglobulin A levels and total protein, hemoglobin in smokeless tobacco chewers and oral submucous fibrosis patients. Contemp Clin Dent 2015;6(Suppl 1):S157-62.
16. Sivaramakrishnan M, Sivapathasundharam B, Jananni M. Evaluation of lactate dehydrogenase enzyme activity in saliva and serum of oral submucous fibrosis patients. J Oral Pathol Med 2015;44(6):449-52.
17. Mohammed F, Manohar V, Jose M, Thapasum AF, Mohamed S, Shamaz BH, et al. Estimation of copper in saliva and areca nut products and its correlation with histological grades of oral submucous fibrosis. J Oral Pathol Med 2015; 44:208–213.
18. Yadav A, Kumar L, Misra N, Deepak U, Shiv Kumar GC. Estimation of serum zinc, copper, and iron in the patients of oral submucous fibrosis. Natl J Maxillofac Surg 2015;6:190–193.
19. Wang YP, Wu YC, Cheng SJ, Chen HM, Sun A, Chang JY. High frequencies of vitamin B12 and folic acid deficiencies and gastric parietal cell antibody positivity in oral submucous fibrosis patients. J Formos. Med Assoc 2015;114(9):813-819.
20. Guruprasad R, Nair PP, Singh M, Singh M, Singh M, Jain A. Serum vitamin C and iron levels in oral submucous fibrosis. Indian J Dent 2014; 5:81–85.
21. Hosthor SS, Mahesh P, Priya SA, Sharada P, Jyotsna M, Chitra S. Quantitative analysis of serum levels of trace elements in patients with oral submucous fibrosis and oral squamous cell carcinoma: a randomized cross-sectional study. J Oral Maxillofac Pathol 2014;18:46–51.
22. Divya VC, Sathasivasubramanian S. Estimation of serum and salivary immunoglobulin G and immunoglobulin A in oral pre-cancer: a study in oral submucous fibrosis and oral lichen planus. J Nat Sci Biol Med 2014;5:90–94.
23. Gharat L, Rathod GP, Kandalgaonkar S. Quantitative estimation of serum fibrinogen degradation product levels in oral premalignant and malignant lesions. J Int Oral Health 2013;5(5): 65–72.
24. Khanna S, Udas AC, Kumar GK, Suvarna S, Karjodkar FR. Trace elements (copper, zinc, selenium and molybdenum) as markers in oral sub mucous fibrosis and oral squamous cell carcinoma. J Trace Elem Med Biol 2013; 27:307-311.
25. Gurudath S, Ganapathy KS, Pai A, Ballal S, Asha ML. Estimation of superoxide dismutase and glutathione peroxidase in oral submucous fibrosis, oral leukoplakia and oral cancer–a comparative study. Asian Pac J Cancer Prev 2012;13:4409–4412.
26. Ayinampudi BK, Narsimhan M. Salivary copper and zinc levels in oral pre-malignant and malignant lesions. J Oral MaxillofacPathol 2012; 16:178-182.
27. Shetty SR, Babu SG, Kumari S, Rao V, Vijay R, Karikal A. Malondialdehyde levels in oral sub mucous fibrosis: a clinicopathological and biochemical study. N Am J Med Sci 2012;4(3):125-128.
28. Tadakamadla J, Kumar S, Mamatha GP. Evaluation of serum copper and iron levels among oral submucous fibrosis patients. Med Oral Patol Oral Cir Bucal. 2011;16(7):1-4.
29. Lee CK, Tsai MT, Lee HC, Chen HM, Chiang CP, Wang YM, et al. Diagnosis of oral submucous fibrosis with optical coherence tomography. J Biomed Opt 2009;14(5):1-7.
30. Rajendran R, Varkey S. Inducible nitric oxide synthase expression is upregulated in oral submucous fibrosis. Indian J Dent Res 2007; 18:94-100.
31. Chung-Hung T, Shun-Fa Y, Yu-Chao C. The upregulation of cystatin C in oral submucous fibrosis. Oral Oncol 2007;43(7):680–685.
32. Khanna SS, Karjodkar FR. Circulating immune complexes and trace elements (copper, iron and selenium) as markers in oral precancer and cancer: a randomised, controlled clinical trial. Head Face Med 2006; 2:33;1-10.
33. Pillai KG, Burde KN. Increased copper level in oral mucosal tissue of patients with submucous fibrosis and who chew areca nut products. West Indian Med J 2005;54(4):270-271.
34. Chiang CP, Hsieh RP, Chen TH, Chang YF, Liu BY, Wang JT et al. High incidence of autoantibodies in Taiwanese patients with oral submucous fibrosis. J Oral Pathol Med 2002;31(7):402-9.
35. Trivedy CR, Warnakulasuriya KA, Peters TJ, Senkus R, Hazarey VK, Johnson NW. Raised tissue copper levels in oral submucous fibrosis. J Oral Pathol Med 2000;29(6):241–248.
36. Haque MF, Meghji S, Khitab U, Harris M. Oral submucous fibrosis patients have altered levels of

cytokine production. J Oral Pathol Med 2000;29(3):123–128

### 22.1.10 Therapuetics and Treatment of OSF

1. Gopinath D, Hui LM, Veettil SK, Balakrishnan Nair A, Maharajan MK. Comparative efficacy of interventions for the management of oral submucous fibrosis: a systematic review and network meta-analysis. J Pers Med. 2022;12(8):1272.
2. Gupta S, Jawanda MK. Laser as a promising non-invasive technique to treat oral submucous fibrosis: a systematic review of the literature. Saudi Dent J. 2021;33(7):413–23.
3. Gondivkar DSM, Gadbail DAR, Sarode DSC, Gondivkar DRS, Patil S, Gaikwad DRN, et al. Treatment outcomes of laser therapy in oral submucous fibrosis—a systematic review. J Oral Biol Craniofac Res. 2020;10:253–8.
4. vander Geer SJ, Reintsema H, Kamstra JI, Roodenburg JLN, Dijkstra PU. The use of stretching devices for treatment of trismus in head and neck cancer patients: a randomized controlled trial. Support Care Cancer. 2020;28:9–11.
5. Kholakiya Y, Jose A, Rawat A, Nagori SA, Jacob S, Roychoudhury A. Surgical management of oral submucous fibrosis with Seagull-nasolabial flap combined with short-term oral pentoxifylline for preventing relapse. J Stomatol Oral Maxillofac Surg. 2020;121(5):512–6.
6. Thakkannavar SS, Naik VV. Histochemical and immunohistochemical analysis of collagen fibers and microvascular density in various grades of oral submucous fibrosis. Iran J Pathol Spring. 2019;14(2):127–34.
7. Xie H, Guo J, Tan B, Wu H. Efficacy of Salvia miltiorrhiza injection combined with steroids in the treatment of oral submucous fibrosis: a meta-analysis of randomized controlled trials. Medicine (Baltimore). 2019;98(27):1–7.
8. Rai A, Kaur M, Gombra V, Hasan S, Kumar N. Comparative evaluation of curcumin and antioxidants in the management of oral submucous fibrosis. J Investig Clin Dent. 2019;10(4):1–9.
9. Lu C, Jian X. Efficacy for combined injection of salvizanolic acid B with triamcinolone acetonide on the treatment of the soft palate with oral submucous fibrosis. Zhong Nan Da XueXue Bao Yi Xue Ban. 2019;44(7):801–4.
10. Li YH, Chang WC, Chiang TE, Lin CS, Chen YW. Mouth-opening device as a treatment modality in trismus patients with head and neck cancer and oral submucous fibrosis: a prospective study. Clin Oral Investig. 2019;23:469–76.
11. Maia AV, Furlan R, Moraes KO, Amaral MS, Medeiros AM, Motta AR. Tongue strength rehabilitation using biofeedback: a case report. Codas. 2019;31:1–7.
12. Khan S, Sinha A, Kumar S, Iqbal H. Oral submucous fibrosis: current concepts on aetiology and management—a review. J Indian Acad Oral Med Radiol. 2018;30:407–11.
13. Li YH, Liu CC, Chiang TE, Chen YW. EZBite open-mouth device: a new treatment option for oral submucous fibrosis-related trismus. J Dent Sci. 2018;13(1):80–1.
14. Saran G, Umapathy D, Misra N, Channaiah SG, Singh P, Srivastava S, et al. A comparative study to evaluate the efficacy of lycopene and curcumin in oral submucous fibrosis patients: a randomized clinical trial. Indian J Dent Res. 2018;29(3):303–12.
15. Qayyum MU, Janjua OS, Ul Haq E, Zahra R. Nasolabial and extended nasolabial flaps for reconstruction in oral submucous fibrosis. J Korean Assoc Oral Maxillofac Surg. 2018;44(4):191–7.
16. Thukral H, Chowdhury SKR, Nagori SA. Surgical management of oral submucous fibrosis using buccal fat pad: a retrospective study of 30 cases. Oral Maxillofac Surg. 2018;22(4):403–8.
17. Dani VB, Patel SH. The effectiveness of therapeutic ultrasound in patients with oral submucosal fibrosis. Indian J Cancer. 2018;55:248–50.
18. Kapre M, Sudhanshu K, editors. Surgery of trismus in oral submucous fibrosis. Singapore: Springer; 2018.
19. Jian XC, Zheng L, Zhu R, Wang BP, Zhou T, Du YX. Clinical effectiveness of salvianolic acid B and triamcinolone acetonide in treatment of oral submucous fibrosis. Zhonghua Kou Qiang Yi Xue Za Zhi. 2017;52(1):16–21.
20. Xiao YC, Jian XC, Zheng L, Zhou C, Du YX. Methods and effects of injection of salvianolic acid B combined with triamcinolone acetonide in the treatment of oral submucous fibrosis. Shanghai Kou Qiang Yi Xue. 2017;26(2):188–92.
21. Daga D, Singh RK, Pal US, Gurung T, Gangwar S. Efficacy of oral colchicine with intralesional hyaluronidase or triamcinolone acetonide in the grade II oral submucous fibrosis. Natl J Maxillofac Surg. 2017;8(1):50–4.
22. Gupta S, Ghosh S, GuptaS SP. Effect of curcumin on the expression of p53, transforming growth factor-β, and inducible nitric oxide synthase in oral submucous fibrosis: a pilot study. J Investig Clin Dent. 2017;8(4):1–6.

23. Yeh MC, Chen KK, Chiang MH, Chen CH, Chen PH, Lee HE, et al. Low-power laser irradiation inhibits arecoline-induced fibrosis: an in vitro study. Int J Oral Sci. 2017;9:38–42.
24. Sadaksharam J, Mahalingam S. Evaluation of oral pentoxifylline in the management of oral submucous fibrosis—an ultrasonographic study. Contemp Clin Dent. 2017;8:200–4.
25. Patil P, Hazarey V, Chaudhari R, Nimbalkar-Patil S. Clinical efficacy of a mouth-exercising device adjunct to local ointment intra-lesional injections and surgical treatment for oral submucous fibrosis: a randomized controlled trial. Asian Pac J Cancer Prev. 2016;17(3):1255–9.
26. Patil PG, Hazarey V, Chaudhari R, Nimbalkar-Patil S. A randomized control trial measuring the effectiveness of a mouth-exercising device for mucosal burning in oral submucous fibrosis. Oral Surg Oral Med Oral Pathol Oral Radiol. 2016;122(6):713–8.
27. Kshirsagar R, Mohite A, Gupta S, Patankar A, Sane V, Raut P. Complications in the use of bilateral inferiorly based nasolabial flaps for advanced oral submucous fibrosis. Natl J Maxillofac Surg. 2016;7(2):115–21.
28. Balaji SM. Versatility of nasolabial flaps for the management of severe trismus in oral submucous fibrosis. Indian J Dent Res. 2016;27(5):492–7.
29. Shah PH, Venkatesh R, More CB, Vassandacoumara V. Comparison of therapeutic efficacy of placental extract with dexamethasone and hyaluronic acid with dexamethasone for oral submucous fibrosis—a retrospective analysis. J Clin Diagn Res. 2016;10(10):ZC63–6.
30. Pentapati KC, Gadicherla S, Smriti K. A randomized double-blind, multiple-arm trial comparing the efficacy of sub- mucosal injections of hyaluronidase, dexamethasone, and combination of dexamethasone and hyaluronidase in the management of oral submucous fibrosis—a commentary. Oral Surg Oral Med Oral Pathol Oral Radiol. 2016;122(6):784.
31. TilakaratneWM ERP, Herath M, Jayasinghe RD, Sitheeque M, Amarasinghe H. Intralesional corticosteroids as a treatment for restricted mouth opening in oral submucous fibrosis. Oral Surg Oral Med Oral Pathol Oral Radiol. 2016;122:224–31.
32. Warnakulasuriya S, Kerr AR. Oral Submucous fibrosis: a review of current management and possible directions for novel therapies. Oral Surg Oral Med Oral Pathol Oral Radiol. 2016;122:232–41.
33. Hazarey VK, Sakrikar AR, Ganvir SM. Efficacy of curcumin in the treatment for oral submucous fibrosis—a randomized clinical trial. J Oral Maxillofac Pathol. 2015;19(2):145–52.
34. Goel S, Ahmed J. A comparative study on efficacy of different treatment modalities of oral submucous fibrosis evaluated by clinical staging in population of southern Rajasthan. J Cancer Res Ther. 2015;11(1):113–8.
35. Srivastava A, Agarwal R, Chaturvedi TP, ChandraASingh OP. Clinical evaluation of the role of tulsi and turmeric in the management of oral submucous fibrosis: a pilot, prospective observational study. J Ayurveda Integr Med. 2015;6(1):45–9.
36. Shah SB, Tauro DP. Clinical and histological basis for the use of nasolabial tissues in the surgical management of oral submucous fibrosis. J Oral MaxillofacSurg. 2015;73(11):2251.e1–2251.e12.
37. Suma GN, Arora MP, Lakhanpal M. Stem cell therapy: a novel treatment approach for oral mucosal lesions. J Pharm Bioallied Sci2015;7(1):2-8.
38. Veedu RA, BalanA SSP. A randomized double-blind, multiple-arm trial comparing the efficacy of submucosal injections of hyaluronidase, dexamethasone, and combination of dexamethasone and hyaluronidase in the management of oral submucous fibrosis. Oral Surg Oral Med Oral Pathol. Oral Radiol. 2015;120(5):588–93.
39. James L, Shetty A, Rishi D, Abraham M. Management of oral submucous fibrosis with injection of hyaluronidase and dexamethasone in grade III oral submucous fibrosis: a retrospective study. J Int Oral Health. 2015;7(8):82–5.
40. Siddiqui IA, Sanna V, Ahmad N, Sechi M, Mukhtar H. Resveratrol nanoformulation for cancer prevention and therapy. Ann N Y Acad Sci. 2015;1348:20–31.
41. Rai A, Datarkar A, Rai M. Is buccal fat pad a better option than nasolabial flap for reconstruction of intraoral defects after surgical release of fibrous bands in patients with oral submucous fibrosis? A pilot study: a protocol for the management of oral submucous fibrosis. J CraniomaxillofacSurg. 2014;42(5):e111–6.
42. Zhang Y, Zhang JJ, Kang WY, Yan WY. Advances of chemical constituents and pharmacological activities of Myristica genus. Zhongguo Zhong Yao Za Zhi. 2014;39:2438–49.
43. Ye X, Zhang J, Lu R, Zhou G. HBO: a possible supplementary therapy for oral potentially malignant disorders. Med Hypotheses. 2014;83:131–6.
44. Patil S, Maheshwari S. Proposed new grading of oral submucous fibrosis based on cheek flexibility. J Clin Exp Dent. 2014;6(3):e255–8.
45. Krishnamoorthy B and M. Khan. Management of oral submucous fibrosis by two different drug regimens: a comparative study. Dent Res J (Isfahan) 2013 Jul;10(4):527-532.

46. Shetty P, Shenai P, Chatra L, Rao PK. Efficacy of spirulina as an antioxidant adjuvant to corticosteroid injection in management of oral submucous fibrosis. Indian J Dent Res. 2013;24:347–50.
47. Alam S, Ali I, Giri KY, Gokulkrishnan S, Natu SS, Faisal M, et al. Efficacy of aloe vera gel as an adjuvant treatment of oral submucous fibrosis. Oral Surg Oral Med Oral Pathol Oral Radiol. 2013;116(6):717–24.
48. Jiang XW, Zhang Y, Yang SK, Zhang H, Lu K, Sun GL. Efficacy of salvianolic acid B combined with triamcinolone acetonide in the treatment of oral submucous fibrosis. Oral Surg Oral Med Oral Pathol Oral Radiol. 2013;115(3):339–44.
49. Bhadage CJ, Umarji HR, Shah K, Välimaa H. Vasodilator isoxsuprine alleviates symptoms of oral submucous fibrosis. Clin Oral Investig. 2013;17(5):1375–82.
50. Patil PG, Patil SP. Novel mouth-exercising device for oral submucous fibrosis. J. Prosthodont. 2012;21:556–60.
51. Chole RH, Gondivkar SM, Gadbail AR, Balsaraf S, Chaudhary S, Dhore SV, et al. Review of drug treatment of oral submucous fibrosis. Oral Oncol. 2012;48(5):393–8.
52. Mehrotra R, Singh HP, Gupta SC, Singh M, Jain S. Pentoxifylline therapy in the management of oral submucous fibrosis. Asian Pac J Cancer Prev. 2011;12(4):971–4.
53. Singh M, Niranjan HS, Mehrotra R, Sharma D, Gupta SC. Efficacy of hydrocortisone acetate/hyaluronidase vs triamcinolone acetonide/hyaluronidase in the treatment of oral submucous fibrosis. Indian J Med Res. 2010;131:665–9.
54. Aziz SR. Lack of reliable evidence for oral submucous fibrosis treatments. Evid Based Dent. 2009;10(1):8–9.
55. Cox S, Zoellner H. Physiotherapeutic treatment improves oral opening in oral submucous fibrosis. J Oral Pathol Med. 2009;38(2):220–6.
56. Lin HJ, Lin JC. Treatment of oral submucous fibrosis by collagenase: effects on oral opening and eating function. Oral Dis. 2007;13(4):407–13.
57. Kumar A, Bagewadi A, Keluskar V, Singh M. Efficacy of lycopene in the management of oral submucous fibrosis. Oral Surg Oral Med Oral Pathol Oral RadiolEndod. 2007;103(2):207–13.
58. Rajendran R, Rani V, Shaikh S. Pentoxifylline therapy: a new adjunct in the treatment of oral submucous fibrosis. Indian J Dent Res. 2006;17:190–8.
59. Haque MF, Meghji S, Nazir R, Harris M. Interferon gamma (IFN-gamma) may reverse oral submucous fibrosis. J Oral Pathol Med. 2001;30(1):12–21.
60. Maher R, Aga P, Johnson NW, Sankaranarayanan R, Warnakulasuriya S. Evaluation of multiple micronutrient supplementation in the management of oral submucous fibrosis in Karachi. Pakistan. Nutr Cancer. 1997;27(1):41–7.
61. Khanna JN, Andrade NN. Oral submucous fibrosis: a new concept in surgical management: report of 100 cases. Int J Oral MaxillofacSurg. 1995;24(6):433–9.
62. Gupta D, Sharma SC. Oral submucous fibrosis–a new treatment regimen. J Oral MaxillofacSurg. 1988;46(10):830–3.

### 22.1.11 Relation and Conversion of OSF to OSCC

1. Saalim M, Sansare K, Karjodkar FR, Johaley S, Ali IK, Sharma SR et al. The prevalence of oral squamous cell carcinoma with oral submucous fibrosis. J Can Res Ther2021;17(6):1510-1514.
2. Shih YH, Chiu KC, Wang TH, Lan WC, Tsai BH, Wu LJ, et al. Effects of melatonin to arecoline-induced reactive oxygen species production and DNA damage in oral squamous cell carcinoma. J Formos Med Assoc. 2021;120:668–78.
3. Pereira T, Surve R, Shetty S, Gotmare S. Qualitative expression of hypoxia-inducible factor-1α in malignant transformation of oral submucous fibrosis: an immunohistochemical study. J Oral MaxillofacPathol. 2020;24:106–12.
4. Joseph I, Elizabeth J, Rao UK, Ranganathan K. Study of Hypoxia-inducible factor-2α expression in the malignant transformation of Oral submucous fibrosis. J Oral Maxillofac Pathol. 2020;24(1):33–9.
5. Meera S, Sarangarajan R. Rajkumar K.8-Isoprostane: a salivary oxidative stress biomarker for oral submucous fibrosis and oral squamous cell carcinoma. J Oral Maxillofac Pathol. 2020;24(2):279–84.
6. Kujan O, Mello FW, Warnakulasuriya S. Malignant transformation of oral submucous fibrosis: a systemic review and meta-analysis. Ora Dis. 2020;00:1–11.
7. Phulari RGS, Dave EJ. A systematic review on the mechanisms of malignant transformation of oral submucous fibrosis. Eur J Cancer Prev. 2020;29(5):470–3.
8. Wadhwan V, Venkatesh A, Reddy V, Malik S. The role of myofibroblasts in the progression of oral submucous fibrosis: a systematic review. J Oral MaxillofacPathol2019;23(2):257-266.

9. Rangaswamy S, Chikkalingaiah RG, Sanjeevarayappa PN, Govindraju P. Carcinoma arising in the background of oral submucous fibrosis. Ann MaxillofacSurg. 2019;9(2):247–52.
10. Hallikeri K, Burde K, Anehosur V, Kulkarni BB, Hiremath SV. p53 polymorphism and association of human papillomavirus in oral submucous fibrosis and oral squamous cell carcinoma: a case-control study. J Oral Maxillofac Pathol. 2019;23:97–103.
11. Siriwardena BS, Jayawardena KL, Senarath NH, Tilakaratne WM. An evaluation of clinical and histopathological aspects of patients with oral submucous fibrosis in the background of oral squamous cell carcinoma. BioMed Res Int. 2018;2018:1–7. ► https://doi.org/10.1155/2018/4154165.
12. Speight PM, Khurram SA, Kujan O. Oral potentially malignant disorders: risk of progression to malignancy. Oral Surg Oral Med Oral Pathol Oral Radiol. 2018;125(6):612–27.
13. Sharma M, Shetty SS, Radhakrishnan R. Oral submucous fibrosis as an overhealing wound: implications in malignant transformation. Recent Pat Anticancer Drug Discov. 2018;13(3):272–91.
14. Bari S, Metgud R, Vyas Z, Tak A. An update on studies on etiological factors, disease progression, and malignant transformation in oral submucous fibrosis. J Cancer Res Ther. 2017;13(3):399–405.
15. Gadbail AR, Chaudhary M, Gawande M, Hande A, Sarode S, Tekade SA, et al. Oral squamous cell carcinoma in the background of oral submucous fibrosis is a distinct clinicopathological entity with better prognosis. J Oral Pathol Med. 2017;46(6):448–53.
16. Chaturvedi P, Malik A, Nair D, Nair S, Mishra A, Garg A, et al. Oral squamous cell carcinoma associated with oral submucous fibrosis have better oncologic outcome than those without. Oral Surg Oral Med Oral Pathol Oral Radiol. 2017;124(3):225–30.
17. Gandhi P, Prasad UC. Evaluation of myofibroblasts in oral submucous fibrosis and oral squamous cell carcinoma: the pathogenesis and correlation. Dent Res J (Isfahan). 2017;14(5):314–20.
18. Mohiuddin S, Fatima N, Hosein S, Hosein M. High risk of malignant transformation of oral submucous fibrosis in Pakistani females: a potential national disaster. J Pak Med Assoc. 2016;66(11):1362–6.
19. Xie X, Jiang Y, Yuan Y, Wang P, Li X, Chen F, et al. MALDI imaging reveals NCOA7 as a potential biomarker in oral squamous cell carcinoma arising from oral submucous fibrosis. Oncotarget. 2016;7:59987–60004.
20. Hegde S, Anuradha A, Asha V. Malignant transformation of oral submucous fibrosis. J Med Radiol Pathol Surg. 2015;1(5):32–6.
21. Chaudhary M, Bajaj S, Bohra S, Swastika N, Hande A. The domino effect: role of hypoxia in malignant transformation of oral submucous fibrosis. J Oral Maxillofac Pathol. 2015;19(2):122–7.
22. Liu B, Shen M, Xiong J, Yuan Y, Wu X, Gao X, et al. Synergistic effects of betel quid chewing, tobacco use (in the form of cigarette smoking), and alcohol consumption on the risk of malignant transformation of oral submucous fibrosis (OSF): a case-control study in Hunan Province, China. Oral SurgOral Med Oral Pathol Oral Radiol. 2015;120:337–45.
23. MishevG DE, Hlushchuk R, Velinov N, Aebersold D, Weinstein F, et al. Prognostic value of matrix metalloproteinases in oral squamous cell carcinoma. BiotechnolBiotechnol Equip. 2014;28:1138–49.
24. Arora R, Adwani D, Naphade M, Bhagat B, Qureshi AQ. Malignant conversion of oral submucous fibrosis in surgically treated case. J Clin Diagn Res. 2014;8:ZD31–2.
25. Shih YH, Chang KW, Chen MY, Yu CC, Lin DJ, Hsia SM, et al. Lysyl oxidase and enhancement of cell proliferation and angiogenesis in oral squamous cell carcinoma. Head Neck. 2013;35:250–6.
26. Chaturvedi P, Vaishampayan SS, Nair S, Nair D, Agarwal JP, Kane SV, et al. Oral squamous cell carcinoma arising in background of oral submucous fibrosis: a clinicopathologically distinct disease. Head Neck. 2013;35(10):1404–9.
27. Ekanayaka RP, Tilakaratne WM. Oral submucous fibrosis: review on mechanisms of pathogenesis and malignant transformation. Oral Surg Oral Med Oral Pathol Oral Radiol. 2016;122(2):192–9.
28. Muttagi SS, Chaturvedi P, Gaikwad R, Singh B, Pawar P. Head and neck squamous cell carcinoma in chronic areca nut chewing Indian women: Case series and review of literature. Indian J Med Paediatr Oncol. 2012;33:32–5.
29. Guo F, Jian XC, Zhou SH, Li N, Hu YJ, Tang ZG. A retrospective study of oral squamous cell carcinomas originated from oral submucous fibrosis. Zhonghua Kou Qiang Yi Xue Za Zhi. 2011;46(8):494–7.
30. Lin KH, Lin CY, Liu CC, Chou MY, Lin JK. Arecoline N-oxide: its mutagenicity and possible role as ultimate carcinogen in areca oral carcinogenesis. J Agric Food Chem. 2011;59:3420–8.
31. Chen PT, Kuan FC, Huang CE, Chen MF, Huang SH, Chen MC, et al. Incidence and patterns of second primary malignancies following oral cavity can-

cers in a prevalent area of betel-nut chewing: a population-based cohort of 26,166 patients in Taiwan. J Clin Oncol. 2011;41(12):1336–43.
32. Chaudhary AK, Pandya S, Mehrotra R, Singh M, Singh M. Role of functional polymorphism of matrix metalloproteinase-2 (-1306 C/T and -168 G/T) and MMP-9 (-1562 C/T) promoter in oral submucous fibrosis and head and neck squamous cell carcinoma in an Indian population. Biomarkers2011;16:577-586.
33. Zhou S, Qu X, Yu Z, Zhong L, Ruan M, Ma C, et al. Survivin as a potential early marker in the carcinogenesis of oral submucous fibrosis. Oral Surg Oral Med Oral PatholOralRadiolEndodontol. 2010;109:575–81.
34. Illeperuma RP, Ryu MH, Kim KY, Tilakaratne WM, Kim J. Relationship of fibrosis and the expression of TGF-ß1, MMP-1, andTIMP-1 with epithelial dysplasia in oral submucous fibrosis. Oral Med Pathol. 2010;15(1):21–8.
35. Tilakaratne WM, Iqbal Z, Teh MT, Ariyawardana A, Pitiyage G, Cruchley A. Upregulation of HIF-1alpha in malignant transformation of oral submucous fibrosis. J Oral Pathol Med. 2008;37:372–7.
36. Zhou SH, Li LL, Jian XC, Wang Y, Chen XQ, Gao X. Molecules of G(2)/M phase and the phosphorylation of survivin in the carcinogenesis of oral submucosal fibrosis. Chin J Stomatol. 2008;43:709–12.
37. Yanjia H, andXinchun J. The role of epithelial-mesenchymal transition in oral squamous cell carcinoma and oral submucous fibrosis. Clin Chim Acta. 2007;383:51–6.
38. Jeng JH, Chang MC, Hahn LJ. Role of areca nut in betel quid-associated chemical carcinogenesis: current awareness and future perspectives. Oral Oncol. 2001;37:477–92.
39. Phukan RK, Ali MS, Chetia CK, Mahanta J. Betel nut and tobacco chewing; potential risk factors of cancer of oesophagus in Assam. India. Br J Cancer. 2001;85(5):661–7.
40. Trivedy C, Warnakulasuriya KA, Tavassoli M, Steingrimsdottir H, Penhallow J, Maher R, Johnson NW. p53 aberrations in oral submucous fibrosis and oral squamous cell carcinoma detected by immunocytochemistry and PCR-SSCP. J Oral Pathol Med. 1998;27(2):72–7.
41. Murti PR, Bhonsle RB, Pindborg JJ, Daftary DK, Gupta PC, Mehta FS. Malignant transformation rate in oral submucous fibrosis over a 17-year period. Community Dent Oral Epidemiol. 1985;13(6):340–1.
42. Pindborg JJ, Murti PR, Bhonsle RB, Gupta PC, Daftary DK, Mehta FS. Oral submucous fibrosis as a precancerous condition. Eur J Oral Sci. 1984;92:224–9.

### 22.1.12 Research Associated with OSF

1. Xu H, Lyu FY, Song JY, Xu YM, Jiang EH, Shang ZJ, Chen LL, Xu Z. Research achievements of oral submucous fibrosis: progress and prospect. Biomed Res Int. 2021;2021
2. Gosavi SR, andTorkadi AA. Serum C-reactive protein in oral submucous fibrosis and oral squamous cell carcinoma: a cross-sectional study. J Oral MaxillofacPathol. 2020;24:46–51.
3. Ray JG, Chatterjee R, Chaudhuri K. Oral submucous fibrosis: a global challenge. Rising incidence, risk factors, management, and research priorities. Periodontol 2000 2019;80(1):200-212.
4. Mantri T, Thete SG, Male V, Yadav R, Grover I, Adsure GR, et al. Study of the role of salivary lactate dehydrogenase in habitual tobacco chewers, oral submucous fibrosis and oral cancer as a biomarker. J Contemp Dent Pract. 2019;20(8):970–3.
5. Vallet SD, Ricard-Blum S. Lysyl oxidases: from enzyme activity to extracellular matrix cross-links. EssaysBiochem. 2019;63:349–64.
6. Tom A, Baghirath V, Krishna B, Ganepalli A, Kumar JV, Mohan SP. Ultrastructural Changes of Collagen in Different Histopathological Grades of Oral Submucous Fibrosis. J Pharm Bioallied Sci. 2019;11:S309–13.
7. Ahmed S, Misra DP, Agarwal V. Interleukin-17 pathways in systemic sclerosis-associated fibrosis. Rheumatol Int. 2019;39(7):1135–43.
8. Yang B, Fu MF, Tang ZG. Rat model with oral submucous fibrosis induced by arecoline and mechanical stimulation. Hua Xi Kou Qiang Yi Xue Za Zhi. 2019;37:260–4.
9. Fang CY, Hsia SM, Hsieh PL, Liao YW, Peng CY, Wu CZ, et al. Slug mediates myofibroblastic differentiation to promote fibrogenesis in buccal mucosa. J Cell Physiol. 2019;234:6721–30.
10. Liu CM, Liao YW, Hsieh PL, Yu CH, Chueh PJ, Lin T, et al. miR-1246 as a therapeutic target in oral submucosa fibrosis pathogenesis. J Formos Med Assoc. 2019;118:1093–8.
11. Panta P, Sarode SC, Sarode GS, Patil S. New directions for oral submucous fibrosis research: whole evaluation for holistic rehabilitation! J. Contemp Dent Pr. 2018;19:901–3.
12. Su TR, Liao YW, Hsieh PL, Tsai LL, Fang CY, Lin T, et al. Butylidenephthalide abrogates the myofibroblasts activation and mesenchymal transdifferentiation in oral submucous fibrosis. Environ Toxicol. 2018;33:686–94.
13. Oscarsson N, Ny L, MolneJ LF, Ricksten SE, Seeman-Lodding H, et al. Hyperbaric oxygen treatment reverses radiation induced pro-fibrotic and

oxidative stress responses in a rat model. Free RadicBiol Med. 2017;103:248–55.
14. Wen QT, Wang T, Yu DH, Wang ZR, Sun Y, Liang CW. Development of a mouse model of arecoline-induced oral mucosal fibrosis. Asian Pac J Trop Med. 2017;10:1177–84.
15. Colak S, Ten Dijke P. Targeting TGF-beta signaling in cancer. Trends Cancer. 2017;3:56–71.
16. Chiang MH, Chen PH, Chen YK, Chen CH, Ho ML, Wang YH. Characterization of a Novel dermal fibrosis model induced by areca nut extract that mimics Oral Submucous Fibrosis. PLoS ONE. 2016;11:1–11.
17. Mari S, Kamath VV, Satelur K, Rajkumar K. Evaluation of transforming growth factor beta1 gene in oral submucous fibrosis induced in Sprague-Dawley rats by injections of areca nut and pan masala (commercial areca nut product) extracts. J Cancer Res. 2016;12:379–85.
18. Huang JL, Lu HH, Lu YN, Hung PS, Lin YJ, Lin CC, et al. Enhancement of the genotoxicity of benzo[a]pyrene by arecoline through suppression of DNA repair in HEp-2 cells. ToxicolVitr. 2016; 33:80–7.
19. Erlewad DM, Mundhe KA, Hazarey VK. Dental Informatics tool "SOFPRO" for the study of oral submucous fibrosis. J Oral MaxillofacPathol. 2016;20(2):194–201.
20. Tsai CH, Lee SS, Chang YC. Hypoxic regulation of plasminogen activator inhibitor-1 expression in human buccal mucosa fibroblasts stimulated with arecoline. J Oral Pathol Med2015; 44: 669–673.
21. Ullah M, Cox S, Kelly E, Moore MA, Zoellner H. Arecoline increases basic fibroblast growth factor but reduces expression of IL-1, IL-6, G-CSF and GM-CSF in human umbilical vein endothelium. J Oral Pathol Med. 2015;44(8): 591–601.
22. Gupta S, Manjunath SM, Jawanda MK, Bharti A. Quantification of Plasma Fibrinogen Degradation Products in Areca Nut Chewers with and without Oral Submucous Fibrosis. J Clin of Diagn Res 2014;8(11):ZC027-ZC030.
23. Kadani M, Satish BN, Maharudrappa B, Prashant KM, Hugar D, Allad U et al. Evaluation of plasma fibrinogen degradation products and total serum protein concentration in oral submucous fibrosis. J Clin Diagn Res 2014;8(5):ZC54-ZC57.
24. Chang NW, Pei RJ, Tseng HC, Yeh KT, Chan HC, Lee MR, et al. Co-treating with arecoline and 4-nitroquinoline 1-oxide to establish a mouse model mimicking oral tumorigenesis. Chem Biol Interact. 2010;183:231–7.
25. Illeperuma RP, Park YJ, Kim J, Jung DW, Tilakaratne WM, et al. Cytokine expression by the treatment of areca nut extract in cultured fibroblasts: comparision between normal oral fibroblasts and hTERT transfected fibroblasts. 15th International Congress on Oral Pathology and Medicine; 2010; Seoul. Korea.
26. Vedeswari CP, Jayachandran S, Ganesan S. In vivo autofluorescence characteristics of pre- and post-treated oral submucous fibrosis: a pilot study. Indian J Dent Res. 2009;20(3):261–7.
27. Haris PS, Balan A, Jayasree RS, Gupta AK. Autofluorescence spectroscopy for the in vivo evaluation of oral submucous fibrosis. Photomed Laser Surg. 2009;27(5):757–61.
28. Lee PH, Chang MC, Chang WH, Wang TM, Wang YJ, Hahn LJ, et al. Prolonged exposure to arecoline arrested human KB epithelial cell growth: regulatory mechanisms of cell cycle and apoptosis. Toxicology. 2006;220:81–9.
29. Chang YC, Hu CC, Lii CK, Tai KW, Yang SH, Chou MY. Cytotoxicity and arecoline mechanisms in human gingival fibroblasts in vitro. Clin Oral Investig. 2001;5(1):51–6.
30. Sharma AK, Gupta R, Gupta HP, Singh AK. Haemodynamic effects of pan masala in healthy volunteers. J Assoc Physicians India. 2000;48(4):400–1.
31. Chang YC, Tai KW, Chou MY, Tseng TH. Synergistic effects of peroxynitrite on arecoline-induced cytotoxicity in human buccal mucosal fibroblasts. Toxicol Lett. 2000;118(1–2):61–8.
32. Marques LJ, Zheng L, Poulakis N, Guzman J, Costabel U. Pentoxifylline inhibits TNF-alpha production from human alveolar macrophages. Am J Respir Crit Care Med. 1999;159:508–11.
33. Kuo MY, Chen HM, Hahn LJ, Hsieh CC, Chiang CP. Collagen biosynthesis in human oral submucous fibrosis fibroblast cultures. J Dent Res. 1995;74:1783–8.

# Supplementary Information



© The Editor(s) (if applicable) and The Author(s), under exclusive license to Springer Nature Switzerland AG 2023
S. Warnakulasuriya, K. Ranganathan (eds.), *Oral Submucous Fibrosis*, Textbooks in Contemporary Dentistry,
https://doi.org/10.1007/978-3-031-12855-4

# Appendix: Prominent Stalwarts in the Study of Oral Submucous Fibrosis

The scientific community can never forget the historical contributions of late Professors Pindborg, Mehta, Schwartz, Lal, and Joshi and the late Sirsat. The work at King's College London led by Prof. Newell Johnson and Prof. Saman Warnakulasuriya and collaborators from India, Sri Lanka, Pakistan, Malaysia, and others provided the basis for present-day understandings of etiology and pathogenesis. Cameos of these distinguished figures follow.

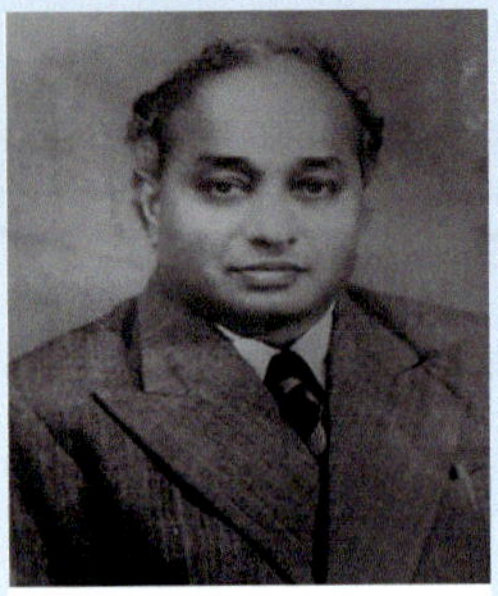

Dr. S.G. Joshi
*(03.01.1908 – 02.12.1954)*

### Dr. S. G. Joshi

Dr. Sadashiv Gopal Joshi was born on January 3, 1908. His schooling and undergraduate course were from Karnataka College, Dharwad. After his interscience examination, he joined Seth G.S. Medical College at Parel, Mumbai. He was a student of the 3rd batch after the college was established. He won gold medals in many subjects during his MBBS course. Postgraduate studies and MS in ENT from KEM Hospital, Mumbai, followed. He established the ENT department in KEM Hospital. He conducted extensive research on the pathology of the inability to open the mouth. He named "submucous fibrosis." He was a pioneer in starting the "fenestration operation" of the ear in India after studying abroad.

He was a keen sports enthusiast and had an immense interest in Indian classical music. He passed away at the young age of 46 years on December 2, 1954, due to a coronary occlusion.

*Biosketch and photo courtesy of Dr Amita Navalkar (granddaughter of late Dr Joshi) and currently Professor of Oral Medicine, Yerela Dental College, Navi Mumbai.*

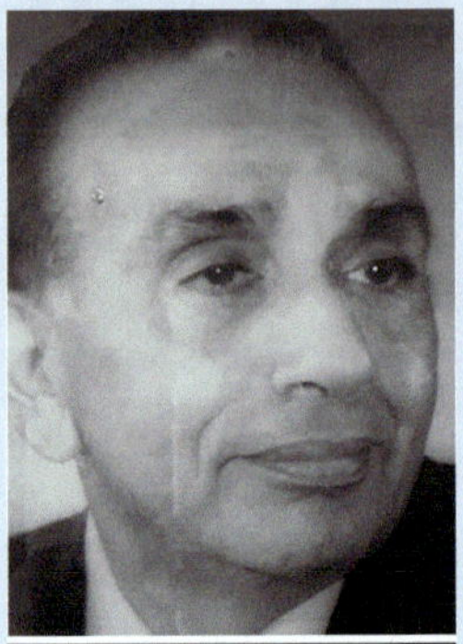

Dr. Fali S Mehta
*(02.04.1923 – 29.08.2004)*

### Dr. Fali S. Mehta

Dr. Fali Mehta was born in Bombay, Maharashtra, on April 2, 1923. He qualified LDSc at Nair Hospital Dental College in 1948. He then traveled to the USA and received his DMD in 1949. He worked with Dr. Irving Glickman from 1949 to 1952. He then returned to Bombay, where he practiced dentistry for more than 50 years. He was actively involved in the wider dental profession including serving as President of the Dental Council of India. He was the principal investigator along with the Late Professor Jens Pindborg and late Dr. James E. Hamner III for the project on tobacco habits and associated lesions in Indian rural populations. He passed away on August 29, 2004.

*Biosketch and photo courtesy Dr. Rushtom Mehta, son.*

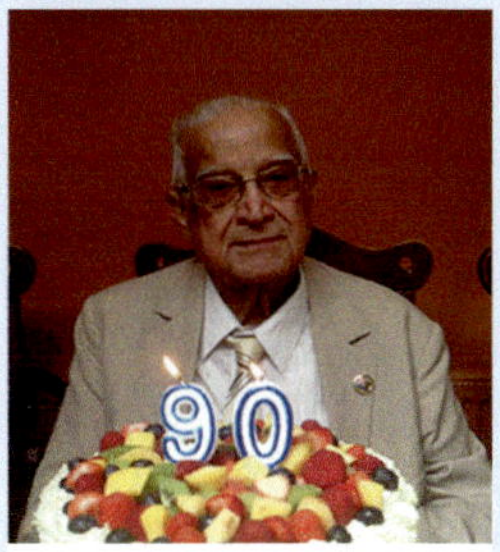

Dr. Daman Lal Sarin
(04.09.1923 – 02.07.2015)

*Celebrating his 90th birthday in 2013*
*Courtesy: Ravi Sarin (Grandson of Late Daman Lal Sarin)*

## Dr. Daman Lal

Dr. Daman Lal Sarin, born in 1923 in undivided Punjab, completed BDS from De' Montmorency Dental College, Lahore, in 1945 and obtained LDS RCS from the Royal College of Surgeons of England a year later. In 1953, while serving at GR Medical College, Gwalior, he published the first detailed cases of previously unreported oral condition—which he coined "diffuse oral submucous fibrosis"—in the Indian population. This is still a landmark contribution. In 1962, he migrated to the United Kingdom and settled in a dental practice at Coventry. He served as a Rotary Foundation Volunteer and had a tremendous journey to treat needy people worldwide, especially refugees from Hong Kong (Vietnam refugees), Kenya, and Guatemala. The Queen of the United Kingdom and associated Commonwealth Territories awarded him the MBE in 1998 for his exemplary charity work as a Rotarian. He died at the age of 92 in 2015 after a very distinguished career. Indeed, he was a true pioneer.

*Biosketch and photo courtesy of Mr. Ravi Sarin, grandson.*

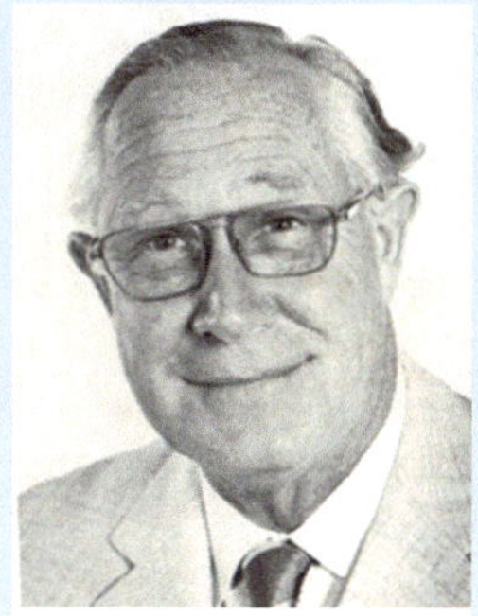

Dr. Jens J Pindborg
(17.08.1921 - 06.08.1995)

## Dr. Jens J. Pindborg

Dr. Pindborg made a mark in oral medicine and pathology in the areas of tumors and HIV infection. He has to his credit over 400 published papers and 20 books. He was the editor of several journals, including the Journal of Oral Pathology and Medicine, Community Dentistry and Oral Epidemiology, Danish Dental Journal, the International Journal of Oral Surgery, and the Journal of Dental Research. Pindborg was a dedicated teacher who delivered lectures worldwide and received honorary doctorates from several universities in Scandinavia and Europe. He died at the age of 73 years after a brief illness. His name will long live on, attached to pathological entities he described including "Pindborg's tumor" and in the gratitude of many who consider him their mentor. He remains a gold standard in oral pathology and medicine.

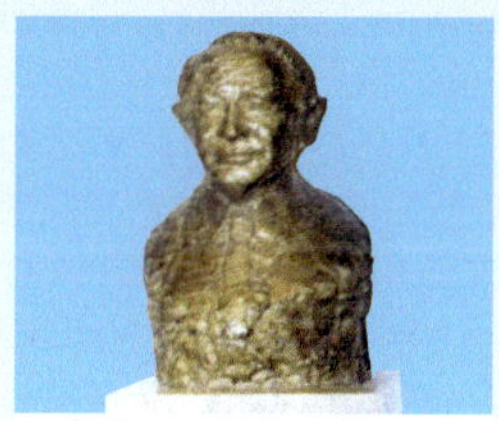

**17 August 1921 - 6 August 1995**
Sculpture of Dr. Jens Pindborg at Royal Dental School,

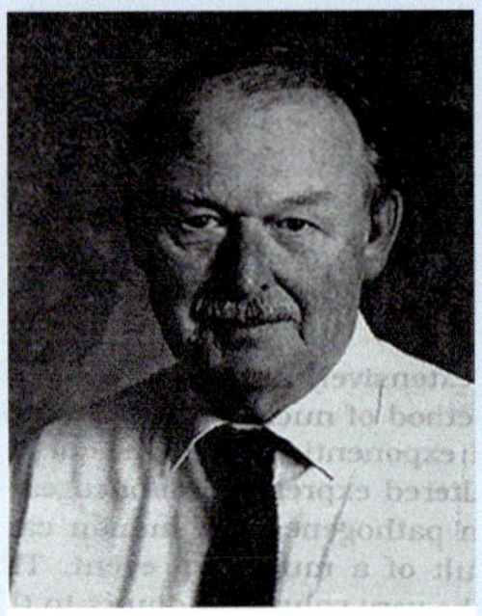

Dr. Christian Werner Van Wyk
*(19.02.1932- 20.04.2003).*

## Dr. Christian Werner Van Wyk

Dr. Christian Werner Van Wyk was born on 19.02.1932 and obtained his BCD from the University of Pretoria (1954), FDS RCS England (1961), and was awarded Ph.D. from the University of Stellenbosch (1972) and DSc for research related to pathoses of the oral mucosa in South Africa (1995). He taught oral pathology at the University of Pretoria (1962–1966), University of Witwatersrand (1967–1970), and University of Stellenbosch (1971–1995). He retired as the Director of the Oral and Dental Research Institute, University of Stellenbosch. He conducted extensive work on oral diseases in South Africa and had 160 research publications and 190 research presentations (40 internationally) in the area of epidemiology, cancer research, animal experimentation, and tissue culture as a model for cancer studies and biocompatibility of dental materials. He, along with Dr. Seedat, was amongst the first to describe areca nut as an etiological agent in the pathogenesis of oral cancer. He visited dental schools in India and gave an oration at the 7th National Conference of the Indian Academy of Oral Pathologists at Nagpur in 1998. Prof. CW Van Wyk, one of the giants of his time, passed away on 20.04.2003.

(*Source Proceedings of 7th National Conference of IAOP Nagpur 1998-South African Dental Journal; June 2003 Vol .58 No. 5.*)

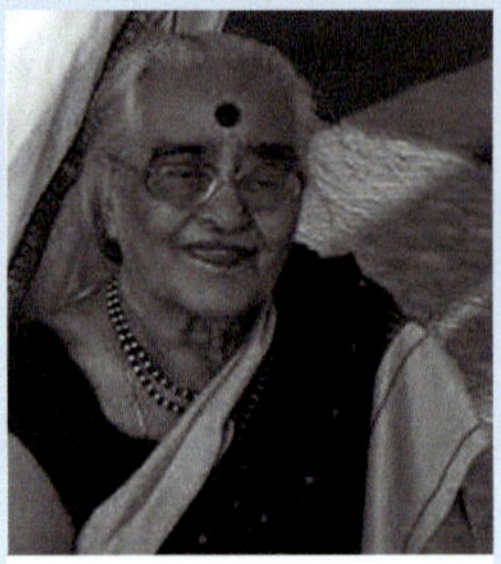

Dr. Satyavati M Sirsat
*(07.10.1925 - 10.07.2010)*

## Dr. Satyavati M. Sirsat

Dr. Sirsat was an Indian scholar and cancer researcher based at what is now known as the Advanced Centre for Treatment, Research and Education in Cancer (ACTREC). She was the first in India to begin an electron microscopy laboratory. She was also the first researcher and Indian student who completed her doctoral studies on submucous fibrosis, at the University of Bombay, in 1958. In collaboration with Professor Pindborg and Padma Bhushan awardee Dr. Vasant Ramji Khanolkar, she studied cases of OSF and developed disease models in Wistar rats. She published extensively on OSF. Dr. Sirsat advised aspiring scientists, "Be honest to your work and true to yourself. Be disciplined. Never disparage the work of your fellow scientists. Be observant—never distort your log or show records to fit a preconceived theory. Above all life is to learn, learn and learn." Dr. Sirsat died from cancer at the age of 84 years in 2010.

## Living Legends

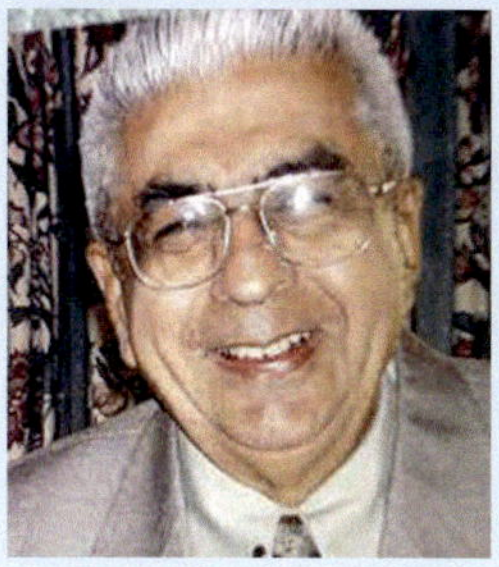

### Dr. Dinesh Daftary

Distinguished oral pathologist, **Dr. Dinesh Daftary**, is one of the first specialists in oral pathology and bacteriology of India (1963), an ex-professor at Nair Hospital Dental College, Mumbai, India. He was a key collaborator with the late Professor J.J. Pindborg for research on oral cancer and "precancer" at the Basic Dental Research Unit, Tata Institute of Fundamental Research, Mumbai, from 1966 to 1996. He published extensively on this topic (42 articles) as well as on wider aspects of oral health (48 articles) as he has always had passion to change the mindset of both the dental and medical professions from "tooth and nothing but tooth and that was the truth" to the holistic concept of oral health. He co-edited "Oral Diseases in the Tropics" published by Oxford University Press. He has received many awards including "Citation of Merit" from the Pierre Fauchard Academy (2014) and the "*Sushruta*" award from the Indian Dental Association for outstanding research (2016). His numerous presentations globally include a keynote at the Royal Society of Medicine, London (1988); panelist in Heidelberg, Germany (1991); and Dr. R. Ahmed oration of the Indian Dental Association (1994). He is a founder member and past president of the Indian Academy of Oral Pathology. He is a founder member of the International Association of Oral Pathology and past associate editor of the Journal of Oral Pathology and Medicine. He has been an active researcher and distinguished clinician for over 60 years and has mentored many younger oral pathologists.

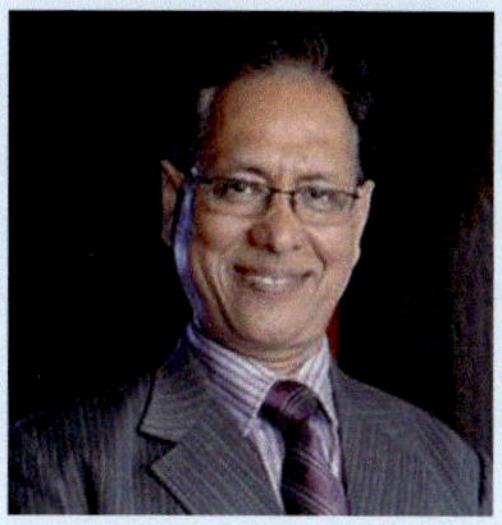

### Dr. Prakash C. Gupta

**Dr. Prakash C. Gupta** is an eminent epidemiologist with a Doctor of Science degree from Johns Hopkins University, USA (1975). He completed MSc from Bombay University in 1965 and was senior research scientist in the TIFR team 1966 to 2004. Currently, he is Director of the Healis Sekhsaria Institute of Public Health, Navi Mumbai. He has an international reputation in tobacco and cancer epidemiology, in advancement of tobacco control policies, and in public health with more than 250 publications in international journals and an H-index of 93 as per Google Scholar. Honors include the Tobacco Free World Award from the Director General, World Health Organization, Geneva, on May 31, 1999, for Outstanding Contributions to Public Health; the Luther Terry Award from the American Cancer Society for exemplary leadership in tobacco control, an outstanding research contribution to the 12th World Conference on Tobacco or Health in Helsinki, Finland, 2003; the *Sushruta* Award from the Indian Dental Association in 2017; and Lifetime Achievement Award from the Foundation for Head and Neck Oncology in 2017. He is listed in the Stanford University top 2% of global scientists in public health with the first rank in India.

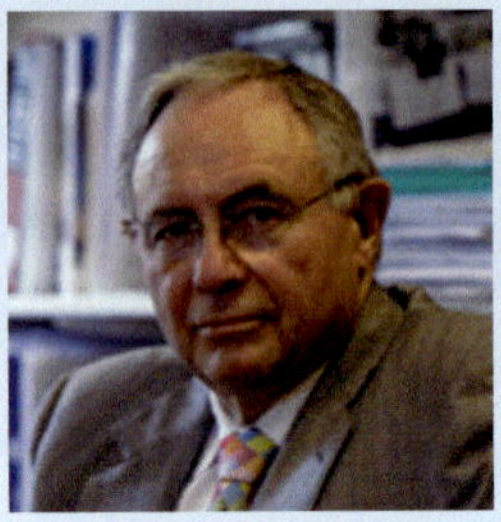

**Emeritus Professor Newell W. Johnson, CMG, FMedSci**

**Professor Newell W. Johnson** is amongst the most cited researchers in the field of dentistry, oral medicine, and pathology: approximately 400 publications, an H-index of 85, and in the Stanford University analysis of the top 2% of scientists in dentistry worldwide. He is an expert in oral cancer, OPMD, dental caries, periodontal diseases, oral manifestations of HIV disease, and other aspects of oral pathology. He has received two Distinguished Scientist Awards from the International Association of Dental Research (in Oral Medicine and Pathology and in Global Oral Health), Honorary Life Membership of the British Societies of Oral and Maxillofacial Pathologists and of Oral Medicine, of the International Association of Oral Pathologists, and has been awarded Companion of the Order of St. Michael and St. George by the Queen of the United Kingdom and of the Commonwealth Territories for his contributions to public health globally. He is a Tomes Medalist of the British Dental Association. A particular pleasure was delivery of Dr. R Ahmed Oration to the Indian Dental Association in 1984. He has facilitated research in the United Kingdom, Australia, Nigeria, Kenya, India, Sri Lanka, Pakistan, Bangladesh, and Papua New Guinea, usually as supervisor to over 35 Ph.D. students. He has served as President of national and international professional societies and was Foundation Dean of the Griffith University School of Dentistry and Oral Health. He continues to be active in education and research across several health sciences. His collaborations with Saman Warnakulasuriya have been extremely productive over many decades.

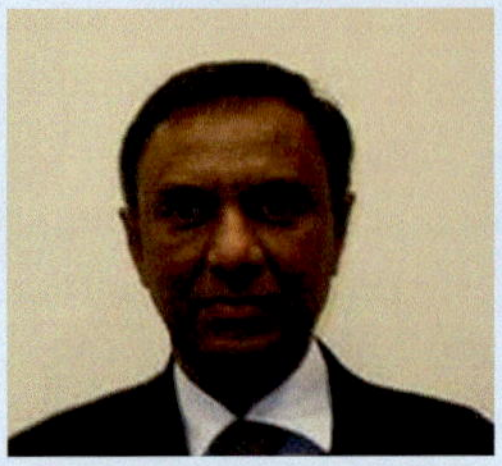

**Emeritus Professor Saman Warnakulasuriya**

**Saman Warnakulasuriya,** Emeritus Professor of Oral Medicine and Experimental Pathology at King's College London, UK, and former Chairman of the Oral Medicine Division at King's College Hospital and Guy's Hospital, London, is listed in the Stanford University as top 2% global scientists. Saman graduated from the University of Peradeniya (then Ceylon) with a first-class honors and obtained fellowships in dentistry from all three Royal Colleges of Surgeons of England, Edinburgh, and Glasgow. He has made major contributions to oral cancer epidemiology, oral medicine, and experimental pathology. He is a stalwart with expertise in the understanding of oral carcinogenesis concerning areca nut and tobacco. His work on smokeless tobacco and areca nut has led to confirmation of these substances as Class I carcinogens by the International Agency on Research on Cancer (IARC). He has been instrumental in reaffirming a Europe-wide ban on the use of smokeless forms of tobacco. He has undertaken extensive research on oral carcinogenesis, oral cancer, and OPMD including aspects ranging from terminology and classification development, epidemiology, molecular cascades, and clinical and histopathological aspects. This is reflected in over 350 publications in PubMed indexed journals with an H-index of 86 of Google Scholar and 28,457 citations. In 2008, Saman was awarded an OBE by her Majesty the Queen of the United Kingdom for his services to medicine. He has also received Distinguished Scientist Awards from the International Association of Dental Research in both Oral Medicine and Pathology (2014) and in Global Oral Health (2021). He plays a leading role in the work of WHO, inter alia as Director of the WHO Collaborating Centre for Oral Cancer based at King's College London and as Chair of ongoing projects for the International Agency for Research on Cancer.

# Index

## A



## B

## C



## D

## E



## F



## G



## H

## N



## O

## P



## Q



## R



## S

## T



## U



## V



## W



## X



## Z

MIX
Papier aus verantwortungsvollen Quellen
Paper from responsible sources
FSC® C105338

If you have any concerns about our products,
you can contact us on
**ProductSafety@springernature.com**

In case Publisher is established outside the EU,
the EU authorized representative is:
**Springer Nature Customer Service Center GmbH**
**Europaplatz 3, 69115 Heidelberg, Germany**

Printed by Libri Plureos GmbH
in Hamburg, Germany